Adrenal Cortex: Pathology and Biology

Adrenal Cortex: Pathology and Biology

Editor: Leroy Finch

AMERICAN
MEDICAL PUBLISHERS
www.americanmedicalpublishers.com

AMERICAN
MEDICAL PUBLISHERS
www.americanmedicalpublishers.com

Cataloging-in-Publication Data

Adrenal cortex : pathology and biology / edited by Leroy Finch.
p. cm.
Includes bibliographical references and index.
ISBN 978-1-63927-853-4
1. Adrenal cortex. 2. Adrenal cortex--Diseases. 3. Adrenal cortex--Diseases--Etiology.
4. Adrenal cortex--Diseases--Diagnosis. 5. Adrenal cortex--Diseases--Treatment. I. Finch, Leroy.
RC659 .A27 2023
616.45--dc23

American Medical Publishers,
41 Flatbush Avenue,
1st Floor, New York,
NY 11217, USA

ISBN 978-1-63927-853-4 (Hardback)

Contents

Preface

The purpose of the book is to provide a glimpse into the dynamics and to present opinions and studies of some of the scientists engaged in the development of new ideas in the field from very different standpoints. This book will prove useful to students and researchers owing to its high content quality.

The term adrenal cortex refers to the outer region and largest part of an adrenal gland. Adrenal cortex is divided into three distinct layers, namely, zona glomerulosa, zona fasciculate, and zona reticularis. The responsibility of each layer is to produce specific hormones. It is also the secondary site for the synthesis of androgens. Zona glomerulosa is the outermost layer of the adrenal cortex. This layer is the main site for the synthesis of aldosterone, a mineralocorticoid. The second zone, zona fasciculata is located between zona glomerulosa and zona reticularis. The basic function of this zone is to produce and secrete glucocorticoids, such as 11-deoxycorticosterone, corticosterone, and cortisol. The major hormone that stimulates cortisol secretion in humans is the ACTH that is released from the anterior pituitary. The third zone, zona reticularis is the innermost layer that produces androgens, namely, dehydroepiandrosterone (DHEA), DHEA sulfate (DHEA-S), and androstenedione (the precursor to testosterone) in humans. This book provides significant information on the pathology and biology of adrenal cortex. It will prove to be immensely beneficial to students and researchers in the field of endocrinology.

At the end, I would like to appreciate all the efforts made by the authors in completing their chapters professionally. I express my deepest gratitude to all of them for contributing to this book by sharing their valuable works. A special thanks to my family and friends for their constant support in this journey.

Editor

1

Adropin Stimulates Proliferation and Inhibits Adrenocortical Steroidogenesis in the Human Adrenal Carcinoma (HAC15) Cell Line

Ewelina Stelcer[1,2,3†], Paulina Milecka[1†], Hanna Komarowska[4], Karol Jopek[1], Marianna Tyczewska[1], Marta Szyszka[1], Marta Lesniczak[1], Wiktoria Suchorska[2,3], Karlygash Bekova[5], Beata Szczepaniak[1], Marek Ruchala[4], Marek Karczewski[6], Tomasz Wierzbicki[7], Witold Szaflarski[1], Ludwik K. Malendowicz[1] and Marcin Rucinski[1]*

[1] Department of Histology and Embryology, Poznan University of Medical Sciences, Poznan, Poland, [2] Radiobiology Lab, Greater Poland Cancer Centre, Poznan, Poland, [3] Department of Electroradiology, Poznan University of Medical Sciences, Poznan, Poland, [4] Department of Endocrinology, Metabolism and Internal Medicine, Poznan University of Medical Sciences, Poznan, Poland, [5] West Kazakhstan Marat Ospanov Medical University, Aktobe, Kazakhstan, [6] Department of General and Transplantation Surgery, Poznan University of Medical Sciences, Poznan, Poland, [7] Department of General, Endocrinological and Gastroenterological Surgery, Poznan University of Medical Sciences, Poznan, Poland

***Correspondence:**
Marcin Rucinski
marcinruc@ump.edu.pl

[†] These authors have contributed equally to this work

Adropin is a multifunctional peptide hormone encoded by the *ENHO* (energy homeostasis associated) gene. It plays a role in mechanisms related to increased adiposity, insulin resistance, as well as glucose, and lipid metabolism. The low adropin levels are strongly associated with obesity independent insulin resistance. On the other hand, overexpression or exogenous administration of adropin improves glucose homeostasis. The multidirectional, adropin-related effects associated with the regulation of metabolism in humans also appear to be attributable to the effects of this peptide on the activity of various elements of the endocrine system including adrenal cortex. Therefore, the main purpose of the present study was to investigate the effect of adropin on proliferation and secretory activity in the human HAC15 adrenal carcinoma cell line. In this study, we obtained several highly interesting findings. First, GPR19, the main candidate sensitizer of adrenocortical cells to adropin, was expressed in HAC15 cells. Moreover, GPR19 expression was relatively stable and not regulated by ACTH, forskolin, or adropin itself. Our findings also suggest that adropin has the capacity to decrease expression levels of steroidogenic genes such as steroidogenic acute regulatory protein (*StAR*) and *CYP11A1*, which then led to a statistically significant inhibition in cortisol and aldosterone biosynthesis and secretion. Based on whole transcriptome study and research involving transforming growth factor (TGF)-β type I receptor kinase inhibitor we demonstrated that attenuation of steroidogenesis caused by adropin is mediated by the TGF-β signaling pathway likely to act through transactivation mechanism. We found that HAC15 cells treated with adropin presented significantly higher proliferation levels than untreated cells. Using specific intracellular inhibitors, we showed that adropin stimulate proliferation via ERK1/2 and AKT dependent signaling pathways. We have also demonstrated that expression of GPR19 is elevated in adrenocortical carcinoma in relation to normal adrenal glands. High level of GPR19 expression in adrenocortical carcinoma may constitute a negative prognostic factor of disease progression.

Keywords: adrenal, adropin, TGF-beta, HAC15, GPR19

INTRODUCTION

Adropin is a peptide hormone encoded by the ENHO (energy homeostasis associated) gene, which is generally expressed in the liver, pancreas, and central nervous system (1). The encoded peptide is composed of 76 amino acids and residues 1-33 (cleaved during secretion) encode a secretory signal peptide sequence (2). This amino acid sequence is characterized by very high interspecies homology: it is identical in mice, rats and humans (3). ENHO expression in the brain is observed in ventromedial and lateral hypothalamic nuclei regulating appetite and autonomic functions. In turn, lower ENHO expression is characteristic in the liver, lung, kidney, ileum, and some endocrine glands. Hepatic ENHO expression is correlated with the expression of genes involved in glucose and lipid metabolism (4, 5). Furthermore, human studies showed that adropin may contribute to cholesterol homeostasis. It was found that in men, plasma adropin concentration is inversely correlated with low-density lipoprotein (LDL-C) cholesterol (6). Physiological serum adropin levels are still poorly defined, however, the adropin concentration in blood depends on a well-defined factors. Low adropin levels are strongly associated with pathological conditions such as insulin resistance, which is independent of the presence of obesity, dyslipidemia, hepatic steatosis, or increased fat mass (7). Overexpression or exogenous administration of adropin improves glucose homeostasis and increases capillary density and blood flow in mouse hind limb ischemia models (8). Moreover, adropin has been reported to have an endothelial protective role through increased eNOS (endothelial nitric oxide synthase) expression. Therefore, it can be assumed that the major function of adropin is to maintain energy homeostasis and insulin response (9). Treatments involving either transgenic overexpression of adropin or systemic adropin treatment clearly attenuate insulin resistance and glucose intolerance in dieting obese mice. In parallel with these observations, adropin knockout mice have been shown to present increased hepatic steatosis, adiposity and insulin resistance (10). By contrast, adropin deficiency correlates with the severity of obesity, dyslipidemia, and insulin resistance (3).

The secretion of adropin into the circulation and its biological effects are still poorly understood. Adropin is an endogenous ligand for GPR19 and adropin-mediated activation of GPR19 stimulates the intracellular MAPK/ERK1/2 signaling pathway, which is essential for the upregulation of E-cadherin and accompanying phenotypic changes in human breast cancer cells (11).

The multidirectional, adropin-related effects associated with the regulation of metabolism in humans also appear to be attributable to the effects of this peptide on the activity of various elements of the endocrine system. The adrenal cortex appears to be among the organs most affected by adropin.

According to the published data, hormonal regulation of adrenal function occurs primarily through activation of G protein-coupled receptors (GPCRs). GPCRs play superior role to many endocrine and neurotransmitter pathways, and their dysfunction contributes to some of the most prevalent human diseases (12). We presume that adropin–next to adiponectin, orexin, leptin, or neuromedin U–constitutes a peptide that affects adrenocortical activity. Given this context, the main purpose of the present study was to investigate the effect of adropin on basic (proliferation) and highly specific (steroidogenesis) biological activity in the HAC15 adrenal carcinoma cell line. The intracellular molecular mechanism of adropin-GPR19 interaction was determined using specific inhibitors and global gene expression study. Finally, the clinical significance of the obtained results was verified by analysis of *ENHO* and *GPR19* gene expression in human normal adrenals in relation to adrenocortical carcinoma.

MATERIALS AND METHODS

Adrenocortical Carcinoma Cell Lines and Treatment

The commercially available HAC15 cell line (ATCC® CRL-3301™, VA, USA) was cultured in a defined medium consisting of DMEM/F-12 without phenol red (Thermo Fisher Scientific, Waltham, MA, USA), 10% Cosmic Calf Serum (Hyclone, GE Healthcare, MA USA), 1% ITS + Premix (Corning, NY, USA), and 1% P/S (Merck Millipore, Darmstadt, Germany). The cells at low passages (p0-p1) underwent starvation in the DMEM/F-12 medium supplemented with 10% charcoal-stripped fetal bovine serum (FBS) (Thermo Fisher Scientific, MA, USA) and 1% P/S for 24 h. Subsequently, the cells were treated with the following compounds: ACTH (Synacthen) 10^{-7} M (Basel, Switzerland), angII 10^{-7} M (Sigma-Aldrich, MO, USA), forskolin 25 μM (Merck Millipore, Germany), and adropin 10^{-8} M (Bachem, Switzerland) for another 24 h. The cells cultured in the medium with 10% charcoal-stripped FBS served as controls. Immediately after 24 h of incubation, the cells and culture media were collected and stored at −80°C for further analysis. The commercially available Y1 cell line (ATCC® CCl-79™, VA, USA) was cultured in defined medium consisting of ATCC-formulated F-12K medium (ATCC® 30-2004™, VA, USA), 2.5% Fetal Bovine Serum (Hyclone, GE Healthcare, MA USA), 15% Donor Horse Serum (Biowest, MO, USA), 1% ITS + Premix (Corning, NY, USA) and 1% P/S (Merck Millipore, Germany).

Primary Human Adrenal Carcinoma (PAC) Cell Culture

Fresh adrenocortical carcinoma tumor samples obtained during surgery treatment, were cut into several small pieces. Adrenal fragments were further dissociated enzymatically in 25 ml of DMEM F12 without phenol red (Thermo Fisher Scientific, MA, USA) medium containing 0.1% type I collagenase (17018029; ThermoFisher Scientific, MA, USA) for 45 min in a 37°C water bath with intermittent mixing. After digestion, the mixture was filtered through a 70 μm sieve. After that tissue was centrifuged at 4°C, 1,200 rpm for 7 min. The cell pellet was resuspended in DMEM F12 medium with an addition of antibiotic-antimycotic solution and 10% FBS (Hyclone, GE Healthcare, MA USA). Primary cell culture were cultivated at 37°C and 5% CO_2 in humidified atmosphere up to 70% confluence. The use of postoperative adrenocortical carcinoma tumor samples for the cell culture has been approved by the Bioethics Committee of PUMS (decision no. 255/15).

Hormone Level Detection

Aldosterone and cortisol concentrations in cell culture media were measured by the ELISA method following the manufacturer's technical protocols (Aldosterone ELISA, cat. no. DE5298 Demeditec Diagnostics GmbH, Kiel, Germany; Cortisol ELISA, cat. no. DEH3388; Corticosterone cat. no. DEV9922 Demeditec Diagnostics GmbH, Kiel, Germany). Absorbance (OD) of each plate well was determined using the Biotek—Synergy 2 microtiter plate reader at 450 nm. Quantitative analysis was carried out using a four-parameter logistic curve (4PL) from "drc" Bioconductor package (13).

Immunofluorescence

The cells were washed tree times with phosphate buffered saline (PBS) solution (Sigma-Aldrich, MO, USA) and fixed for 20–25 min in 100% methanol. Then, they were rinsed with PBS supplemented with 1% bovine serum albumin (BSA) (Sigma-Aldrich, MO, USA). Then the cells were incubated in PBS containing 1% BSA and 0.2% Triton X-100 (Sigma-Aldrich, MO, USA) for 30 min. After this time, the cells were washed tree times with PBS + 1% BSA. The cells were incubated overnight at 4°C with the following primary antibodies: GPR-19 (ab123014, Abcam, UK) (1:200); CYP11B2 (ab167413, Abcam, UK) (1:250); StAR (8449S, Cell Signaling Technology, MA, USA) (1:250); and CYP11A1 (14217S, Cell Signaling Technology, MA, USA) (1:800). All of primary antibodies were diluted in PBS containing 1% BSA and 0.2% Triton X-100. After incubation with the primary antibodies, the cells were rinsed with PBS + 1% BSA. A secondary antibody–rabbit polyclonal antibody (1:500) (711-546-152) (Jackson ImmunoResearch, PA, USA)–was diluted with PBS+ 1% BSA and incubated for 1 h at 37°C in the dark. Then the cells were washed with PBS+ 1% BSA and stained for 5 min with diamidino-2-phenylindole dye (DAPI) solution (Sigma-Aldrich, MO, USA) in water (1:10,000). Before undergoing microscope analysis, the cells were washed three times with PBS. The acquisition was done using confocal laser scanning microscopy (Olympus FV10i with dedicated 60x water-immersion objective). Z-stack images were collected using Olympus FV10-ASW software. The same laser power (40% for Alexa Fluor® 488 and 12% for DAPI) was used for all images. Densitometric analysis was performed using ImageJ software (ImageJ 1.5q, Wayne Rasband, National Institutes of Health, USA) according to The Open Lab Book protocol (https://theolb.readthedocs.io/en/latest/imaging/measuring-cell-fluorescence-using-imagej.html). The images were measured by fluorescence using the green channel color range. Three images from each group were evaluated. The software was used to calculate integrated density from ten randomly selected areas of 40/40 pixels. Background fluorescence was determined for each image. The corrected total cell fluorescence (CTCF) values were calculated according to the following formula: CTCF = integrated density–(selected area X mean background fluorescence). All CTCF sets ($N = 30$/group) are shown on the graph and statistically analyzed (Mann–Whitney *U*-test).

Western Blot Analysis

Total proteins for the Western blot analysis were extracted from the HAC15 cells 24 h after treatment. Cells were collected, washed with PBS, and homogenized with RIPA buffer (ThermoFisher Scientific, MA, USA). After centrifugation at 13,000 rpm at 4°C for 30 min, the supernatant was transferred into new tubes. The concentration of the protein sample was measured using the Pierce BCA Protein Assay Kit (23225, MA, USA). Fifteen micrograms of total protein of each cell extract was resolved by Tris/Glycine/Sodium dodecyl sulfate polyacrylamide gel electrophoresis and transferred to a polyvinylidinedifluoride membrane (1704156, Bio-Rad, CA, USA). Non-specific binding was blocked by incubation in 5% non-fat milk in Tris-buffered saline and Tween 20 at room temperature for 1 h. Blots were then probed overnight at 4°C with anti-GPR 19 1 μg/ml (ab 123014 abcam, UK) and anti-GPADH 1:1000 (5174S, Cell Signaling Technology, MA, USA). Immunoreactive bands were then probed for 1 h at room temperature with the appropriate horseradish peroxidase (HRP)-conjugated secondary anti-Rabbit IgG-HRP 1:2000 (7074S, Cell Signaling Technology, MA, USA). Protein bands were detected by WesternBright Quantum HRP substrate (Advansta, CA, USA) and imaged using a ChemiDoc Imaging Systems (Biorad, CA, USA).

RNA Extraction

Total RNA isolation was performed according to the modified Chomczynski method with TRI Reagent (Sigma-Aldrich, MO, USA) and the RNeasy Mini Elute Cleanup Kit (Qiagen, Hilden, Germany) in accordance with the manufacturer's instructions. The concentration of isolated RNA was determined by spectrophotometric measurement of absorbance at 260 nm. The purity of the extracted RNA was calculated using an absorbance ratio of 260/280 nm (NanoDrop spectrophotometer, Thermo Scientific, MA, USA). The integrity and quality of the isolated RNA was examined with the Agilent 2100 Bioanalyzer (Agilent Technologies, Inc., Santa Clara, CA, USA). The received RNA integrity numbers (RINs) varied from 8.5 to 10, with an average of 9.2. RNA samples were diluted to 50 ng/μl. One-hundred ng of RNA was dedicated to the microarray study. The remaining total RNA was utilized for the validation of microarray results by qPCR.

Reverse Transcriptase-PCR and qPCR Analysis

The reverse transcriptase (RT) reaction was carried out using the iScript™ cDNA synthesis kit (Bio-Rad, CA, USA) in a total volume of 20 ul. One μg of total RNA was incubated with Oligo(dT) as primer for 40 min, at a temperature of 45°C. Real-time PCR reactions were carried out using the LightCycler® 480 Probes Master (Roche, Switzerland) and pair of specific primers and probes designed with the Universal Probe Library software (Roche Diagnostics, Switzerland). RT-qPCR reactions were carried out under the following thermal conditions: 10-min denaturation step for the Taq DNA polymerase activation, then by a two-step amplification program repeated 40 times: denaturation at 95°C for 30 s followed by annealing and extension at 64°C for 60 s. The cycle threshold values obtained for the genes of interest were normalized to hypoxanthine-guanine phosphoribosyltransferase gene (HPRT), which previous studies have shown to be one of the most stable reference genes in the adrenal gland (14). The expression level for each examined gene was determined using the formula $-2^{\Delta\Delta ct}$. The reaction was carried out in triplicate for each of analyzed genes.

Microarray Expression Study

The microarray study was performed as described in detail elsewhere (15–18). The total RNA isolated previously was pooled into four samples per group (control, ACTH, forskolin and adropin) treated as described above (see *Cell culture and Treatment* section). The protocol including *in vitro* transcription, biotin labeling, and cDNA fragmentation was performed using the Affymetrix GeneChip IVT Express Kit (Affymetrix, Santa Clara, CA, USA). Then the biotin labeled cDNA were hybridized with the Affymetrix Gene Chip Human Genome U219 microarrays together with appropriate internal controls. The hybridization was performed in the AccuBlockTM Digital Dry Bath hybridization oven (Labnet International, Inc., Edison, NJ, USA) at 45°C for 16 h. Subsequently, the microarrays were washed and stained by means of the Affymetrix GeneAtlas Fluidics Station (Affymetrix, Santa Clara, CA, USA). The microarrays were scanned using the Imaging Station of the GeneAtlas System. Initial analysis of the scanned microarrays was carried out with Affymetrix GeneAtlas TM Operating Software.

Analysis of Microarray Data

For all bioinformatic analyses we used R statistical programming language supplemented with relevant Bioconductor libraries. Background correction, normalization with calculation of the normalized expression values was carried out by the robust multiarray average (RMA) normalization method implemented in the "Affy" library (19). Biological annotation was obtained from the "oligo" library and combined with the normalized expression data set (20). Differential expression was calculated using linear models for microarray data from the "limma" library (21). The selection criteria for a differentially expressed genes (DEGs) based on a absolute fold change >2 and a $p < 0.05$. Technical description with raw and normalized data files were deposited in the Gene Expression Omnibus (GEO) repository at the National Center for Biotechnology Information (http://www.ncbi.nlm.nih.gov/geo/) under the GEO accession number: GSE150775.

Assignment of Differentially Expressed Genes to Appropriate Gene Ontology Biological Process (GO BP)

ENTREZ ids with fold change values of differentially expressed genes were subjected to gene ontology enrichment analysis using the "clusterProfiler" library (22). The analysis was performed separately for each comparison. Reference GO annotation data was obtained directly from the human annotation library "org.Hs.eg.db." Enriched GO BP terms were visualized as a heatmap in relation to expression levels of relevant DEGs.

Gene Set Enrichment Analysis (GSEA)

GSEA was used to identify the level of depletion or enrichment in gene expression between two compared groups within pre-defined gene sets (GO terms, pathways). The method employs the Kolmogorov–Smirnov statistical test to determine significantly depleted or enriched gene sets (23). Analysis was carried out using the "FGSEA" Bioconductor library (24). Normalized fold change values from all of the genes were $\log_2$ transformed and sorted. Then using signal-to-noise ratio with 10,000 time permutation, enrichment scores (ESs) were calculated for all of predefined gene set from the Reactome database (from the Molecular Signatures Database) (25, 26). Obtained ESs were normalized by their gene set size. For each of depleted/enriched terms, the p-value was adjusted by FDR. Gene sets with adj. $p < 0.05$ were uploaded to Cytoscape (v. 3.7.2) to generate enrichment map with links between significantly-enriched processes (27, 28). Enriched terms were clustered and annotated using the AutoAnnotate v1.3.2 Cytoscape plugin (29). From the selected gene sets, the genes with the highest impact on the analyzed biological process that contributed the most to the enriched signal were extracted. These genes with their fold change values were visualized in Cytoscape.

RT-qPCR Validation of Microarray Data

Real Time-PCR reactions were performed using the PrimePCR™ Custom Plates (Bio-Rad, CA, USA) and the specific synthesized primers for each gene: tissue factor pathway; jun proto-oncogene (*JUN*); histone cluster 1; H2bm (*HIST1H2BM*); arrestin domain containing 3 (*ARRCD3*); and kinesin family member 20A (*KIF20A*). The cDNA samples were analyzed for genes of interest and for the reference gene HPRT. The expression level for each target gene was calculated as $-2^{\Delta\Delta ct}$. The reaction was performed in triplicate for the gene of interest. The result of the validation is presented in the **Supplementary Figure 1**.

Inhibiting TGF-β Type I Receptor Kinase for Hormone Level Detection

To inhibit the TGF-β type I receptor (TβRI) kinase in the HAC15 cell line, we used the LY-364947 (Merck Millipore, Germany) in a final concentration of 10 μM. Prior to adropin treatment, cells were subjected to the influence of the TβRI kinase inhibitor for 1 h. Next, HAC15 cells were incubated with adropin for 24 h, using the following variants: HAC15+ DMSO (control); HAC15 + inhibitor dissolved in DMSO; HAC15+adropin+ DMSO; and HAC15+ inhibitor dissolved in DMSO +adropin. Finally, aldosterone and cortisol secretion rates were determined.

BrdU Cytometry Analysis

After 24 h of treatment, the cells were removed from 6-well plates with 1 mM EDTA (Sigma-Aldrich, MO, USA). After detachment, cells were centrifuged and resuspended in fresh medium. Cells were counted by means of the MOXI Z automated cell counter (4×10^5 cells were used for the analysis). According to manufacturer instructions, cells were fixed and permeabilised. Then, the cells were washed and stained with PerCP-Cy™5.5 Anti-BrdU antibody (51-9007682, BD Biosciences, NJ, USA). Data acquisition was performed with a multiparameter flow cytometer (CytoFLEX; Beckman Coulter, IN, USA) and results were analyzed with FlowJo software (FlowJo, LLC, OR, USA). Statistical significance was calculated on the basis of Student's t-test, with significance levels set at $p < 0.05$.

RTCA Cell Proliferation Assay. Identification of Potential Adropin-Dependent Signaling Pathways Using Specific Inhibitors

To verify the effect of adropin on the proliferation rate of HAC15 cells together with the identification of the intracellular mechanism, we applied an electrical impedance-based cell proliferation assay, named Real-Time Cell Analyser (RTCA, Roche Applied Science, GmbH, Penzberg, Germany). The RTCA system detects fluctuations in electrical impedance on the integrated sensory electrodes located at the bottom of the chamber's 16-hole slide plates (E-Plate 16), which are covered by dividing cells. Electrical impedance is measured at 15-min intervals throughout the cultivation period. The main RTCA readout is the "Cell Index" –a measurable parameter corresponding to the relative change in electrical impedance depending on the rate of proliferation or apoptosis of the cultivated cells. The influence of adropin on HAC15 cell proliferation was studied in two independent experiments. In the first one it was examined whether adropin stimulates HAC15 cell proliferation through ERK1/2 and PI3/AKT dependent signaling pathway. HAC15 cells were cultivated in the following experimental groups: (1) control (2) adropin (10^{-8}M) (3) PI3/AKT inhibitor–LY294002 (10^{-7}M), (4) MEK1/2-dependent inhibitor of ERK1/2–U0126 (10^{-7}M), (5) adropin (10^{-8}M) + LY294002 (10^{-7}M), (6) adropin (10^{-8}M) + U0126 (10^{-7}M). The second experiment examined the potential role of TGF-dependent pathway in the regulation of HAC15 cell proliferation affected by ardopin. An analogous experimental model was used here as in the experiments on the inhibition of TGF-β type I receptor kinase for hormone level detection, including following groups: (1) control, (2) adropin (10^{-8}M), (3) LY-364947 (10 μM), (4) adropin (10^{-8}M) + LY-364947 (10 μM).

Each experimental group was seeded in the eight E-plate wells to a final volume of 200 μl per well. The cell index was normalized (normalized cell index) at time of examined substances administration using software from the same manufacturer (RTCA Software, v. 1.2, November 2009). HAC15 cells were cultivated with examined substances per approximately 50 h. Each experiment was repeated ≥ three times.

Normal Adrenal and Adrenocortical Carcinoma Samples

Human adrenocortical carcinoma samples were obtained from the 13 patients qualified for adrenalectomy. Normal adrenal glands ($N = 13$) were collected during the kidney transplantation procedure. After surgical removal, adrenal fragments of size 0.5 cm^3 were immediately immersed in RNA Later Storage Solution (Sigma-Aldrich, Missouri, USA) to stabilize and protect intracellular RNA. Then samples were stored at −70°C until RNA isolation, reverse transcription and qPCR analysis were carried out. The research protocol was approved by the Bioethics Committee of PUMS (decision No. 255/15). Written consent was obtained from adrenalectomized patients as well as from kidney donors.

Analysis of The Cancer Genome Atlas (TCGA) Dataset

Clinical description file and RNAseq counts for 92 cases of adrenocortical carcinoma were obtained from public TCGA database (30) using FireBrowse server (http://gdac.broadinstitute.org/) (31). Normalization of raw counts was done with voom algorithm from "Limma" package (21). Log transformed, normalized expression data for *ENHO* and *GPR19* gene were retrieved from the whole adrenocortical carcinoma expression dataset. The obtained data was divided in two separate populations with high and low expression of the *ENHO* and *GPR19*. The median value was taken as a cut-off point, so the expression of the examined genes above the median was assigned to the high expression group, while the samples with expression below the median was included in the low expression group. The groups were compared by Kaplan–Meier survival analysis. Survival plots with lograng p-value estimation were performed using "survival" R library (32) in relation to death event according to clinical description file.

RESULTS

The Adropin Precursor Gene ENHO and Its Receptor (GPR19) Are Expressed in the HAC15 Adrenocortical Cell Line. Expression of the Analyzed Genes Is Relatively Stable and Not Significantly Regulated by ACTH, Forskolin, or Adropin Itself

QPCR analysis revealed expression of the adropin precursor gene (ENHO) and the adropin receptor (GPR19) in the HAC15 cell line. We also sought to determine whether this expression is regulated by the most commonly used adrenal steroidogenesis stimulators such as ACTH at a concentration of 10^{-7} M and 25 μM forskolin. Incubation for 24 h with these substances did not significantly alter the expression of the genes. We also verified the effect of adropin on the expression of the *ENHO* and *GPR19* receptor genes. Analogously to ACTH and forskolin, 24 h incubation in 10^{-8}M adropin did not affect the expression of those genes (**Figure 1A**). We also confirmed GPR19 expression at the protein level using immunofluorescence (**Figure 1B**) and western blot (**Figure 1C**). Immuofluorescence staining revealed that GPR19 expression is mainly localized within cytoplasmic vesicles and cell membranes (**Figure 1B**). Semi-quantitative analysis of GPR19 expression at protein level confirmed that its expression is not regulated by the all of examined substances (**Figure 1C**).

Adropin Inhibits Basal Secretion of Aldosterone and Glucocorticoids in HAC15, Y1 and PAC Cells

To analyse the effect of adropin on secretion of the main adrenocortical hormones, we utilized three different cell culture models: two adrenocortical carcinoma cell lines derived from human (HAC15), and mouse (Y1) as well as primary human adrenal carcinoma (PAC) cell culture. Approximately 70% confluent HAC15, Y1 and PAC cells seeded in 96-well plate were treated with 10^{-8} M adropin for 24 h. In all of studied cell culture models, we observed that adropin cause a significant inhibition in aldosterone and glucocorticoid secretion. In each of the analyzed cells, we noticed strong stimulation of adrenocortical hormone secretion by ACTH or forskolin, that served as a positive control. As the current research focuses mainly on the human adrenal glands, detailed results for the HAC15 cell line are presented below.

Adropin significantly reduced median aldosterone (211.4 pg/ml) and cortisol (110.21 ng/ml) secretion compared to the relevant control groups (aldosterone = 506.5 pg/ml, cortisol = 352.06 ng/ml). In both cases forskolin and ACTH were used as positive controls. Unlike H295R cells, HAC15 cells are an adrenocortical cell line with an active ACTH receptor denominated MC2R; however, the response of these cells to ACTH is relatively weak, as our results demonstrate: 24 h incubation of HAC15 cells with 10^{-7} M ACTH led to a weak stimulation of aldosterone secretion (median = 612.35 pg/ml). ACTH-stimulated cortisol secretion increased slightly (median = 383.51 ng/ml). Forskolin is a potent cAMP-dependent pathway activator, the main trigger of adrenocortical steroidogenesis and incubation of HAC15 cells with 25 μM forskolin led to rapid stimulation of both aldosterone (median = 1181.62 pg/ml) and cortisol (median = 691.37 ng/ml) secretion (**Figure 2A**).

Adropin Inhibits AngII or Forskolin Stimulated Secretion of Aldosterone and Cortisol in HAC15 Cells

In further studies, we examined whether the inhibitory effect of adropin on adrenocortical hormones secretion could also occur after stimulation of HAC15 cells with angiotensin 2 (**Figure 3A**) or forskolin (**Figure 3B**). As expected, the secretion of the studied adrenocortical hormones was significantly increased under the influence of angII or forskolin in relation to the untreated control group. Adropin significantly reduced angII-stimulated median aldosterone (523 pg/ml) and cortisol (216 ng/ml) secretion compared to angII stimulated cells (aldosterone = 588 pg/ml, cortisol = 383 ng/ml). A similar pattern of adrenocortical hormone secretion was observed regarding to forskolin-stimulated HAC15 cells, where adropin significantly decreased forskolin-stimulated aldosterone and cortisol secretion (aldosterone = 867 pg/ml, cortisol = 380 ng/ml) in relation to forskolin-stimulated cells (aldosterone = 769 pg/ml, cortisol = 530 ng/ml).

Inhibitory Effect of Adropin on Adrenocortical Steroidogenesis Occurs by Decreasing the Expression of Rate-Limiting Genes for the Initial Steps of Steroid Biosynthesis

The steroidogenic acute regulatory protein (StAR) and side-chain cleavage enzyme (CYP11A1) catalyze the first, rate-limiting step of steroidogenesis. StAR enables cholesterol translocation into the inner mitochondrial membrane (IMM), where CYP11A1 transforms cholesterol to pregnenolone. To assess the relative changes in *StAR* and *CYP11A1* gene expression following adropin treatment, we performed relative QPCR using specific primers. Additionally, we extracted normalized data from a microarray study of the genes. According to the QPCR, 24 h incubation of HAC15 cells with adropin resulted in a statistically significant decrease in expression of *StAR* and the *CYP11A1* gene (44 and 45% from baseline values, respectively) (**Figure 4**). *StAR* and *CYP11A1* gene expression presented a similar profile in the microarray study, although statistically insignificant compared to controls. As expected, forskolin strongly stimulated the expression of *StAR* and *CYP11A1*, which were, respectively, 3.23 and 2.48 times higher than controls. Similarly, ACTH was also stimulative, but only with the QPCR method, where ACTH increased *StAR* expression by 1.63 and *CYP11A1* expression by 1.74. Adropin did not affect expression of the *CYP11B2* gene encoding aldosterone synthase; only forskolin induced a significant stimulation of *CYP11B2* expression (20.54-fold increase).

Next, we performed semi-quantitative analysis of StAR, CYP11A1 and CYP11B2 expression at the protein level using immunofluorescence. The use of identical experimental conditions and the same laser power for fluorochrome excitation allowed us to evaluate signal intensity and consequently to perform semi-quantitative analysis of StAR, CYP11A1 and CYP11B2 expressed in HAC15 cells subjected to 24 h ACTH, forskolin, or adropin stimulation. Representative images and a summary graph with statistical analyses are presented in **Figure 5**. In general, the expression profiles of StAR, CYP11A1 and CYP11B2 proteins correspond to the expression profile of their respective genes. Our data show that 24 h of adropin incubation with HAC15 cells led to a 2.88-fold decrease in StAR protein expression vs. the control group

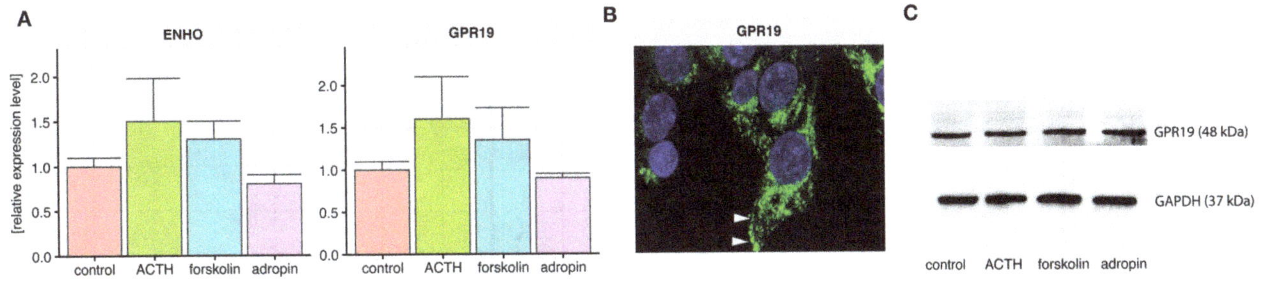

FIGURE 1 | Relative expression levels of the adropin precursor gene *ENHO* and the adropin receptor *GPR19* in HAC15 cells. **(A)** Real time qPCR study in untreated (control) cells and cells incubated with ACTH, forskolin, and adropin for 24 h ($N = 4$/group). Statistical differences were determined by Mann–Whitney U non-parametric test compared to controls. Both the expression of *ENHO* and *GPR19* did not differ significantly from the control group. **(B)** GPR19 immunoreactivity in untreated HAC15 cells. The reaction was detected in cytoplasmic vesicles and cell membranes (indicated by white arrows). **(C)** Semi-quantitative analysis of GPR19 expression at protein level using western blot method.

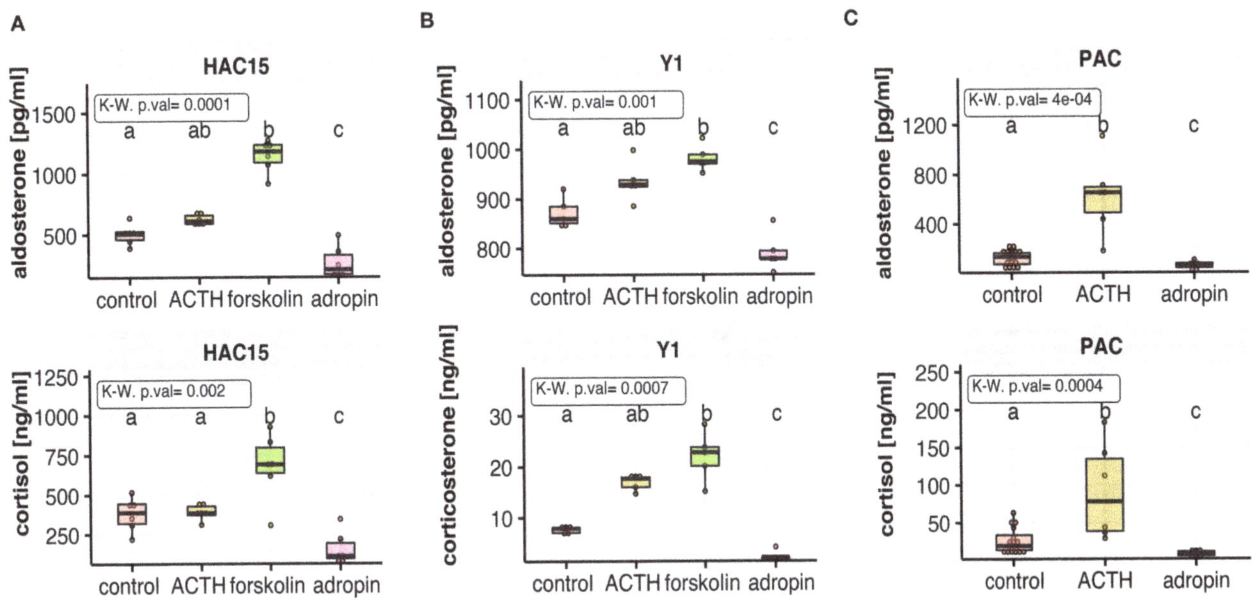

FIGURE 2 | The effect of adropin on aldosterone and cortisol or corticosterone secretion in the following cell culture models: human adrenal carcinoma (HAC15) cell line **(A)**, mouse adrenocortical tumor (Y1) cell line **(B)** and primary human adrenal carcinoma (PAC) cell culture **(C)**. All of studied cells were exposed to adropin for 24 h. ACTH or forskolin treated cells were used as a positive controls. Results are presented as medians with IQR. Statistical differences were determined by Kruskal–Wallis test followed by Dunn's *post hoc* test. Groups sharing the same letter are not significantly different according to Dunn's test.

(median CTCF 1,447 vs. 4,177, respectively). Adropin also inhibited expression of the CYP11A1 protein, leading to 1.49-fold decrease in CYP11A1 expression vs. controls (median CTCF, 4,264 vs. 6,357). Adropin did not significantly alter CYP11B2 expression vs. controls (median CTCF = 5,083 vs. 5,880, respectively). Incubation of HAC15 cells with ACTH led to 1.23-fold increase in StAR protein expression (median CTCF = 5,169) and 2.8-fold increase in CYP11A1 (median CTCF = 17,801), without a significant effect on CYP11B2 protein expression (median CTCF = 6,010). Forskolin caused a significant increase in expression of StAR, CYP11A1 and CYP11B2 proteins, leading to a 3.2-, 2.26- and 1.49-fold increase in their expression, respectively (median CTCF values: StAR = 13,648, CYP11A1 = 14,377, and CYP12B2 = 8,756).

Adropin Moderately Alters the Transcriptomic Profile of HAC15 Cells

The Affymterix Gene Chip Human Genome U219 Array Strips used in the current study allowed for the simultaneous examination of gene expression of 19,285 human transcripts. The transcriptome study was performed 24 h after adding ACTH, forskolin, or adropin to the culture medium. The transcriptomic profile was compared to the group of untreated cells (controls). The general profile of transcriptome changes is shown as a

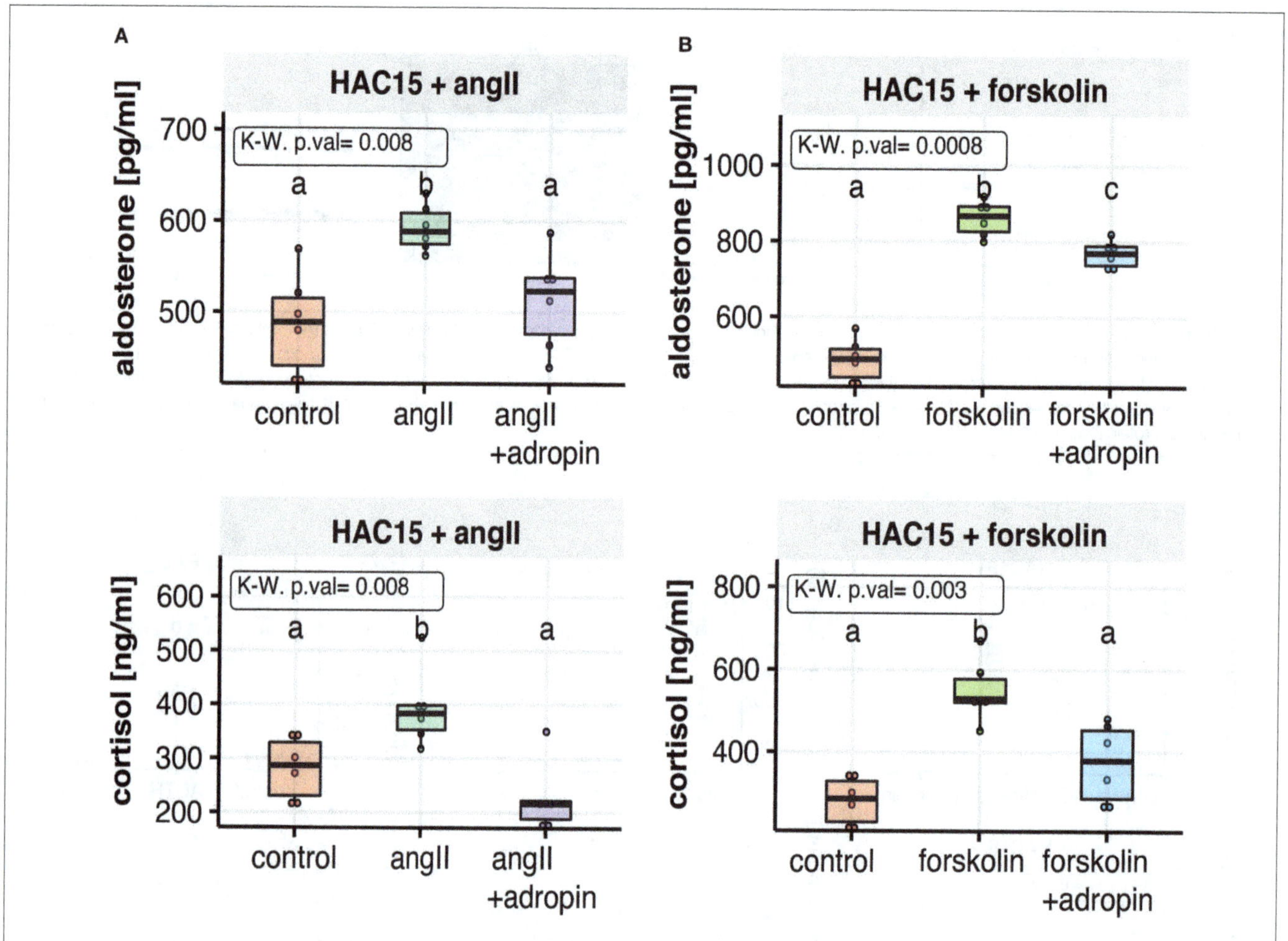

FIGURE 3 | The effect of adropin on angII **(A)** or forskolin **(B)** stimulated aldosterone and cortisol secretion in the human adrenal carcinoma (HAC15) cell line exposed to adropin for 24 h. Results are presented as medians with IQR. Statistical differences were determined by Kruskal–Wallis test followed by Dunn's *post hoc* test. Groups sharing the same letter are not significantly different according to Dunn's test.

volcano plot (**Figure 6**). We assumed the following selection criteria for DEG: an expression |fold difference| (absolute value)> 2 and $p \leq 0.05$. According to these criteria, only three genes were significantly upregulated after ACTH treatment, while 136 genes were upregulated and 61 downregulated by forskolin. Adropin caused a decrease in the expression of 6 genes and an increase in 31 genes. Genes with significant changes and the highest fold values are marked by their symbols on the volcano plot graphs. Adropin significantly altered expression in the following genes: histone cluster 1; H2BM (*HIST1H2BM*; fold = −3.19); nuclear factor of kappa light polypeptide gene enhancer in B-cells inhibitor; zeta (*NFKBIZ*, fold = 2.38); glycerol phosphocholine phosphodiesterase GDE1 homolog (*GPCPD1*, fold = 2.3); protein disulfide isomerase family A, member 6 (*PDIA6*, fold = 3.05); TPT1 antisense RNA 1 (*TPT1-AS1*, fold = 2.59); RNA, U5B small nuclear 1 (*RNU5B-1*, fold = 2.31); zinc finger protein 248 (*ZNF248*, fold = 2.31); jun proto-oncogene (*JUN*, fold = 2.77); piccolo presynaptic cytomatrix protein (*PCLO*, fold = 2.46); and solute carrier family 16, member 6 (*SLC16A6*, fold = 2.46)

After studying the steroidogenesis-related genes, we found that adropin decreased the expression of these genes. Although the fold values in some of the genes were below the cut-off threshold, there was an evident trend showing the capacity of adropin to inhibit steroidogenesis-related gene expression (**Figure 7**).

Adropin Exerts a Significant Effect on the Genes Involved in the TGF Beta Signaling Pathway

To determine the biological processes most likely to be regulated by adropin, we analyzed enrichment in the relevant ontological groups from the GO BP database. We performed a similar analysis for forskolin. Whole sets of differentially expressed genes (197 for forskolin vs. controls; 37 for adropin

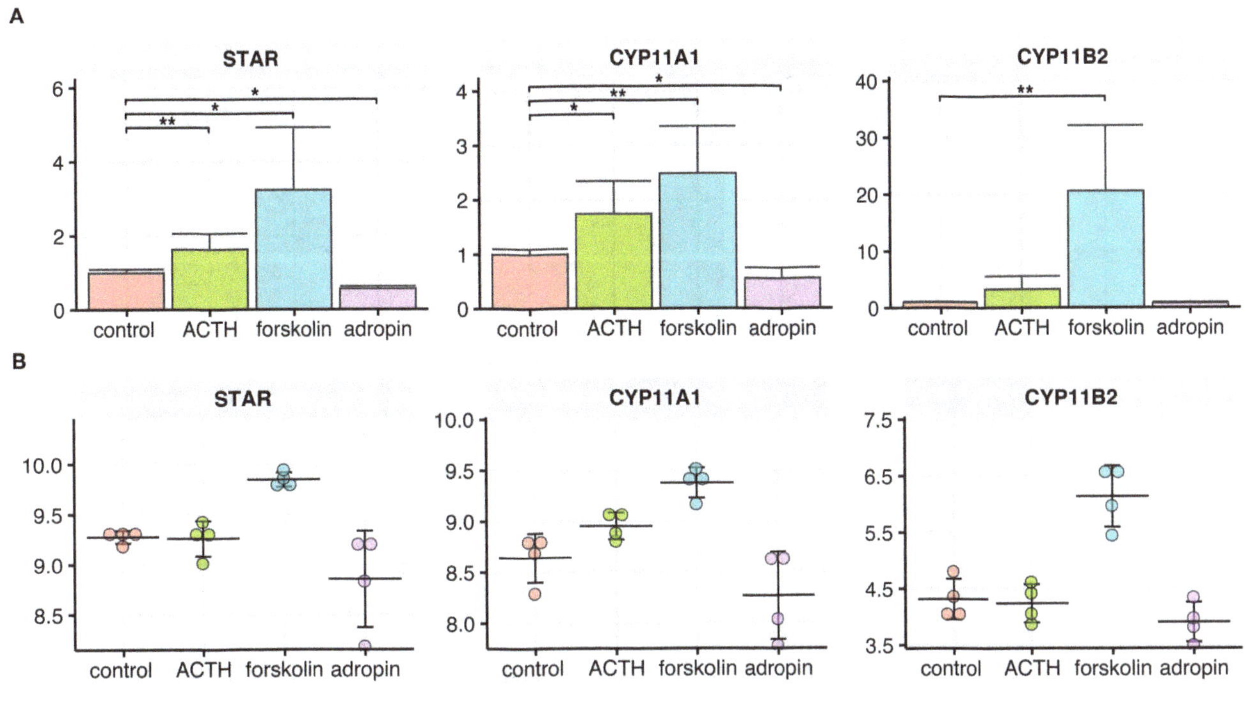

FIGURE 4 | Relative expression levels of *CYP11A1*, *CYP11B2* and *StAR* genes in the HAC15 cell line after 24 h incubation with ACTH, forskolin, and adropin vs. controls (untreated cells). **(A)** Real time QPCR study ($N = 4$/group). Statistical differences were determined by the Mann–Whitney U non-parametric test compared to controls. $^{*}p < 0.05$; $^{**}p < 0.01$. **(B)** Normalized expression values extracted from the microarray data set ($N = 4$/group).

vs. controls) were subjected to gene ontology enrichment analysis using ClusterProfiler. The result of this analysis is shown as a heatmap (**Figure 8**). The results show that adropin activated 30 different biological processes, most of which ($N = 15$) were related to processes involved in cell cycle regulation, including the following: "signal transduction involved in G2 DNA damage checkpoint"; "positive regulation of endothelial cell proliferation"; "G2 DNA damage checkpoint" "regulation of cell cycle checkpoint"; "mitotic spindle assembly checkpoint" "negative regulation of mitotic metaphase/anaphase transition"; "negative regulation of metaphase/anaphase transition of cell cycle"; "negative regulation of chromosome separation." Another significant cluster of gene ontology terms concerned the regulation of immune response process: "positive regulation of leukocyte differentiation"; "inflammatory response to wounding"; "positive regulation of T-helper 17 type immune response"; "regulation of T-helper 17 cell differentiation"; "T-helper 17 type immune response"; "T-helper 17 cell differentiation."

The above analysis of ontological groups was carried out in the relatively small group of adropin-regulated genes that met the assumed cut-off criteria (fold > 2, $p < 0.05$), which explains why the ontological groups presented in **Figure 8** consist of a small number of genes. This suggests that the transcriptome profile affected by 24 h incubation of HAC15 cells with adropin may be regulated in a limited manner, as evidenced by the fact that most genes did not pass the cut-off criteria. Therefore, we decided to rely on GSEA based on the ranking of all genes regardless of the assumed cut-off values. In this analysis, the fold change values of all genes were $\log_2$ transformed and ranked according to their logFC value. Next, these values were used for a 10,000 time permutation test to calculate the enrichment score (ES) within predefined gene sets from the Reactome database. Enrichment scores were normalized by their gene set size and presented as a normalized enrichment score (NES) in which positive NES values indicate that the process is stimulated by adropin. Gene sets with adjusted $p < 0.05$ were exported to Cytoscape software to generate links between significantly enriched processes (Enrichment Map) (**Figure 9A**). The largest cluster of enriched terms were related to "TGF beta signaling," for which we found five significant enrichment terms: "Signaling by TGF beta family members" (NES = 1.81, adj. $p = 0.042$); "TGF beta receptor signaling activates SMADs" (NES = 1.86, adj. $p = 0.036$); "Signaling by TGF beta receptor complex" (NES = 1.92, adj. $p = 0.037$); "SMAD2 SMAD3:SMAD4 heterotrimer regulates transcription" (NES = 1.83, adj. $p = 0.041$); and "Downregulation of TGF beta receptor signaling" (NES = 1.95, adj. $p = 0.036$). Interaction network between genes with the highest impact on "TGF beta signaling" enriched terms are presented in **Figure 9B**. The expression of all presented genes increased under the influence of adropin stimulation, suggesting that this peptide

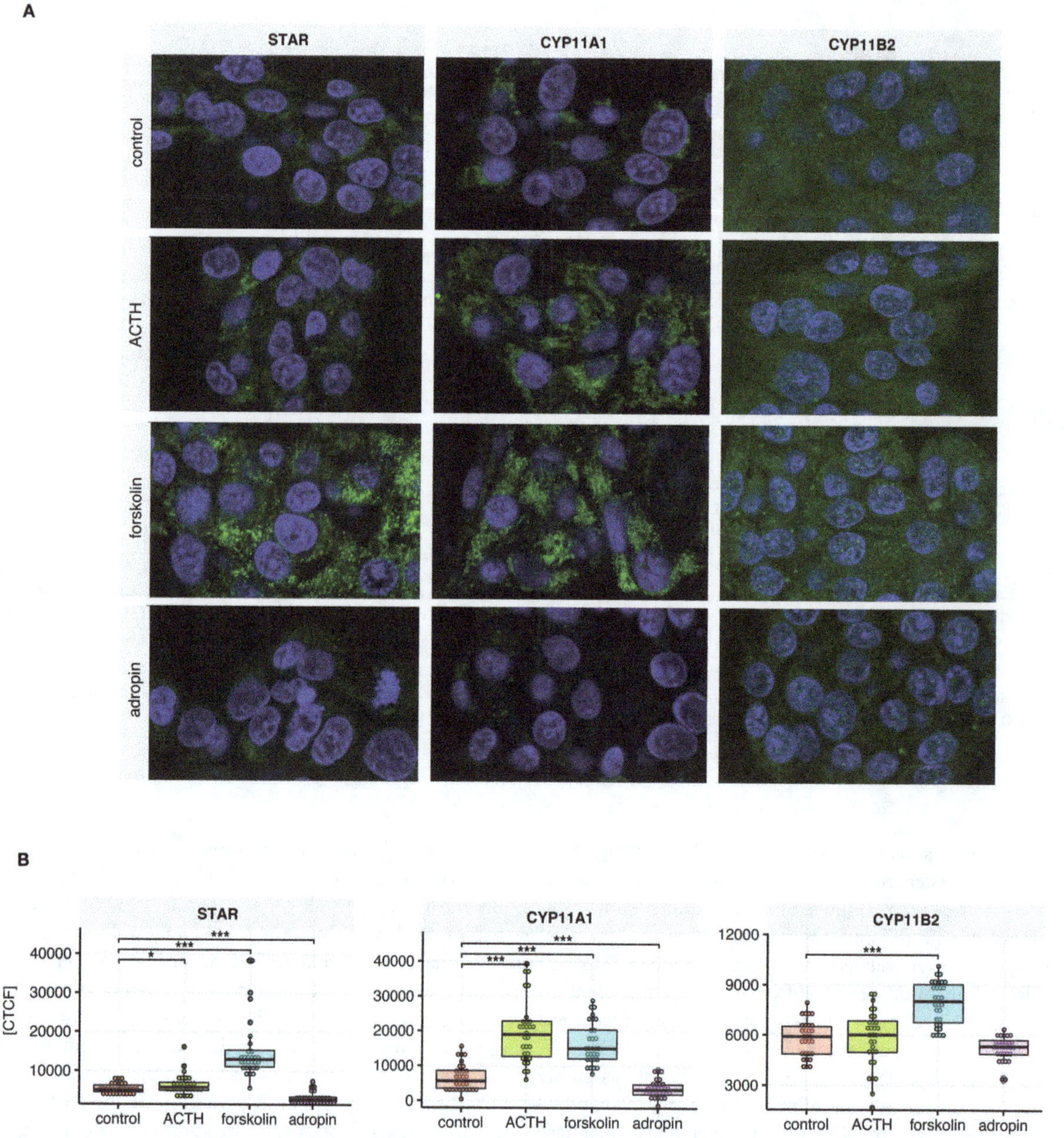

FIGURE 5 | StAR, CYP11A1, CYP11B2 immunoreactivity in untreated HAC15 cells (controls) and cells incubated with ACTH, forskolin and adropin for 24 h. **(A)** Representative images of the HAC15 cells from each group, where the positive reaction of antibody binding was visualized in green, while the cell nuclei were stained in blue with DAPI. **(B)** Densitometric analysis of the fluorescence intensity (*N* =3 0/group). Statistical differences were determined by the Mann–Whitney U non-parametric test compared to controls. $^{*}p < 0.05$; $^{***}p < 0.001$. CTCF indicates corrected total cell fluorescence.

affects physiological function of HAC15 cells via a TGF beta-dependent pathway.

Adropin Inhibits Adrenocortical Steroidogenesis via TGF Beta Mediated Pathway

The experiment was conducted on 70% confluent HAC15 cells seeded in 96-well plates. In order to inhibit the TGF beta-dependent cell response, the TβRI kinase inhibitor was given to appropriate groups (I) and then the HAC15 cells were incubated for 1 h. Next, adropin was administered. The results are shown in **Figure 10**. The inhibitor itself had no significant effect on median aldosterone (188.68 pg/ml) and cortisol (208.54 ng/ml) secretion compared to controls (aldosterone =195.59 pg/ml, cortisol = 141.49 ng/ml). As noted above, adropin significantly reduced median aldosterone (102.6 pg/ml) and cortisol secretion (104.4 ng/ml). However, in the group in which TGF-beta signaling was inhibited by adropin administration, this effect

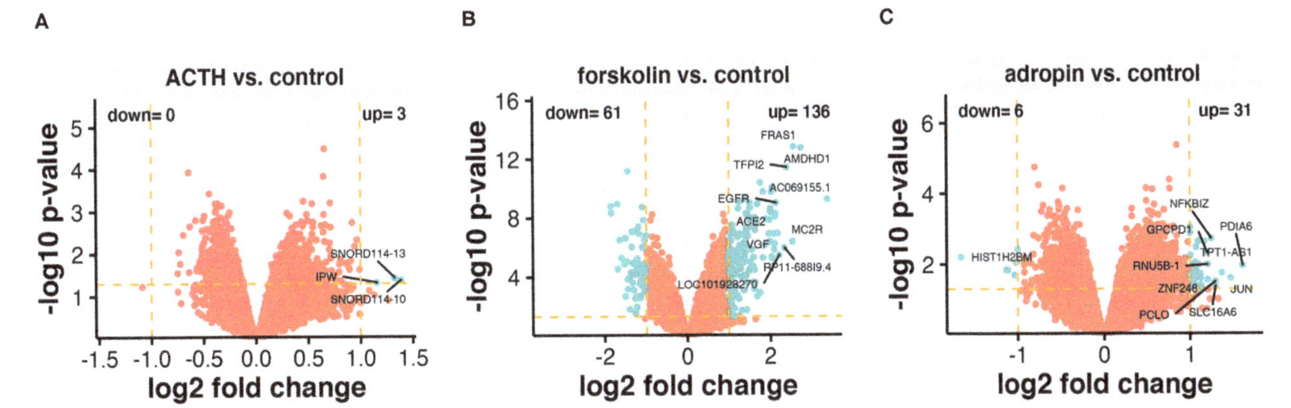

FIGURE 6 | Total gene expression profile of the HAC15 cell line after 24 h incubation with ACTH **(A)**, forskolin **(B)**, and adropin **(C)** compared to control (untreated) cells. Each dot represents a mean value of the single gene expression ($n = 4$/group). Dotted lines indicate cut-off values (two-fold change in expression and $p < 0.05$ with FDR correction). The red dots represent the genes below the cut-off limit. The turquoise color marks upregulated and downregulated genes. Ten genes with the highest differences within fold change values were labeled with the appropriate gene symbols.

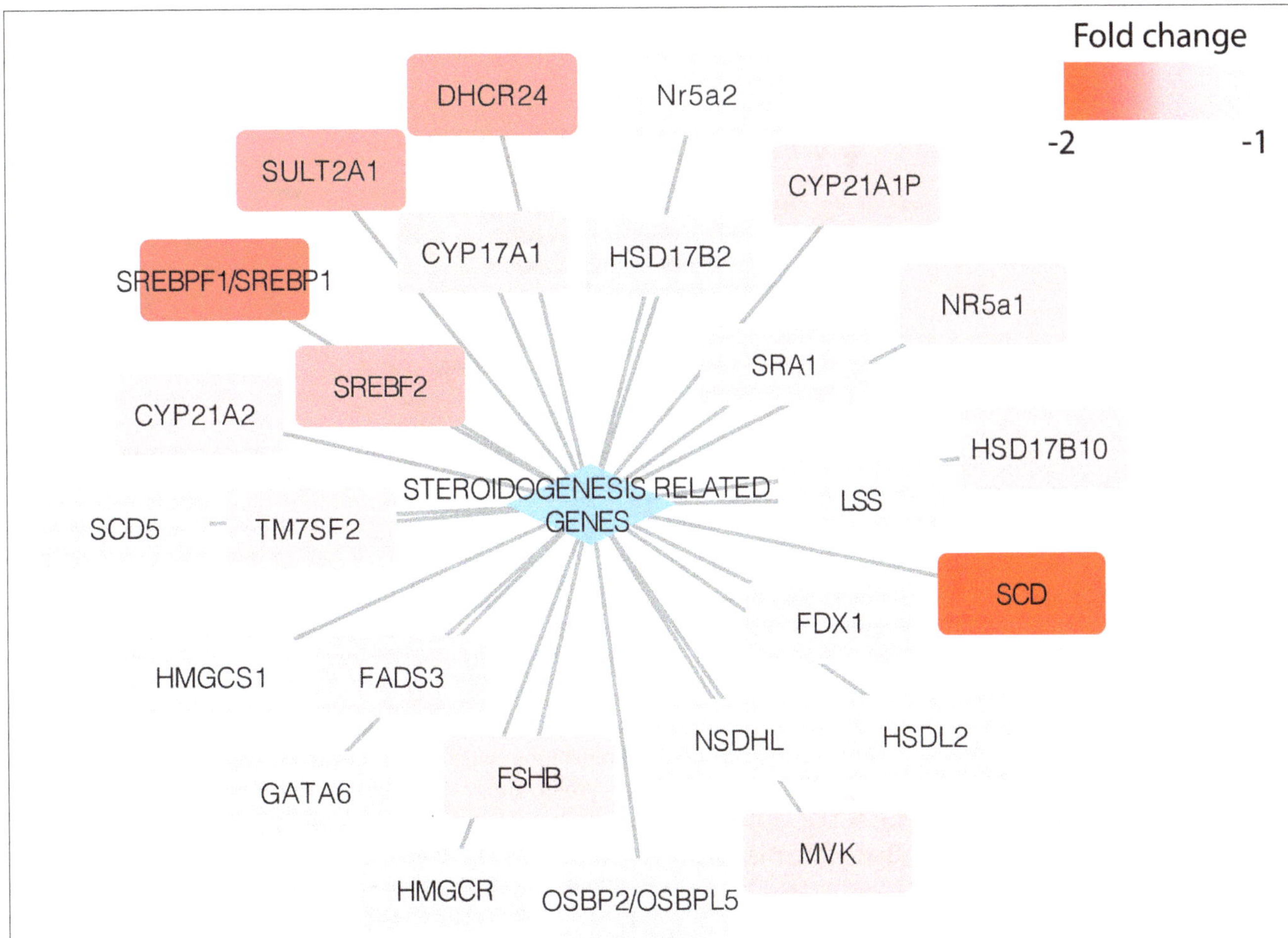

FIGURE 7 | Expression of steroidogenesis-related genes in the HAC15 cell line after 24 h incubation with adropin compared to control (untreated) cells. Appropriate fold change values are marked in red.

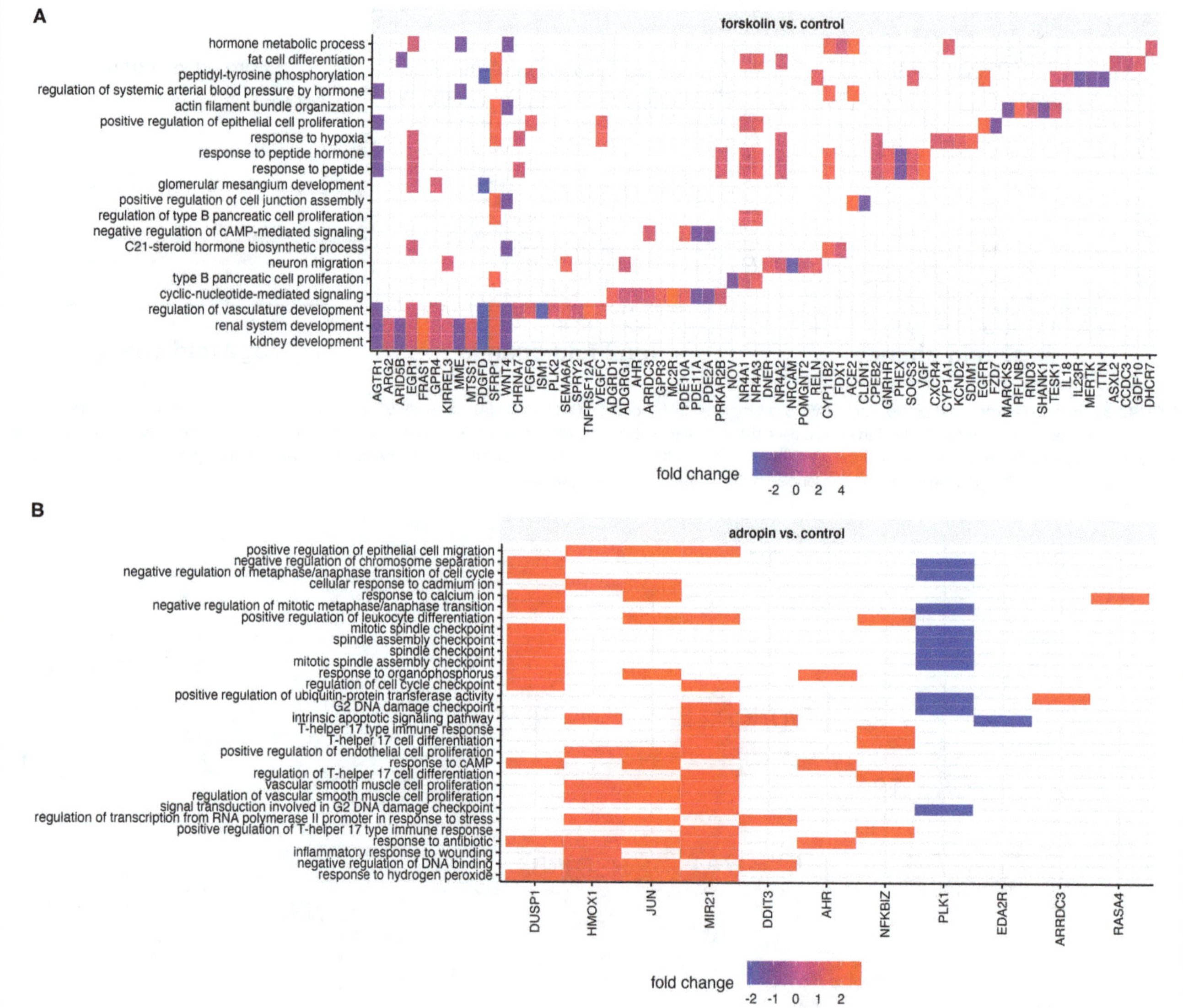

FIGURE 8 | Heatmap of overrepresented gene sets from GO BP (gene ontology–biological process) database, regulated by forskolin **(A)** and adropin **(B)** compared to the control group. The graphs show only the GO groups above the established cut-off criteria (adjusted $p < 0.05$). Fold change values for each DEG were mapped with the appropriate color. Gene symbols of DEGs are shown on the x scale.

was either completely absent for aldosterone (205.68 pg/ml) or it resulted an increase of cortisol secretion (283.96 ng/ml). These results confirm that adropin has the capacity to inhibit adrenocortical steroidogenesis of HAC15 cells via the TGF-β mediated pathway.

Adropin Stimulates the Proliferative Activity of HAC15 Cells via ERK1/2 and AKT, Independently of TGF Beta Mediated Pathway

The effect of 10^{-8}M adropin on the proliferation of HAC15 cells was determined by two independent methods. First, we applied flow cytometry method involving cell labeling with BrdU (**Figure 11A**). The measurement was made -at 24 and 48 h after peptide administration. At 24 h post-adropin administration, we observed no significant changes in the number of HAC15 cells vs. the untreated control group; however, after 48 h, the proliferation rate of HAC15 cells incubated with adropin had increased significantly (**Figure 11A**). The second method of proliferation rate testing based on impedance measurement of proliferating cells using the xCelligence (RTCA). This method enables continuous, real-time proliferation assessment, measured in 15-min intervals. Within 50 h from adropin administration we observed again its stimulatory effect on proliferation (**Figure 11B**) To verify whether the adropin stimulatory effect on HAC15 cells proliferation depends on ERK1/2 and AKT activation, we perform RTCA analysis in the presence of pharmacological MEK1/2-dependent inhibitor

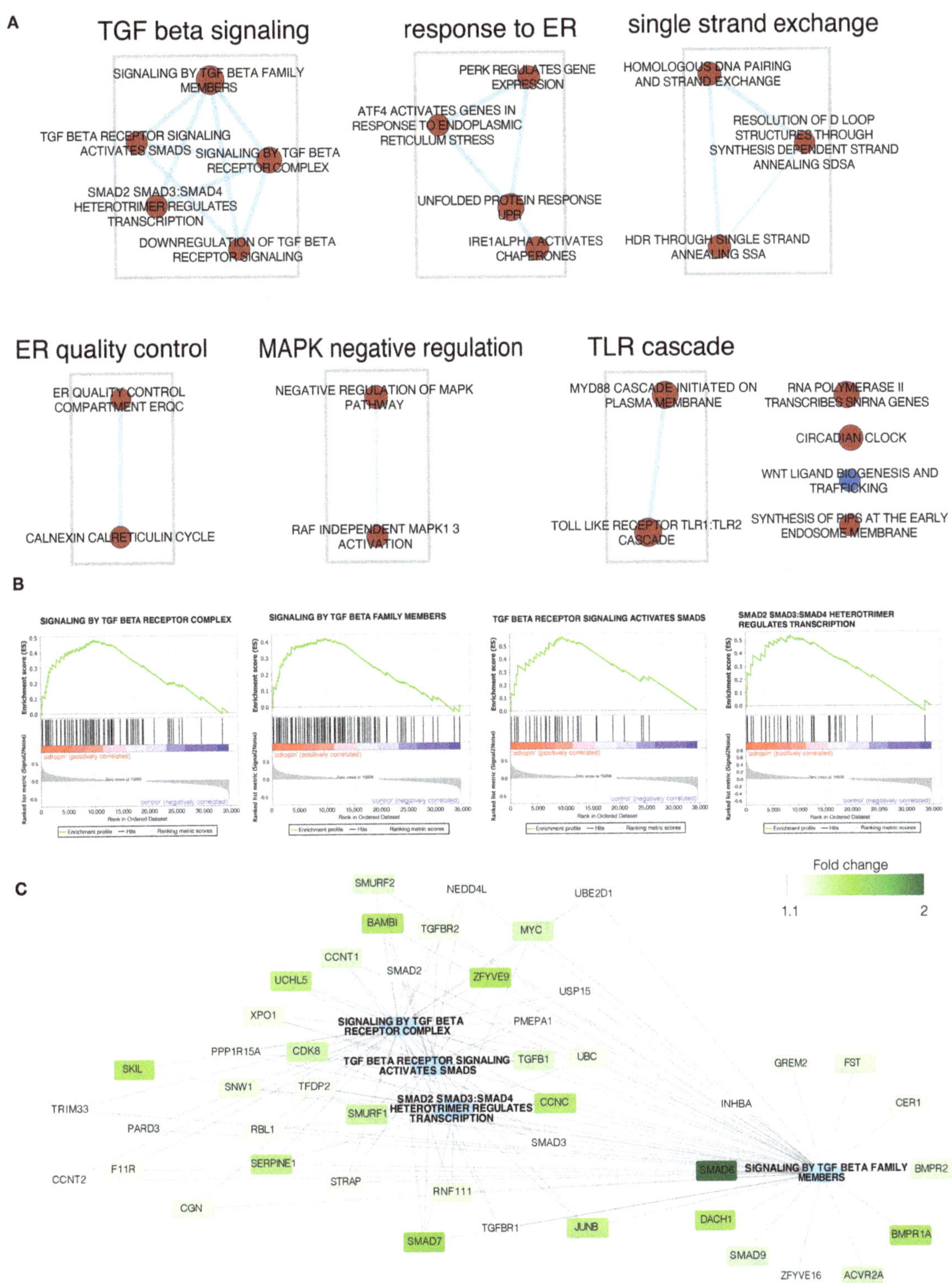

FIGURE 9 | Gene set enrichment analysis affected by adropin compared to control group. **(A)** Enrichment map of gene sets regulated by adropin (red = activated, blue = inhibited). The thickness of the connecting line corresponds to the level of gene matching to individual terms. **(B)** Enrichment plot of: "Signaling by TGF beta receptor complex," "Signaling by TGF beta family members," "TGF beta receptor signaling activated by SMADs," "SMAD2 SMAD3:SMAD4 heterotrimer regulates transcription." Each of the graphs shows the positive value of the enrichment score (ES) indicating activation of genes forming these processes under the influence of adropin. **(C)** Interaction network between genes with the highest impact on the biological processes analyzed. Fold change values for individual genes are marked by color scale.

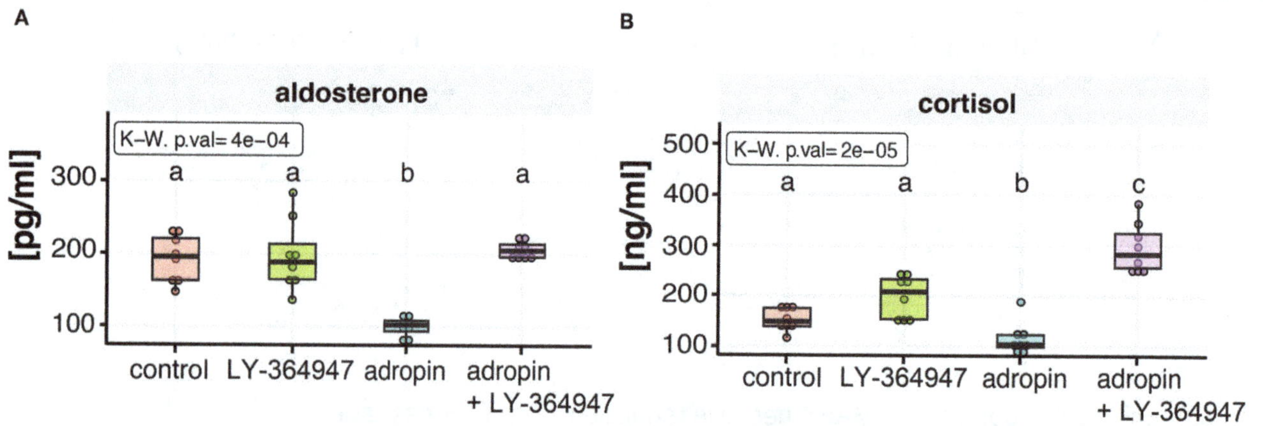

FIGURE 10 | Effect of TGF beta signaling inhibitor (LY-364947) on adropin dependent aldosterone **(A)** and cortisol **(B)** inhibition in HAC15 cells. Approximately 70% confluent HAC15 cells seeded in 96-well plates were incubated with LY-364947 for 1 h prior to subsequent 24 h adropin treatment. Aldosterone and cortisol secretion rates were statistically evaluated by the Kruskal–Wallis test followed by Dunn's *post hoc* test. Groups sharing the same letter are not significantly different according to Dunn's test.

of ERK1/2 (U0126) and PI3/AKT inhibitor (LY294002). We have also investigated the potential role of TGF beta-dependent pathway in HAC15 cells proliferation using LY-364947 inhibitor (**Figure 11B**). In the presence of ERK1/2 and PI3/AKT inhibitors, adropin induced HAC15 cells proliferation was completely inhibited (adropin + U0126 and adropin + LY294002 in relation to adropin group on **Figure 11B** left side). On the other hand, the presence of LY-364947 in the culture medium did not significantly suppress the stimulating effects of adropin (adropin + LY-364947 in relation to adropin group on **Figure 11B** right side). These data suggest that adropin stimulate HAC15 cells via ERK1/2 and AKT dependent mechanism independently of TGF beta mediated pathway.

GPR19 Expression Is Elevated in Human Adrenocortical Carcinoma. High Level of GPR19 Could Constitute a Negative Prognostic Factor of Disease Progression

Due to the significant stimulatory role of the adropin-GPR19 system in the proliferation of human derived adrenocortical carcinoma cell line (HAC15), mediated by ERK1/2 and AKT dependent mechanism, we undertook the analysis regarding the clinical significance of the obtained results. According GEPIA (Gene Expression Profiling Interactive Analysis) (33) web server for cancer and normal gene expression profiling based on RNA-seq data, expression of *GPR19* in normal human organs is the highest in brain and testis. These observations are consistent with the data deposited in the NCBI database (https://www.ncbi.nlm.nih.gov/gene/2842). According to GEPIA and NCBI data, expression of *GPR19* in normal adrenal gland is relatively low, but it' s strongly rising in adrenal carcinoma (0.37 in normal adrenal vs. 9.69 in adrenal carcinoma according to GEPIA) (**Figure 12A**). Expression analysis of our normal adrenal samples in relation to adrenocortical carcinoma ($N = 13$/group) showed that the expression of the adropin precursor gene–*ENHO* was not regulated in the study groups (**Figure 12B**). Expression of *GPR19* was significantly increased in adrenocortical carcinoma, which is in line with previously reported GEIPA data. According Kaplan–Meier survival analysis of data received from TCGA, expression of *ENHO* gene do not have a significant impact on the survival profile of patients with adrenocortical carcinoma (logrank $p = 0.27$) (**Figure 12C**), however elevated expression of *GPR19* leads to a statistically significant decrease in survival (logrank $p = 0.0008$), suggesting that high expression of *GPR19* could constitute a negative prognostic factor of disease progression.

DISCUSSION

Adropin is a newly identified metabolic hormone expressed inter alia in the liver and brain. It plays a role in mechanisms related to increased adiposity, insulin resistance, as well as glucose and lipid metabolism (1). Adropin is a secretory signal peptide which has been shown to alter whole body glucose and lipid metabolism after administration in mice and rats, and it also activates signaling pathways involved in glucose and lipid metabolism in mammalian cell lines (34, 35).

To verify our hypothesis that adropin plays an important role in adrenocortical hormone biosynthesis, we selected the human adrenal cell model based on the HAC15 cell line because HAC15 cells secrete mineralocorticoids, glucocorticosteroids, and adrenal androgens. While numerous experiments have been carried out on NCI-H295 cells, our *in vitro* research model with HAC15 cells seems to be more valuable because, unlike NCI-H295 cells, HAC15 adrenocortical cells react to some extent to corticotropin stimulation and also have good forskolin response (36, 37).

The current study has several objectives: (1) to determine the impact of adropin on the proliferation rate of HAC15 adrenocortical cells with analysis of ERK1/2, AKT signaling pathway contribution in this process, (2) to evaluate the role of the adropin in the regulation of primary physiological function

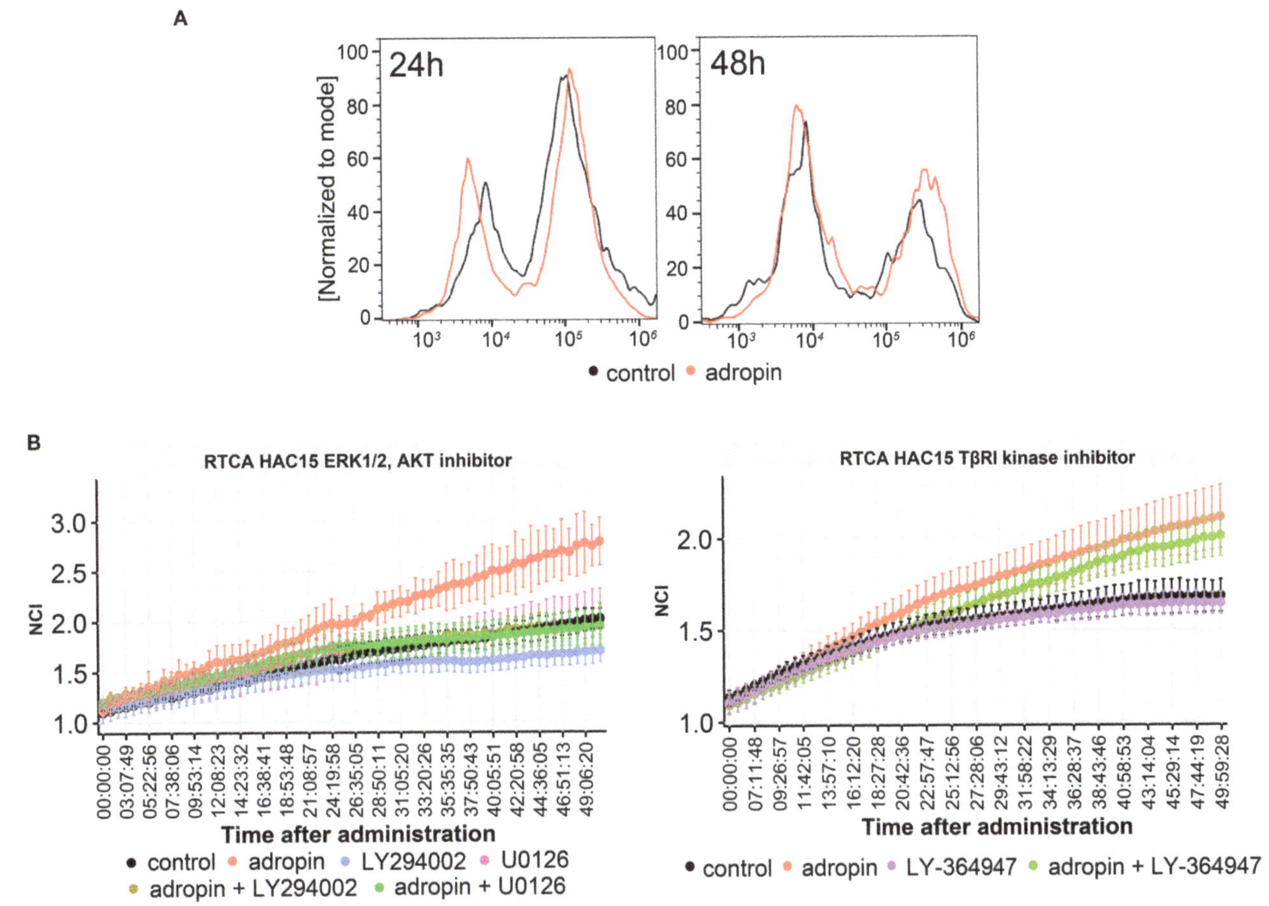

FIGURE 11 | The role of adropin in HAC15 cell proliferation. **(A)** Flow cytometry study on the contribution of adropin (10^{-8} M concentration) in stimulation of HAC15 cell proliferation, measured at 24 and 48 h after peptide administration. **(B)** Effect of ERK 1/2, AKT and TBRI kinase inhibitors on adropin-induced HAC15 cell proliferation using xCelligence Real-Time Cell Analyzer–RTCA **(B)**. The RTCA chart presents mean normalized cell index (NCI) +-SD.

in adrenocortical cells (i.e., mineralocorticoid and glucocorticoid secretion), (3) to examine the response of HAC15 adrenocortical cells to treatment with adropin, forskolin, and ACTH at the gene and protein level, (4) to assess how administration of adropin changes the expression of key genes involved in steroidogenesis, and (5) to evaluate clinical significance of the obtained results by analysis of *ENHO* and *GPR19* gene expression in human normal adrenals in relation to adrenocortical carcinoma.

To our knowledge, the current study is the first to examine the direct effect of adropin on the regulation of adrenocortical steroidogenesis. We have shown that exposure to adropin significantly inhibits the basal and angII or forskolin stimulated secretion of aldosterone and cortisol by HAC15 cells. Adropin reduced also the secretion of adrenocortical hormones in Y1-mouse adrenocortical carcinoma cell lines as well as in primary human adrenal carcinoma cell culture, proving its universal mechanism of inhibiting the secretion of adrenal hormones from tumor derived adrenocortical cells. Thus, adropin belongs to the group of biologically active peptides that directly inhibit adrenocortical steroidogenesis. Other peptides in this group include bursal anti-steroidogenic peptide (BASP) (38); atrial natriuretic peptide (ANP) (39); B-type natriuretic peptide (BNP) (40); and thyrotropin (TRH) (41).

We also proved that adropin-mediated adrenal steroidogenesis inhibition occurs by suppressing expression of the StAR protein and CYP11A1 gene, which are involved in the initial stages of steroidogenesis. The steroidogenic acute regulatory protein (StAR) and side-chain cleavage enzyme (CYP11A1) catalyze the first and rate-limiting step of steroidogenesis. StAR enables cholesterol translocation into the inner mitochondrial membrane (IMM), where CYP11A1 transforms cholesterol to pregnenolone (42).

We also evaluated the molecular aspects of inhibition of steroidogenesis by adropin in HAC15 cells through global gene expression analysis using a microarray approach. HAC15 cells exposed to adropin showed altered expression of genes that regulate biological processes such as cell cycle regulation and immune response; however, the overall expression profile was characterized by a relatively weak modulation, which is reflected by a low number of genes above the cut-off values

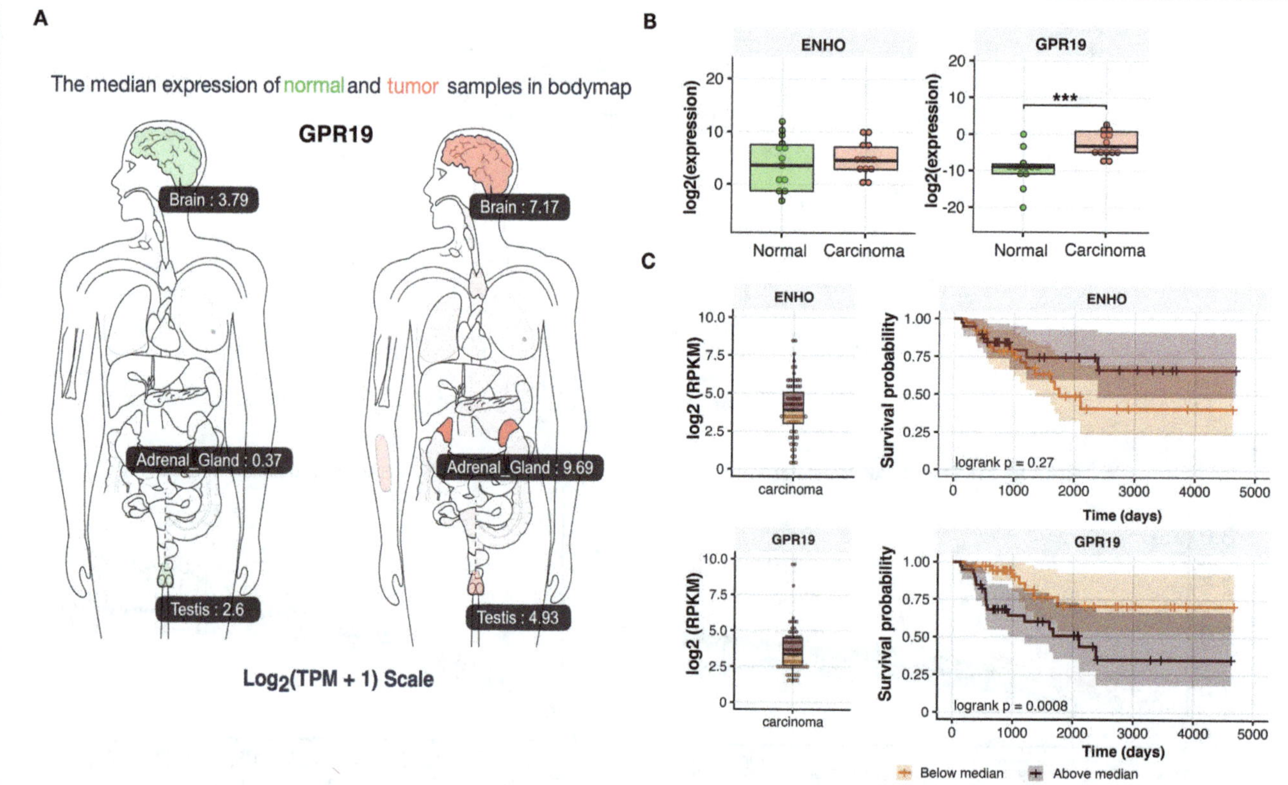

FIGURE 12 | Expression of *ENHO* and *GPR19* in clinical samples. **(A)** Profile of *GPR19* expression in normal and tumor samples from GEPIA (Gene Expression Profiling Interactive Analysis) database. **(B)** Expression of *ENHO* and *GPR19* in normal and tumor samples of human adrenal gland. **(C)** Kaplan–Meier survival analysis of 92 cases of adrenocortical carcinoma obtained from TCGA database. Expression data for *ENHO* and *GPR19* were divided into group with high (above median) and low expression (bellow median). Statistical differences were determined by the Mann–Whitney U non-parametric test compared to normal adrenals. $^{***}p < 0.001$.

in the volcano plot. Further analysis with GSEA revealed that adropin induces the expression of a gene cluster associated with the TGF-β signaling pathway. This observation allowed us to suggest that adropin-mediated inhibition of steroidogenesis may occur through the activation of the TGF-β signaling pathway. Accordingly, TGFβ appears to be a negative regulator of adrenocortical steroidogenesis. In this context, other studies have shown that TGFβ inhibits adrenal hormone biosynthesis in sheep (43) and bovine primary cultures of adrenocortical cells (44). Furthermore, Liakos et al. observed that TGFβ1 significantly inhibits forskolin-induced steroid 11β-hydroxylase activity and CYP11B1 mRNA levels, as well as angiotensin II-induced aldosterone synthase activity and CYP11B2 mRNA levels in the human adrenocortical tumor cell line NCI-H295R (45). Another study demonstrated that TGF-β1 inhibits progesterone and estradiol production by trophoblast cells; however, these inhibitory effects were diminished if the cholesterol transport and aromatization steps were bypassed, suggesting that the action of TGF-β1 on steroid production is exerted at the level of cholesterol transport and aromatase activity (46). Consistent with these reports, other studies have confirmed that TGF-β1 downregulates StAR expression and decreases progesterone production in cultured human granulosa cells (47). Treatment with TGF-β1 activates the Smad2/3 and ERK1/2 signaling pathways. Based on siRNA-mediated knockdown approaches and pharmacological inhibitors, those authors showed that activation of the Smad3 and ERK1/2 signaling pathways are needed for the TGF-β1–induced downregulation of StAR expression and a decrease in progesterone production. These results provide important insights into the molecular mechanisms that mediate TGF-β1–regulated StAR expression and progesterone production (47). Park et al. (48) found that the inhibitory effect of TGF-β1 on testicular steroidogenesis occurs through the cross-talk of TGF-b1/ALK5-activated Smad3 with orphan nuclear receptor Nur77. Consequently, Smad3 indirectly regulates the promoter activity of steroidogenic genes. These findings provide a molecular mechanism for TGF-β1-mediated repression of testosterone production in testicular Leydig cells (48).

Adrenocortical cells possess TGFβ1 receptors (mainly type I: TGFBR1 and type III: TGFBR3), which increase in number in response to ACTH treatment. Binding of mature TGFβ1 to its adrenocortical cell receptors causes numerous intracellular biochemical events resulting in inhibited cortisol production. Two important targets negatively regulated by TGFβ1 are angiotensin II receptors and the steroid 17a-hydroxylase (cytochrome P-45017) enzyme (49).

Currently, it is accepted that adropin exerts its biological role through activation of the GPR19 receptor, which belongs to the G-protein-coupled receptor family (GPCR) (50). The current model of GPCR signaling includes three main pathways: (1) the classical pathway, where appropriate ligand binding leads to downstream activation of G protein and other effector molecules, (2) arrestin signaling via ligand-regulated scaffolds (51), and (3) transactivation of protein serine/threonine kinase receptors (PS/TKRs), including TGFBR1, through the receptors of GPCR agonists, a mechanism first described by Ullrich in 1996 (52, 53). Our results suggest that adropin exerts its inhibitory effect on HAC15 cell steroidogenesis by binding to the GPR19 receptor and then stimulating the TGF-β-dependent pathway via transactivation. Based on experiments using the TGFβl kinase inhibitor, we confirmed that attenuation of steroidogenesis caused by adropin is mediated by the TGF-β signaling pathway, confirming the adropin-dependent transactivation mechanism. Other GPCR agonists such as thrombin (54), factor X (55), LPA (56) and endothelin-1 (57) lead to time-dependent activation of the TGF-β dependent signaling pathway. Previous research has shown that in vascular smooth muscle cells thrombin transactivation of the TGFBR1 based on cytoskeletal reorganization that activates Ras homolog member A (RhoA)/Rho-associated, coiled-coil containing protein kinase (ROCK) signaling, triggering the activation of integrin-dependent signaling and finally activating the large latent complex which holds TGF-β near the cell surface with the potential for activation of TGFBR1 (54, 58). Although our microarray study showed that adropin did not affect the expression of the RhoA/ROCK genes in the HAC15 cells, their expression was relatively high (data not shown), indicating that this intracellular mechanism of TGFBR1 transactivation may also occur in the HAC15 cell line. However, this hypothesis requires further study for confirmation.

We used the GSEA approach to identify numerous genes with increased expression due to activation of the TGF-β dependent pathway; however, we also identified genes that lead to increased TGF-β signaling pathway activity. Previous research has shown that silencing the dachshund family transcription factor 1 (DACH1) in H295R cells increases aldosterone production by suspending the TGF-β signaling pathway, whereas overexpression of DACH1 caused decreasing in aldosterone biosynthesis by activating the TGF-β dependent pathway (59). In the context of our study, incubation of HAC15 cells with adropin significantly stimulated DACH1 gene expression (fold = 1.64, adj. $p = 0.04$), which in turn may boost the inhibitory effect of TGF-β on HAC15 cell steroidogenesis.

The available published data indicate that adropin exerts a stimulating effect on the proliferative activity of a variety of cells. Among other mechanisms, it has been shown that adropin stimulates 3T3-L1 (fibroblasts) and rat primary preadipocyte cell proliferation via the ERK1/2 and AKT signaling pathways. (34). Adropin stimulate proliferation in mesenchymal-like MDA-MB-231 cells by MAPK/ERK1/2 signaling pathway which is essential for the upregulation of E-cadherin and accompanying phenotypic changes in human breast cancer cells (11). Moreover, adropin upregulates—both *in vitro* and *in vivo*—the expression of eNOS in endothelial cells. Furthermore, endothelial cells exposed to adropin show increased proliferation and migration, higher capillary-like tube formation rates, decreased permeability, and less TNF-alpha induced apoptosis (8). By contrast, Sato et al. demonstrated that in human aortic smooth muscle cells (HASMCs), adropin suppressed cell migration and proliferation without inducing apoptosis *via* ERK1/2 and Bax downregulation (60). It is important to emphasize that our results showed that exposing HAC15 cells to adropin stimulates the proliferative activity of HAC15 cells via ERK1/2 and AKT mediated pathway (**Figure 11B**). Moreover, the stimulatory effect of adropin on the proliferation of these cells was long-lasting, persisting throughout the entire time (50 h after administration) the cells were cultured in the presence of the peptide.

Because of stimulatory effect of the adropin on proliferation of human derived adrenocortical carcinoma cell line occurred via ERK1/2 and AKT dependent mechanism, we decided to analyse the clinical significance of the obtained results. According to the GEPIA data and our results, the expression of GPR19 was significantly elevated in adrenocortical carcinoma in relation to normal adrenal. Considering the stimulatory roles of adropin on HAC15 cell proliferation, we can assume that elevated expression of the GPR19 may indirectly cause a speed-up rate of proliferation in adrenocortical carcinoma. This suggestion seems to be confirmed in Kaplan–Meier survival analysis of 91 adrenocortical carcinoma samples from TCGA database. Increased expression of GPR19 leads to a statistically significant decrease in survival, suggesting that high expression of GPR19 could constitute a negative prognostic factor of adrenocortical carcinoma disease progression, however this aspect require further studies.

Most of the results discussed in this paper are based on experiments involving the administration (both *in vivo* and *in vitro*) of exogenous adropin. The physiological role of this peptide in the body remains an open question. Experiments on adropin knockout mice (AdrKO) provide some information in this respect, with published data showing that adropin prevents insulin resistance, dyslipidemia, impaired glucose tolerance, and loss of T lymphocytes (3, 61). The role of GPR19, the putative adropin receptor, is also debatable and not fully understood. In this respect, Martin (62) performed a study to evaluate agonist-independent constitutive signaling of several GPCR receptors. Using this method, the GPR19 receptor was classified as a "non-responder," with "revealed patterns that suggest either a lack of constitutive signaling or an unresolved triggering condition (i.e., agonist dependent)" (62). The identification of a specific adropin antagonist would possible provide a better understanding of the role of this peptide in cells, organs, and in the entire body.

CONCLUSIONS

In this study, we investigated the influence of exogenous adropin on proliferation and steroidogenesis in the human HAC15 adrenal carcinoma cell line. We found that exposing HAC15 cells to adropin decrease the secretion of aldosterone and cortisol by HAC15 cells. This effect was accompanied by inhibition of both StAR and CYP11A1 expression. Bioinformatic analysis based on microarray data suggests that adropin-mediated inhibition of adrenocortical hormone biosynthesis involves activation of the TGF-β signaling pathway likely to act through transactivation mechanism. We also found that HAC15 cells treated with adropin presented significantly higher proliferation rate than untreated cells. Using specific intracellular inhibitors, we showed that adropin stimulated proliferation occurs via ERK1/2 and AKT dependent signaling pathways. GPR19 expression was elevated in human adrenocortical carcinoma in relation to normal adrenals. High level of GPR19 could constitute a negative prognostic factor of disease progression.

AUTHOR CONTRIBUTIONS

ES, PM, and HK invented and designed the experiments, performed the experiments, analyzed the data, and prepared the manuscript. KJ performed the microarray experiments. MT and MS performed the experiments and performed QPCR. ML and WSu performed the experiments. BS and KB performed the experiments and analyzed the data. MRuch, MK, and TW designed the experiments and performed the experiments. WSz designed the experiments, performed the experiments, analyzed the data, prepared graphical presentation, and prepared the manuscript. LM invented and designed the experiments, analyzed the data, and prepared the manuscript. MRuci invented and designed the experiments, analyzed the data, prepared graphical presentation, and prepared the manuscript. All authors contributed to the article and approved the submitted version.

FUNDING

This research was supported by: Opus Grant program of the National Science Center No. UMO-2017/25/B/NZ4/00065. KB (WKMOMU) and WSz (PUMS) were supported by the Social Health Insurance Project, Republic of Kazakhstan (Contract No. SHIP-2.3/CS-02).

SUPPLEMENTARY MATERIAL

Supplementary Figure 1 | Expression of ARRDC3, JUN, HIST1H2BM and KIF20A genes in the HAC15 cell line after 24 h of incubation with ACTH, forskolin and adropin versus control (untreated) cells. Real time QPCR study ($N = 4$/group). Statistical differences were determined by the Mann–Whitney U non-parametric test compared to controls. $^*p < 0.05$; $^{**}p < 0.01$.

REFERENCES

1. Kumar KG, Trevaskis JL, Lam DD, Sutton GM, Koza RA, Chouljenko VN, et al. Identification of adropin as a secreted factor linking dietary macronutrient intake with energy homeostasis and lipid metabolism. *Cell Metab.* (2008) 8:468–81. doi: 10.1016/j.cmet.2008.10.011
2. Wang S, Gao Y, Liu G, Deng D, Chen R, Zhang Y, et al. Molecular cloning, characterization and expression of the energy homeostasis-associated gene in piglet. *J Zhejiang Univ Sci B.* (2015) 16:524–32. doi: 10.1631/jzus.B1400260
3. Ganesh Kumar K, Zhang J, Gao S, Rossi J, McGuinness OP, Halem HH, et al. Adropin deficiency is associated with increased adiposity and insulin resistance. *Obesity.* (2012) 20:1394–402. doi: 10.1038/oby.2012.31
4. Jasaszwili M, Billert M, Strowski MZ, Nowak KW, Skrzypski M. Adropin as a fat-burning hormone with multiple functions—review of a decade of research. *Molecules.* (2020) 25:1–12. doi: 10.3390/molecules25030549
5. Butler AA, Zhang J, Price CA, Stevens JR, Graham JL, Stanhope KL, et al. Low plasma adropin concentrations increase risks of weight gain and metabolic dysregulation in response to a high-sugar diet in male nonhuman primates. *J Biol Chem.* (2019) 294:9706–19. doi: 10.1074/jbc.RA119.007528
6. Ghoshal S, Stevens JR, Billon C, Girardet C, Sitaula S, Leon AS, et al. Adropin: an endocrine link between the biological clock and cholesterol homeostasis. *Mol Metab.* (2018) 8:51–64. doi: 10.1016/j.molmet.2017.12.002
7. Choi HN, Yim JE. Plasma adropin as a potential marker predicting obesity and obesity-associated cancer in korean patients with type 2 diabetes mellitus. *J Cancer Prev.* (2018) 23:191–6. doi: 10.15430/JCP.2018.23.4.191
8. Lovren F, Pan Y, Quan A, Singh KK, Shukla PC, Gupta M, et al. Adropin is a novel regulator of endothelial function. *Circulation.* (2010) 18:25–32. doi: 10.1161/CIRCULATIONAHA.109.931782
9. Yang C, DeMars KM, Candelario-Jalil E. Age-dependent decrease in adropin is associated with reduced levels of endothelial nitric oxide synthase and increased oxidative stress in the rat brain. *Aging Dis.* (2018) 9:322–30. doi: 10.14336/AD.2017.0523
10. Gao S, McMillan RP, Zhu Q, Lopaschuk GD, Hulver MW, Butler AA. Therapeutic effects of adropin on glucose tolerance and substrate utilization in diet-induced obese mice with insulin resistance. *Mol Metab.* (2015) 4:310–24. doi: 10.1016/j.molmet.2015.01.005
11. Rao A, Herr DR. G protein-coupled receptor GPR19 regulates E-cadherin expression and invasion of breast cancer cells. *Biochim Biophys Acta - Mol Cell Res.* (2017) 1864:1318–27. doi: 10.1016/j.bbamcr.2017.05.001
12. Ramanjaneya M, Karteris E, Chen J, Rucinski M, Ziolkowska A, Ahmed N, et al. QRFP induces aldosterone production via PKC and T-type calcium channel-mediated pathways in human adrenocortical cells: evidence for a novel role of GPR103. *Am J Physiol Endocrinol Metab.* (2013) 305:E1049–58. doi: 10.1152/ajpendo.00191.2013
13. Ritz C, Baty F, Streibig JC, Gerhard D. Dose-response analysis using R. *PLoS ONE.* (2015) 10:e0146021. doi: 10.1371/journal.pone.0146021
14. Rucinski M, Malendowicz LK. Precerebellin-related genes and precerebellin 1 peptide in endocrine glands of the rat - Pattern of their expression. *Int J Mol Med.* (2009) 23:113–9. doi: 10.3892/ijmm_00000108
15. Szyszka M, Paschke L, Tyczewska M, Jopek K, Celichowski P, Milecka P, et al. Analysis of transcriptome, selected intracellular signaling pathways, proliferation and apoptosis of LNCaP cells exposed to high leptin concentrations. *Int J Mol Sci.* (2019) 20:1–25. doi: 10.3390/ijms20215412
16. Jopek K, Tyczewska M, Ramanjaneya M, Szyszka M, Celichowski P, Milecka P, et al. Effect of ACTH and HCG on the expression of gonadotropin-inducible ovarian transcription factor 1 (Giotl) gene in the rat adrenal gland. *Int J Mol Sci.* (2018) 19:1–21. doi: 10.3390/ijms19082285
17. Jopek K, Tyczewska M, Celichowski P, Malendowicz LK, Rucinski M. Transcriptome profile in unilateral adrenalectomy-induced compensatory adrenal growth in the rat. *Int J Mol Sci.* (2018) 19:1–17. doi: 10.3390/ijms19041111
18. Jopek K, Celichowski P, Szyszka M, Tyczewska M, Milecka P, Malendowicz LK, et al. Transcriptome profile of rat adrenal evoked by gonadectomy and testosterone or estradiol replacement. *Front Endocrinol.* (2017) 8:1–16. doi: 10.3389/fendo.2017.00026
19. Gautier L, Cope L, Bolstad BM, Irizarry RA. Affy - analysis of affymetrix genechip data at the probe level. *Bioinformatics.* (2004) 20:307–15. doi: 10.1093/bioinformatics/btg405
20. Carvalho BS, Irizarry RA. A framework for oligonucleotide microarray preprocessing. *Bioinformatics.* (2010) 26:2363–7. doi: 10.1093/bioinformatics/btq431
21. Ritchie ME, Phipson B, Wu D, Hu Y, Law CW, Shi W, et al. Limma powers differential expression analyses for RNA-sequencing and microarray studies. *Nucleic Acids Res.* (2015) 43:gkv007. doi: 10.1093/nar/gkv007
22. Yu G, Wang LG, Han Y, He QY. ClusterProfiler: an R package for comparing biological themes among gene clusters. *Omi A J Integr Biol.* (2012) 16:284–7. doi: 10.1089/omi.2011.0118

23. Mootha VK, Daly MJ, Patterson N, Hirschhorn JN, Groop LC, Altshuler D. Reply to "Statistical concerns about the GSEA procedure." *Nat Genet.* (2004) 36:663. doi: 10.1038/ng0704-663b
24. Sergushichev AA. An algorithm for fast preranked gene set enrichment analysis using cumulative statistic calculation. *bioRxiv [Preprint].* (2016). doi: 10.1101/060012
25. Liberzon A, Birger C, Thorvaldsdóttir H, Ghandi M, Mesirov JP, Tamayo P. The molecular signatures database hallmark gene set collection. *Cell Syst.* (2015) 1:417–25. doi: 10.1016/j.cels.2015.12.004
26. Subramanian A, Tamayo P, Mootha VK, Mukherjee S, Ebert BL, Gillette MA, et al. Gene set enrichment analysis: a knowledge-based approach for interpreting genome-wide expression profiles. *Proc Natl Acad Sci USA.* (2005) 102:15545–50. doi: 10.1073/pnas.0506580102
27. Bader GD, Isserlin R, Merico D, Voisin V. Enrichment Map - a Cytoscape app to visualize and explore OMICs pathway enrichment results. *F1000Res.* (2014) 3:1–9. doi: 10.12688/f1000research.4536.1
28. Shannon P, Markiel A, Ozier O, Baliga NS, Wang JT, Ramage D, et al. Cytoscape: a software environment for integrated models of biomolecular interaction networks. *Genome Res.* (2003) 13:2498–504. doi: 10.1101/gr.1239303
29. Kucera M, Isserlin R, Arkhangorodsky A, Bader GD. AutoAnnotate: a Cytoscape app for summarizing networks with semantic annotations [version 1; referees: 2 approved]. *F1000Res.* (2016) 5:1–14. doi: 10.12688/f1000research.9090.1
30. Weinstein JN, Collisson EA, Mills GB, Shaw KRM, Ozenberger BA, Ellrott K, et al. The cancer genome atlas pan-cancer analysis project. *Nat Genet.* (2013) 35:1113–20. doi: 10.1038/ng.2764
31. Deng M, Brägelmann J, Kryukov I, Saraiva-Agostinho N, Perner S. FirebrowseR: An R client to the broad institute's firehose pipeline. *Database.* (2017) 2016:1–6. doi: 10.1093/database/baw160
32. Therneau TM. *survival: A Package for Survival Analysis in R.* R package version 2.37.7. R Packag version 238 (2014).
33. Tang Z, Li C, Kang B, Gao G, Li C, Zhang Z. GEPIA: a web server for cancer and normal gene expression profiling and interactive analyses. *Nucleic Acids Res.* (2017) 45:W98–102. doi: 10.1093/nar/gkx247
34. Jasaszwili M, Wojciechowicz T, Billert M, Strowski MZ, Nowak KW, Skrzypski M. Effects of adropin on proliferation and differentiation of 3T3-L1 cells and rat primary preadipocytes. *Mol Cell Endocrinol.* (2019) 496:110532. doi: 10.1016/j.mce.2019.110532
35. Marczuk N, Cecerska-Heryc E, Jesionowska A, Dolegowska B. Adropin - physiological and pathophysiological role. *Postepy Hig Med Dosw.* (2016) 70:981–8. doi: 10.5604/17322693.1220082
36. Wang T, Rainey WE. Human adrenocortical carcinoma cell lines. *Mol Cell Endocrinol.* (2012) 351:58–65. doi: 10.1016/j.mce.2011.08.041
37. Rainey WE, Saner K, Schimmer BP. Adrenocortical cell lines. *Mol Cell Endocrinol.* (2004) 228:23–38. doi: 10.1016/j.mce.2003.12.020
38. Byrd JA, Dean CE, Fossum TW, Hargis BM. Effect of bursal anti-steroidogenic peptide (BASP) on cortisol biosynthesis in ACTH-stimulated canine adrenocortical carcinoma cells *in vitro. Vet Immunol Immunopathol.* (1995) 47:35–42. doi: 10.1016/0165-2427(94)05388-9
39. Cherradi N. Atrial Natriuretic Peptide Inhibits Calcium-Induced Steroidogenic Acute Regulatory Protein Gene Transcription in Adrenal Glomerulosa Cells. *Mol Endocrinol.* (1998) 12:962–972. doi: 10.1210/mend.12.7.0132
40. Liang F, Kapoun AM, Lam A, Damm DL, Quan D, O'Connell M, et al. B-type natriuretic peptide inhibited angiotensin II-stimulated cholesterol biosynthesis, cholesterol transfer, and steroidogenesis in primary human adrenocortical cells. *Endocrinology.* (2007) 148:3722–3729. doi: 10.1210/en.2006-1599
41. Neri G, Malendowicz LK, Andreis P, Nussdorfer GG. Thyrotropin-releasing hormone inhibits glucocorticoid secretion of rat adrenal cortex:*in vivo* and *in vitro* studies. *Endocrinology.* (1993) 133:511–4. doi: 10.1210/endo.133.2.8393765
42. Gallo-Payet N. Adrenal and extra-adrenal functions of ACTH. *J Mol Endocrinol.* (2016) 56:T135–56. doi: 10.1530/JME-15-0257
43. Rainey WE, Viard I, Mason JI, Cochet C, Chambaz EM, Saez JM. Effects of transforming growth factor beta on ovine adrenocortical cells. *Mol Cell Endocrinol.* (1988) 60:189–98. doi: 10.1016/0303-7207(88)90178-5
44. Hotta M, Baird A. Differential effects of transforming growth factor type β on the growth and function of adrenocortical cells *in vitro. Proc Natl Acad Sci USA.* (1986) 83:7795–9. doi: 10.1073/pnas.83.20.7795
45. Liakos P, Lenz D, Bernhardt R, Feige JJ, Defaye G. Transforming growth factor β1 inhibits aldosterone and cortisol production in the human adrenocortical cell line NCI-H295R through inhibition of CYP11B1 and CYP11B2 expression. *J Endocrinol.* (2003) 176:69–82. doi: 10.1677/joe.0.1760069
46. Luo S. Transforming growth factor-beta1 inhibits steroidogenesis in human trophoblast cells. *Mol Hum Reprod.* (2002) 8:318–25. doi: 10.1093/molehr/8.4.318
47. Fang L, Chang HM, Cheng JC, Leung PCK, Sun YP. TGF-β1 downregulates StAR expression and decreases progesterone production through smad3 and ERK1/2 signaling pathways in human granulosa cells. *J Clin Endocrinol Metab.* (2014) 99:E2234–43. doi: 10.1210/jc.2014-1930
48. Park E, Song CH, Park J Il, Ahn RS, Choi HS, Ko CM, Transforming growth factor-β1 signaling represses testicular steroidogenesis through cross-talk with orphan nuclear receptor Nur77. *PLoS ONE.* (2014) 9:e104812. doi: 10.1371/journal.pone.0104812
49. Feige JJ, Cochet C, Savona C, Shi DL, Keramidas M, Defaye G, et al. Transforming growth factor ß1: an autocrine regulator of adrenocortical steroidogenesis. *Endocr Res.* (1991) 17:267–79. doi: 10.1080/07435809109027201
50. Tapa D, hStoner MW, Zhang M, Xie B, Manning JR, Guimaraes D, et al. Adropin regulates pyruvate dehydrogenase in cardiac cells via a novel GPCR-MAPK-PDK4 signaling pathway. *Redox Biol.* (2018) 18:25–32. doi: 10.1016/j.redox.2018.06.003
51. Lefkowitz RJ, Shenoy SK. Transduction of receptor signals by β-arrestins. *Science.* (2005) 308:512–7. doi: 10.1126/science.1109237
52. Daub H, Weiss FU, Wallasch C, Ullrich A. Role of transactivation of the EGF receptor in signalling by G-protein-coupled receptors. *Nature.* (1996) 379:557–60. doi: 10.1038/379557a0
53. Burch ML, Ballinger ML, Yang SNY, Getachew R, Itman C, Loveland K, et al. Thrombin stimulation of proteoglycan synthesis in vascular smooth muscle is mediated by protease-activated receptor-1 transactivation of the transforming growth factor βtype I receptor. *J Biol Chem.* (2010) 285:26798–26805. doi: 10.1074/jbc.M109.092767
54. Chaplin R, Thach L, Hollenberg MD, Cao Y, Little PJ, Kamato D. Insights into cellular signalling by G protein coupled receptor transactivation of cell surface protein kinase receptors. *J Cell Commun Signal.* (2017) 11:117–125. doi: 10.1007/s12079-017-0375-9
55. Scotton CJ, Krupiczojc MA, Königshoff M, Mercer PF, Lee YCG, Kaminski N, et al. Increased local expression of coagulation factor X contributes to the fibrotic response in human and murine lung injury. *J Clin Invest.* (2009) 119:2550–63. doi: 10.1172/JCI33288
56. Xu MY, Porte J, Knox AJ, Weinreb PH, Maher TM, Violette SM, et al. Lysophosphatidic acid induces αvβ36 integrin-mediated TGF-β activation via the LPA2 receptor and the small G protein Gαq. *Am J Pathol.* (2009) 174:1264–79. doi: 10.2353/ajpath.2009.080160
57. Jain R, Shaul PW, Borok Z, Willis BC. Endothelin-1 induces alveolar epithelial-mesenchymal transition through endothelin type A receptor-mediated production of TGF-β1. *Am J Respir Cell Mol Biol.* (2007) 37:38–47. doi: 10.1165/rcmb.2006-0353OC
58. Burch ML, Getachew R, Osman N, Febbraio MA, Little PJ. Thrombin-mediated proteoglycan synthesis utilizes both protein-tyrosine kinase and serine/threonine kinase receptor transactivation in vascular smooth muscle cells. *J Biol Chem.* (2013) 288:7410–9. doi: 10.1074/jbc.M112.400259
59. Zhou J, Shaikh LH, Neogi SG, Mcfarlane I, Zhao W, Figg N, et al. DACH1, a zona glomerulosa selective gene in the human adrenal, activates transforming growth factor-β signaling and suppresses aldosterone secretion. *Hypertension.* (2015) 65:1103–1110. doi: 10.1161/HYP.0000000000000025
60. Sato K, Yamashita T, Shirai R, Shibata K, Okano T, Yamaguchi M, et al. Adropin contributes to anti-atherosclerosis by suppressing monocyte-endothelial cell adhesion and smooth muscle cell proliferation. *Int J Mol Sci.* (2018) 19:1–16. doi: 10.3390/ijms19051293
61. Chen S, Zeng K, Liu QC, Guo Z, Zhang S, Chen XR, et al. Adropin deficiency worsens HFD-induced metabolic defects. *Cell Death Di.s.* (2017) 8:e3008. doi: 10.1038/cddis.2017.362
62. Martin AL, Steurer MA, Aronstam RS. Constitutive activity among orphan class-A G protein coupled receptors. *PLoS ONE.* (2015) 10:e0138463. doi: 10.1371/journal.pone.0138463

2

Functional Zonation of the Adult Mammalian Adrenal Cortex

Gavin P. Vinson *

School of Biological and Chemical Sciences, Queen Mary University of London, London, UK

Correspondence:
Gavin P. Vinson
g.p.vinson@qmul.ac.uk

The standard model of adrenocortical zonation holds that the three main zones, glomerulosa, fasciculata, and reticularis each have a distinct function, producing mineralocorticoids (in fact just aldosterone), glucocorticoids, and androgens respectively. Moreover, each zone has its specific mechanism of regulation, though ACTH has actions throughout. Finally, the cells of the cortex originate from a stem cell population in the outer cortex or capsule, and migrate centripetally, changing their phenotype as they progress through the zones. Recent progress in understanding the development of the gland and the distribution of steroidogenic enzymes, trophic hormone receptors, and other factors suggests that this model needs refinement. Firstly, proliferation can take place throughout the gland, and although the stem cells are certainly located in the periphery, zonal replenishment can take place within zones. Perhaps more importantly, neither the distribution of enzymes nor receptors suggest that the individual zones are necessarily autonomous in their production of steroid. This is particularly true of the glomerulosa, which does not seem to have the full suite of enzymes required for aldosterone biosynthesis. Nor, in the rat anyway, does it express MC2R to account for the response of aldosterone to ACTH. It is known that in development, recruitment of stem cells is stimulated by signals from within the glomerulosa. Furthermore, throughout the cortex local regulatory factors, including cytokines, catecholamines and the tissue renin-angiotensin system, modify and refine the effects of the systemic trophic factors. In these and other ways it more and more appears that the functions of the gland should be viewed as an integrated whole, greater than the sum of its component parts.

Keywords: glomerulosa, fasciculata, reticularis, X-Zone, cell proliferation, cell migration, cortisol, aldosterone

INTRODUCTION—THE STANDARD MODEL

The nature and significance of the zonation of the mammalian adrenal cortex has attracted considerable interest during the fifteen decades following the first description of its three main zones, zona glomerulosa, zona fasciculata, and zona reticularis, by Arnold (1866). Later, Gottschau (1883) was the first to suggest that adrenocortical cells originate in the outer part of the gland, and migrate centripetally, thus becoming phenotypically glomerulosa, then fasciculata and reticularis in sequence. Zwemer et al. (1938) illustrated a direct lineage of cortical cells from the connective tissue capsule. Before the functions of the gland were understood, studies were directed to further descriptions of adrenocortical morphology and development, in mammals and other vertebrates (Dostoiewsky, 1886; Rabl, 1891; Wiesel, 1902). By the 1940s it was clear that the adrenal cortex, as well as the medulla, is crucially involved in the response to stress, and further, that secretions of the cortex fell into three functional classes: androgens, and what Selye and Jensen were the first to call mineralocorticoids and glucocorticoids (Selye, 1946; Selye and Jensen, 1946). Coupled with the observable changes in appearance and abundance of the zones in different physiological situations it then became apparent that the different zones had different functions, and androgens, mineralocorticoids, and glucocorticoids were now thought to be products of the zona reticularis, zona glomerulosa, and zona fasciculata respectively (Vines, 1938; Swann, 1940; Chester Jones, 1957; Deane, 1962). Moreover, their regulation was different, and though the inner adrenocortical zones, fasciculata and reticularis, were dependent on an intact pituitary and the secretion of ACTH, the glomerulosa was not (Chester Jones, 1957; Deane, 1962; Vinson, 2003). Later, the essential role of the renin-angiotensin system in the regulation of aldosterone was elucidated (Gross, 1958; Laragh et al., 1960; Carpenter et al., 1961), though other factors, possibly many, are also involved (Vinson et al., 1992b; Ehrhart-Bornstein et al., 1998; Mulrow, 1999; Vinson, 2003).

Together, such evidence has led to the development of what may be thought of as the Standard Model of adrenocortical zonation:

(i) Adrenocortical cells arise in the outer part of the gland and migrate centripetally, with changes in phenotype as they progress from the glomerulosa through the fasciculata to the reticularis, where they undergo apoptosis.
(ii) Each of the three main differentiated zones secretes a specific profile of steroid hormones.
(iii) Each of the zones is under separate and independent regulatory control.

There have, however, always been gaps in interpretation that have scarcely been addressed. Among these is the challenge of unraveling the mechanisms underlying the profound changes of phenotype that the cells undergo during their lifespan. Again, but less frequently considered, what drives cell migration in the mature gland? Additionally, and rarely addressed: what is the significance of the zonal arrangement—what advantage is conferred by the configuration of the different zones as concentric shells?

It is the purpose of this review to examine both whether the Standard Model remains compatible with the literature of the last few years, and also whether there are now clues to these additional problems.

WHAT DO WE MEAN BY ADRENOCORTICAL ZONATION?

It is important to define the terms we use. Zonation is a descriptive term, which has been applied by different observers to mean sometimes quite different things. Without a strict, generally adhered-to definition, it is most appropriate to go back to the pioneers of the terminology, and follow their usage. Since the earliest descriptors of adrenocortical zonation were morphological and topographical, and these alone were used for 70–80 years, it follows that, without a contrary formal decision, agreed perhaps by a caucus of international exponents of the field, zonation remains defined by cellular morphology and topology alone (**Figures 1, 2**).

The names of the three main zones are descriptive of the arrangement of their cells. Thus, the zona glomerulosa is so called because the whorls or baskets of cells that compose it somewhat recall the glomeruli of the kidney (Latin *glomus*, ball) though this is more apparent in some species (e.g., the dog) than others (rat, human). The cells of the zona fasciculata lie in parallel radial cords, and the name stems originally from the Roman symbol of office, the *fasces* or bundle of birch rods (etymologically the same origin, incidentally, as *fascist*), cf. the anatomical term *fascicle* (bundle of nerves or muscle fibers), while the cords of cells of the reticularis form a network (Latin: *rete*). Essentially, the smaller, more densely staining glomerulosa cells are characterized by their lamelliform cristae, whereas the larger and paler fasciculata cells have tubulo-vesicular cristae. The reticularis cells retain tubulo-vesicular cristae, and are again more densely staining and smaller than fasciculata cells. Lipid distribution varies with the state of stimulation, but in general is greater in the inner zones. These criteria have been reviewed on many occasions (Chester Jones, 1957; Deane, 1962; Neville and O'Hare, 1981; Vinson et al., 1992b).

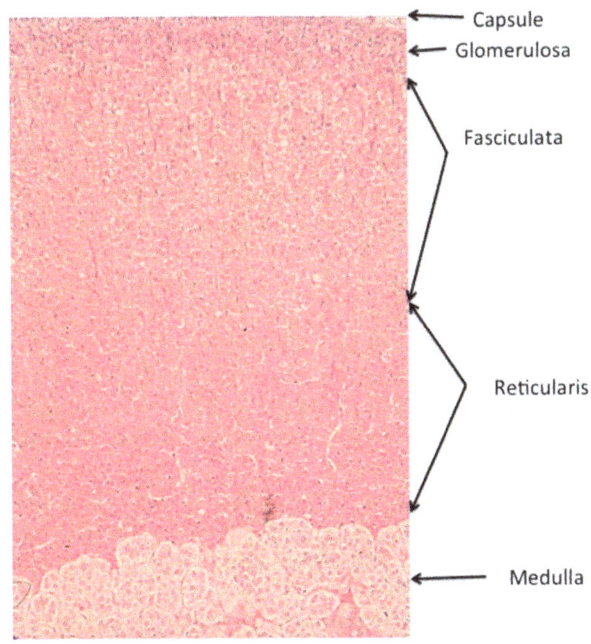

FIGURE 1 | Zonation of the Wistar rat adrenal cortex. The main zones of the cortex. The arrangement of the concentric bands of cells is representative of most mammal species, though there is some species variation. In the adult human gland, the glomerulosa is sparse and confined to discrete islets, whereas in others, such as the dog, the glomerulosa is much more marked, with large whorls of cells justifying the comparison with the renal glomerulus. Additional zones may occur in other species, including the X zone in the mouse gland, and the fetal zone in the developing and newborn human gland (See Chester Jones, 1957; Deane, 1962; Neville and O'Hare, 1981; Vinson et al., 1992b).

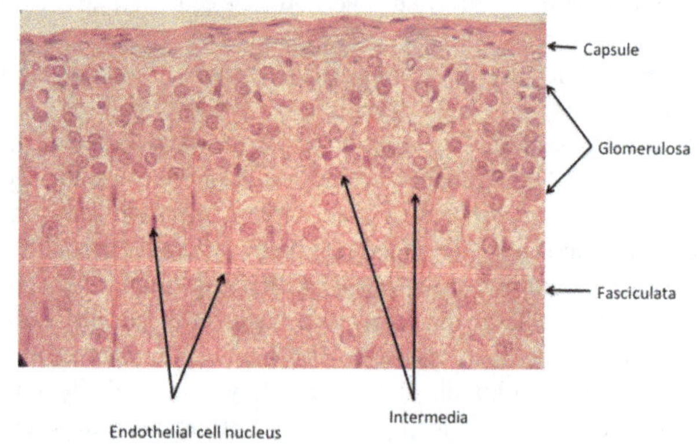

FIGURE 2 | Higher power view of the capsule/glomerulosa/outer fasciculata view of the rat adrenal cortex. Note that in this tissue from an ~2 month old animal, the zona intermedia is very sparse. There is a marked differentiation between the glomerulosa and the fasciculata, emphasizing the precision with which the signals that determine positioning of the different cell types must operate (see text).

Thus, zonation is not described by function, nor by the presence of this or that steroid product, or molecular marker. As it happens, and as this article will make clear, function follows morphology/topology only partially. For example, in the rat adrenal, only outer zona glomerulosa cells express CYP11B2 (see **Table 1** for abbreviations) in sodium sufficient animals, and the inner glomerulosa does not. The non-CYP11B2-containing glomerulosa region was first called the white or undifferentiated zone (ZU) (Mitani et al., 1994, 1995), while others have called it the "zona intermedia" (Engeland and Levay-Young, 1999; Ulrich-Lai et al., 2006). This is confusing, because the term zona intermedia was previously applied to a morphologically distinct flattened cell type, quite different from the glomerulosa, that is limited to a very few cells at the glomerulosa-fasciculata border (Cater and Lever, 1954; Chester Jones, 1957; Deane, 1962; Nussdorfer, 1986). Indeed Cater and Lever (Cater and Lever, 1954) report it as absent from 2 month old rat adrenals, while it is very marked in older animals. It is sparsely evident in the illustration in **Figure 2**. It should be noted that these descriptions apply to the rat adrenal, and the presence of a discrete ZU in other species is not clear (see below).

Similarly, others have interpreted, and used, CYP11B2 as a "highly specific zona glomerulosa marker" (Freedman et al., 2013). It isn't, since (as noted above) it is expressed by only a small population of glomerulosa cells.

In yet another re-writing of the literature on adrenocortical zonation, some authors appear to define the zona reticularis, not on the basis of its morphology, but as the site of DHEA and androstenedione production. Defined in this way, the rat adrenal, it is claimed, does not contain a zona reticularis (de Joussineau et al., 2012; Pihlajoki et al., 2015), when it quite obviously does!—see **Figure 1**—moreover reticularis cells have been isolated from rat adrenals, their steroidogenic potential analyzed, and even shown to produce androstenedione, albeit in small amounts (Bell et al., 1978, 1979), see also (Pignatelli et al., 2006).

TABLE 1 | Abbreviations used.

ACTH	Adrenocorticotrophic hormone, corticotrophin
AgRP	Agouti-related peptide
AKR1B7	Aldo-keto reductase family 1 member B7
AKR1C3	Aldo-keto reductase family 1 member C3, type 5 17β-HSD
ANP	Atrial natriuretic peptide
AP-1	Activator protein 1 (c-fos, c-jun heterodimeric transcription factor)
APCC	Aldosterone producing cell clusters
ARNTL	Aryl hydrocarbon receptor nuclear translocator-like protein 1, =BMAL
AsP	Adrenal secretory protease
AT1R	Angiotensin II type 1 receptor
AZ1	Adrenocortical zonation factor
BMAL	basic helix-loop-helix/PER-ARNT-SIM (bHLH/PAS) transcription factor, = ARNTL, MOP3
BMP	Bone morphogenetic protein
3β-HSD	3β-hydroxysteroid dehydrogenase
11β-HSD	11β-hydroxysteroid dehydrogenase
20α-HSD	20α-hydroxysteroid dehydrogenase
18-OH-DOC	18-hydroxydeoxycorticosterone
BrdU	Bromodeoxyuridine
c-AMP	cyclic adenosine monophosphate
c-fos	See AP1
c-jun	See AP1
CLOCK	Circadian Locomotor Output Cycle Kaput gene
CRF	Corticotrophin releasing factor
Cry2	Cryptochrome circadian clock 2 gene
Cyt B5	Cytochrome B5
CYP2D16	Cytochrome $P450_{2D16}$
CYP11A	Cytochrome $P450_{scc}$(cholesterol side chain cleavage)
CYP11B1	Cytochrome $P450_{11B1}$(11β-hydroxylase)
CYP11B2	Cytochrome $P450_{11B2}$ (aldosterone synthase)
CYP17	Cytochrome $P450_{17}$(17-hydroxylase)
CYP21	Cytochrome $P450_{21}$(21-hydroxylase)
Dab-2	Disabled homolog-2, = DOC2, C9, p96/p67
DACH-1	Dachshund family transcription factor
DAX1	Dosage sensitive reversal adrenal hypoplasia critical region, chromosome X, = NrOb1
DHCR24	24 dehydrocholesterol reductase, seladin-1
DHEA	Dehydroepiandrosterone
Eph	Ephrin receptor
ERK	Extracellular signal regulated kinase, = MAPK
bFGF	basic Fibroblast growth factor
GATA	GATA sequence binding transcription factor
Gli1	Glioblastoma 1
Grx	Glutaredoxin
GPCR	G protein coupled receptor
IGIF	Interferon-γ inducing factor = IL 18 or IL-1γ
IGF	Insulin-like growth factor
IL	Interleukin
IP3	Inositol trisphosphate
IZA	Inner zone antigen, = PGRMC-1, Sigma 2 receptor
Ki67	Antigen K67, = MKI67

(Continued)

TABLE 1 | Continued

LEF1	Lymphoid enhancer-binding factor 1
LHR	Luteinizing hormone receptor
MC2R/MC5R	Melanocortin receptor 2/5 (ACTH/ melanotrophin receptors respectively)
MAPK	Mitogen activated protein kinase, =ERK
MnSOD	Manganese euperoxide dismutase
MRAP	Melanocortin-2-receptor accessory protein
α-MSH	α-melanocyte stimulating hormone
Nek2	NMA (never in mitosis gene a) related expressed kinase 2
NGFIB	nerve growth factor induced clone B;
NPY	Neuropeptide Y
Notch1,2	Notch (Drosophila) homolog 1,2
NOV	Nephroblastoma overexpressed, = CCN3
NURR-1	Nur-related factor 1
OAT	Organic anion transporter
OATP	Organic anion transporter polypeptide
ODC	Ornithine decarboxylase
Per	Period component of Per/Tim (timeless) heterodimer
Pik3c2g	Phosphatidylinositol-4-phosphate 3-kinase C2 domain-containing gamma polypeptide gene
PKC	Protein kinase C
Prkar1α	Type 1 α-regulatory subunit of cAMP dependent protein kinase
PPARγ	Peroxisome proliferator activated receptorγ
Pref1	Preadipocyte factor 1, = dlk1 (delta like homolog 1)
Prx	Peroxiredoxin
ROS	Reactive oxygen species
R26 YFP	Rosa 26 yellow fluorescent protein
Rev-Erbα)	Nuclear receptor subfamily 1, group D, member 1, NR1D1
SCN	Suprachiasmatic nucleus
SF1	Steroidogenic factor 1 (also AD4BP, NR5A1)
Shh	Sonic hedgehog (hedgehog signaling pathway component)
SLC27A2	Solute carrier family 27 (fatty acid transporter), member 2
StAR	Steroidogenic acute regulatory protein
SULT2A1	Steroid sulfotransferase
TASK1,3	TWIK-related acid-sensitive K^+channels, KCNK3 and 9 (members of family of two-pore domain potassium channels)
TGFβ	Transforming growth factor
TNF	Tumor necrosis factor
Trx	Thioredoxin
TrxR	Thioredoxin reductase
TSPAN12	Tetraspanin 12
Ucn3	Urocortin 3
VIP	Vasoactive intestinal peptide
Wnt	Wingless related integration site
ZU	Undifferentiated zone

ORIGIN OF THE ADRENAL CORTEX, CELL PROLIFERATION, AND MIGRATION

The adrenal cortex originates from a section of the coelomic epithelium, firstly as part of the SF1-expressing adrenogonadal primordium, then separating as the adrenal anlage into approximately its ultimate location, ventrolateral to the dorsal aorta. At this site, it is invaded by cells from the neural crest, and eventually becomes encapsulated as the discrete adrenal gland (Xing et al., 2015). An interplay between the transcription factors SF1 and Dax1 determines the extent to which steroidogenic enzymes are induced, and adrenocortical cells become differentiated: Dax 1, as a co-repressor of SF1, sustains the pluripotential stem cell-like phenotype (Xing et al., 2015).

In the established cortex, the central concept that there is a stem cell population located in the capsule or immediate subcapsular region (Zwemer et al., 1938; Lombardo and Cortesini, 1988) has largely been supported by evidence from several types of experiment that track the fate of labeled cells.

Earlier studies followed labeled cells after the pulse administration of tritiated thymidine in the rat (Wright, 1971; Wright et al., 1973; Zajicek et al., 1986), latterly BrdU was used in mice (Chang et al., 2013). These gave broadly similar results, showing initial labeling in the outer part of the gland, with centripetal migration and phenotype change at a rate of 13–20 μm per day in the mouse adrenal (Chang et al., 2013), reaching the medulla after 104 days from initial labeling in the rat gland (Zajicek et al., 1986). Others have used transgenic mice bearing the 21OH/LacZ gene (Morley et al., 1996) or other constructs (Walczak and Hammer, 2015). Using 21OH/LacZ transgenic mice gives typical results in that mice bearing this transgene develop stripes of beta-gal staining cells in the adrenal extending from the capsule to the medulla, consistent with the concept of an outer region of proliferation with subsequent inward migration. It has to be said that the staining is not consistent with the distribution of 21-hydroxylase in the normal mouse adrenal, which is present only as a trace in the glomerulosa, though strongly expressed in the adrenal inner zones (Chang et al., 2013). Similar radial distribution of labeled cells has shown such lineages in mice bearing for example *shh^{gfpcre};R26-YFP* cells: *shh* is highly transcribed in the outer cortex in the mouse (though only in the ZU in the rat), so this parallels the results obtained with 21OH/LacZ. A similar cell lineage is seen in mice with the *Gli1-creT2 R26-X* label: *Gli1* is normally transcribed in the inner capsule in cells that apparently represent stem cells. Since the capsular expression of Gli1 is induced by shh signaling, this suggests what King and co-authors call a bootstrapping loop, by which the recruitment of new cortical cells from the capsule is stimulated, and both *shh* and *Gli1* cells are transformed into other cell types throughout the cortex (King et al., 2009). In fact this process is reinforced by the glomerulosa specific Dlk1 (also known as Pref-1), a member of the Notch family, which is co-expressed with shh in the rat, and, like shh, also signals to the capsule, inducing Gli-1 transcription and cortical cell recruitment (Guasti et al., 2013b; Finco et al., 2015). In mouse adrenals regenerating after dexamethasone treatment, fasciculata cells were similarly shown to be formed directly from CYP11B2-Cre-bearing zona glomerulosa cells in an SF-1 dependent process (Freedman et al., 2013), although the possibility of an intermediate shh-expressing form does not seem to be excluded.

There is often some ambiguity in such studies in that although the Standard Model is supported, alternative lineages are not necessarily excluded. Thus, fasciculata cells may be formed in the mouse adrenal from sources independent of the glomerulosa (Freedman et al., 2013). That proliferation may occur at various sites in the gland (Payet et al., 1980; Kirillov and Popova, 1985; McEwan et al., 1996, 1999) does not of itself counter the view that the stem cells are capsular or subcapsular. However, there is some additional complexity revealed by the timed appearance of BrdU labeled cells following pulse labeling in the mouse adrenal cortex that suggests there may be variation in the fates of individual cells (Chang et al., 2013), for example, some cells may be retained in the glomerulosa. Perhaps this may be expected from the evidence of the expanded glomerulosa, and CYP11B2 expression, that results from a low sodium diet or angiotensin II treatment (McEwan et al., 1996, 1999). In control mice, Ki67 staining showed proliferation predominantly in the glomerulosa and also in the outer fasciculata, where it was significantly increased by a pulse of ACTH. These fasciculata cells also expressed 21-hydroxylase, whereas the BrdU and Ki67 stained glomerulosa cells were steroidogenically inert, confirming that proliferation occurs in differentiated as well as partially differentiated cells (Chang et al., 2013).

Another example of such ambiguity is found in rats, where the compensatory hypertrophy following unilateral adrenalectomy may depend on proliferation in the fasciculata (Engeland et al., 2005) thus 5 days after enucleation proliferation may occur in both the glomerulosa and the inner part of the regenerating fasciculata, and after 10–28 days in the outer fasciculata (Ennen et al., 2005). Different sources of cells may also arise in other experimental conditions, for example in the Prkar1a knockout mouse, there is a strong ACTH-independent centrifugal expansion of corticosterone secreting cells, apparently from the X-zone (Sahut-Barnola et al., 2010; de Joussineau et al., 2012). All these potential sites for proliferation and migration of cells are indicated in **Figure 3**.

The assumption that, since adrenocortical cells originate in the outer part of the gland, and migrate centripetally, apoptosis is essentially a reticularis event, also requires re-examination, and it now appears that apoptosis occurs throughout all three zones in humans (Wolkersdorfer and Bornstein, 1998), and in the rat (Petrovic-Kosanovic et al., 2013). Like the cortex-wide proliferation that has been described, this presumably confers flexible tissue remodeling at all levels in the gland. ACTH inhibits apoptosis, thus stabilizing cortical structure *in vivo* (Carsia et al., 1996; Thomas et al., 2004), and *in vitro* according to some authors (Carsia et al., 1996) although not according to others, who describe ACTH-induced apoptosis in cultured rat cells (Mattos et al., 2011).

MAINTENANCE OF ZONAL DIFFERENTIATION

Here zonal differentiation implies the anatomical and functional features that distinguish the cells of the different zones. As emphasized above, and will be seen in **Table 2**, functional differences are not always definitive, many properties may be shared. Nevertheless, it is remarkable how the differentiation between glomerulosa and fasciculata, for example, is maintained (cf. **Figures 1, 2**). The selection and maintenance of cellular phenotype clearly depends on location within the gland. Thus, the three adrenocortical zones always occupy the same relative position, glomerulosa outermost, reticularis innermost, adjacent

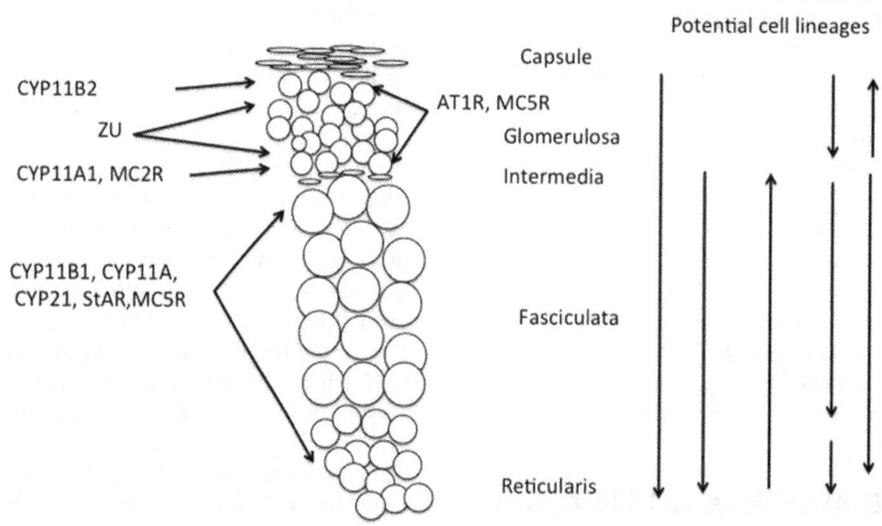

FIGURE 3 | Schematic showing distribution of melanocortin receptors and steroidogenic enzymes in the outer adrenal cortex of the rat (cf. Figure 1). This illustrates that cellular interaction appears to be required to explain both the synthesis of aldosterone and its regulation by ACTH, thus requiring modification of the Standard Model of adrenocortical zonation. Vertical arrows indicate potential origins of proliferation and direction of migration of adrenocortical cells. Although the stem cell population is usually held to be in the capsular/subcapsular region, evidence for all of these possible sites for subsequent proliferation has been reported, (see text and Kim and Hammer, 2007; Chang et al., 2013; Freedman et al., 2013).

TABLE 2 | Characteristics of zonal function in (a) rat (b) mouse, and (c) human adult adrenal glands.

(a) Rat				
Factor/Gene	**Glomerulosa**	**Fasciculata/**	**Reticularis**	**References**
STEROIDOGENESIS				
CYP11A	+/−?	+ + +		Roskelley and Auersperg, 1990; Halder et al., 1998; Mitani et al., 1999; Guasti et al., 2013b; but see Engeland and Levay-Young (1999)
CYP11B1	−	+ + +	+/−	Ho and Vinson, 1993; Halder et al., 1998; Mitani et al., 1999
CYP11B2	+	−		Halder et al., 1998; Peters et al., 1998; Mitani et al., 1999
CYP21	+/−	+ + +		Chang et al., 2011, 2013
3β-HSD	+	+ + +		Dupont et al., 1991; Engeland and Levay-Young, 1999; Pignatelli et al., 1999
11β-HSD1	−	−	+	Shimojo et al., 1996
11β-HSD2	−	++	++	Smith et al., 1997; Atanassova and Koeva, 2012
StAR	−	+ + +		Peters et al., 1998, 2007
RECEPTORS				
ATR1	+ + +	−	−	Lehoux et al., 1997
MC2R	+/− Inner ZU,	+ + +	+/−	Gorrigan et al., 2011
MRAP	+/− see text	+ + +	+/−	
MRAP2	=/−	+/−	+/−	
MC5R	+ + +	+		Griffon et al., 1994; van der Kraan et al., 1998
ZONAL HOMEOSTASIS				
Shh	+ + +	−		Guasti et al., 2011, 2013b
Pref-1/dlk1	+ + +	−		Halder et al., 1998; Raza et al., 1998; Whitworth and Vinson, 2000
NEUROTRANSMITTER				
VIP	+	−		Holzwarth et al., 1987; Bernet et al., 1994
NPY	+	−		Holzwarth et al., 1987; Bernet et al., 1994; Renshaw and Hinson, 2001
Catecholamines	+	−		Holzwarth et al., 1987; Bornstein and Ehrhart-Bornstein, 1992
CYTOKINES				
IGIF	−	+ + +	++	Conti et al., 1997
*IL-6	+			Judd and MacLeod, 1992
*TNF	+			Judd and MacLeod, 1995
GROWTH FACTORS				
Prorenin	+	++	+	Ho and Vinson, 1998
bFGF	+	+		Chambaz et al., 1994; Ho and Vinson, 1995, 1997
IGF	+	+		
TGFβ	−	−		
SIGNALING				
ANP	+ + +	−		Lai et al., 2000
AgRP	−	+ + +	+ + +	Bicknell et al., 2000
Prorenin	−	+		Ho and Vinson, 1998
MAPK:ERK-1, ERK-2	++	−		McNeill et al., 1998; McNeill and Vinson, 2000; Vinson et al., 2000; Guasti et al., 2013b
SF-1	++	++		Raza et al., 1998
Dab2	+ + +	−		Romero et al., 2007
Nek 2b	+	+ + +	−	de Mendonca et al., 2014
Notch1	+ + +	++	+	
Notch2	+capsule	−	−	
Notch3	+ + +	++	+	
DETOXIFICATION				
**MnSOD*	−	++		Raza and Vinson, 2000
CLOCK GENES				
PER 1	(?)	+ + + (reticularis)		Fahrenkrug et al., 2008
PER 2 Bmal 1				

(Continued)

TABLE 2 | Continued

Factor/Gene	Glomerulosa	Fasciculata/	Reticularis	References
OTHER				
IZA	–	+++	++	Barker et al., 1992; Halder et al., 1998; Vendeira et al., 1999; Raza et al., 2001
OAT1	–	++		Beery et al., 2003
Oatp1,2	–	++		
Oatp3	++	–		
AsP	+++	+		Bicknell et al., 2001
EphA2, EphA2, EphA3	++	–		Brennan et al., 2008
Spexin	+++	++	++	Rucinski et al., 2010

*Release from incubated glomerulosa cells **immunoblotting

(b) Mouse

Factor/Gene	Glomerulosa	Fasciculata/Reticularis	X-Zone	References
STEROIDOGENESIS				
CYP11B1	–	+++	– (?)	Mukai et al., 2003; King et al., 2009
CYP11B2	+++	–		
20α-HSD	–	–	++	Hershkovitz et al., 2007
3β-HSD	+++	+++	–	
CYP21	+/–	+++		Chang et al., 2013
RECEPTORS				
ATR1	+++	–	–	Huang et al., 2013
SIGNALING				
Shh	+++	–		King et al., 2009
Dax1	+++	–		Kim et al., 2009
				Mukai et al., 2002; Scheys et al., 2011
GATA4/GATA6 GATA4 in outer capsule only	+++			
β-catenin	+++	+/–		Tevosian et al., 2015
				Pihlajoki et al., 2015
CLOCK GENES				
Bmal1, CLOCK, Cry2	+++	++		Oster et al., 2006
Per1, Per2, Per3, Rev-Erbα				
Pik3c2g	–	–	+++	Pihlajoki et al., 2013
DETOXIFICATION				
AKR1B7	–?	++		Aigueperse et al., 2001; Martinez et al., 2001
Grx 1	+/–	+++	+	Godoy et al., 2011
Grx 2,5	++	+	++	
Prx 1,4,5	+	+++	+	
Prx 3	+	+	++	
Trx 1,2	+	+++	+	
TrxR2	+	–	+	
Other				
AZ-1	+++	++(?)	++(?)	Mukai et al., 2003; Bastida et al., 2007; Li et al., 2007
ODC	+++	++	–	

(c) Human

Factor/Gene	Glomerulosa	Fasciculata	Reticularis	References
STEROIDOGENESIS				
CYP11B1	–	+++	+++	Nishimoto et al., 2010
CYP11B2	+	–	–	

(Continued)

TABLE 2 | Continued

Factor/Gene	Glomerulosa	Fasciculata/	Reticularis	References
†CYP11A		+++	+++	Rege et al., 2014
CYP17		+++	+++	Nishimoto et al., 2010
CYPB5		+	+++	Rainey et al., 2002
SULT2A1		+	+++	Rainey and Nakamura, 2008
3β-HSD	+	+++	+/−	Nishimoto et al., 2010; but see Rainey et al. (2002)
†*3β-HSD2*		+++	+	Rege et al., 2014
†*AKR1C3*		+		
ZONAL HOMEOSTASIS				
DACH1	+	+++		Zhou et al., 2015
BMP4	+++	++	+	Rege et al., 2015
SIGNALING				
*†*LEF1*		+++	+/−	Rege et al., 2014
*†*NOV*		+++	+/−	
†*SLC27A2*		+	+++	
†*TSPAN12*		+	+++	
NGFIB	+++	++		Bassett et al., 2004b
Nurr-1	+++	+		
PPARγ	++	+		Uruno et al., 2011
Ucn3	+	+		Fukuda et al., 2005
CRF1	+/−	++	++	
CRF2	+/−	++	++	
LHR		+/−	+	Pabon et al., 1996
DETOXIFICATION				
Seladin	−	+++	+++	Battista et al., 2009
†*AKR1C3*		+	+++	Rege et al., 2014

This table lists some of the genes and gene products that have been used to define the different functions of the zones of the adrenal cortex, mostly using either immunocytochemistry (shown in normal text) or in situ hybridization (in italics). It is by no means exhaustive, many more components have been listed, notably when cDNA arrays have been used, (e.g., de Mendonca et al., 2014; Nishimoto et al., 2014; Tyczewska et al., 2014). Plus signs (+) indicate presence, minus signs (−) absence. The number of + signs gives a rough indication of the abundance of signal under control conditions, i.e., with no special treatment. Naturally all of these values may change, sometimes enormously, if neutral physiological regimes are perturbed.

Also reported in glomerulosa, but data not provided.

†*Transcriptome profiling.*

to the medulla, and the fasciculata between. How can this be achieved? As discussed further below, differentiated zonal function is maintained by systemic factors, including (in experimental animals at least) angiotensin II, potassium ions and α-MSH in the glomerulosa, and ACTH in the fasciculata and reticularis. At the same time these activators are clearly not the originating stimuli for differentiation since their receptors are already zonally distributed in order for them to have a zonally specific response—they therefore reinforce the actions of existing morphogens. An example of how this can be disturbed is given by experiments in which the disruption of the tandem potassium channels TASK1 and TASK3 gives rise to extended expression of CYP11B2 in the mouse fasciculata, resulting in aldosterone secretion that is insensitive to sodium intake, though sensitive to ACTH regulation. This is only true of females, so this unprecedented chaotically unzoned hypersecretion of aldosterone is remediable by testosterone treatment (Heitzmann et al., 2008). In contrast to the action of testosterone, which tends to restore the normal zonal, i.e., exclusively glomerulosa, distribution of CYP11B2, inactivation of the Cav2.3 calcium channel in $TASK1^{-/-}$ mice reduces aldosterone to normal levels, but leaves CYP11B2 in the fasciculata (El Wakil, 2013).

So, if systemic factors cannot be responsible for localization of cell type and the organization of the zones, these must instead depend on factors within the gland. It may be speculated what such factors might be. We have previously considered these to be of three types, morphogens or paracrine agents produced within the gland, growth factors that essentially amplify the morphogenic signal, and transcription factors (Vinson and Ho, 1998; Vinson, 2003). In essence this is illustrated by the action of shh in upregulating Gli1, or the Wnt/catenin systems, described more fully below.

The concept that morphogens, secreted by a fixed source, diffuse along a concentration gradient to inform more or less remote cells of their position, and trigger appropriate responses, is sometimes difficult to envisage, because of the randomness of diffusion, and its susceptibility to local variation due for example to tissue inhomogeneity (Lander, 2013), and, in the case of the adrenal, also because of the relatively massive centripetal blood flow (Vinson et al., 1985b; Vinson and Hinson, 1992). The actions of morphogen gradients have been most widely studied in the context of limb development and regeneration in mice and other vertebrates. In mice, for example, bone morphogenetic proteins, BMPs, which are closely related to the TGF family, stimulate local growth and regeneration (Urist, 1965; Reddi, 1998; Bandyopadhyay et al., 2006; Tsuji et al., 2006; Yu et al., 2012) and have been primarily recognized for their roles in stimulating chondrogenesis and osteogenesis. However, they are also important in other tissues including the prostate (Thomas et al., 1998) breast and prostate cancer (Buijs et al., 2010), and in the pituitary and other components of the reproductive system (Shimasaki et al., 2004). Here wnt and shh signaling is crucial, as in the early development of the adrenal (below). In the limb, induction of shh is brought about by retinoic acid, which generates positional information at various stages in development (Tickle, 2006). This is achieved with a robustness that is remarkable, given the inherent variation in retinoic acid availability, depending as it does on dietary sources. But retinoic acid gradients may not depend solely on release and diffusion, but additionally on sites of degradation, as in the zebrafish brain (White et al., 2007; Schilling et al., 2012). It is possible that this applies to other morphogens, which could be critical when not only morphogen concentration but the duration of target cell exposure is critical, as in the mouse limb response to shh (Tickle, 2006). Crucially, it is thought that sharp boundaries between different cell types, such as found in the adrenal cortex, can still be achieved in the presence of a fluctuating and shallow morphogen gradient, by means of various mechanisms that depend in part on cell plasticity and in part on intercellular signaling. In other systems, these may include for example the retinoic acid-sensitive autoactivating genes Krox 20 and Hoxb1 that are mutually inhibitory in the zebrafish hindbrain (Zhang et al., 2012). Other mechanisms of noise-induced switching have been described (Schilling et al., 2012). Nevertheless, interfering with gap junctions affects positional clarity (Tickle, 2006), so direct cell-cell signaling is also involved (Lander, 2013).

With regard to the adrenal, it is clear that the same morphogens may play a role as in vertebrate limb regeneration, notably Wnt, Shh and BMPs. BMPs are expressed in all zones of the human adrenal cortex, but particularly the glomerulosa (see **Table 2**). Additionally, in H295R cells, BMP4 suppresses CYP17 RNA and protein, and DHEA secretion (Rege et al., 2015). In contrast, overexpression of the transcription factor DACH1 activates TGFβ and canonical Wnt signaling pathways, thereby suppressing CYP11B2 and aldosterone secretion (Zhou et al., 2015). Considerable advances in recent years have highlighted the particular importance of the Wnt/catenin system (MacDonald et al., 2009). Secreted Wnt glycoproteins bind to GPCRs of the *frizzled* family, bringing about increased cell content of the coactivator β-catenin, now known to be essential for the differentiation of SF1 positive adrenocortical cells from the adrenal capsule, and for their proliferation (Kim et al., 2008, 2009). The Wnt/catenin signaling system is involved in adrenocortical development in other ways also, by interaction with the nuclear receptor Dax1 and inhibin, both of which modulate adrenal/gonadal selection. Dax1is induced by SF1, but inhibits SF1 stimulated gene transcription (Ito et al., 1997; Yu et al., 1998). DAX1 is prominent in the subcapsular region in the mouse adrenal (but completely absent from the X-zone) (Mukai et al., 2002), together with β-catenin (Pihlajoki et al., 2015). Inhibin-α, which suppresses gonadal phenotype, is induced by SF1 and β-catenin (Gummow et al., 2003). The overall outcome of these effects in combination, is both to establish the adrenocortical fate of the subcapsular cells, while maintaining their further developmental plasticity (Wood and Hammer, 2010; Simon and Hammer, 2012). This, in effect, defines the glomerulosa (Berthon et al., 2012). SF1 is absolutely required for the development of the gland, and for the cell redifferentiation associated with centripetal migration (Freedman et al., 2013).

The search for stimulators of migration has however so far produced meager results. It is possible that the extracellular matrix may be involved: in bovine adrenal cells, laminin secretion is regulated by ACTH, and, in Boyden chamber experiments, laminin acted as a chemoattractant in promoting adrenal cell migration. However, the distribution of laminin is uniform throughout the cortex, and therefore seems unlikely to promote adrenocortical cell cellular migration (Pellerin et al., 1997). Other extracellular matrix proteins, including fibronectin and collagens I and IV, have been shown to affect steroidogenic enzyme expression in rat adrenal cells in culture, and in particular to modulate basal and ACTH stimulated steroid secretion (Otis et al., 2007). Additionally, rat glomerulosa cells secrete fibronectin, which promotes proliferation, while angiotensin II interferes with this process at the level of integrin binding, thus inhibiting proliferation while enhancing steroidogenesis (Otis et al., 2008).

Equally, how the inward migration of cells is achieved while the position of the zones relative to each other remains constant also continues to be a matter of some mystery. It is possible to speculate that various mechanisms might play a role. It is entirely possible that structures within the gland external to the adrenocortical cells themselves provide positional information. Such structures could include the neural network or elements of the vasculature, which though not necessarily visible in conventional microscopy are nevertheless important components both of which affect adrenocortical function (**Figure 4**; Vinson and Hinson, 1992; Vinson et al., 1994) and may be independent of ACTH (Bocian-Sobkowska et al., 1997). Alternatively, the relative positions of the capsule, external to the cortex, and of the inner medulla might suggest that a morphogenetic landscape could be generated by signals from these two poles. Certainly medullary products can affect inner cortical function (Ehrhart-Bornstein et al., 2000; Haidan et al., 2000). Or, another possibility is that positional information is provided by the adrenocortical cells themselves. Cortical cells, arranged as they are in cords traversing the cortex, themselves provide a polarity, indeed each cell may have an apical and a basal pole. Clearly this is true at least of some of them: cells of the outermost glomerulosa layer (which express both CYP11B2, AT1R, and MC5R) about the capsule at one pole, and other, perhaps less differentiated cells at the base. The innermost glomerulosa cells in the ZU abut either true zona intermedia or outer fasciculata cells, while the innermost reticularis cells

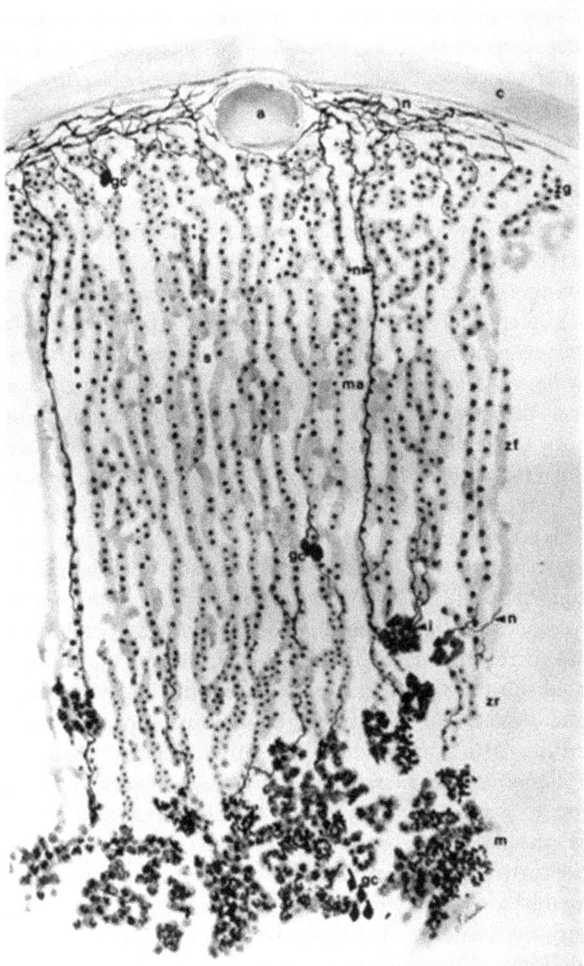

FIGURE 4 | General arrangement of the vasculature and innervation of the rat adrenal cortex. Most nerves are located in the capsular (c) and subcapsular region, with arborization around the vasculature, including arterioles (a) and around the cells of the glomerulosa (zg). Nerve fibers are rare in the fasciculata (zf), but some traverse the width of the zone, often associated with medullary arteries (ma, 6–8 per gland), which specifically supply the medulla. Most of the blood reaching the medulla passes centripetally through the sinuses, which, in contrast to the thicker walled medullary arteries, are bordered by a single layer of very attenuated endothelial cells (cf. **Figure 2**). Near the medulla (m) a few short nerve fibers reach the reticularis (zr) from islets of chromaffin cells (i) in the inner cortex and from the medulla itself. There is now considerable evidence that products from both neural tissue and vasculature can affect corticosteroid secretion. They may also provide positional information for migrating and transforming cortical cells (see text). Drawing by Bridget Landon. Reproduced with permission from Vinson et al. (1994).

lie directly adjacent to the medulla in the rat: in other species, such as the postpubertal male mouse there may be a band of connective tissue around the medulla. Such cell-cell contact is known to be important in positional information in other tissues (Tickle, 2006; Lander, 2013). The Eph/ephrin forward-reverse signaling system provides a possible mechanism for such cellular orientation and migration within the zones, and elements of the system have been demonstrated in the rat adrenal cortex. In particular, EphA2 is strongly transcribed in the rat glomerulosa, and responds to the physiological stimuli of a low sodium diet, captopril, or betamethasone treatment in a manner that suggests association with cell phenotype (Brennan et al., 2008).

FUNCTIONAL ZONATION OF THE ADRENAL CORTEX

A summary of some of the components expressed in the zones of the rat mouse and human cortex is given in **Table 2**. The Standard Model of adrenocortical zonation, as summarized in the Introduction, interprets functional zonation in terms of steroid hormone output alone. It is quite evident that in fact many other adrenocortical cell products are zone specific, and functional zonation is not just about steroids. Many of these other zonally organized functions, such as receptors and signaling pathways that transduce trophic hormone action, can be considered to complement the steroidogenic function. Others, such as clock genes, or enzymes metabolizing xenobiotics, may not be quite so easily accommodated in this way.

Although the same corticosteroids, cortisol, corticosterone, and aldosterone (though not usually all three) appear throughout the non-mammalian vertebrates, functional zonation of the adrenal cortex is a universal feature in mammals alone. While the appearance of the zones in different mammalian species may vary, aspects of their function do not. Thus, it is clear that the CYP11B2 catalyzed production of aldosterone is invariably limited to a population of cells in the zona glomerulosa, and CYP11B1 generates cortisol (or corticosterone in rats, mice, and some other species) predominantly in the fasciculata, and to a lesser extent, in the reticularis. Though this is consistent with the Standard Model, it is nevertheless now clear that some qualification is required.

The qualification arises because the extent of *de novo* steroidogenesis that can be unequivocally associated with each zone is limited. The human adrenal, for example, is complex. Here the well-defined CYP11B2-expressing glomerulosa seen in young individuals gives way in advancing years to a sparse glomerulosa generally confined to scattered islets (Neville and O'Hare, 1981; Aiba and Fujibayashi, 2011), interspersed by cells that may be analogous to those of the rat ZU [and are called the "progenitor zone" by Aiba and Fujibayashi (2011)], but which express 3β-HSD. Later, CYP11B2 expressing cell clusters (APCC) develop at the glomerulosa/fasciculata border, and extend into the fasciculata (Aiba and Fujibayashi, 2011; Nishimoto et al., 2015): these appear from the age of about 30 years. These additional sites of aldosterone production, arising as a consequence of somatic mutation of ion channels, are common in normal subjects, but the authors hypothesize that they predispose to primary aldosteronism (Nishimoto et al., 2015).

In the rat zona glomerulosa, starkly, of the steroidogenic enzymes only CYP11B2 is at all strongly expressed, and that only in the outermost glomerulosa: other required components for complete steroidogenesis, including CYP11A and CYP21 are barely detectable (**Table 2**), as is StAR according to some authors

(Peters et al., 1998, 2007), but not others (Lehoux et al., 1998; Tyczewska et al., 2014). 3β-HSD appears to be present in all zones in the rat, as it is in the mouse (**Table 2**) though it is not expressed in the glomerulosa of the bovine adrenal (Ishimura and Fujita, 1997) while in humans it is relatively sparse in the glomerulosa according to some authors (Nishimoto et al., 2010), but not others (Rainey et al., 2002). Guasti et al. (2013a) located CYP11A in the inner undifferentiated zone (ZU) of the rat adrenal zona glomerulosa, quite clearly—indeed by definition—not a site of CYP11B2 expression, which, as noted, is normally confined to a very few cells in the outer glomerulosa. Notably, this site of CYP11A expression coincides with an intense signal for MC2R mRNA, otherwise apparently lacking in the rat glomerulosa (Gorrigan et al., 2011). The intensity of MC2R mRNA staining in this region is not inconsistent with the observations of Gallo-Payet and Escher (1985) who found greater ACTH binding in the glomerulosa than other zones, but who did not distinguish between CYP11B2 expressing and non-expressing glomerulosa cells. Also contrary to expectation, StAR and CYP11A are not always co-expressed. Thus not only does the inner ZU site of CYP11A not coincide with CYP11B2, with the caveats above in mind, it does not here coincide with StAR either: Peters and colleagues have consistently demonstrated StAR expression throughout the fasciculata, but, in untreated animals, hardly at all in any of the morphologically distinct smaller glomerulosa cells in the rat, including the ZU (Peters et al., 1998, 2007).

SF1 though is very definitely present throughout the adrenal cortex (Morohashi et al., 1994; Raza et al., 1998). Although SF1 is absolutely required for the development of the gland and its steroidogenic capacity (Lala et al., 1992; Parker and Schimmer, 1993; Parker et al., 1995; Freedman et al., 2013), its role must be very different in the cells of the different zones. Thus, although exposure to high SF1 inhibits CYP11B2 expression (Ye et al., 2009), the presence of SF1 in the glomerulosa is required not only for functional CYP11B2, but also for the glomerulosa-fasciculata cell type transformation that is a feature of adrenal cell centripetal migration and redifferentiation (Freedman et al., 2013).

In contrast to the glomerulosa, all fasciculata cells strongly express all of the enzymes required for glucocorticoid production enzymes, CYP11A1, CYP21, CYP11B1, 3β-HSD, and StAR, together with, in human (and other species') glands, CYP17 as well. These components are also present in the reticularis though (with the possible exception of CYP17) in lower abundance.

This then raises the question: how is aldosterone produced in the rat and human gland, if the entire required suite of enzymes and StAR are not co-expressed? Twenty years ago, we suggested that (at least) two cell types are required for aldosterone synthesis and secretion in the rat adrenal (Vinson et al., 1995; Vinson, 2004). The evidence for this is primarily that in the rat the efficient production of aldosterone *in vitro* requires an intact gland, and as it is disrupted, from whole tissue, first to separated zones, then to enzyme dispersed cells, aldosterone yields *in vitro* are progressively diminished, whereas corticosterone output is unchanged, and 18-OH-DOC, a major product of the fasciculata in the rat (Tait et al., 1970; Nonaka and Okamoto, 1991; Okamoto and Nonaka, 1992), is increased (Vinson et al., 1985a). Together with other evidence this suggested 18-OH-DOC might be an aldosterone precursor in this species (Vinson et al., 1992a, 1995; Vinson, 2004). Objections may be raised on the basis that the hemiketal structure of 18-OH-DOC is stable, and not easily converted, that the blood flow is centripetal, hence precluding steroid movement from inner zone to the glomerulosa, and that conversion of exogenous precursors is invariably inefficient. However, tracer 18-OH-DOC is certainly converted to aldosterone by rat glomerulosa tissue, and is sensitive to sodium status (Fattah et al., 1977). How it could reach the glomerulosa *in vivo* remains open to speculation, but if we accept that shh and wnt diffuse centrifugally (see above), there seems no reason why other substances should not. Or there may be cell-cell transport: it is not the proteolytic enzmes used in cell dispersal methods that diminishes aldosterone output, but the physical disruption of the capsular tissue (Raven et al., 1983). Finally, in the rat 18-OH-DOC circulates at concentrations sufficient to be utilized as substrate (Vinson, 2004).

It is not suggested that the same mechanism would necessarily operate in any species other than the rat, which seems to be unique in that 18-OH-DOC is a major product of the fasciculata. Nevertheless, in this connection it is intriguing that in the human gland there exist more obvious mechanisms for the transfer of steroid substrate or other products from the inner zones to the glomerulosa. First, there are arteriovenous loops which derive from the cortical arterioles in the capsule region, pass through the glomerulosa and fasciculata, but then loop back to the outer cortex to a site near their origin. Secondly, as the adrenal vein leaves the gland, the cortex is inverted and wraps around the vein as the cortical cuff, which retains its zonation, (though inverted). Here the blood supply is from the arteriae comitantes in the wall of the vein. Drainage from this region is through vessels from the medulla through the cortex (i.e., from reticularis to the fasciculata and glomerulosa), thence to the central vein (**Figure 5**) (Dobbie and Symington, 1966; Neville and O'Hare, 1981). Finally, in older subjects, CYP11B2 expressing aldosterone producing cell clusters project into the fasciculata (Nishimoto et al., 2015), providing the possibility of much more intimate contact between the different cell types.

A more specific function for the reticularis has sometimes seemed to be less clear cut, especially in those species in which 17-hydroxylase (CYP17) is sparse, but in the human, and some other species, it is the major source of C_{19} steroids, especially dehydroepiandrosterone, both as the free steroid and as the sulfate. This general concept has been strengthened by methods developed to separate individual cell types, and assess their steroid output *in vitro*, and most recently by microdissection and transcriptome profiling (see **Table 2**). Notably, these methods have shown that CYP11A1 (side chain cleavage) and CYP17 (17-hydroxylase) gene transcripts are similar in the human fasciculata and reticularis, but Cyt B5A, sulfotransferase SULT2A1, and 17β-HSD (aldo-ketose reductase AKR1C3) are significantly more prominent in the reticularis (Rainey et al., 2002; Rege et al., 2014). The combined activity of these components accounts for the characteristic secretion of large amounts of DHEAS by the reticularis: Cyt B5 has been recognized as an important regulator of CYP17, and its presence is required for the efficient side chain

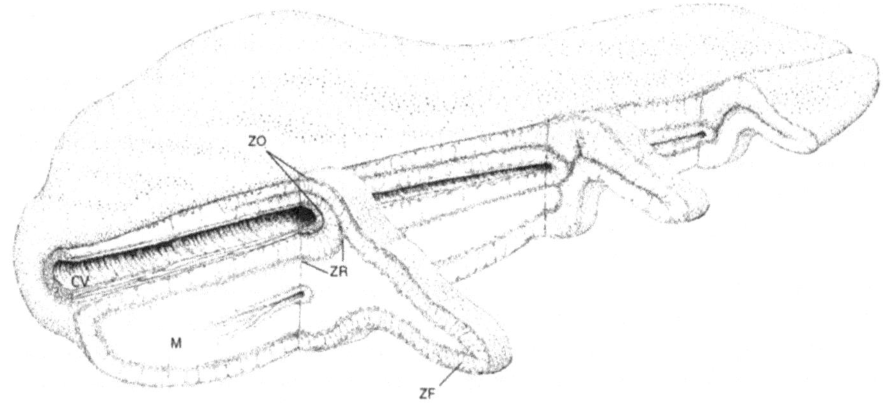

FIGURE 5 | General structure of the human adrenal gland showing the cortical cuff. The inward folding adjacent to the central vein results in a doubling of the cortical thickness and the juxtaposition in this region of the inner zona glomerulosa and the central vein. C, cortex; M, medulla; ZG, zona glomerulosa; ZF, zona fasciculata; ZR, zona reticularis; CV, central vein. Drawing by B. Landon. Figure reproduced with permission from Vinson and Hinson (1992).

cleavage activity of CYP17, though not for its 17α-hydroxylase function (Hall, 1991; Lee-Robichaud et al., 1995; Soucy and Luu-The, 2002). Cyt B5 acts through allosteric action rather than (as originally thought) provision of the second electron required for side chain cleavage (Auchus et al., 1998; Akhtar et al., 2005). It is the heightened secretion of DHEA and DHEAS by the reticularis that incurs the onset of adrenarche in humans (Belgorosky et al., 2008).

How then is androstenedione, the second most abundant androgen secreted by the human adrenal, actually synthesized? As we now see, in the human gland, the fasciculata cell expresses 3β-HSD, but the reticularis only a trace. On the other hand, the fasciculata expresses relatively little Cyt B5, required for C_{21} steroid side chain cleavage, whereas the reticularis expresses a lot. Perhaps interaction between the cell types, as postulated for aldosterone biosynthesis above, provides an answer, with transfer of DHEA from the reticularis to the fasciculata for the final stage of 3β-HSD catalyzed dehydrogenation/isomerization to give the Δ^4-3-ketone configuration of androstenedione.

Zonation in the adrenal cortex of the mouse is more complex than the broad divisions into glomerulosa, fasciculata, and reticularis, usually taken as the mammalian norm, because of the additional presence of an inner zone, the X-zone, that is only apparent in the prepubertal animals of both sexes, and in the nulliparous adult female. It does not appear to be responsive to ACTH, and it has been suggested that it is supported by LH (Chester Jones, 1955). It involutes at puberty in the male mouse, and at first pregnancy in the female leaving a band of connective tissue between the reticularis and the medulla. Its involution is exquisitely sensitive to testosterone, and although from more recent studies it appears that involution precedes the increase in blood testosterone associated with puberty in the male (Hershkovitz et al., 2007), involution does not occur in castrates, and castration of adult males results in the development of a secondary X-zone lying outside the connective tissue residue of the original (Chester Jones, 1955, 1957). The function of the X-zone has remained largely obscure, though it is known to express 20α-hydroxysteroid dehydrogenase, but not 3β-hydroxysteroid dehydrogenase, which occurs widely throughout the rest of the cortex (Hershkovitz et al., 2007). To some extent the lack of data regarding this zone is compounded by the wide variation in its appearance, indeed in some inbred laboratory animals, notably the DDD strain, the extent of X-zone vacuolation suggests the presence of little functional tissue at all (Suto, 2012).

Other components that have a clear zonal distribution are enzymes that are thought to protect the gland against toxic products associated with a high degree of cytochrome P450 activity. Thus the aldo-keto reductase-like enzyme, AKR1B7 disposes of isocaproic aldehyde, the byproduct of CYP11A1 mediated cholesterol side chain cleavage, and manganese superoxide dismutase may protect against free radicals arising from leaky mitochondrial cytochrome P450 activity, Both of these enzymes are expressed in inner adrenocortical zones (in mouse and rat respectively) (Sahut-Barnola et al., 2000; Martinez et al., 2001; Raza et al., 2005), but not in the glomerulosa. In this context, seladin-1 (DHCR24), highly expressed in human and rat fasciculata cells, may be involved in oxidative stress management, and use of a specific seladin-1 inhibitor enhances ROS formation in response to ACTH (Battista et al., 2009). It may also be involved in specific regulation of DHEA secretion (see below).

The multifunctional protein that we originally called the Inner Zone Antigen (IZA) because it is present in the rat adrenocortical fasciculata and reticularis but not glomerulosa (Laird et al., 1988; Barker et al., 1992) was later identified with the so-called progesterone receptor membrane component 1 (PGRMC1) (Min et al., 2004; Cahill, 2007), and is now also designated as the sigma 2 receptor (Xu et al., 2011; Zeng et al., 2016). In the rat adrenal this protein specifically supports 21-hydroxylation (Laird et al., 1988; Min et al., 2005). The inner zone distribution of all three of these components, AKR1B7, MnSOD, IZA/PGRMC1/Sigma2, and their absence from the glomerulosa is entirely consistent with the view that the glomerulosa is not a significant site of *de novo* steroidogenesis.

Another metabolic function of the adrenal has been described that has a distinct zonal distribution, this is the capacity for xenobiotic metabolism conferred by CYP2D16, a member of the CYP2D cytochrome P450 subfamily, in the reticularis of the guinea pig (Martin and Black, 1983; Black et al., 1989; Jiang et al., 1996; Yuan et al., 1998, 2001). CYP2D16 increases with age, and is more abundant in males than in females, there are also strain differences (Huang et al., 1996). In contrast to CYP17, which is enhanced, CYP2D16 is diminished by ACTH treatment (Yuan et al., 1998), as is 21-hydroxylase in the reticularis, but not in the outer zones (Colby et al., 1992). It is also bimodally distributed in that it is abundant in the majority of individual animals, but low in others (Colby et al., 2000). CYP2D isoforms themselves have 21-hydroxylase activity however, and are responsible for this function in the rat brain (Kishimoto et al., 2004). Type 5 17β-HSD, another member of the aldo-keto reductase family, also designated AKR1C3, is prominently transcribed in the human reticularis (Rege et al., 2014). Its function, presumably, is the reduction of 17-ketosteroids, such as androstenedione to testosterone (Nakamura et al., 2009). Conceivably it may also be protective, perhaps, like CYP2D16, metabolizing xenobiotics or (like AKR1B7) metabolizing isocaproic aldehyde. Interestingly, in other cell types, AKR1C3 also suppresses cell differentiation (Desmond et al., 2003).

Also not directly part of the corticosteroid synthesizing apparatus are the clock genes, which are zonally distributed, though quite differently, in rat and mouse adrenals. Thus *Per 1, Per 2,* and *Bmal 1* are most strongly expressed in the reticularis in rats, but, together with other clock genes (see **Table 2**) in glomerulosa and fasciculata in mice. Their expression depends on clock time, and is instrumental in maintaining the circadian rhythm inherent in corticosteroid secretion, in conjunction with hypothalamic/pituitary input (and in turn its regulation by the SCN clock system) and SCN regulated autonomic innervation (Ishida et al., 2005; Chung S. et al., 2011; Leliavski et al., 2015).

The secretion of endogenous ouabain is also zonal, in that bovine glomerulosa cells secrete several times as much as fasciculata cells, both under control conditions, and also when stimulated by angiotensin II or ACTH (Laredo et al., 1995). The presence of signaling molecules NOV, SCL27A2, and TSPAN12, not previously associated with adrenal function, and their differential transcription in the zones of the human adrenal cortex (Rege et al., 2014; see **Table 2**) also add to the view that our understanding of zonation is far from complete.

REGULATION OF ADRENOCORTICAL ZONATION

Trophic Regulation of Zonal Function

In part, the maintenance of the differentiated cortex follows the activation of specific signaling pathways. Glomerulosa steroidogenic function, that is the expression of CYP11B2 and the final stage of aldosterone synthesis, for example, is induced by (among other factors) angiotensin II stimulation, via angiotensin type 1 receptors (ATR1a and b) resulting in the activation of calcium mediated signaling pathways, whereas the fasciculata, CYP11B1 expression and cortisol/corticosterone production are ACTH dependent, modulated by the melanocortin type 2 receptor (MC2R) acting through cAMP formation.

Regulation of the Glomerulosa

Angiotensin II, the potassium ion and ACTH are the most widely studied regulators of aldosterone secretion and glomerulosa function. They have both acute effects and longer term trophic actions.

There is ample evidence that angiotensin II supports glomerulosa structure and aldosterone secretion in a manner which parallels that of dietary sodium restriction: this topic has been reviewed on many occasions, and need not be repeated here (Mulrow, 1999; Hattangady et al., 2012; Bollag, 2014). The potassium ion also has direct stimulatory actions, both on acute secretion of aldosterone (Haning et al., 1970; Aguilera and Catt, 1978), and, longer term, in induction of CYP11B2 (Tremblay et al., 1992; Yagci et al., 1996). Its action is mediated through voltage gated calcium channels (Haning et al., 1970; Aguilera and Catt, 1986; Kenyon et al., 1991) but also may require the presence of angiotensin II, perhaps generated by the intra-adrenal RAS, as well (Yamaguchi et al., 1990; Tremblay et al., 1992; Gupta et al., 1995; Vinson et al., 1998), certainly the actions of angiotensin II and potassium ions are linked (Shepherd et al., 1991).

ACTH, has long been recognized as an acute stimulator of aldosterone secretion (Haning et al., 1970; Aguilera and Catt, 1978; Braley et al., 1992; Williams, 2005; Hattangady et al., 2012; Bollag, 2014). In the rat, this presents an enigma, how is this achieved?—given what we now know about the distribution of MC2R and CYP11A expressing cell types, which in the glomerulosa are seemingly confined to the inner ZU and do not coincide with CYP11B2 (Gorrigan et al., 2011; Guasti et al., 2013a). But glomerulosa preparations, such as used by many authors (Haning et al., 1970; Aguilera and Catt, 1978; Braley et al., 1992; Williams, 2005) clearly will contain both CYP11B2 and CYP11A/MC2R-expressing cell types, as well as, usually, some fasciculata cells as well. This raises the possibility of cell-cell interaction, developed further below.

Chronically, on the other hand, ACTH does not support the glomerulosa cell phenotype, but instead downregulates CYP11B2, induces CYP11B1, and in these and other ways imposes the fasciculata phenotype instead (Aguilera et al., 1981; Ho and Vinson, 1993; Ni et al., 1995; Mitani et al., 1996). Though aldosterone secretion is also sensitive to ACTH stimulation (Hattangady et al., 2012), MC2R inactivated mice have normal glomerulosa, but greatly involuted fasciculata (Chida et al., 2007), whereas POMC knock-out may disrupt the adrenal entirely (see below). This may be attributed to the additional loss of α-MSH which in rats acts specifically on the glomerulosa in which MC5R abound (van der Kraan et al., 1998; Liakos et al., 2000): α-MSH acting on MC5R is 10 times more potent than ACTH (1-39), and 100 times more than γ-MSH in stimulating cAMP (Griffon et al., 1994). There is however a problem in that α-MSH stimulation of aldosterone production by the rat adrenal is not convincingly linked to cAMP, which is only stimulated at high α-MSH concentrations, whereas IP3 and PKC pathways are activated at lower levels (Kapas et al., 1992, 1994); others have suggested that a further MSH receptor remains to be discovered (Bicknell et al., 2000). In hypophysectomised rats, α-MSH, not ACTH is the POMC product that restores aldosterone secretion and its response to sodium depletion (Shenker et al., 1985), cf. (Vinson et al., 1980; Costa et al., 2011).

Downstream of the increased intracellular calcium evoked by potassium or angiotensin II, the orphan nuclear receptors Nurr1 and NFGFIB are both implicated in CYP11B2 expression, which also responds to COUP, SF-1 and CREB through promoter sites (Bassett et al., 2004b,c). NFGFIB, somewhat more widespread through the (human) cortex than Nurr1 (see **Table 2**), also mediates the expression of 3β-HSD2, which converts the Δ^5,3β-hydroxy configuration of 17α-hydroxypregnenolone or DHEA to the corresponding Δ^4,3-ketones (Bassett et al., 2004a,d). Angiotensin II also inhibits CYP17 expression, via PKC and src-kinase mediated pathways.

Many other factors have been found to modulate aldosterone secretion, at least under experimental conditions, these include particularly the neurotransmitters (Torda et al., 1988; Janossy et al., 1998; Vinson, 2003; Whitworth et al., 2003) cytokines, which are also produced within the gland (Judd and MacLeod, 1992; Ehrhart-Bornstein et al., 1998; Judd, 1998; Call et al., 2000), vascular products, including endothelins, nitric oxide, and adrenomedullin (Hinson and Kapas, 1998; Delarue et al., 2004), and adipokines (Willenberg et al., 2008).

Actions of ACTH on Adrenal Proliferation and Zonation

The earliest observations on the effects of hypophysectomy and ACTH treatment on adrenal form and function, showing the absolute dependence of the inner adrenocortical zones, but not the glomerulosa, on an intact functioning pituitary, was borne out by later experiments using specific gene knockout methods. First, the elimination of POMC products, including ACTH, was shown to prevent the complete development of the adrenal gland. In one study, the adrenals of POMC$^{-/-}$ mice were not macroscopically discernable, and both corticosterone and aldosterone were undetectable (Yaswen et al., 1999). However, in another report, although both fasciculata and reticularis/X-zone were greatly reduced in the mutant animals, the glomerulosa was relatively unaffected, and this was reflected in the milder effect on circulating aldosterone, while corticosterone was virtually eliminated (Coll et al., 2004). The administration of ACTH restored both circulating corticosterone (but not aldosterone) and adrenocortical structure to normal (Coll et al., 2004). In a later study, MC2R$^{-/-}$ animals were also shown to have normal glomerulosa structure, but greatly reduced inner adrenocortical zones, combined with undetectable plasma corticosterone while aldosterone was reduced by two thirds (Chida et al., 2007). These effects, of POMC [at least in the (Coll et al., 2004) study] and MC2R knockout, appear accurately to reproduce the actions of hypophysectomy (Chester Jones, 1957; Deane, 1962; Vinson, 2003). It is curious that the rat adrenal also expresses AgRP, an α-MSH antagonist (Yang et al., 1999) but only in the fasciculata and reticularis, and not the glomerulosa (Bicknell et al., 2000): in the mouse, the agouti locus is associated with X-zone, but not reticularis, morphology (Tanaka et al., 1994, 2006).

Other studies suggest that even within the zona fasciculata different areas may respond differently to chronic stress, which induced hyperplasia in the outer fasciculata, and hypertrophy in the inner fasciculata, while glomerulosa cell size was reduced (Ulrich-Lai et al., 2006).

Peptides derived from pro-γ-MSH, a 16kD fragment from the N-terminus of the POMC molecule secreted by the pituitary, that do not contain the γ-MSH sequence are thought to have a role in stimulating adrenocortical proliferation (Estivariz et al., 1982, 1988) and POMC 1-28 in particular has been shown to have this activity. An adrenal serine protease, designated AsP, which is thought to generate mitogenic peptides from pro-γ-MSH at the adrenocortical cell surface, has been characterized (Bicknell et al., 2001; Bicknell, 2003). Support for this concept has been provided by some subsequent authors, who found that POMC 1-28 stimulated adrenocortical proliferation in dexamethasone or hypophysectomised rats, though primarily in the glomerulosa (Torres et al., 2010; Mendonca and Lotfi, 2011), but others found it had no effect on adrenal growth in POMC$^{-/-}$ mice, although there was a good response to ACTH (Coll et al., 2006). In contrast, *in vitro*, rat POMC 1-28 stimulated proliferation in cultured rat glomerulosa and fasciculata/reticularis cells, but ACTH was inhibitory (Mattos et al., 2011). The discrepancy between the stimulatory actions of ACTH on adrenal cell proliferation *in vivo* and its inhibitory actions *in vitro* is difficult to resolve. It is possible that other tissue components, such as the vasculature (**Figure 4**), absent from cell cultures, are required for the proliferative actions of ACTH *in vivo* (Thomas et al., 2004).

Although dependence on ACTH is paramount, other factors are known to modulate fasciculata cell secretory activity, including cytokines, which are differentially produced throughout the cortex, and have specific actions on individual cell types (Spangelo et al., 1995; Judd, 1998; Koldzic-Zivanovic et al., 2006; Woods and Judd, 2008), and neurotransmitters (Ehrhart-Bornstein et al., 2000). The possibility of medullary, neural and vascular regulation of cortical function is emphasized by the intimate relationship between these adrenal gland components (**Figure 4**).

Regulation of the Reticularis

The control of adrenal androgen secretion is problematic, in that although supported by ACTH, secretion of androstenedione and DHEA is dissociated from cortisol under some conditions, and particularly during adrenarche which has led some authors to postulate additional pituitary or other factors (McKenna et al., 1997; l'Allemand and Biason-Lauber, 2000), and, more recently, melatonin was found to stimulate DHEA release from cultured adrenals of the solitary hamster *Phodopus sungorus* (Rendon et al., 2015). However, the factors causing the increase of adrenal androgen secretion during adrenarche are largely unknown, as are those causing the later decline, or adrenopause (Dharia and Parker, 2004; Bird, 2012) leading some authors to postulate the importance of intra-adrenal factors; these could include growth factors (l'Allemand and Biason-Lauber, 2000), cytokines or even steroids. Cortisol stimulates DHEA secretion in H295R cells by inhibiting 3β-HSD (Topor et al., 2011), DHEA modulates chromaffin cell proliferation and differentiation (Chung K. F. et al., 2011) and LH receptors are present in human fasciculata and reticularis, albeit at a low level (Pabon et al., 1996; Rao, 2010). However, another provocative finding in this regard is that inhibition of seladin-1, which is strongly expressed in the fasciculata and reticularis of the human adrenal, specifically inhibits the ACTH induced secretion of DHEA in human adrenal cells, while having no effect on cortisol output (Battista et al., 2009). This awaits physiological interpretation.

THE SIGNIFICANCE OF ADRENOCORTICAL ZONATION—HOW DOES THE STANDARD MODEL STAND UP?

That adrenocortical cells arise in the capsular or subcapsular region of the gland and migrate inwards is now virtually unchallenged. That proliferation can occur throughout the gland is also clear, but does not affect the main thesis, even given there appear to be exceptional situations in which migration may be reversed.

It is also clear that the distribution of enzymes and other components between the zones show sharp phenotypic differences between the glomerulosa and the fasciculata, and slightly less sharp differences between the fasciculata and the reticularis, hence the inwardly migrating cells undergo more or less profound phenotypic changes in their lifespan. What remains unclear is how this is achieved, although recent advances in our understanding of the role of morphogens such as wnt and shh give some powerful guides: these go a long way to explaining how the glomerulosa becomes differentiated from the capsule. Remaining to be determined is how the fasciculata becomes distinct from the glomerulosa, or the reticularis from the fasciculata. What morphogens are involved here?

As well as the speculation that they could conceivably be products of neural or vascular components of the gland (**Figure 4**), one school of thought holds that it could be the steroid products themselves. From *in vitro* studies, and on the basis that there may be a gradient of steroids from the outer to the inner part of the cortex, Hornsby and colleagues postulated that this results in high concentrations of steroids in the inner zones, which, by acting as pseudosubstrates, could directly compromise cytochrome P450 structure and function, in this way perhaps inhibiting hydroxylase activity in the reticularis, for example (Hornsby, 1987). Though this is contrary to the usual concept of morphogen diffusion which posits a decrease in concentration with distance from the source, it acquires new life, and a new mechanism, with the characterization of GR in the human adrenal cortex, particularly in the reticularis (Paust et al., 2006).

That the individual zones have defined steroidogenic roles is clear. Whether they are completely autonomous is less so. Rather, because of the paucity of other steroidogenic enzymes in the CYP11B2 expressing cells of the glomerulosa, it is arguable that the substrate for CYP11B2 must come from the fasciculata, and the different ways this could occur are via cell-cell contact, or by uptake from the general circulation, as presumably is the case for extra-adrenal CYP11B2 thought by some to be expressed in the vasculature and other tissues (Hatakeyama et al., 1996; Taves et al., 2011; though not by others, MacKenzie et al., 2012) or by diffusion. Similarly, the production of androstenedione by the human gland would seem, on the basis of the zonal distribution of enzymes possibly to be a reflection of the availability of DHEA from the reticularis to 3β-HSD in the fasciculata.

If that is the case, then the regulation of these secretory products must also reflect co-operation between zones. Given the distribution of mRNA coding for MC2R in the rat adrenal, in the inner ZU, and fasciculata/reticularis but not in the CYP11B2 region of the glomerulosa (Gorrigan et al., 2011), the well-recognized stimulation of aldosterone secretion by ACTH is otherwise difficult to explain. Of course it is still possible that it is the MC5R in the glomerulosa to which ACTH binds. The actions of angiotensin II and α-MSH on aldosterone secretion in the rat are equally difficult to understand, because the appropriate receptors, AT1R and MC5R respectively, do not appear to coincide with CYP11A1, thus cholesterol side chain cleavage, the recognized site in the pathway for stimulation of steroid hormone secretion, seemingly cannot be directly affected by these agents (**Figure 3**).

Taken together, all this evidence seems to suggest it may be mistaken to think of the adrenal cortex, or even the whole adrenal gland, as simply a collection of different types of cells, each independently performing its role in isolation. Rather we should think of these different cell types as acting in concert. We have understood for some time now that there are intraadrenal mechanisms that modify and refine the signals from the systemic regulators. These comprise medullary products, cytokines, the adrenal renal-angiotensin system, among others, and have been reviewed elsewhere (Ehrhart-Bornstein et al., 1998). Extending this has been conceptually problematic in view of the apparently confounding effect of the blood flow through the gland, which would seemingly limit the action any cell might have on other than its closest neighbors by secreted products.

We now know that secreted products from adrenocortical cells can indeed pervade the gland through diffusion, and this has been demonstrated by the wnt-catenin and shh-Gli signaling systems. So if it is possible for these products then there is no reason why it cannot be the case for others, including perhaps catecholamines, cytokines, and the steroids themselves. This may give a partial explanation for the architecture of the gland, one of the problems posed at the start of this article—why are the zones arranged as concentric spheres? One answer may be that this has the potential to maximize the likelihood of diffused products arriving at their targets. If we take as an example the secretion of shh from its origin in the ZU, random walk diffusion to its target in the inner capsule is better achieved when the capsule completely envelops the glomerulosa than it would be if the system were more open, or composed of sheets, like a mesentery or secretory epithelium.

In addition, there is absolutely no reason to suppose the steroids themselves do not move between the zones, as substrates or modifiers. How else can we explain how aldosterone or androstenedione are synthesized? And, given that MC2R and CYP11A1 are expressed in the ZU and fasciculata, but not the CYP11B2 expressing cells of the rat glomerulosa, how else can we explain how ACTH has its undoubted action on aldosterone secretion, other than by the enhanced provision of steroid substrates from the ZU or the fasciculata to the CYP11B2 cells in the glomerulosa?

Like the human body itself, the function of the adrenal gland is an integrated whole, much greater than the sum of its parts. We should aim to think of it that way.

AUTHOR CONTRIBUTIONS

GV researched and wrote this article.

ACKNOWLEDGMENTS

I am most grateful to Drs. Peter King and Leonardo Guasti, of the Centre for Endocrinology, William Harvey Research Institute, Queen Mary University of London, London EC1M 6BQ, for their careful reading of the manuscript and for their helpful comments and suggestions.

REFERENCES

1. Aguilera, G., and Catt, K. J. (1978). Loci of action of regulators of aldosterone biosynthesis in isolated glomerulosa cells. *Endocrinology* 104, 1046–1052. doi: 10.1210/endo-104-4-1046
2. Aguilera, G., and Catt, K. J. (1986). Participation of voltage-dependent calcium channels in the regulation of adrenal glomerulosa function by angiotensin II and potassium. *Endocrinology* 118, 112–118. doi: 10.1210/endo-118-1-112
3. Aguilera, G., Fujita, K., and Catt, K. J. (1981). Mechanisms of inhibition of aldosterone secretion by adrenocorticotropin. *Endocrinology* 108, 522–528. doi: 10.1210/endo-108-2-522
4. Aiba, M., and Fujibayashi, M. (2011). Alteration of subcapsular adrenocortical zonation in humans with aging: the progenitor zone predominates over the previously well-developed zona glomerulosa after 40 years of age. *J. Histochem. cytochem.* 59, 557–564. doi: 10.1369/0022155411404071
5. Aigueperse, C., Val, P., Pacot, C., Darne, C., Lalli, E., Sassone-Corsi, P., et al. (2001). SF-1 (steroidogenic factor-1), C/EBPbeta (CCAAT/enhancer binding protein), and ubiquitous transcription factors NF1 (nuclear factor 1) and Sp1 (selective promoter factor 1) are required for regulation of the mouse aldose reductase- like gene (AKR1B7) expression in adrenocortical cells. *Mol. Endocrinol.* 15, 93–111. doi: 10.1210/mend.15.1.0577
6. Akhtar, M. K., Kelly, S. L., and Kaderbhai, M. A. (2005). Cytochrome b(5) modulation of 17a-hydroxylase and 17-20 lyase (CYP17) activities in steroidogenesis. *J. Endocrinol.* 187, 267–274. doi: 10.1677/joe.1.06375
7. Arnold, J. (1866). Ein beitrag zu der feineren structur und demchemismus der nebennieren. *Virchows Archiv Pathologie, Anatomie, Physiologie* 39, 64–117. doi: 10.1007/BF01979887
8. Atanassova, N., and Koeva, Y. (2012). "Hydroxysteroid dehydrogenases - biological role and clinical importance - review, Chapter 6," *in Dehydrogenases,* ed R. A. Canuto (Intech), 115–164.
9. Auchus, R. J., Lee, T. C., and Miller, W. L. (1998). Cytochrome b5 augments the 17,20-lyase activity of human P450c17 without direct electron transfer. *J. Biol. Chem.* 273, 3158–3165. doi: 10.1074/jbc.273.6.3158
10. Bandyopadhyay, A., Tsuji, K., Cox, K., Harfe, B. D., Rosen, V., and Tabin, C. J. (2006). Genetic analysis of the roles of BMP2, BMP4, and BMP7 in limb patterning and skeletogenesis. *PLoS Genet.* 2:e216. doi: 10.1371/journal.pgen.0020216
11. Barker, S., Laird, S. M., Ho, M. M., Vinson, G. P., and Hinson, J. P. (1992). Characterisation of a rat adrenocortical inner zone specific antigen and identification of a putative precursor. *J. Mol. Endocr.* 9, 95–102. doi: 10.1677/jme.0.0090095
12. Bassett, M. H., Suzuki, T., Sasano, H., de Vries, C. J. M., Jimenez, P. T., Carr, B. R., et al. (2004a). The orphan nuclear receptor NGFIB regulates transcription of 3 beta-hydroxysteroid dehydrogenase - Implications for the control of adrenal functional zonation. *J. Biol. Chem.* 279, 37622–37630. doi: 10.1074/jbc.M405431200
13. Bassett, M. H., Suzuki, T., Sasano, H., White, P. C., and Rainey, W. E. (2004b). The orphan nuclear receptors NURR1 and NGFIB regulate adrenal aldosterone production. *Mol. Endocrinol.* 18, 279–290. doi: 10.1210/me.2003-0005
14. Bassett, M. H., White, P. C., and Rainey, W. E. (2004c). The regulation of aldosterone synthase expression. *Mol. Cell. Endocrinol.* 217, 67–74. doi: 10.1016/j.mce.2003.10.011
15. Bassett, M. H., White, P. C., and Rainey, W. E. (2004d). A role for the NGFI-B family in adrenal zonation and adrenocortical disease. *Endocr. Res.* 30, 567–574. doi: 10.1081/ERC-200043715
16. Bastida, C. M., Cremades, A., Castells, M. T., Lopez-Contreras, A. J., Lopez-Garcia, C., Sanchez-Mas, J., et al. (2007). Sexual dimorphism of ornithine decarboxylase in the mouse adrenal: influence of polyamine deprivation on catecholamine and corticoid levels. *Am. J. Physiol. Endocrinol. Metab.* 292, E1010–E1017. doi: 10.1152/ajpendo.00316.2006
17. Battista, M. C., Roberge, C., Martinez, A., and Gallo-Payet, N. (2009). 24- dehydrocholesterol reductase/seladin-1: a key protein differentially involved in adrenocorticotropin effects observed in human and rat adrenal cortex. *Endocrinology* 150, 4180–4190. doi: 10.1210/en.2009-0410
18. Beery, E., Middel, P., Bahn, A., Willenberg, H. S., Hagos, Y., Koepsell, H., et al. (2003). Molecular evidence of organic ion transporters in the rat adrenal cortex with adrenocorticotropin-regulated zonal expression. *Endocrinology* 144, 4519–4526. doi: 10.1210/en.2002-221001
19. Belgorosky, A., Baquedano, M. S., Guercio, G., and Rivarola, M. A. (2008). Adrenarche: postnatal adrenal zonation and hormonal and metabolic regulation. *Horm. Res.* 70, 257–267. doi: 10.1159/000157871
20. Bell, J. B., Gould, R. P., Hyatt, P. J., Tait, J. F., and Tait, S. A. (1978). Properties of rat adrenal zona reticularis cells: preparation by gravitational sedimentation. *J. Endocrinol.* 77, 25–41. doi: 10.1677/joe.0.0770025
21. Bell, J. B., Gould, R. P., Hyatt, P. J., Tait, J. F., and Tait, S. A. (1979). Properties of rat adrenal zona reticularis cells: production and stimulation of certain steroids. *J. Endocrinol.* 83, 435–447. doi: 10.1677/joe.0.0830435
22. Bernet, F., Bernard, J., Laborie, C., Montel, V., Maubert, E., and Dupouy, J. P. (1994). Neuropeptide-Y (NPY)- and vasoactive-intestinal-peptide (VIP)-induced aldosterone secretion by rat capsule/glomerular zone could be mediated by catecholamines via b(1) adrenergic-receptors. *Neurosci. Lett.* 166, 109–112. doi: 10.1016/0304-3940(94)90852-4
23. Berthon, A., Martinez, A., Bertherat, J., and Val, P. (2012). Wnt/beta-catenin signalling in adrenal physiology and tumour development. *Mol. Cell. Endocrinol.* 351, 87–95. doi: 10.1016/j.mce.2011.09.009
24. Bicknell, A. B. (2003). Identification of a serine protease involved with the regulation of adrenal growth. *Ann. N.Y. Acad. Sci.* 994, 118–122. doi: 10.1111/j.1749-6632.2003.tb03170.x
25. Bicknell, A. B., Lomthaisong, K., Gladwell, R. T., and Lowry, P. J. (2000). Agouti related protein in the rat adrenal cortex: implications for novel autocrine mechanisms modulating the actions of pro-opiomelanocortin peptides. *J. Neuroendocrinol.* 12, 977–982. doi: 10.1046/j.1365-2826.2000.0 0543.x
26. Bicknell, A. B., Lomthaisong, K., Woods, R. J., Hutchinson, E. G., Bennett, H. P., Gladwell, R. T., et al. (2001). Characterization of a serine protease that cleaves pro-gamma-melanotropin at the adrenal to stimulate growth. *Cell* 105, 903–912. doi: 10.1016/S0092-8674(01)00403-2
27. Bird, I. M. (2012). In the zone: understanding zona reticularis function and its transformation by adrenarche. *J. Endocrinol.* 214, 109–111. doi: 10.1530/JOE- 12-0246
28. Black, V. H., Barilla, J. R., and Martin, K. O. (1989). Effects of age, adrenocorticotropin, and dexamethasone on a male-specific cytochrome P450 localized in the inner zone of the guinea pig adrenal. *Endocrinology* 124, 2494–2248. doi: 10.1210/endo-124-5-2494

29. Bocian-Sobkowska, J., Malendowicz, L. K., and Wozniak, W. (1997). Comparative stereological studies on zonation and cellular composition of adrenal glands of normal and anencephalic human fetuses. II. Cellular composition of the gland. *Histol. Histopathol.* 12, 391–399.
30. Bollag, W. B. (2014). Regulation of aldosterone synthesis and secretion. *Compr. Physiol.* 4, 1017–1055. doi: 10.1002/cphy.c130037
31. Bornstein, S. R., and Ehrhart-Bornstein, M. (1992). Ultrastructural evidence for a paracrine regulation of the rat adrenal cortex mediated by the local release of catecholamines from chromaffin cells. *Endocrinology* 131, 3126–3318.
32. Braley, L. M., Adler, G. K., Mortensen, R. M., Conlin, P. R., Chen, R., Hallahan, J., et al. (1992). Dose effect of adrenocorticotropin on aldosterone and cortisol biosynthesis in cultured bovine adrenal glomerulosa cells: *in vitro* correlate of hyperreninemic hypoaldosteronism. *Endocrinology* 131, 187–194.
33. Brennan, C. H., Chittka, A., Barker, S., and Vinson, G. P. (2008). Eph receptors and zonation in the rat adrenal cortex. *J. Endocrinol.* 198, 185–191. doi: 10.1677/JOE-08-0084
34. Buijs, J. T., Petersen, M., van der Horst, G., and van der Pluijm, G. (2010). Bone morphogenetic proteins and its receptors; therapeutic targets in cancer progression and bone metastasis? *Curr. Pharm. Des.* 16, 1291–1300. doi: 10.2174/138161210791033987
35. Cahill, M. A. (2007). Progesterone receptor membrane component 1: an integrative review. *J. Steroid Biochem. Mol. Biol.* 105, 16–36. doi: 10.1016/j.jsbmb.2007.02.002
36. Call, G. B., Husein, O. F., McIlmoil, C. J., Adams, A., Heckmann, R. A., and Judd, A.
37. M. (2000). Bovine adrenal cells secrete interleukin-6 and tumor necrosis factor *in vitro*. *Gen. Comp. Endocrinol.* 118, 249–261. doi: 10.1006/gcen.2000.7458
38. Carpenter, C. C., Davis, J. O., and Ayers, C. R. (1961). Relation of renin, angiotensin II, and experimental renal hypertension to aldosterone secretion. *J. Clin. Invest.* 40, 2026–2042. doi: 10.1172/JCI104429
39. Carsia, R. V., Macdonald, G. J., Gibney, J. A., Tilly, K. I., and Tilly, J. L. (1996). Apoptotic cell death in the rat adrenal gland: an *in vivo* and *in vitro* investigation. *Cell Tissue.Res.* 283, 247–254. doi: 10.1007/s004410050535
40. Cater, D. B., and Lever, J. D. (1954). The zona intermedia of the adrenal cortex; a correlation of possible functional significance with development, morphology and histochemistry. *J. Anat.* 88, 437–454.
41. Chambaz, E. M., Cochet, C., Souchelnitskiy, S., Defaye, G., and Feige, J. J. (1994). Growth-factors and pericellular components as a local signaling relay in the action of systemic hormones. *Horm. Res.* 42, 35–38. doi: 10.1159/000184142
42. Chang, S. P., Morrison, H. D., Nilsson, F., Kenyon, C. J., West, J. D., and Morley, S. D. (2013). Cell proliferation, movement and differentiation during maintenance of the adult mouse adrenal cortex. *PLoS ONE* 8:e81865. doi: 10.1371/journal.pone.0081865
43. Chang, S. P., Mullins, J. J., Morley, S. D., and West, J. D. (2011). Transition from organogenesis to stem cell maintenance in the mouse adrenal cortex. *Organogenesis* 7, 267–280. doi: 10.4161/org.7.4.18060
44. Chester Jones, I. (1955). Role of the adrenal cortex in reproduction. *Br. Med. Bull.* 11, 156–160.
45. Chester Jones, I. (1957). *The Adrenal Cortex*. Cambridge: University Press. Chida, D., Nakagawa, S., Nagai, S., Sagara, H., Katsumata, H., Imaki, T., et al. (2007). Melanocortin 2 receptor is required for adrenal gland development, steroidogenesis, and neonatal gluconeogenesis. *Proc. Natl. Acad. Sci. U.S.A.* 104, 18205–18210. doi: 10.1073/pnas.0706953104
46. Chung, K. F., Qin, N., Androutsellis-Theotokis, A., Bornstein, S. R., and Ehrhart- Bornstein, M. (2011). Effects of dehydroepiandrosterone on proliferation and differentiation of chromaffin progenitor cells. *Mol. Cell. Endocrinol.* 336, 141–148. doi: 10.1016/j.mce.2010.11.028
47. Chung, S., Son, G. H., and Kim, K. (2011). Circadian rhythm of adrenal glucocorticoid: its regulation and clinical implications. *Biochim. Biophys. Acta* 1812, 581–591. doi: 10.1016/j.bbadis.2011.02.003
48. Colby, H. D., Huang, Y., Jiang, Q., and Voigt, J. M. (2000). Bimodal expression of CYP2D16 in the guinea pig adrenal cortex. *Pharmacology* 61, 78–82. doi: 10.1159/000028384
49. Colby, H. D., Levitt, M., Pope, M. R., and Johnson, P. B. (1992). Differential effects of adrenocorticotropic hormone on steroid hydroxylase activities in the inner and outer zones of the guinea pig adrenal cortex. *J. Steroid Biochem. Mol. Biol.* 42, 329–335. doi: 10.1016/0960-0760(92)90136-7
50. Coll, A. P., Challis, B. G., Yeo, G. S., Snell, K., Piper, S. J., Halsall, D., et al. (2004). The effects of proopiomelanocortin deficiency on murine adrenal development and responsiveness to adrenocorticotropin. *Endocrinology* 145, 4721–4727. doi: 10.1210/en.2004-0491
51. Coll, A. P., Fassnacht, M., Klammer, S., Hahner, S., Schulte, D. M., Piper, S., et al. (2006). Peripheral administration of the N-terminal pro-opiomelanocortin fragment 1-28 to Pomc-/- mice reduces food intake and weight but does not affect adrenal growth or corticosterone production. *J. Endocrinol.* 190, 515–525. doi: 10.1677/joe.1.06749
52. Conti, B., Jahng, J. W., Tinti, C., Son, J. H., and Joh, T. H. (1997). Induction of interferon-gamma inducing factor in the adrenal cortex. *J. Biol. Chem.* 272, 2035–2037. doi: 10.1074/jbc.272.4.2035
53. Costa, J. L., Forbes, S., Brennan, M. B., and Hochgeschwender, U. (2011). Genetic modifications of mouse proopiomelanocortin peptide processing. *Mol. Cell.*
54. *Endocrinol.* 336, 14–22. doi: 10.1016/j.mce.2010.12.032
55. de Joussineau, C., Sahut-Barnola, I., Levy, I., Saloustros, E., Val, P., Stratakis, C. A., et al. (2012). The cAMP pathway and the control of adrenocortical development and growth. *Mol. Cell. Endocrinol.* 351, 28–36. doi: 10.1016/j.mce.2011.10.006
56. de Mendonca, P. O., Costa, I. C., and Lotfi, C. F. (2014). The involvement of Nek2 and Notch in the proliferation of rat adrenal cortex triggered by POMC-derived peptides. *PLoS ONE* 9:e108657. doi: 10.1371/journal.pone.0108657
57. Deane, H. W. (1962). "The anatomy, chemistry, and physiology of adrenocortical tissue," in *Handbuch der Experimentalle Pharmakologie*, Vol. 14 (Berlin: Springer), 1–85.
58. Delarue, C., Conlon, J. M., Remy-Jouet, I., Fournier, A., and Vaudry, H. (2004). Endothelins as local activators of adrenocortical cells. *J. Mol. Endocrinol.* 32, 1–7. doi: 10.1677/jme.0.0320001
59. Desmond, J. C., Mountford, J. C., Drayson, M. T., Walker, E. A., Hewison, M., Ride,
60. J. P., et al. (2003). The aldo-keto reductase AKR1C3 is a novel suppressor of cell differentiation that provides a plausible target for the non-cyclooxygenase- dependent antineoplastic actions of nonsteroidal anti-inflammatory drugs. *Cancer Res.* 63, 505–512.
61. Dharia, S., and Parker, C. R. Jr. (2004). Adrenal androgens and aging. *Semin. Reprod. Med.* 22, 361–368. doi: 10.1055/s-2004-861552
62. Dobbie, J. W., and Symington, T. (1966). The human adrenal gland with special reference to the vasculature. *J. Endocrinol.* 34, 479–489. doi: 10.1677/joe.0.0340479
63. Dostoiewsky, A. (1886). Ein Beitrag zur mikroskopischen Anatomie der Nebennieren bei Säugethieren. *Archiv für mikroskopische Anatomie* 27, 272–296. doi: 10.1007/BF02955421
64. Dupont, E., Rheaume, E., Simard, J., Luu-The, V., Labrie, F., and Pelletier, G. (1991). Ontogenesis of 3 beta-hydroxysteroid dehydrogenase/delta 5-delta 4 isomerase in the rat adrenal as revealed by immunocytochemistry and in situ hybridization. *Endocrinology* 129, 2687–2292. doi: 10.1210/endo-129-5-2687
65. Ehrhart-Bornstein, M., Haidan, A., Alesci, S., and Bornstein, S. R. (2000). Neurotransmitters and neuropeptides in the differential regulation of steroidogenesis in adrenocortical-chromaffin co-cultures. *Endocr. Res.* 26, 833–842. doi: 10.3109/07435800009048606
66. Ehrhart-Bornstein, M., Hinson, J. P., Bornstein, S. R., Scherbaum, W. A., and Vinson, G. P. (1998). Intraadrenal interactions in the regulation of adrenocortical steroidogenesis. *Endocr. Rev.* 19, 101–143. doi: 10.1210/edrv.19.2.0326
67. El Wakil, A. (2013). Inactivation of Cav3.2 T-type calcium channels regulates partially ectopic aldosterone [production in Task1 knckout mice without correcting their adrenocortical zonation pattern. *Egypt J. Exp. Biol.* 9, 95–100.
68. Engeland, W. C., Ennen, W. B., Elayaperumal, A., Durand, D. A., and Levay-Young, B. K. (2005). Zone-specific cell proliferation during compensatory adrenal growth in rats. *Am. J. Physiol. Endocrinol.metab.* 288, E298–E306. doi: 10.1152/ajpendo.00307.2004
69. Engeland, W. C., and Levay-Young, B. K. (1999). Changes in the glomerulosa cell phenotype during adrenal regeneration in rats. *Am. J. Physiol.* 276, R1374– R1182.
70. Ennen, W. B., Levay-Young, B. K., and Engeland, W. C. (2005). Zone-specific cell proliferation during adrenocortical regeneration after enucleation in rats. *Am. J.Physiol. Endocrinol. Metab.* 289, E883–E891. doi: 10.1152/ajpendo.00031.2005 Estivariz, F. E., Iturriza, F., McLean, C.,

Hope, J., and Lowry, P. J. (1982). Stimulation of adrenal mitogenesis by N-terminal proopiocortin peptides. *Nature* 297, 419–422. doi: 10.1038/297419a0

71. Estivariz, F. E., Morano, M. I., Carino, M., Jackson, S., and Lowry, P. J. (1988). Adrenal regeneration in the rat is mediated by mitogenic N-terminal pro-opiomelanocortin peptides generated by changes in precursor processing in the anterior pituitary. *J. Endocrinol.* 116, 207–216. doi: 10.1677/joe.0.11 60207
72. Fahrenkrug, J., Hannibal, J., and Georg, B. (2008). Diurnal rhythmicity of the canonical clock genes Per1, Per2 and Bmal1 in the rat adrenal gland is unaltered after hypophysectomy. *J. Neuroendocrinol.* 20, 323–329. doi: 10.1111/j.1365- 2826.2008.01651.x
73. Fattah, D. I., Whitehouse, B. J., and Vinson, G. P. (1977). Biosynthesis of Aldosterone from 18-hydroxylated precursors by rat adrenal tissue *in vitro*. *J. Endocrinol.* 75, 187–195. doi: 10.1677/joe.0.0750187
74. Finco, I., LaPensee, C. R., Krill, K. T., and Hammer, G. D. (2015). Hedgehog signaling and steroidogenesis. *Annu. Rev. Physiol.* 77, 105–129. doi: 10.1146/annurev-physiol-061214-111754
75. Freedman, B. D., Kempna, P. B., Carlone, D. L., Shah, M. S., Guagliardo, N. A., Barrett, P. Q., et al. (2013). Adrenocortical zonation results from lineage conversion of differentiated zona glomerulosa cells. *Dev. Cell* 26, 666–673. doi: 10.1016/j.devcel.2013.07.016
76. Fukuda, T., Takahashi, K., Suzuki, T., Saruta, M., Watanabe, M., Nakata, T., et al. (2005). Urocortin 1, urocortin 3/stresscopin, and corticotropin-releasing factor receptors in human adrenal and its disorders. *J. Clin. Endocrinol. Metab.* 90, 4671–4678. doi: 10.1210/jc.2005-0090
77. Gallo-Payet, N., and Escher, E. (1985). Adrenocorticotropin receptors in rat adrenal glomerulosa cells. *Endocrinology* 117, 38–46. doi: 10.1210/endo-117- 1-38
78. Godoy, J. R., Funke, M., Ackermann, W., Haunhorst, P., Oesteritz, S., Capani, F., et al. (2011). Redox atlas of the mouse.immunohistochemical detection of glutaredoxin-, peroxiredoxin-, and thioredoxin-family proteins in various tissues of the laboratory mouse. *Biochim. Biophys. Acta* 1810, 2–92. doi: 10.1016/j.bbagen.2010.05.006
79. Gorrigan, R. J., Guasti, L., King, P., Clark, A. J., and Chan, L. F. (2011). Localisation of the melanocortin-2-receptor and its accessory proteins in the developing and adult adrenal gland. *J. Mol. Endocrinol.* 46, 227–232. doi: 10.1530/JME-11-0011 Gottschau, M. (1883). Struktur und embryonale Entwicklung der Nebennieren bei Säugetieren. *Arch. Anat. Physiol. Lpz.* 9, 412–458.
80. Griffon, N., Mignon, V., Facchinetti, P., Diaz, J., Schwartz, J. C., and Sokoloff, P. (1994). Molecular cloning and characterization of the rat fifth melanocortin receptor. *Biochem. Biophys. Res. Commun.* 200, 1007–1014. doi: 10.1006/bbrc.1994.1550
81. Gross, F. (1958). Renin und Hypertensin: Physiologische oder pathologische Wirkstoffe. *Klin Wochenschr* 36, 693–706. doi: 10.1007/BF01493136
82. Guasti, L., Candy Sze, W. C., McKay, T., Grose, R., and King, P. J. (2013a). FGF signalling through Fgfr2 isoform IIIb regulates adrenal cortex development. *Mol. Cell. Endocrinol.* 371, 182–188. doi: 10.1016/j. mce.2013.01.014
83. Guasti, L., Cavlan, D., Cogger, K., Banu, Z., Shakur, A., Latif, S., et al. (2013b). Dlk1 up-regulates Gli1 expression in male rat adrenal capsule cells through the activation of beta1 integrin and ERK1/2. *Endocrinology* 154, 4675–4684. doi: 10.1210/en.2013-1211
84. Guasti, L., Paul, A., Laufer, E., and King, P. (2011). Localization of Sonic hedgehog secreting and receiving cells in the developing and adult rat adrenal cortex. *Mol. Cell. Endocrinol.* 336, 117–122. doi: 10.1016/j. mce.2010.11.010
85. Gummow, B. M., Winnay, J. N., and Hammer, G. D. (2003). Convergence of Wnt signaling and steroidogenic factor-1 (SF-1) on transcription of the rat inhibin alpha gene. *J. Biol. Chem.* 278, 26572–26579. doi: 10.1074/jbc. M212677200
86. Gupta, P., Francosaenz, R., and Mulrow, P. J. (1995). Locally generated angiotensin-II in the adrenal-gland regulates basal, corticotropin-stimulated, and potassium-stimulated aldosterone secretion. *Hypertension* 25, 443–448. doi: 10.1161/01.HYP.25.3.443
87. Haidan, A., Bornstein, S. R., Liu, Z., Walsh, L. P., Stocco, D. M., and Ehrhart-Bornstein, M. (2000). Expression of adrenocortical steroidogenic acute regulatory (StAR) protein is influenced by chromaffin cells. *Mol. Cell. Endocrinol.* 165, 25–32. doi: 10.1016/S0303-7207(00)00267-7
88. Halder, S. K., Takemori, H., Hatano, O., Nonaka, Y., Wada, A., and Okamoto, M. (1998). Cloning of a membrane-spanning protein with epidermal growth factor- like repeat motifs from adrenal glomerulosa cells. *Endocrinology* 139, 3316–3328. doi: 10.1210/en.139.7.3316
89. Hall, P. F. (1991). Cytochrome P-450 C21scc: one enzyme with two actions: hydroxylase and lyase. *J. Steroid Biochem. Mol. Biol.* 40, 527–532. doi: 10.1016/0960-0760(91)90272-7
90. Haning, R., Tait, S. A. S., and Tait, J. F. (1970). *In vitro* effects of ACTH, angiotensins, serotonin, and potassium on steroid output and conversion of corticosterone to aldosterone by isolated adrenal cells. *Endocrinology* 87, 1147–1167. doi: 10.1210/endo-87-6-1147
91. Hatakeyama, H., Miyamori, I., Takeda, Y., Yamamoto, H., and Mabuchi, H. (1996). The expression of steroidogenic enzyme genes in human vascular cells. *Biochem. Mol. Biol. Int.* 40, 639–645. doi: 10.1080/15216549600201233
92. Hattangady, N. G., Olala, L. O., Bollag, W. B., and Rainey, W. E. (2012). Acute and chronic regulation of aldosterone production. *Mol. Cell. Endocrinol.* 350, 151–162. doi: 10.1016/j.mce.2011.07.034
93. Heitzmann, D., Derand, R., Jungbauer, S., Bandulik, S., Sterner, C., Schweda, F., et al. (2008). Invalidation of TASK1 potassium channels disrupts adrenal gland zonation and mineralocorticoid homeostasis. *EMBO J.* 27, 179–187. doi: 10.1038/sj.emboj.7601934
94. Hershkovitz, L., Beuschlein, F., Klammer, S., Krup, M., and Weinstein, Y. (2007). Adrenal 20alpha-hydroxysteroid dehydrogenase in the mouse catabolizes progesterone and 11-deoxycorticosterone and is restricted to the X-zone. *Endocrinology* 148, 976–988. doi: 10.1210/en.2006-1100
95. Hinson, J. P., and Kapas, S. (1998). The role of endothelial cell products in the regulation of adrenocortical function: actions of endothelin, nitric oxide, adrenomedullin and PAMP. *Horm. Metab. Res.* 30, 334–340. doi: 10.1055/s- 2007-978894
96. Ho, M. M., and Vinson, G. P. (1993). 11 beta-Hydroxylase gene expression in the rat adrenal cortex. *J. Endocrinol.* 139, 301–306. doi: 10.1677/joe.0. 1390301
97. Ho, M. M., and Vinson, G. P. (1995). Endocrine control of the distribution of basic fibroblast growth- factor, insulin-like growth-factor-i and transforming growth factor- beta(1) messenger-rnas in adult-rat adrenals using nonradioactive in- situ hybridization. *J. Endocrinol.* 144, 379–387. doi: 10.1677/joe.0.1440379
98. Ho, M. M., and Vinson, G. P. (1997). Peptide growth factors and the adrenal cortex.
99. *Microsc. Res. Tech.* 36, 558–568. Ho, M. M., and Vinson, G. P. (1998). Transcription of (pro)renin mRNA in the rat adrenal cortex, and the effects of ACTH treatment and a low sodium diet. *J. Endocrinol.* 157, 217–223. doi: 10.1677/joe.0.1570217
100. Holzwarth, M. A., Cunningham, L. A., and Kleitman, N. (1987). The role of adrenal nerves in the regulation of adrenocortical functions. *Ann. N.Y. Acad. Sci.* 512, 449–464. doi: 10.1111/j.1749-6632.1987.tb24980.x
101. Hornsby, P. J. (1987). Physiological and pathological effects of steroids on the function of the adrenal cortex. *J. Steroid Biochem.* 27, 1161–1171. doi: 10.1016/0022-4731(87)90203-2
102. Huang, Y., Jiang, Q., Voigt, J. M., Debolt, K. M., and Colby, H. D. (1996). Strain differences in adrenal CYP2D16 expression in guinea pigs. Relationship to xenobiotic metabolism. *Biochem. Pharmacol.* 52, 1925–1929. doi: 10.1016/S0006-2952(96)00665-X
103. Huang, Z., Ohno, N., Terada, N., Saitoh, Y., Chen, J., and Ohno, S. (2013). Immunohistochemical detection of angiotensin II receptors in mouse cerebellum and adrenal gland using "*in vivo* cryotechnique". *Histochem. Cell Biol.* 140, 477–490. doi: 10.1007/s00418-013-1084-y
104. Ishida, A., Mutoh, T., Ueyama, T., Bando, H., Masubuchi, S., Nakahara, D., et al. (2005). Light activates the adrenal gland: timing of gene expression and glucocorticoid release. *Cell Metab.* 2, 297–307. doi: 10.1016/j. cmet.2005. 09.009
105. Ishimura, K., and Fujita, H. (1997). Light and electron microscopic immunohistochemistry of the localization of adrenal steroidogenic enzymes. *Microsc. Res. Tech.* 36, 445–453.
106. Ito, M., Yu, R., and Jameson, J. L. (1997). DAX-1 inhibits SF-1-mediated transactivation via a carboxy-terminal domain that is deleted in adrenal hypoplasia congenita. *Mol. Cell. Biol.* 17, 1476–1483. doi: 10.1128/ MCB.17.3.1476
107. Janossy, A., Orso, E., Szalay, K. S., Juranyi, Z., Beck, M., Vizi, E. S., et al. (1998). Cholinergic regulation of the rat adrenal zona glomerulosa. *J. Endocrinol.* 157, 305–315. doi: 10.1677/joe.0.1570305
108. Jiang, Q., Huang, Y., Voigt, J. M., DeBolt, K. M., Kominami, S., Takemori, S., et al. (1996). Differential effects of adrenocorticotropin *in vivo* on

cytochromes P4502D16 and P450c17 in the guinea pig adrenal cortex. *Endocrinology* 137, 4811–4486. doi: 10.1210/en.137.11.4811
109. Judd, A. M. (1998). Cytokine expression in the rat adrenal cortex. *Horm. Metab. Res.* 30, 404–410. doi: 10.1055/s-2007-978905
110. Judd, A. M., and MacLeod, R. M. (1992). Adrenocorticotropin increases interleukin-6 release from rat adrenal zona glomerulosa cells. *Endocrinology* 130, 1245–1254.
111. Judd, A. M., and MacLeod, R. M. (1995). Differential release of tumor necrosis factor and IL-6 from adrenal zona glomerulosa cells *in vitro*. *Am. J. Physiol.* 268, E114–E120.
112. Kapas, S., Orford, C. D., Barker, S., Vinson, G. P., and Hinson, J. P. (1992). Studies on the intracellular mechanism of action of alpha-melanocyte-stimulating hormone on rat adrenal zona glomerulosa. *J. Mol. Endocrinol.* 9, 47–54. doi: 10.1677/jme.0.0090047
113. Kapas, S., Purbrick, A., Barker, S., Vinson, G. P., and Hinson, J. P. (1994). Alpha-melanocyte-stimulating hormone-induced inhibition of angiotensin II receptor-mediated events in the rat adrenal zona glomerulosa. *J. Mol. Endocrinol.* 13, 95–104. doi: 10.1677/jme.0.0130095
114. Kenyon, C. J., Shepherd, R. M., Fraser, R., Pediani, J. D., and Elder, H. Y. (1991). The role of potassium and other ions in the control of aldosterone synthesis. *Endocr. Res.* 17, 225–236. doi: 10.1080/07435809109027199
115. Kim, A. C., Barlaskar, F. M., Heaton, J. H., Else, T., Kelly, V. R., Krill, K. T., et al. (2009). In search of adrenocortical stem and progenitor cells. *Endocr. Rev.* 30, 241–263. doi: 10.1210/er.2008-0039
116. Kim, A. C., and Hammer, G. D. (2007). Adrenocortical cells with stem/progenitor cell properties: recent advances. *Mol. Cell. Endocrinol.* 265–266, 10–16. doi: 10.1016/j.mce.2006.12.028
117. Kim, A. C., Reuter, A. L., Zubair, M., Else, T., Serecky, K., Bingham, N. C., et al. (2008). Targeted disruption of beta-catenin in Sf1-expressing cells impairs development and maintenance of the adrenal cortex. *Development* 135, 2593–2602. doi: 10.1242/dev.021493
118. King, P., Paul, A., and Laufer, E. (2009). Shh signaling regulates adrenocortical development and identifies progenitors of steroidogenic lineages. *Proc. Natl. Acad. Sci. U.S.A.* 106, 21185–21190. doi: 10.1073/pnas.09094 71106
119. Kirillov, O. I., and Popova, S. B. (1985). Adrenal cortex of rat: diurnal variation of nuclear volumes and mitotic index of cells in zona fasciculata. *Exp. Clin*
120..Endocrinol. 86, 375–337. doi: 10.1055/s-0029-1210514
121. Kishimoto, W., Hiroi, T., Shiraishi, M., Osada, M., Imaoka, S., Kominami, S., et al. (2004). Cytochrome P450 2D catalyze steroid 21-hydroxylation in the brain. *Endocrinology* 145, 699–705. doi: 10.1210/en.2003-1109
122. Koldzic-Zivanovic, N., Tu, H., Juelich, T. L., Rady, P. L., Tyring, S. K., Hudnall, S. D., et al. (2006). Regulation of adrenal glucocorticoid synthesis by interleukin- 10: a preponderance of IL-10 receptor in the adrenal zona fasciculata. *Brain Behav. Immun.* 20, 460–468. doi: 10.1016/j.bbi.2005.09.003
123. Lai, F. J., Shin, S. J., Lee, Y. J., Lin, S. R., Jou, W. Y., and Tsai, J. H. (2000).
124. Up-regulation of adrenal cortical and medullary atrial natriuretic peptide and gene expression in rats with deoxycorticosterone acetate-salt treatment. *Endocrinology* 141, 325–332. doi: 10.1210/en.141.1.325
125. Laird, S. M., Vinson, G. P., and Whitehouse, B. J. (1988). Monoclonal antibodies against rat adrenocortical cell antigens. *Acta Endocrinol.* 119, 420–426. doi: 10.1530/acta.0.1190420
126. Lala, D. S., Rice, D. A., and Parker, K. L. (1992). Steroidogenic factor I, a key regulator of steroidogenic enzyme expression, is the mouse homolog of fushi tarazu-factor I. *Mol. Endocrinol.* 6, 1249–1258.
127. l'Allemand, D., and Biason-Lauber, A. (2000). Intra-adrenal regulation of androgen synthesis. *Eur. J. Clin. Invest.* 30(Suppl. 3), 28–33. doi: 10.1046/j.1365- 2362.2000.0300s3028.x
128. Lander, A. D. (2013). How cells know where they are. *Science* 339, 923–927. doi: 10.1126/science.1224186
129. Laragh, J. H., Angers, M., Kelly, W. G., and Lieberman, S. (1960). Hypotensive agents and pressor substances. The effect of epinephrine, norepinephrine, angiotensin II, and others on the secretory rate of aldosterone in man. *JAMA* 174, 234–240. doi: 10.1001/jama.1960.03030030014003
130. Laredo, J., Hamilton, B. P., and Hamlyn, J. M. (1995). Secretion of endogenous ouabain from bovine adrenocortical cells: role of the zona glomerulosa and zona fasciculata. *Biochem. Biophys. Res. Commun.* 212, 487–493. doi: 10.1006/bbrc.1995.1996
131. Lee-Robichaud, P., Wright, J. N., Akhtar, M. E., and Akhtar, M. (1995). Modulation of the activity of human 17 alpha-hydroxylase-17,20-lyase (CYP17) by cytochrome b5: endocrinological and mechanistic implications. *Biochem. J.* 308, 901–998. doi: 10.1042/bj3080901
132. Lehoux, J. G., Bird, I. M., Briere, N., Martel, D., and Ducharme, L. (1997). Influence of dietary sodium restriction on angiotensin II receptors in rat adrenals. *Endocrinology* 138, 5238–5547. doi: 10.1210/en.138.12.5238
133. Lehoux, J. G., Fleury, A., and Ducharme, L. (1998). The acute and chronic effects of adrenocorticotropin on the levels of messenger ribonucleic acid and protein of steroidogenic enzymes in rat adrenal *in vivo*. *Endocrinology* 139, 3913–3922. doi: 10.1210/en.139.9.3913
134. Leliavski, A., Dumbell, R., Ott, V., and Oster, H. (2015). Adrenal clocks and the role of adrenal hormones in the regulation of circadian physiology. *J. Biol. Rhythms* 30, 20–34. doi: 10.1177/0748730414553971
135. Li, D., Mukai, K., Suzuki, T., Suzuki, R., Yamashita, S., Mitani, F., et al. (2007). Adrenocortical zonation factor 1 is a novel matricellular protein promoting integrin-mediated adhesion of adrenocortical and vascular smooth muscle cells. *FEBS J.* 274, 2506–2522. doi: 10.1111/j.1742-4658.2007.05786.x
136. Liakos, P., Chambaz, E. M., Feige, J. J., and Defaye, G. (2000). Expression and regulation of melanocortin receptor-5 (MC5-R) in the bovine adrenal cortex. *Mol. Cell. Endocrinol.* 159, 99–107. doi: 10.1016/S0303-7207(99)00196-3
137. Lombardo, L. D., and Cortesini, C. (1988). The origin and differentiation of adrenocortical cells in rats with portacaval shunt. A structural and ultrastructural study. *Histol. Histopathol.* 3, 163–171.
138. MacDonald, B. T., Tamai, K., and He, X. (2009). Wnt/beta-catenin signaling: components, mechanisms, and diseases. *Dev. Cell* 17, 9–26. doi: 10.1016/j.devcel.2009.06.016
139. MacKenzie, S. M., Connell, J. M., and Davies, E. (2012). Non-adrenal synthesis of aldosterone: a reality check. *Mol. Cell. Endocrinol.* 350, 163–167. doi: 10.1016/j.mce.2011.06.026
140. Martin, K. O., and Black, V. H. (1983). Effects of age and adrenocorticotropin on microsomal enzymes in guinea pig adrenal inner and outer cortices. *Endocrinology* 112, 573–559. doi: 10.1210/endo-112-2-573
141. Martinez, A., Aigueperse, C., Val, P., Dussault, M., Tournaire, C., Berger, M., et al. (2001). Physiological functions and hormonal regulation of mouse vas deferens protein (AKR1B7) in steroidogenic tissues. *Chem. Biol. Interact.* 130–132, 903–917. doi: 10.1016/S0009-2797(00)00244-1
142. Mattos, G. E., Jacysyn, J. F., Amarante-Mendes, G. P., and Lotfi, C. F. (2011). Comparative effect of FGF2, synthetic peptides 1-28 N-POMC and ACTH on proliferation in rat adrenal cell primary cultures. *Cell Tissue Res.* 345, 343–356. doi: 10.1007/s00441-011-1220-8
143. McEwan, P. C., Lindop, G. B., and Kenyon, C. J. (1996). Control of cell-proliferation in the rat adrenal-gland *in-vivo* by the renin-angiotensin system. *Am. J. Physiol. 34, E*192–E198.
144. McEwan, P. E., Vinson, G. P., and Kenyon, C. J. (1999). Control of adrenal cell proliferation by AT1 receptors in response to angiotensin II and low-sodium diet. *Am. J. Physiol.* 276, E303–E309.
145. McKenna, T. J., Fearon, U., Clarke, D., and Cunningham, S. K. (1997). A critical review of the origin and control of adrenal androgens. *Baillieres Clin. Obstet. Gynaecol.* 11, 229–248. doi: 10.1016/S0950-3552(97)80035-1
146. McNeill, H., Puddefoot, J. R., and Vinson, G. P. (1998). MAP kinase in the rat adrenal gland. *Endocr. Res.* 24, 373–380. doi: 10.3109/07435809809032617 McNeill, H., and Vinson, G. P. (2000). Regulation of MAPK activity in response
147. to dietary sodium in the rat adrenal gland. *Endocr. Res.* 26, 879–883. doi: 10.3109/07435800009048612
148. Mendonca, P. O., and Lotfi, C. F. (2011). The proliferative effect of synthetic N- POMC(1-28) peptides in rat adrenal cortex: a possible role for cyclin E. *Mol. Cell. Endocrinol.* 336, 156–161. doi: 10.1016/j.mce.2010.12.012
149. Min, L., Strushkevich, N. V., Harnastai, I. N., Iwamoto, H., Gilep, A. A., Takemori, H., et al. (2005). Molecular identification of adrenal inner zone antigen as a heme-binding protein. *Febs J.* 272, 5832–5843. doi: 10.1111/j.1742- 4658.2005.04977.x
150. Min, L., Takemori, H., Nonaka, Y., Katoh, Y., Doi, J., Horike, N., et al. (2004). Characterization of the adrenal-specific antigen IZA (inner zone antigen) and its role in the steroidogenesis. *Mol. Cell. Endocrinol.* 215, 143–148. doi: 10.1016/j.mce.2003.11.025
151. Mitani, F., Miyamoto, H., Mukai, K., and Ishimura, Y. (1996). Effects of long- term stimulation of ACTH-secretion and angiotensin- II-secretion on the rat adrenal-cortex. *Endocr. Res.* 22, 421–431. doi: 10.1080/07435809609043728
152. Mitani, F., Mukai, K., Miyamoto, H., Suematsu, M., and Ishimura, Y.

(1999). Development of functional zonation in the rat adrenal cortex. *Endocrinology* 140, 3342–3353. doi: 10.1210/en.140.7.3342

153. Mitani, F., Ogishima, T., Miyamoto, H., and Ishimura, Y. (1995). Localization of p450aldo and p45011-beta in normal and regenerating rat adrenal-cortex. *Endocr. Res.* 21, 413–423. doi: 10.3109/07435809509030457

154. Mitani, F., Suzuki, H., Hata, J. I., Ogishima, T., Shimada, H., and Ishimura, Y. (1994). A novel cell layer without corticosteroid-synthesizing enzymes in rat adrenal-cortex - histochemical detection and possible physiological-role. *Endocrinology* 135, 431–438.

155. Morley, S. D., Viard, I., Chung, B. C., Ikeda, Y., Parker, K. L., and Mullins, J. J. (1996). Variegated expression of a mouse steroid 21-hydroxylase/beta-galactosidase transgene suggests centripetal migration of adrenocortical cells. *Mol. Endocrinol.* 10, 585–598.

156. Morohashi, K., Iida, H., Nomura, M., Hatano, O., Honda, S., Tsukiyama, T., Niwa, O., Hara, T., Takakusu, A., Shibata, Y., and et al. (1994). Functional difference between Ad4BP and ELP, and their distributions in steroidogenic tissues. *Mol. Endocrinol.* 8, 643–653.

157. Mukai, K., Mitani, F., Nagasawa, H., Suzuki, R., Suzuki, T., Suematsu, M., et al. (2003). An inverse correlation between expression of a preprocathepsin B-related protein with cysteine-rich sequences and steroid 11beta - hydroxylase in adrenocortical cells. *J. Biol. Chem.* 278, 17084–17092. doi: 10.1074/jbc.M301477200

158. Mukai, T., Kusaka, M., Kawabe, K., Goto, K., Nawata, H., Fujieda, K., et al. (2002). Sexually dimorphic expression of Dax-1 in the adrenal cortex. *Genes Cells* 7, 717–729. doi: 10.1046/j.1365-2443.2002.00556.x

159. Mulrow, P. J. (1999). Angiotensin II and aldosterone regulation. *Regul. Pept.* 80, 27–32. doi: 10.1016/S0167-0115(99)00004-X

160. Nakamura, Y., Hornsby, P. J., Casson, P., Morimoto, R., Satoh, F., Xing, Y., et al. (2009). Type 5 17beta-hydroxysteroid dehydrogenase (AKR1C3) contributes to testosterone production in the adrenal reticularis. *J. Clin. Endocrinol. Metab.* 94, 2192–2198. doi: 10.1210/jc.2008-2374

161. Neville, A. M., and O'Hare, M. J. (1981). *The Human Adrenal Cortex*. Berlin: Springer-Verlag.

162. Ni, H., Mune, T., Morita, H., Daidoh, H., Hanafusa, J., Shibata, T., et al. (1995). Inhibition of aldosterone turn-off phenomenon following chronic adrenocorticotropin treatment with *in vivo* administration of antiglucocorticoid and antioxidants in rats. *Eur. J. Endocrinol.* 133, 578–584. doi: 10.1530/eje.0.1330578

163. Nishimoto, K., Harris, R. B., Rainey, W. E., and Seki, T. (2014). Sodium deficiency regulates rat adrenal zona glomerulosa gene expression. *Endocrinology* 155, 1363–1372. doi: 10.1210/en.2013-1999

164. Nishimoto, K., Nakagawa, K., Li, D., Kosaka, T., Oya, M., Mikami, S., et al. (2010). Adrenocortical zonation in humans under normal and pathological conditions. *J. Clin. Endocrinol. Metab.* 95, 2296–2305. doi: 10.1210/jc.2009-2010

165. Nishimoto, K., Tomlins, S. A., Kuick, R., Cani, A. K., Giordano, T. J., Hovelson, D. H., et al. (2015). Aldosterone-stimulating somatic gene mutations are common in normal adrenal glands. *Proc. Natl. Acad. Sci. U.S.A.* 112, E4591–E4599. doi: 10.1073/pnas.1505529112

166. Nonaka, Y., and Okamoto, M. (1991). Functional expression of the cDNAs encoding rat 11-b-hydroxylase [cytochrome-p450(11-b)] and aldosterone synthase [cytochrome-p450(11-b, aldo)]. *Eur. J. Biochem.* 202, 897–902. doi: 10.1111/j.1432-1033.1991.tb16449.x

167. Nussdorfer, G. G. (1986). Cytophysiology of the adrenal cortex. *Int. Rev. Cytol.* 98, 1–405.

168. Okamoto, M., and Nonaka, Y. (1992). Molecular-biology of rat steroid 11-b-hydroxylase [p450(11-b)] and aldosterone synthase [p450(11-b, aldo)]. *J. Steroid Biochem. Mol. Biol.* 41, 415–419. doi: 10.1016/0960-0760(92)90367-R

169. Oster, H., Damerow, S., Kiessling, S., Jakubcakova, V., Abraham, D., Tian, J., et al. (2006). The circadian rhythm of glucocorticoids is regulated by a gating mechanism residing in the adrenal cortical clock. *Cell Metab.* 4, 163–173. doi: 10.1016/j.cmet.2006.07.002

170. Otis, M., Campbell, S., Payet, M. D., and Gallo-Payet, N. (2007). Expression of extracellular matrix proteins and integrins in rat adrenal gland: importance for ACTH-associated functions. *J. Endocrinol.* 193, 331–347. doi: 10.1677/JOE-07- 0055

171. Otis, M., Campbell, S., Payet, M. D., and Gallo-Payet, N. (2008). In adrenal glomerulosa cells, angiotensin II inhibits proliferation by interfering with fibronectin-integrin signaling. *Endocrinology* 149, 3435–3445. doi: 10.1210/en.2008-0282

172. Pabon, J. E., Li, X., Lei, Z. M., Sanfilippo, J. S., Yussman, M. A., and Rao, C. V. (1996). Novel presence of luteinizing hormone/chorionic gonadotropin receptors in human adrenal glands. *J. Clin. Endocrinol. Metab.* 81, 2397–2400.

173. Parker, K. L., and Schimmer, B. P. (1993). Transcriptional regulation of the adrenal steroidogenic enzymes. *Trends Endocrinol. Metab.* 4, 46–50. doi: 10.1016/S1043-2760(05)80014-1

174. Parker, K. L., Ikeda, Y., and Luo, X. (1995). The nuclear receptor sf-1 acts at multiple levels of endocrine development. *Mol. Biol. Cell* 6:1344.

175. Paust, H. J., Loeper, S., Else, T., Bamberger, A. M., Papadopoulos, G., Pankoke, D., et al. (2006). Expression of the glucocorticoid receptor in the human adrenal cortex. *Exp. Clin. Endocrinol. Diabetes* 114, 6–10. doi: 10.1055/s-2005-873007

176. Payet, N., Lehoux, J. G., and Isler, H. (1980). Effect of ACTH on the proliferative and secretory activities of the adrenal glomerulosa. *Acta Endocr.* 93, 365–374. doi: 10.1530/acta.0.0930365

177. Pellerin, S., Keramidas, M., Chambaz, E. M., and Feige, J. J. (1997). Expression of laminin and its possible role in adrenal cortex homeostasis. *Endocrinology* 138, 1321–1137. doi: 10.1210/en.138.3.1321

178. Peters, B., Clausmeyer, S., Obermuller, N., Woyth, A., Kranzlin, B., Gretz, N., et al. (1998). Specific regulation of StAR expression in the rat adrenal zona glomerulosa. *an in situ* hybridization study. *J. Histochem. Cytochem.* 46, 1215–1221. doi: 10.1177/002215549804601101

179. Peters, B., Teubner, P., Clausmeyer, S., Puschner, T., Maser-Gluth, C., Wrede, H. J., et al. (2007). StAR expression and the long-term aldosterone response to high- potassium diet in Wistar-Kyoto and spontaneously hypertensive rats. *Am. J. Physiol. Endocrinol. Metab.* 292, E16–E23. doi: 10.1152/ajpendo.00454.2005

180. Petrovic-Kosanovic, D., Ajdzanovic, V., Cakic-Milosevic, M., Koko, V., and Milosevic, V. (2013). The effects of acute heat stress on proliferative and apoptotic processes in the rat adrenal cortex. *Arch. Biol. Sci.* 65, 905–909. doi: 10.2298/ABS1303905K

181. Pignatelli, D., Bento, M. J., Maia, M., Magalhaes, M. M., Magalhaes, M. C., and Mason, J. I. (1999). Ontogeny of 3beta-hydroxysteroid dehydrogenase expression in the rat adrenal gland as studied by immunohistochemistry. *Endocr. Res.* 25, 21–27. doi: 10.1080/07435809909066126

182. Pignatelli, D., Xiao, F., Gouveia, A. M., Ferreira, J. G., and Vinson, G. P. (2006). Adrenarche in the rat. *J. Endocrinol.* 191, 301–308. doi: 10.1677/joe.1.06972 Pihlajoki, M., Dorner, J., Cochran, R. S., Heikinheimo, M., and Wilson, D. B.

183. (2015). Adrenocortical zonation, renewal, and remodeling. *Front. Endocrinol.* 6:27. doi: 10.3389/fendo.2015.00027

184. Pihlajoki, M., Gretzinger, E., Cochran, R., Kyronlahti, A., Schrade, A., Hiller, T., et al. (2013). Conditional mutagenesis of Gata6 in SF1-positive cells causes gonadal-like differentiation in the adrenal cortex of mice. *Endocrinology* 154, 1754–1767. doi: 10.1210/en.2012-1892

185. Rabl, H. (1891). Die Entwicklung und Structur der Nebennieren bei den Vögeln. *Archiv für mikroskopische Anatomie* 38, 492–523. doi: 10.1007/BF02954398 Rainey, W. E., and Nakamura, Y. (2008). Regulation of the adrenal androgen biosynthesis. *J. Steroid Biochem. Mol. Biol.* 108, 281–286. doi: 10.1016/j.jsbmb.2007.09.015

186. Rainey, W. E., Carr, B. R., Sasano, H., Suzuki, T., and Mason, J. I. (2002). Dissecting human adrenal androgen production. *Trends Endocrinol. Metab.* 13, 234–239. doi: 10.1016/S1043-2760(02)00609-4

187. Rao, C. V. (2010). Human adrenal LH/hCG receptors and what they could mean for adrenal physiology and pathology. *Mol. Cell. Endocrinol.* 329, 33–36. doi: 10.1016/j.mce.2010.05.012

188. Raven, P. W., McCredie, E., McAuley, M., and Vinson, G. P. (1983). Origins of the differences in function of rat adrenal zona glomerulosa cells incubated as intact tissue and as collagenase-prepared cell suspensions. *Cell Biochem. Funct.* 1, 17–24. doi: 10.1002/cbf.290010104

189. Raza, F. S., Okamoto, M., Takemori, H., and Vinson, G. P. (2005). Manganese superoxide dismutase activity in the rat adrenal. *J. Endocrinol.* 184, 77–84. doi: 10.1677/joe.1.05755

190. Raza, F. S., Puddefoot, J. R., and Vinson, G. P. (1998). Pref-1, SF- 1 and adrenocortical zonation. *Endocr. Res.* 24, 977–981. doi: 10.3109/07435809809032720

191. Raza, F. S., Takemori, H., Tojo, H., Okamoto, M., and Vinson, G. P. (2001). Identification of the rat adrenal zona fasciculata/reticularis specific protein, inner zone antigen (IZAg), as the putative membrane progesterone receptor. *Eur. J. Biochem.* 268, 2141–2147. doi: 10.1046/j.1432-1327.2001.02096.x

192. Raza, F. S., and Vinson, G. P. (2000). Adrenocortical expression of MnSOD. *Endocr. Res.* 26, 959–963. doi: 10.3109/07435800009048623
193. Reddi, A. H. (1998). Role of morphogenetic proteins in skeletal tissue engineering and regeneration. *Nat. Biotechnol.* 16, 247–252. doi: 10.1038/nbt0398-247
194. Rege, J., Nakamura, Y., Wang, T., Merchen, T. D., Sasano, H., and Rainey, W. E. (2014). Transcriptome profiling reveals differentially expressed transcripts between the human adrenal zona fasciculata and zona reticularis. *J. Clin. Endocrinol. Metab.* 99, E518–E527. doi: 10.1210/jc.2013-3198
195. Rege, J., Nishimoto, H. K., Nishimoto, K., Rodgers, R. J., Auchus, R. J., and Rainey, W. E. (2015). Bone Morphogenetic Protein-4 (BMP4): a paracrine regulator of human adrenal C19 steroid synthesis. *Endocrinology* 156, 2530–2540. doi: 10.1210/en.2014-1942
196. Rendon, N. M., Rudolph, L. M., Sengelaub, D. R., and Demas, G. E. (2015). The agonistic adrenal: melatonin elicits female aggression via regulation of adrenal androgens. *Proc. Biol. Sci.* 282:20152080. doi: 10.1098/rspb.2015.2080
197. Renshaw, D., and Hinson, J. P. (2001). Neuropeptide Y and the adrenal gland: a review. *Peptides.* 22, 429–438. doi: 10.1016/S0196-9781(01)00353-9
198. Romero, D. G., Yanes, L. L., de Rodriguez, A. F., Plonczynski, M. W., Welsh, B. L., Reckelhoff, J. F., et al. (2007). Disabled-2 is expressed in adrenal zona glomerulosa and is involved in aldosterone secretion. *Endocrinology* 148, 2644–2652. doi: 10.1210/en.2006-1509
199. Roskelley, C. D., and Auersperg, N. (1990). Density separation of rat adrenocortical cells: morphology, steroidogenesis, and P-450scc expression in primary culture. *In.Vitro.Cell Dev. Biol.* 26, 493–501. doi: 10.1007/BF02624091
200. Rucinski, M., Porzionato, A., Ziolkowska, A., Szyszka, M., Macchi, V., De Caro, R., et al. (2010). Expression of the spexin gene in the rat adrenal gland and evidences suggesting that spexin inhibits adrenocortical cell proliferation. *Peptides* 31, 676–682. doi: 10.1016/j.peptides.2009.12.025
201. Sahut-Barnola, I., de Joussineau, C., Val, P., Lambert-Langlais, S., Damon, C., Lefrancois-Martinez, A. M., et al. (2010). Cushing's syndrome and fetal features resurgence in adrenal cortex-specific Prkar1a knockout mice. *PLoS Genet.* 6:e1000980. doi: 10.1371/journal.pgen.1000980
202. Sahut-Barnola, I., Lefrancois-Martinez, A. M., Jean, C., Veyssiere, G., and Martinez, A. (2000). Adrenal tumorigenesis targeted by the corticotropin-regulated promoter of the aldo-keto reductase AKR1B7 gene in transgenic mice. *Endocr. Res.* 26, 885–898. doi: 10.3109/07435800009048613
203. Scheys, J. O., Heaton, J. H., and Hammer, G. D. (2011). Evidence of adrenal failure in aging Dax1-deficient mice. *Endocrinology* 152, 3430–3439. doi: 10.1210/en.2010-0986
204. Schilling, T. F., Nie, Q., and Lander, A. D. (2012). Dynamics and precision in retinoic acid morphogen gradients. *Curr. Opin. Genet. Dev.* 22, 562–569. doi: 10.1016/j.gde.2012.11.012
205. Selye, H. (1946). The general adaptation syndrome and the diseases of adaptation. *J. Clin. Endocrinol. Metab.* 6, 117–230. doi: 10.1210/jcem-6-2-117
206. Selye, H., and Jensen, H. (1946). The chemistry of the hormones. *Ann. Rev. Biochem.* 15, 347–360. doi: 10.1146/annurev.bi.15.070146.002023
207. Shenker, Y., Villareal, J. Z., Sider, R. S., and Grekin, R. J. (1985). Alpha-melanocyte-stimulating hormone stimulation of aldosterone secretion in hypophysectomized rats. *Endocrinology* 116, 138–141. doi: 10.1210/endo-116- 1-138
208. Shepherd, R. M., Fraser, R., Nichols, D. J., and Kenyon, C. J. (1991). Efflux of potassium-ions in angiotensin-II-stimulated bovine adrenocortical-cells. *J. Endocrinol.* 128, 297–304. doi: 10.1677/joe.0.1280297
209. Shimasaki, S., Moore, R. K., Otsuka, F., and Erickson, G. F. (2004). The bone morphogenetic protein system in mammalian reproduction. *Endocr. Rev.* 25, 72–101. doi: 10.1210/er.2003-0007
210. Shimojo, M., Whorwood, C. B., and Stewart, P. M. (1996). 11 beta-Hydroxysteroid dehydrogenase in the rat adrenal. *J. Mol. Endocrinol.* 17, 121–130. doi: 10.1677/jme.0.0170121
211. Simon, D. P., and Hammer, G. D. (2012). Adrenocortical stem and progenitor cells: implications for adrenocortical carcinoma. *Mol. Cell. Endocrinol.* 351, 2–11. doi: 10.1016/j.mce.2011.12.006
212. Smith, R. E., Li, K. X., Andrews, R. K., and Krozowski, Z. (1997). Immunohistochemical and molecular characterization of the rat 11 beta-hydroxysteroid dehydrogenase type II enzyme. *Endocrinology* 138, 540–547.
213. Soucy, P., and Luu-The, V. (2002). Assessment of the ability of type 2 cytochrome b5 to modulate 17,20-lyase activity of human P450c17. *J. Steroid Biochem. Mol. Biol.* 80, 71–75. doi: 10.1016/S0960-0760(01)00171-6
214. Spangelo, B. L., Judd, A. M., Call, G. B., Zumwalt, J., and Gorospe, W. C. (1995). Role of the cytokines in the hypothalamic-pituitary-adrenal and gonadal axes. *Neuroimmunomodulation* 2, 299–312. doi: 10.1159/000097209
215. Suto, J. (2012). Quantitative trait locus mapping of genes associated with vacuolation in the adrenal X-zone of the DDD/Sgn inbred mouse. *BMC Genet.* 13:95. doi: 10.1186/1471-2156-13-95
216. Swann, G. (1940). The pituitary-adrenocortical relationship. *Physiol.Rev.* 20, 493–521.
217. Tait, S. A., Schulster, D., Okamoto, M., Flood, C., and Tait, J. F. (1970). Production of steroids by *in vitro* superfusion of endocrine tissue. II. steroid output from bisected whole, capsular and decapsulated adrenals of normal intact, hypophysectomized and hypophysectomized-nephrectomized rats as a function of time of superfusion. *Endocrinology* 86, 360–382. doi: 10.1210/endo- 86-2-360
218. Tanaka, S., Kuwahara, S., Nishijima, K., Ohno, T., and Matsuzawa, A. (2006). Genetic association of mutation at agouti locus with adrenal x zone morphology in BALB/c mice. *Exp. Anim.* 55, 343–347. doi: 10.1538/expanim.55.343
219. Tanaka, S., Nishimura, M., and Matsuzawa, A. (1994). Genetic association between agouti locus and adrenal X zone morphology in SM/J mice. *Acta Anat.* 149, 170–113. doi: 10.1159/000147573
220. Taves, M. D., Gomez-Sanchez, C. E., and Soma, K. K. (2011). Extra-adrenal glucocorticoids and mineralocorticoids: evidence for local synthesis, regulation, and function. *Am. J. Physiol. Endocrinol. Metab.* 301, E11–E24. doi: 10.1152/ajpendo.00100.2011
221. Tevosian, S. G., Jimenez, E., Hatch, H. M., Jiang, T., Morse, D. A., Fox, S. C., et al. (2015). Adrenal development in mice requires GATA4 and GATA6 transcription factors. *Endocrinology* 156, 2503–2517. doi: 10.1210/en.2014-1815
222. Thomas, M., Keramidas, M., Monchaux, E., and Feige, J. J. (2004). Dual hormonal regulation of endocrine tissue mass and vasculature by adrenocorticotropin in the adrenal cortex. *Endocrinology* 145, 4320–4329. doi: 10.1210/en.2004-0179
223. Thomas, R., Anderson, W. A., Raman, V., and Reddi, A. H. (1998). Androgen- dependent gene expression of bone morphogenetic protein 7 in mouse prostate. *Prostate* 37, 236–245.
224. Tickle, C. (2006). Making digit patterns in the vertebrate limb. *Nat. Rev. Mol. Cell. Biol.* 7, 45–53. doi: 10.1038/nrm1830
225. Topor, L. S., Asai, M., Dunn, J., and Majzoub, J. A. (2011). Cortisol stimulates secretion of dehydroepiandrosterone in human adrenocortical cells through inhibition of 3betaHSD2. *J. Clin. Endocrinol. Metab.* 96, E31–E39. doi: 10.1210/jc.2010-0692
226. Torda, T., Cruciani, R. A., and Saavedra, J. M. (1988). Localization of neuropeptide Y binding sites in the zona glomerulosa of the bovine adrenal gland. *Neuroendocrinology* 48, 207–210. doi: 10.1159/000125010
227. Torres, T. E., de Mendonca, P. O., and Lotfi, C. F. (2010). Synthetic modified N- POMC(1-28) controls *in vivo* proliferation and blocks apoptosis in rat adrenal cortex. *Cell Tissue Res.* 341, 239–250. doi: 10.1007/s00441-010-0998-0
228. Tremblay, A., Parker, K. L., and Lehoux, J. G. (1992). Dietary potassium supplementation and sodium restriction stimulate aldosterone synthase but not 11 beta-hydroxylase P-450 messenger ribonucleic acid accumulation in rat adrenals and require angiotensin II production. *Endocrinology* 130, 3152–3318. Tsuji, K., Bandyopadhyay, A., Harfe, B. D., Cox, K., Kakar, S., Gerstenfeld, L., et al. (2006). BMP2 activity, although dispensable for bone formation, is required for the initiation of fracture healing. *Nat. Genet.* 38, 1424–1429. doi: 10.1038/ng1916
229. Tyczewska, M., Rucinski, M., Ziolkowska, A., Szyszka, M., Trejter, M., Hochol- Molenda, A., et al. (2014). Enucleation-induced rat adrenal gland regeneration: expression profile of selected genes involved in control of adrenocortical cell proliferation. *Int. J. Endocrinol.* 2014:130359. doi: 10.1155/2014/130359
230. Ulrich-Lai, Y. M., Figueiredo, H. F., Ostrander, M. M., Choi, D. C., Engeland, W. C., and Herman, J. P. (2006). Chronic stress induces adrenal hyperplasia and hypertrophy in a subregion-specific manner. *Am. J. Physiol. Endocrinol. Metab.* 291, E965–E973. doi: 10.1152/ajpendo.00070.2006
231. Urist, M. R. (1965). Bone: formation by autoinduction. *Science* 150, 893–899. doi: 10.1126/science.150.3698.893

232. Uruno, A., Matsuda, K., Noguchi, N., Yoshikawa, T., Kudo, M., Satoh, F., et al. (2011). Peroxisome proliferator-activated receptor- suppresses CYP11B2 expression and aldosterone production. *J. Mol. Endocrinol.* 46, 37–49. doi: 10.1677/JME-10-0088

233. van der Kraan, M., Adan, R. A., Entwistle, M. L., Gispen, W. H., Burbach, J. P., and Tatro, J. B. (1998). Expression of melanocortin-5 receptor in secretory epithelia supports a functional role in exocrine and endocrine glands. Endocrinology 139, 2348–2355. doi: 10.1210/en.139.5.2348

234. Vendeira, P., Pignatelli, D., Neves, D., Magalhaes, M. M., Magalhaes, M. C., and Vinson, G. P. (1999). Effects of prolonged infusion of basic fibroblast growth factor and IGF-I on adrenocortical differentiation in the autotransplanted adrenal: an immunohistochemical study. J. Endocrinol. 162, 21–29. doi: 10.1677/joe.0.1620021

235. Vines, H. W. C. (1938). "The adreno-genital syndrome: some histological observations,"in The Adrenal Cortex and Intersexuality, eds L. R. Broster, C. Allen, H. W. C. Vines, J. Patterson, A. W. Greenwood, G. F. Marrian, and G. C. Butler (London: Chapman and Hall), 137–197.

236. Vinson, G. P. (2003). Adrenocortical zonation and ACTH. Microsc. Res. Tech. 61, 227–239. doi: 10.1002/jemt.10331

237. Vinson, G. P. (2004). Glomerulosa function and aldosterone synthesis in the rat. Mol. Cell. Endocrinol. 217, 59–65. doi: 10.1016/j.mce.2003.10.010

238. Vinson, G. P., Firth, K. M., McNeill, H. M., and Puddefoot, J. R. (2000). "Differentiation of function in the zones of the rat adrenal cortex," in Molecular Steroidogenesis, eds M. Okamoto, Y. Ishimura, and H. Nawata (Tokyo: Universal Academy Press, Inc.), 205–208.

239. Vinson, G. P., and Hinson, J. P. (1992). "Blood flow and hormone secretion in the adrenal gland," in The Adrenal Gland, 2nd Edn., ed V. H. T. James (New York, NY: Raven Press), 71–86.

240. Vinson, G. P., Hinson, J. P., and Raven, P. W. (1985a). The relationship between tissue preparation and function; methods for the study of control of aldosterone secretion: a review. Cell. Biochem. Funct. 3, 235–253. doi: 10.1002/cbf.290030402

241. Vinson, G. P., Hinson, J. P., and Toth, I. E. (1994). The neuroendocrinology of the adrenal cortex. J. Neuroendocr. 6, 235–246. doi: 10.1111/j.1365-2826.1994.tb00578.x

242. Vinson, G. P., and Ho, M. M. (1998). Origins of zonation: the adrenocortical model of tissue development and differentiation. Clin. Exp. Pharmacol. Physiol. 25, S91–S96. doi: 10.1111/j.1440-1681.1998.tb02308.x

243. Vinson, G. P., Ho, M. M., and Puddefoot, J. R. (1998). Adrenocortical zonation and the adrenal renin-angiotensin system. Endocr. Res. 24, 677–686. doi: 10.3109/07435809809032669

244. Vinson, G. P., Laird, S. M., Hinson, J. P., and Teja, R. (1992a). Origin of aldosterone in trypsin-stimulated rat adrenal zona glomerulosa incubations. J. Endocrinol. 135, 125–133. doi: 10.1677/joe.0.1350125

245. Vinson, G. P., Pudney, J. A., and Whitehouse, B. J. (1985b). The mammalian adrenal circulation and the relationship between adrenal blood flow and steroidogenesis. J. Endocrinol. 105, 285–294. doi: 10.1677/joe.0.1050285

246. Vinson, G. P., Teja, R., Ho, M. M., and Puddefoot, J. R. (1995). A two cell type theory for aldosterone biosynthesis: the roles of 11b-hydroxylase and aldosterone synthase, and a high capacity, tightly binding steroid carrier (TBSC) for 18-hydroxydeoxycorticosterone. J. Endocrinol. 144, 359–368. doi: 10.1677/joe.0.1440359

247. Vinson, G. P., Whitehouse, B. J., Dell, A., Etienne, T., and Morris, H.

248. R. (1980). Characterisation of an adrenal zona glomerulosa stimulating component of posterior pituitary extracts as a-MSH. Nature 284, 464–467. doi: 10.1038/284464a0

249. Vinson, G. P., Whitehouse, B. J., and Hinson, J. P. (1992b). The Adrenal Cortex. Englewood Heights, NJ: Prentice-Hall.

250. Walczak, E. M., and Hammer, G. D. (2015). Regulation of the adrenocortical stem cell niche: implications for disease. Nat. Rev. Endocrinol. 11, 14–28. doi: 10.1038/nrendo.2014.166

251. White, R. J., Nie, Q., Lander, A. D., and Schilling, T. F. (2007). Complex regulation of cyp26a1 creates a robust retinoic acid gradient in the zebrafish embryo. PLoS Biol. 5:e304. doi: 10.1371/journal.pbio.0050304

252. Whitworth, E. J., Kosti, O., Renshaw, D., and Hinson, J. P. (2003). Adrenal neuropeptides: regulation and interaction with ACTH and other adrenal regulators. Microsc. Res. Tech. 61, 259–267. doi: 10.1002/jemt.10335

253. Whitworth, E., and Vinson, G. P. (2000). Zonal differentiation in the rat adrenal cortex. Endocr. Res. 26, 973–998. doi: 10.3109/07435800009048625

254. Wiesel, J. (1902). Beiträge zur Anatomie und Entwickelung der menschlichen Nebenniere. Anatomische Hefte 19, 483–522. doi: 10.1007/BF02298163

255. Willenberg, H. S., Schinner, S., and Ansurudeen, I. (2008). New mechanisms to control aldosterone synthesis. Horm. Metab. Res. 40, 435–441. doi: 10.1055/s- 2008-1065336

256. Williams, G. H. (2005). Aldosterone biosynthesis, regulation, and classical mechanism of action. Heart Fail. Rev. 10, 7–13. doi: 10.1007/s10741-005-2343-3 Wolkersdorfer, G. W., and Bornstein, S. R. (1998). Tissue remodelling in the adrenal gland. Biochem. Pharmacol. 56, 163–171. doi: 10.1016/S0006-2952(98)00067-7

257. Wood, M. A., and Hammer, G. D. (2010). Adrenocortical stem and progenitor cells: unifying model of two proposed origins. Mol. Cell. Endocrinol. 336, 206–212. doi: 10.1016/j.mce.2010.11.012

258. Woods, A. M., and Judd, A. M. (2008). Interleukin-4 increases cortisol release and decreases adrenal androgen release from bovine adrenal cells. Domes.t Anim. Endocrinol. 34, 372–382. doi: 10.1016/j.domaniend.2007.10.004

259. Wright, N. A. (1971). Cell proliferation in the prepubertal male rat adrenal cortex: an autoradiographic study. J. Endocrinol. 49, 599–609. doi: 10.1677/joe.0.0490599

260. Wright, N. A., Voncina, D., and Morley, A. R. (1973). An attempt to demonstrate cell migration from the zona glomerulosa in the prepubertal male rat adrenal cortex. J. Endocrinol. 59, 451–459. doi: 10.1677/joe.0.0590451

261. Xing, Y., Lerario, A. M., Rainey, W., and Hammer, G. D. (2015). Development of adrenal cortex zonation. Endocrinol. Metab. Clin. North. Am. 44, 243–274. doi: 10.1016/j.ecl.2015.02.001

262. Xu, J., Zeng, C., Chu, W., Pan, F., Rothfuss, J. M., Zhang, F., et al. (2011). Identification of the PGRMC1 protein complex as the putative sigma-2 receptor binding site. Nat. Commun. 2, 380. doi: 10.1038/ncomms1386

263. Yagci, A., Oertle, M., Seiler, H., Schmid, D., Campofranco, C., and Muller, J. (1996). Potassium induces multiple steroidogenic enzymes in cultured rat zona glomerulosa cells. Endocrinology 137, 2406–2214. doi: 10.1210/en.137. 6.2406

264. Yamaguchi, T., Naito, Z., Stoner, G. D., Franco Saenz, R., and Mulrow, P. J. (1990). Role of the adrenal renin-angiotensin system on adrenocorticotropic hormone- and potassium-stimulated aldosterone production by rat adrenal glomerulosa cells in monolayer culture. Hypertension 16, 635–641. doi: 10.1161/01.HYP.16.6.635

265. Yang, Y. K., Thompson, D. A., Dickinson, C. J., Wilken, J., Barsh, G. S., Kent, S. B., et al. (1999). Characterization of Agouti-related protein binding to melanocortin receptors. Mol. Endocrinol. 13, 148–155. doi: 10.1210/mend.13.1.0223

266. Yaswen, L., Diehl, N., Brennan, M. B., and Hochgeschwender, U. (1999). Obesity in the mouse model of pro-opiomelanocortin deficiency responds to peripheral melanocortin. Nat. Med. 5, 1066–1070. doi: 10.1038/12506

267. Ye, P., Nakamura, Y., Lalli, E., and Rainey, W. E. (2009). Differential effects of high and low steroidogenic factor-1 expression on CYP11B2 expression and aldosterone production in adrenocortical cells. Endocrinology 150, 1303–1309. doi: 10.1210/en.2008-0667

268. Yu, L., Han, M., Yan, M., Lee, J., and Muneoka, K. (2012). BMP2 induces segment-specific skeletal regeneration from digit and limb amputations by establishing a new endochondral ossification center. Dev. Biol. 372, 263–273. doi: 10.1016/j.ydbio.2012.09.021

269. Yu, R. N., Ito, M., and Jameson, J. L. (1998). The murine Dax-1 promoter is stimulated by SF-1 (steroidogenic factor-1) and inhibited by COUP-TF (chicken ovalbumin upstream promoter-transcription factor) via a composite nuclear receptor-regulatory element. Mol. Endocrinol. 12, 1010–1022. doi: 10.1210/mend.12.7.0131

270. Yuan, B. B., Tchao, R., Funae, Y., Voigt, J. M., and Colby, H. D. (1998). Effects of ACTH administration on zonation of the guinea pig adrenal cortex. Mol. Cell. Endocrinol. 146, 129–136. doi: 10.1016/S0303-7207(98)00189-0

271. Yuan, B. B., Tchao, R., Voigt, J. M., and Colby, H. D. (2001). Maturational changes in CYP2D16 expression and xenobiotic metabolism in adrenal glands from male and female guinea pigs. Drug metab. Dispos. 29, 194–119.

272. Zajicek, G., Ariel, I., and Arber, N. (1986). The streaming adrenal cortex: direct evidence of centripetal migration of adrenocytes by estimation of cell turnover rate. J. Endocrinol. 111, 477–482. doi: 10.1677/joe.0.1110477

273. Zeng, C., Garg, N., and Mach, R. H. (2016). The PGRMC1 protein level correlates with the binding activity of a sigma-2 fluorescent probe (SW120) in rat brain cells. Mol. Imaging Biol. 18, 172–179. doi: 10.1007/s11307-015-0891-z

274. Zhang, L., Radtke, K., Zheng, L., Cai, A. Q., Schilling, T. F., and Nie, Q. (2012). Noise drives sharpening of gene expression boundaries in the zebrafish hindbrain. Mol. Syst. Biol. 8:613. doi: 10.1038/msb.2012.45

275. Zhou, J., Shaikh, L. H., Neogi, S. G., McFarlane, I., Zhao, W., Figg, N., et al. (2015). DACH1, a zona glomerulosa selective gene in the human adrenal, activates transforming growth factor-beta signaling and suppresses aldosterone secretion. Hypertension 65, 1103–1110. doi: 10.1161/HYP.0000000000000025

276. Zwemer, R., Wotton, R., and Norkus, M. (1938). A study of corticoadrenal cells. Anat. Rec. 72, 249–263. doi: 10.1002/ar.1090720210

3

Comparative Effect of ACTH and Related Peptides on Proliferation and Growth of Rat Adrenal Gland

Claudimara Ferini Pacicco Lotfi and Pedro O. R. de Mendonca*

Department of Anatomy, Institute of Biomedical Science, University of São Paulo, São Paulo, Brazil

***Correspondence:**
Claudimara Ferini Pacicco Lotfi
clotfi@usp.br

Pro-opiomelanocortin (POMC) is a polypeptide precursor known to yield biologically active peptides related to a range of functions. These active peptides include the adrenocorticotropic hormone (ACTH), which is essential for maintenance of adrenal growth and steroidogenesis, and the alpha-melanocyte stimulation hormone, which plays a key role in energy homeostasis. However, the role of the highly conserved N-terminal region of POMC peptide fragments has begun to be unraveled only recently. Here, we review the cascade of events involved in regulation of proliferation and growth of murine adrenal cortex triggered by ACTH and other POMC-derived peptides. Key findings regarding signaling pathways and modulation of genes and proteins required for the regulation of adrenal growth are summarized. We have outlined the known mechanisms as well as future challenges for research on the regulation of adrenal proliferation and growth triggered by these peptides.

Keywords: adrenal growth, ACTH, N-POMC, proliferation, cell cycle

INTRODUCTION

The primary function of the adrenal cortex is to produce steroids. Each zone of the adrenal cortex synthesizes different steroids in response to endocrine and paracrine stimuli. Adrenal function and maintenance of adrenal size are associated with regulation of adrenocortical growth, a topic that has been covered by other studies (1, 2). This review summarizes our understanding of growth regulators of the murine adrenal and highlights the action of adrenocorticotropic hormone (ACTH) and N-terminal peptides of pro-opiomelanocortin (N-POMC) in the control of proliferation and maintenance of the adrenal cortex.

PRO-OPIOMELANOCORTIN IN MURINE

Pomc is a gene that belongs to the opioid/orphanin family. It is a highly conserved gene found from agnathan fish to mammals (3). In murines, this gene encodes a prohormone of 235 amino acids produced mainly by corticotropic cells in the pituitary gland. Post-translational processing at specific sites results in production of various smaller peptides, including peptide hormones with a range of physiological functions (**Figure 1**). In addition to the pituitary gland, POMC peptides are found in a diverse range of tissues, including the hypothalamus, skin, lung, gut, and pancreas (4). POMC transcripts found in these tissues are not full length, resulting in low levels of protein (5), and its function is not clear. POMC peptides in the circulation are derived mainly from the pituitary, and thus, the peptides produced in peripheral tissues act in an autocrine or paracrine way. The enzymes

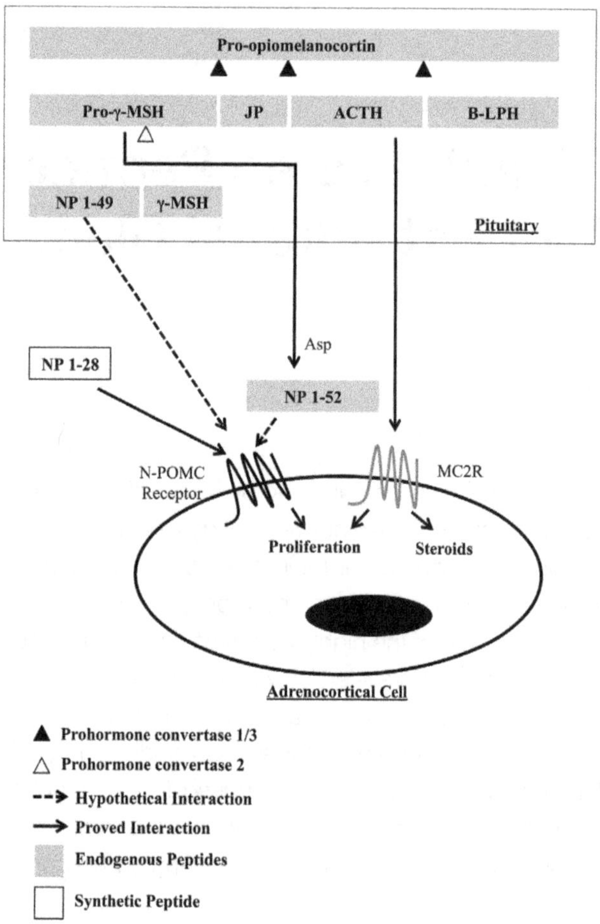

FIGURE 1 | Processing of POMC in the murine pituitary, highlighting the resulting peptides that act in the proliferation of adrenocortical cells. γ-MSH, gamma-melanocyte-stimulating hormone; JP, joining peptide; ACTH, adrenocorticotropic hormone; B-LPH, beta-lipotropin; NP, N-terminal peptides of pro-opiomelanocortin; Asp, adrenal serine protease.

responsible for cleavage of POMC are called prohormone convertases (PC) and are of two types, PC1 and PC2. In the anterior lobe of the pituitary, the action of PC1 generates the main four POMC-derived peptides: the N-terminal peptide 1–74 (N-POMC 1–74 or pro-gamma-MSH), the joining peptide (JP), ACTH, and beta-lipotrophin (β-LPH). In the intermediate lobe, ACTH is cleaved by PC2 to produce alpha-melanocyte-stimulating hormone (α-MSH) and the corticotrophin-like intermediate peptide (CLIP); β-LPH is completely processed to γ-LPH and β-endorphin; and pro-gamma-MSH is cleaved to generate γ1- or γ3-MSH and N-POMC 1–49. γ1-MSH is found in humans but not in murines, as the cleavage site (a dibasic residue pair required for processing γ3-MSH into γ1-MSH) is missing in rodents (6). γ-MSH appears to potentiate the steroidogenic effect of ACTH in the adrenal gland, but the exact form of the peptide (γ1, γ2, or γ3) that produces this effect is still unclear (7). Currently, the concept of tissue-specific cleavage of POMC is acceptable, at least in the adrenal gland, where a serine-protease has been cloned and is responsible for cleaving the pro-gamma-MSH into a 52-residue peptide (8). The family of G-protein-coupled receptors named melanocortin receptors (composed of five members) is responsible for intermediating the action of POMC peptides.

PROLIFERATIVE ADRENAL CORTEX RESPONSES TO ACTH

The 39-amino acid peptide ACTH is the primary regulator of adrenal gland growth, maintenance, and function. Due to the actions of corticotropin-releasing hormone (CRH), arginine vasopressin, and other secretagogues, ACTH stimulates the pituitary corticotroph cells to release ACTH (9). ACTH binds to specific high-affinity receptors [melanocortin receptor 2 (MC2R)] located on the surface of adrenal cortical cells, stimulating the production of cortisol and corticosterone in murines, which in turn suppresses ACTH-releasing factors. ACTH increases rat adrenal weight by inducing both hyperplasia and hypertrophy in specific zones. In fact, administration of chronic exogenous ACTH in rats induces hyperplasia and hypertrophy in the outer and inner zona fasciculata, respectively (10), and results in a 70% increase of adrenal mass in rats (11). This phenomenon is also seen in knockout mice for both glucocorticoid and dopamine receptors showing elevated levels of circulating ACTH (12, 13). On the other hand, low levels of ACTH, such as those seen in animals submitted to hypophysectomy (14) or treated with dexamethasone (15), result in adrenal atrophy. When adrenal growth occurs to compensate for unilateral adrenalectomy in hypophysectomized rats, neither a decrease in circulating corticosterone nor elevated ACTH levels are observed (16), suggesting the action of neural mediation or other POMC-derived peptides.

MOLECULAR MECHANISMS IMPLICATED IN ACTH ADRENOCORTICAL GROWTH

Abundant data relating to the signaling triggered by ACTH have been provided by experiments performed in cultured normal and tumoral adrenocortical cells. However, the *in vitro* action of ACTH on signaling pathways involved with adrenocortical growth is controversial and seems to depend on the cell type, the state of the responding cell, and other environmental signals from extracellular matrices (17, 18).

ACTH *In Vitro*

In support of the mitogenic or antimitogenic action of ACTH, there are studies analyzing the regulation of ERK/MAPK and related pathways, in different cell types. In quiescent Y1 mouse adrenocortical tumor cells, the molecular mechanisms of cell cycle control comprise two contrasting control pathways for 1-nM ACTH treatment: (1) a mitogenic effect *via* induction of the *fos* and *jun* gene families and weak activation of ERK/MAPK; and (2) a cAMP/PKA-mediated antimitogenic mechanism comprising Akt pathway deactivation, cMyc degradation, and $p27^{Kip1}$ induction (17, 19, 20). However, the ability of activate the ERK/MAPK was not interrupted in the cAMP-resistant mutant Y1 cells (Kin-8 cells) stimulated by ACTH, indicating the PKA not mediate the mitogenic action of ACTH (21). Arola and collaborators (22) also found an ACTH-inducible biphasic growth effect in rat adrenocortical cells in primary culture, in which a 7–70 nM ACTH-mitogenic effect transduced through the cAMP-mediated system and an ACTH-antimitogenic took place *via* a cAMP-independent pathway.

In another study performed with Y1 cells, the authors observed the inhibition of ERK/MAPK and c-Jun N-terminal kinases pathways through a PKC and Ca^{2+}-dependent pathway (23), which favors an antimitogenic action of ACTH. In agreement, it was demonstrated by Bey and collaborators (24) that in Y1 cells, MAPK phosphatase-1 is a component of the ACTH signaling cascade, suggesting that ACTH can downregulate MAPKs. The antimitogenic and pro-apoptotic action of ACTH was reinforced in normal adrenal cells. In rat adrenocortical cells in primary culture, treatment for 3 days with 1-nM ACTH-induced apoptosis, activation of PKA/CREB but not ERK, and expression of c-Fos protein (25, 26). Also in support to antimitogenic action of ACTH, in bovine adrenocortical cells, angiotensin II activate MAPK after 5 min of treatment (EC50 = 0.1 nM), whereas ACTH does not stimulate ERK (27). Moreover, in rat adrenal zona glomerulosa cells, ERK activation blocked cell proliferation (28, 29).

In another widely used cellular model, the H295 human adrenocortical tumor cell line, which shares similarities with cells of the zona glomerulosa, ACTH stimulates ERK/MAPK signaling. However, in H295 cells, it has been described that MAPK stimulation by 100-nM ACTH depends on receptor internalization (30). On the other hand, in MC2R-transfected human embryonic kidney cells (31), 1-nM ACTH induces ERK phosphorylation that is partially PKA dependent. However, arrestin-coupled internalization does not involve any level of ACTH-dependent ERK phosphorylation (32). In summary, the analysis of signaling pathways involving the action of ACTH on different cell types and *in vitro* conditions gives support for an antimitogenic action of ACTH.

ACTH *In Vivo*

In research involving depletion of the hypothalamic–pituitary–adrenal (HPA) axis using *in vivo* models with various approaches such as enucleation-induced adrenal regeneration (33), dexamethasone (Dex) treatment, and hypophysectomy, most but not all of the evidence converges on existing signals and pathways related to a mitogenic effect of ACTH.

Early response genes in the Fos and Jun gene families that form the transcriptional factor AP-1 and stimulate cellular proliferation (34) are induced by both ACTH and FGF2 infused in the rat adrenal gland *in situ* or in the adrenal cortex of hypophysectomized rats (35, 36). In enucleation-induced rat adrenal gland regeneration, the Fos gene was unregulated in the first 2 days of regeneration, while after 5 days of enucleation, downregulation of the Fos and Jun genes was observed (37).

Although it has been proposed that ACTH induces SAPK/JNK signaling activation and ERK/MAPK inhibition *in vivo* (23), results of chronic ACTH treatment in Dex-treated rats showed that ACTH is able to induce a sustained and progressive increase in ERK activation and proliferating cell nuclear antigen (PCNA) expression in all adrenal zones (38).

Other findings link the proliferative action of ACTH in Dex-treated rats with regulation of the cyclin-dependent kinase inhibitors (CDKIs) p27Kip1 and p57Kip2 in a time- and site-specific manner. A study shows that after Dex treatment, most of the cells expressed p27Kip1 but not p57Kip2. Subsequent ACTH treatment suppressed p27Kip1 expression and induced p57Kip2, while PCNA-expressing cells appeared mainly around the zona glomerulosa (39). Other cell-cycle regulators are also implicated in ACTH adrenocortical growth of Dex-treated rats. Besides increasing p27Kip1 expression, inhibition of the HPA axis downregulates cyclin D2 and D3 expression in the adrenal cortex. ACTH increases cyclin E and D3 expression, while it reduces expression of p27Kip1 protein in the outer and inner fraction preparations of adrenal cortex, respectively (40, 41). Moreover, the cell-cycle regulation is time dependent and zone specific. More recently, the Nek2 gene and its protein, together with the Notch gene, have also been shown to be involved in the cell cycle regulation triggered by ACTH (42).

The extracellular matrix (ECM) contributes to the regulation of cell proliferation and cell differentiation and therefore has a role in embryonic development and adult tissue homeostasis. Feige and colleagues have described the composition and expression of ECM components in the adult adrenal gland (43, 44). From the periphery to the center of the gland, the authors observed differential expression of fibronectin and laminin, which can be associated with specific activities of the cell components of the zones. However, studies conducted by the Gallo-Payet group show that ECM modulates basal and ACTH-induced cell functions, with fibronectin and collagen I and IV favoring steroid secretion, while laminin promotes proliferation (18). These findings illustrate the importance of the morphological changes associated with ACTH.

Despite the *in vivo* evidence that ACTH is the only factor that stimulates adrenal growth, other studies point in a different direction. As briefly described above, there are considerable data showing that ACTH inhibited growth of adrenal cells *in vitro*. In addition, Rao and colleagues (45) showed that rats treated with antiserum against ACTH had significant reduction of blood corticosteroids levels but did not exhibit adrenal atrophy. These and other results, which have been described in comprehensive reviews of the last 60 years of POMC research (46, 47), suggest that another factor distinct from ACTH has the ability to promote adrenal growth.

PROLIFERATIVE ADRENAL CORTEX RESPONSES TO N-POMC PEPTIDES

In 1980, Estivariz and colleagues (48) extracted and purified pro-gamma-MSH from human pituitaries and showed that this peptide could not prevent adrenal atrophy in hypophysectomized rats. However, smaller N-POMC peptides (without the γ3-MSH portion) produced by trypsin digestion of pro-gamma-MSH or extracted from pituitary glands proved to be potent mitogens both *in vivo* and *in vitro*. In this section, we present information on the proliferative effect of the most important N-POMC peptides.

N-POMC 1–28

N-POMC 1–28 was first isolated from human pituitary glands and later characterized as an extraction artifact (49). Even though N-POMC 1–28 is not an endogenous peptide, it has been extensively used to show the mitogenic effect of the N-POMCs. Moreover, the first 28 amino acids of the N-terminal portion of POMC have been shown to be essential to the triggering of adrenal cell proliferation. The mitogenic activity of N-POMC 1–28 has been demonstrated *in vivo* in murine models (40, 50, 51) and *in vitro* in Y1, NCI-H295R, and rat primary culture cells (26, 52, 53). Peripheral delivery of this peptide in *Pomc* KO mice does not promote any alterations in the adrenal gland (54) but may prevent atrophy of regenerating adrenal glands after hypophysectomy (55). These findings mean that besides promoting mitosis, this peptide may prevent apoptosis of adrenal cells. Indeed, our group has shown the anti-apoptotic effect of N-POMC 1–28 in adrenal glands of hypophysectomized rats (51). However, the molecular mechanisms underlying this effect are not clear. The positions of two disulfide bridges (between cysteine residues 2–24 and 8–20) seem to be essential to its biological activity (56).

N-POMC 1–49

N-POMC 1–49 is an endogenous peptide produced and secreted by the intermediary lobe of the pituitary. It is one of the products from the cleavage of pro-gamma-MSH into smaller peptides. *In vitro* studies have shown that this peptide may promote proliferation of Y1 and NCI-H295R cells (52, 53). However, *in vivo* studies have shown that N-POMC 1–49 does not increase adrenal weight in fetal sheep when infused for 48 h (57). Interestingly, the presence of an O-linked glycan seems to be crucial for its proliferative effect. However, cleavage of pro-gamma-MSH in the pituitary occurs only if the O-linked glycan is not present in the molecule, resulting in an N-POMC 1–49 without the glycan [reviewed in Bicknell and Lowry (58)]. Clearly, the present data are controversial, and more assays must be done before it can be concluded that N-POMC 1–49 is the natural N-POMC peptide involved in adrenal proliferation and maintenance.

Pro-Gamma-MSH

Pro-gamma-MSH is considered to be an active fragment found in the bloodstream at the same levels as ACTH (59). When infused into sheep fetus, this N-POMC peptide increased adrenal weight (57). However, as mentioned before, when administered in hypophysectomized rats, no effect on the adrenal weight was observed (60). Since the mitogenic peptides are located in the N-terminal portion of pro-gamma-MSH, a hypothesis of post-secretional cleavage occurring at the level of specific tissues has emerged. Indeed, Bicknell and collaborators (8) characterized a serine protease they named AsP (adrenal serine protease) that is present in the ECM of adrenal cells and is responsible for cleaving pro-gamma-MSH. The cleavage releases a peptide of 52 residues that induces proliferation of adrenal cortical cells. Moreover, Asp is capable of cleaving small basic substrates (e.g., arginine–arginine, lysine–arginine, etc.), generating N-POMC 1–49. These findings suggest the existence of an endogenous mitogenic N-POMC peptide, but no consensus about its identity has been reached.

THE MOLECULAR MECHANISM INVOLVED IN THE N-POMC PROLIFERATIVE EFFECT

The proliferative effect of N-POMC peptides has been established since the beginning of the 1980s, but its mechanism has begun to be unveiled only recently. The first study on this topic, conducted by Fassnacht and colleagues (52), concluded that N-POMC 1–28 promotes cell proliferation in NCI-H295R, Y1, and primary cultures of bovine adrenocortical cells by triggering a rapid activation of the ERK/MAPK but not the APK/JNK or p38 pathways. Pepper and Bicknell (53) corroborated those findings and showed that the upstream ERK regulators c-RAF and MEK were activated in Y1 and NCI-H295R cells treated with N-POMC 1–28 or N-POMC 1–49. In 2011, Mattos and collaborators (26) showed that ERK1/2 was activated in primary cultures of rat adrenocortical cells treated with N-POMC 1–28.

In 2014, we performed a PCR array to evaluate the effect of N-POMC 1–28 on the expression of key genes related to the control of the cell cycle. The genes *Nek2* and *Notch* were upregulated after treatment, suggesting that the proliferative effect of this peptide might be mediated by these genes (42). Additional research is needed to further elucidate the molecular mechanisms involved in the proliferative effect of N-POMC.

A fundamental question that has yet to be definitively answered is the identification of the receptor through which N-POMC peptides elicit their effects on adrenal growth. There have been two unsuccessful attempts to identify such a receptor (53, 58). In 2014, we joined efforts with Bicknell's group and proposed a new approach to identifying this receptor. We cloned the most expressed orphan G-protein-coupled receptors in the rat adrenal gland and performed a magnetic cell separation assay using the N-POMC peptide attached to magnetic beads. A likely candidate for the N-POMC receptor was identified, confirmed by ligand-binding assays, and shown to be capable of activating the ERK pathway after stimulation with N-POMC. Further experiments are now been conducted to characterize *in vivo* and *in vitro* this potential adrenal N-POMC receptor. Final confirmation of the identity of the adrenal N-POMC receptor is essential for the understanding of cell proliferation in adrenocortical cells.

CONCLUSION

In this paper, we summarize the current state of knowledge of the roles of ACTH and N-POMC in the proliferation of murine adrenal cells. We identify gaps in knowledge and describe conflicting results that need to be further investigated in order to fully understand the biology of this phenomenon. Examples of such urgently needed studies include gene array assays and pathway analysis to provide more data on the molecular mechanisms triggered by N-POMC peptides as well as to confirm the identity of the natural endogenous mitogenic N-POMC peptide. A holistic and interdisciplinary approach will be required, as none of these peptides or hormones act alone in nature. On the contrary, they trigger a net of responses and activate dozens of pathways simultaneously. When we begin to examine this phenomenon from a holistic perspective, we may come to truly understand the proliferative effect of these peptides.

AUTHOR CONTRIBUTIONS

The authors CL and PM contributed to the conception and design work.

ACKNOWLEDGMENTS

We would like to thank past and present students from the laboratory who have contributed to the work summarized in this mini-review, in particular Rozana B. F. Baccaro, Gabriele Ebling Mattos, Thompson E. Pavan Torres, and Ismael Cabral Costa.

FUNDING

CL received funding from Fundação de Amparo à Pesquisa do Estado de São Paulo (Fapesp, the State of São Paulo Research Foundation), from Conselho Nacional de Desenvolvimento Científico e Tecnológico (CNPq, National Council for Scientific and Technological Development), and from Pró-Reitoria de Pesquisa da Universidade de São Paulo (Dean's Office of the University of São Paulo for Research Projects); PM is recipient of a scholarship from FAPESP.

REFERENCES

1. Whitworth EJ, Kosti O, Renshaw D, Hinson JP. Adrenal neuropeptides: regulation and interaction with ACTH and other adrenal regulators. *Microsc Res Tech* (2003) **61**(3):259–67. doi:10.1002/jemt.10335
2. Hoeflich A, Bielohuby M. Mechanisms of adrenal gland growth: signal integration by extracellular signal regulated kinases1/2. *J Mol Endocrinol* (2009) **42**(3):191–203. doi:10.1677/JME-08-0160
3. Kawauchi H, Takahashi A, Abe K. Gamma-melanotropin is not present in an N-terminal peptide of salmon proopiocortin. *Int J Pept Protein Res* (1981) **18**(3):223–7. doi:10.1111/j.1399-3011.1981.tb02975.x
4. Smith AI, Funder JW. Proopiomelanocortin processing in the pituitary, central nervous system, and peripheral tissues. *Endocr Rev* (1988) **9**(1):159–79. doi:10.1210/edrv-9-1-159
5. Lacaze-Masmonteil T, de Keyzer Y, Luton JP, Kahn A, Bertagna X. Characterization of proopiomelanocortin transcripts in human nonpituitary tissues. *Proc Natl Acad Sci U S A* (1987) **84**(20):7261–5. doi:10.1073/pnas.84.20.7261
6. Jackson S, Salacinski P, Hope J, Lowry PJ. An investigation of N-terminal pro-opiocortin peptides in the rat pituitary. *Peptides* (1983) **4**(4):431–8. doi:10.1016/0196-9781(83)90045-1
7. Harmer SC, Bicknell AB. Role of gamma-MSH peptides in the regulation of adrenal steroidogenesis. *Peptides* (2005) **26**(10):1944–51. doi:10.1016/j.peptides.2004.11.028
8. Bicknell AB, Lomthaisong K, Woods RJ, Hutchinson EG, Bennett HP, Gladwell RT, et al. Characterization of a serine protease that cleaves pro-gamma-melanotropin at the adrenal to stimulate growth. *Cell* (2001) **105**(7):903–12. doi:10.1016/S0092-8674(01)00403-2
9. Watanabe T, Oki Y, Ort DN. Kinetic actions and interactions of arginine vasopressin, angiotensin-II, and oxytocin on adrenocorticotropin secretion by rat anterior pituitary cells in the microperifusion system. *Endocrinology* (1989) **125**(4):1921–31. doi:10.1210/endo-125-4-1921
10. Ulrich-Lai YM, Figueiredo HF, Ostrander MM, Choi DC, Engeland WC, Herman JP. Chronic stress induces adrenal hyperplasia and hypertrophy in a subregion-specific manner. *Am J Physiol Endocrinol Metab* (2006) **291**(5):E965–73. doi:10.1152/ajpendo.00070.2006
11. Nussdorfer GG, Rebuffat P, Mazzocchi G, Belloni AS, Meneghelli V. Investigations on adrenocortical mitochondria turnover. I. Effect of chronic treatment with ACTH on the size and number of rat zona fasciculada mitochondria. *Cell Tissue Res* (1974) **150**(1):79–94.
12. Cole TJ, Blendy JA, Monaghan AP, Krieglstein K, Schmid W, Aguzzi A, et al. Targeted disruption of the glucocorticoid receptor gene blocks adrenergic chromaffin cell development and severely retards lung maturation. *Genes Dev* (1995) **9**(13):1608–21. doi:10.1101/gad.9.13.1608
13. Saiardi A, Borrelli E. Absence of dopaminergic control on melanotrophs leads to Cushing's-like syndrome in mice. *Mol Endocrinol* (1998) **12**(8):1133–9. doi:10.1210/me.12.8.1133
14. Jones IC, Roby CC. Some aspects of zonation and function of the adrenal cortex. I. The effects of hypophysectomy on the adrenal cortex of the adult male mouse. *J Endocrinol* (1954) **10**(3):245–50. doi:10.1677/joe.0.0100266
15. Wright NA, Appleton D. The action of dexamethasone on the adrenal cortex. *J Endocrinol* (1972) **53**(3):xxxvii.
16. Engeland WC, Shinsako J, Dallman MF. Corticosteroids and ACTH are not required for compensatory adrenal growth. *Am J Physiol* (1975) **229**(5):1461–4.
17. Rocha KM, Forti FL, Lepique AP, Armelin HA. Deconstructing the molecular mechanism of cell cycle control in a mouse adrenocortical cell line: roles of ACTH. *Microsc Res Tech* (2003) **61**(3):268–74. doi:10.1002/jemt.10336
18. Otis M, Campbell S, Payet MD, Gallo-Payet N. Expression of extracellular matrix proteins and integrins in rat adrenal gland: importance for ACTH-associated functions. *J Endocrinol* (2007) **193**(3):331–47. doi:10.1677/JOE-07-0055
19. Lotfi CF, Todorovic Z, Armelin HA, Schimmer BP. Unmasking a growth-promoting effect of the adrenocorticotropic hormone in Y1 mouse adrenocortical tumor cells. *J Biol Chem* (1997) **272**(47):29886–91. doi:10.1074/jbc.272.47.29886
20. Lotfi CF, Armelin HA. c-Fos protein is a mediator in mitogenic response to ACTH. *Endocr Res* (1998) **24**(3–4):421–4. doi:10.3109/07435809809032626
21. Le T, Schimmer BP. The regulation of MAPKs in Y1 mouse adrenocortical tumor cells. *Endocrinology* (2001) **142**(10):4282–7. doi:10.1210/endo.142.10.8441
22. Arola J, Heikkilä P, Kahri AI. Biphasic effect of ACTH on growth of rat adrenocortical cells in primary culture. *Cell Tissue Res* (1993) **271**(1):169–76. doi:10.1007/BF00297555
23. Watanabe G, Pena P, Albanese C, Wilsbacher LD, Young JB, Pestell RG. Adrenocorticotropin induction of stress-activated protein kinase in the adrenal cortex in vivo. *J Biol Chem* (1997) **272**(32):20063–9. doi:10.1074/jbc.272.32.20063
24. Bey P, Gorostizaga AB, Maloberti PM, Lozano RC, Poderoso C, Cornejo Maciel F, et al. Adrenocorticotropin induces mitogen-activated protein kinase phosphatase 1 in Y1 mouse adrenocortical tumor cells. *Endocrinology* (2003) **144**(4):1399–406. doi:10.1210/en.2002-220987
25. Mattos GE, Lotfi CF. Differences between the growth regulatory pathways in primary rat adrenal cells and mouse tumor cell line. *Mol Cell Endocrinol* (2005) **245**(1–2):31–42. doi:10.1016/j.mce.2005.10.001
26. Mattos GE, Jacysyn JF, Amarante-Mendes GP, Lotfi CF. Comparative effect of FGF2, synthetic peptides 1-28 N-POMC and ACTH on proliferation in rat adrenal cell primary cultures. *Cell Tissue Res* (2011) **345**(3):343–56. doi:10.1007/s00441-011-1220-8
27. Chabre O, Cornillon F, Bottari SP, Chambaz EM, Vilgrain I. Hormonal regulation of mitogen-activated protein kinase activity in bovine adrenocortical cells: cross-talk between phosphoinositides, adenosine 3',5'-monophosphate, and tyrosine kinase receptor pathways. *Endocrinology* (1995) **136**(3):956–64. doi:10.1210/en.136.3.956
28. Otis M, Campbell S, Payet MD, Gallo-Payet N. Angiotensin II stimulates protein synthesis and inhibits proliferation in primary cultures of rat adrenal glomerulosa cells. *Endocrinology* (2005) **146**(2):633–42. doi:10.1210/en.2004-0935
29. Otis M, Gallo-Payet N. Role of MAPKs in angiotensin II-induced steroidogenesis in rat glomerulosa cells. *Mol Cell Endocrinol* (2007) **265-266**:126–30. doi:10.1016/j.mce.2006.12.008

30. Janes ME, Chu KM, Clark AJ, King PJ. Mechanisms of adrenocorticotropin-induced activation of extracellularly regulated kinase 1/2 mitogen-activated protein kinase in the human H295R adrenal cell line. *Endocrinology* (2008) **149**(4):1898–905. doi:10.1210/en.2007-0949
31. Sebag JA, Hinkle PM. Regulation of G protein-coupled receptor signaling: specific dominant-negative effects of melanocortin 2 receptor accessory protein 2. *Sci Signal* (2010) **3**(116):ra28. doi:10.1126/scisignal.2000593
32. Roy S, Roy SJ, Pinard S, Taillefer LD, Rached M, Parent JL, et al. Mechanisms of melanocortin-2 receptor (MC2R) internalization and recycling in human embryonic kidney (hek) cells: identification of Key Ser/Thr (S/T) amino acids. *Mol Endocrinol* (2011) **25**(11):1961–77. doi:10.1210/me.2011-0018
33. Holzwarth MA, Shinsako J, Dallman MF. Adrenal regeneration. Time course, effect of hypothalamic hemi-islands and response to unilateral adrenalectomy. *Neuroendocrinology* (1980) **31**(3):168–76. doi:10.1159/000123069
34. Angel P, Karin M. The role of Jun, Fos and the AP-1 complex in cell-proliferation and transformation. *Biochim Biophys Acta* (1991) **1072**(2–3):129–57.
35. Baccaro RB, Mendonça PO, Torres TE, Lotfi CF. Immunohistochemical Jun/Fos protein localization and DNA synthesis in rat adrenal cortex after treatment with ACTH or FGF2. *Cell Tissue Res* (2007) **328**(1):7–18. doi:10.1007/s00441-006-0352-8
36. Torres TE, Lotfi CF. Distribution of cells expressing Jun and Fos proteins and synthesizing DNA in the adrenal cortex of hypophysectomized rats: regulation by ACTH and FGF2. *Cell Tissue Res* (2007) **329**(3):443–55. doi:10.1007/s00441-007-0436-0
37. Tyczewska M, Rucinski M, Ziolkowska A, Szyszka M, Trejter M, Hochol-Molenda A, et al. Enucleation-induced rat adrenal gland regeneration: expression profile of selected genes involved in control of adrenocortical cell proliferation. *Int J Endocrinol* (2014) **2014**:130359. doi:10.1155/2014/130359
38. Ferreira JG, Cruz C, Vinson GP, Pignatelli D. ACTH modulates ERK phosphorylation in the adrenal gland in a time-dependent manner. *Endocr Res* (2007) **30**(4):661–6. doi:10.1081/ERC-200043952
39. Kobayashi H, Kambe F, Imai T, Hibi Y, Kikumori T, Ohmori S, et al. Differential expression of cyclin-dependent kinase inhibitors, p27Kip1 and p57Kip2, by corticotropin in rat adrenal cortex. *J Endocrinol* (2006) **189**(3):671–9. doi:10.1677/joe.1.06419
40. Mendonça PO, Lotfi CF. The proliferative effect of synthetic N-POMC(1-28) peptides in rat adrenal cortex: a possible role for cyclin E. *Mol Cell Endocrinol* (2011) **336**(1–2):156–61. doi:10.1016/j.mce.2010.12.012
41. de Mendonca PO, Liria CW, Machini MT, Lotfi CF. N-POMC1-28 increases cyclin D expression and inhibits P27(kip1) in the adrenal cortex. *Mol Cell Endocrinol* (2013) **371**(1–2):166–73. doi:10.1016/j.mce.2012.11.017
42. de Mendonca PO, Costa IC, Lotfi CF. The involvement of Nek2 and Notch in the proliferation of rat adrenal cortex triggered by POMC-derived peptides. *PLoS One* (2014) **9**(10):e108657. doi:10.1371/journal.pone.0108657
43. Pellerin S, Keramidas M, Chambaz EM, Feige JJ. Expression of laminin and its possible role in adrenal cortex homeostasis. *Endocrinology* (1997) **138**(3):1321–7. doi:10.1210/en.138.3.1321
44. Feige JJ, Keramidas M, Chambaz EM. Hormonally regulated components of the adrenocortical cell environment and the control of adrenal cortex homeostasis. *Horm Metab Res* (1998) **30**(6–7):421–5. doi:10.1055/s-2007-978908 Review
45. Rao AJ, Long JA, Ramachandran J. Effects of antiserum to adrenocorticotropin on adrenal growth and function. *Endocrinology* (1978) **102**(2):371–8. doi:10.1210/endo-102-2-371
46. Lowry P. 60 years of POMC: purification and biological characterisation of melanotrophins and corticotrophins. *J Mol Endocrinol* (2015). doi:10.1530/JME-15-0260
47. Bicknell AB. N-terminal POMC peptides and adrenal growth. *J Mol Endocrinol* (2016). doi:10.1530/JME-15-0269
48. Estivariz FE, Hope J, McLean C, Lowry PJ. Purification and characterization of a gamma-melanotropin precursor from frozen human pituitary glands. *Biochem J* (1980) **191**(1):125–32. doi:10.1042/bj1910125
49. McLean C, Hope J, Salacinski P, Estivariz F, Lowry PJ. Purification and characterization of amino-terminal pro-opiocortin peptides from human pituitary glands. *Biosci Rep* (1981) **1**(11):843–9. doi:10.1007/BF01114817
50. Lowry PJ, Silas L, McLean C, Linton EA, Estivariz FE. Pro-gamma-melanocyte-stimulating hormone cleavage in adrenal gland undergoing compensatory growth. *Nature* (1983) **306**(5938):70–3. doi:10.1038/306070a0
51. Torres TE, de Mendonça PO, Lotfi CF. Synthetic modified N-POMC(1-28) controls in vivo proliferation and blocks apoptosis in rat adrenal cortex. *Cell Tissue Res* (2010) **341**(2):239–50. doi:10.1007/s00441-010-0998-0
52. Fassnacht M, Hahner S, Hansen IA, Kreutzberger T, Zink M, Adermann K, et al. N-terminal proopiomelanocortin acts as a mitogen in adrenocortical tumor cells and decreases adrenal steroidogenesis. *J Clin Endocrinol Metab* (2003) **88**(5):2171–9. doi:10.1210/jc.2002-021318
53. Pepper DJ, Bicknell AB. The stimulation of mitogenic signaling pathways by N-POMC peptides. *Mol Cell Endocrinol* (2009) **300**(1–2):77–82. doi:10.1016/j.mce.2008.09.021
54. Coll AP, Fassnacht M, Klammer S, Hahner S, Schulte DM, Piper S, et al. Peripheral administration of the N-terminal pro-opiomelanocortin fragment 1-28 to Pomc-/- mice reduces food intake and weight but does not affect adrenal growth or corticosterone production. *J Endocrinol* (2006) **190**(2):515–25. doi:10.1677/joe.1.06749
55. Estivariz FE, Carino M, Lowry PJ, Jackson S. Further evidence that N-terminal pro-opiomelanocortin peptides are involved in adrenal mitogenesis. *J Endocrinol* (1988) **116**(2):201–6. doi:10.1677/joe.0.1160201
56. Denef C, Roudbaraki M, Van Bael A. Growth and differentiation factors derived from the N-terminal domain of pro-opiomelanocortin. *Clin Exp Pharmacol Physiol* (2001) **28**(3):239–43. doi:10.1046/j.1440-1681.2001.03421.x
57. Ross JT, Bennett HP, James S, McMillen IC. Infusion of N-proopiomelanocortin-(1-77) increases adrenal weight and messenger ribonucleic acid levels of cytochrome P450 17alpha-hydroxylase in the sheep fetus during late gestation. *Endocrinology* (2000) **141**(6):2153–8. doi:10.1210/en.141.6.2153
58. Bicknell AB, Lowry PJ. Adrenal growth is controlled by expression of specific pro-opiomelanocortin serine protease in the outer adrenal cortex. *Endocr Res* (2002) **28**(4):589–95. doi:10.1081/ERC-120016971
59. Chan JS, Seidah NG, Chrétien M. Measurement of N-terminal (1-76) of human proopiomelanocortin in human plasma: correlation with adrenocorticotropin. *J Clin Endocrinol Metab* (1983) **56**(4):791–6. doi:10.1210/jcem-56-4-791
60. Estivariz FE, Iturriza F, McLean C, Hope J, Lowry PJ. Stimulation of adrenal mitogenesis by N-terminal proopiocortin peptides. *Nature* (1982) **297**(5865):419–22. doi:10.1038/297419a0

4

Transcriptome Profile of Rat Adrenal Evoked by Gonadectomy and Testosterone or Estradiol Replacement

Karol Jopek, Piotr Celichowski, Marta Szyszka, Marianna Tyczewska, Paulina Milecka, Ludwik K. Malendowicz and Marcin Rucinski*

Department of Histology and Embryology, Poznan University of Medical Science, Poznan, Poland

***Correspondence:**
Ludwik K. Malendowicz
lkm@ump.edu.pl

Sex differences in adrenal cortex structure and function are well known in different species. In the rat, they are manifested as larger adrenal cortex and higher corticosterone secretion by females compared with males. These sex differences depend, among others, on functioning of the hypothalamic-pituitary-adrenal axis (HPA). In this aspect, it is widely accepted that testosterone exerts an inhibitory and estradiol stimulatory effect on the said axis. The molecular bases of these sex-related differences are poorly understood. Therefore, we performed studies aimed to demonstrate the effect of testosterone and estradiol on the expression of differentially regulated genes in rat adrenal gland. The classical method applied in the study—gonadectomy and gonadal hormone replacement—allows obtaining results suggesting a physiological role of the tested hormone (testosterone or estradiol) in the regulation of the specific genes. Adult male and female rats were either gonadectomized or sham operated. Half of orchiectomized rats were replaced with testosterone while ovariectomized ones with estradiol. Transcriptome was identified by means of Affymetrix® Rat Gene 2.1 ST Array. Differentially expressed genes were analyzed by means of DAVID web-based bioinformatic tools and confirmed by means of Gene Set Enrichment Analysis. For selected genes, validation of the results was performed using QPCR. Performed experiments have provided unexpected results. Contrary to expectations, in orchiectomized rats, testosterone replacement stimulates expression of numerous genes, mainly those associated with lipids and cholesterol metabolism. However, in ovariectomized animals, estradiol replacement inhibits the expression of genes, mainly those involved in intracellular signaling pathways. The physiological relevance of these findings awaits further research.

Keywords: rat, adrenal gland, transcriptome, global gene profiling, functional annotation clustering, gonadectomy, testosterone, estradiol

INTRODUCTION

Sex-related differences in the structure and function of the adrenal cortex of mature rats are well recognized. These differences are the result of the action of sex hormones on the various components of the hypothalamic-pituitary-adrenal axis (HPA). The results of studies on the effects of gonadectomy and sex hormone replacement on the rat adrenal cortex suggest that estrogens stimulate and androgens inhibit the HPA axis function. The results of these studies are presented in many comprehensive monographs and textbooks (1–7). It is important to note that in gonadectomized animals sex hormones exert generalized response, not limited to HPA axis only. For example, they regulate the levels of corticosteroid-binding globulins (CBG) (8–11) as well as corticosterone biological half-time (12–14). CBG is involved in the mechanism of steroid hormone action by keeping steroids in circulation, and therefore controlling the availability of unbound hormones for their targets. In the rat, CBG levels are notably higher in females. Orchiectomy (ORX) resulted in 60–70% increase in CBG levels, while ovariectomy (OVX) had no effect (8, 15). Of interest, in the rat, estradiol effect on CBG is mediated via thyroid gland. Furthermore, biological half-life of corticosterone in adult male rats is ca. two times longer than in females (12, 16). Also, the metabolic clearance rate of corticosterone is markedly higher in female than male rats (17, 18).

The above-described sex differences in the structure and functions of the rat adrenal cortex probably depend on differences in the gene expression of this gland. However, to our knowledge, no studies are available on the effects of estradiol or testosterone on transcriptome profile of the rat adrenal gland. Regarding this, recently we have shown that in adult rat adrenal cortex, the differentially expressed genes that are significantly enriched included genes involved in steroid hormone metabolism, and their expression levels in females were significantly higher compared with those in the male rat (19). Generally, if compared with males, in the female rats higher expression levels of genes involved directly in steroid hormone synthesis were accompanied by lower expression levels of genes regulating basal cell functions. To our knowledge, only one publication on global gene profiling refers to the effect of testosterone on the expression of genes in the adrenal gland and it relates to the mouse (20). In this research, however, authors administered testosterone into intact female mice. Comparison between females and females treated with testosterone revealed 94 differentially regulated genes, with 23 being upregulated and 71 downregulated. The observed changes in gene expression authors combine with the disappearance of the X zone of the mouse adrenal cortex. It should be emphasize that this experimental model is not a physiological one.

In the present study, to demonstrate the effect of estradiol and testosterone on the expression of differentially regulated genes in rat adrenal gland, we applied experimental model considered in endocrinology as the "gold standard." Dual control, it means removal of the gonads and replacement with the appropriate hormone allows obtaining results suggesting a physiological role of the tested hormone (estradiol or testosterone) in the regulation of the specific genes. Performed experiments have provided unexpected results. Contrary to expectations, in orchiectomized rats, testosterone replacement stimulates expression of numerous genes, mainly associated with lipids and lipid metabolism. However, in ovariectomized animals, estradiol replacement inhibits the expression of genes, mainly those involved in intracellular signaling pathways.

In the present study, to demonstrate the effect of estradiol and testosterone on the expression of differentially regulated genes in rat adrenal gland, we applied the classical method used to study endocrine glands, it means "remove and replace" (gonadectomy and gonadal hormone replacement). Performed experiments have provided unexpected results. Contrary to expectations, in orchiectomized rats, testosterone replacement stimulates expression of numerous genes, mainly associated with lipids and lipid metabolism. However, in ovariectomized animals, estradiol replacement inhibits the expression of genes, mainly those involved in intracellular signaling pathways.

MATERIALS AND METHODS

Animals and Experiments

Adult female and male Wistar rats (12 weeks old; body weight: 120–150 g) were obtained from the Laboratory Animals Breeding Center, Department of Toxicology, Poznan University of Medical Sciences, Poznan, Poland. Animals were kept under standardized conditions of light (14:10 h light–dark cycle, illumination onset 06.00) at constant temperature (23°C) with free access to standard food pellets and water. All experiments were carried out between 10 and 11 am. All procedures described herein were approved by the Local Ethics Committee for Animal Research (Poznan, Poland), permission number: LKE—11/2015. All possible efforts have been done to minimize the number of animals and their suffering.

Rats were gonadectomized or sham operated under ketamine (100 mg/kg, i.p.) and xylazine (10 mg/kg, i.p.) anesthesia. ORX was performed via scrotal access while OVX by two dorsolateral incisions. Fourteen days after surgery, half of ORX rats was replaced with testosterone (s.c. injection of Testoviron-Depot, Schering AG, Berlin, 5 mg/100 g body weight), while half of OVX animals with estradiol (s.c. injection of Estradiol-Depot, Jenapharm, 0.5 mg/100 g body weight). Doses of administered depo hormones were based on previous reports (21–24). It is believed that from both compounds either testosterone or estradiol are liberated slowly, providing a physiological hormone levels in gonadectomized rats. As emphasized by Schulte-Beerbühl and Nieschlag (24), increasing the dose of injected testosterone esters appears not to influence the maximal concentrations of testosterone in the blood but rather the duration of the effect. Moreover, administration of depo compounds allows to avoid the stress evoked by daily administration of the tested substances. After 2 weeks (4 weeks post surgery), rats were decapitated. Adrenal glands were collected to RNAlader and stored in −70°C for further analyses. Seminal vesicles and uteri were also collected and weighed.

Corticosterone, Cholesterol, and Lipoproteins Detection

Serum corticosterone levels were determined by means of ELISA kit (ELISA Demeditec kit). Serum total cholesterol, lipoproteins, and triglycerides concentrations were evaluated by means of Roche Cobas Integra 400+ system.

RNA Extraction

Total RNA was extracted from samples of entire adrenals using TRI Reagent (Sigma, St. Louis, MO, USA) and RNeasy MinElute cleanup Kit (Qiagen, Hilden, Germany). The amount of total mRNA was determined from the optical density at 260 nm, and the RNA purity was estimated using the 260/280 nm absorption ratio (higher than 1.8) (NanoDrop spectrophotometer, Thermo Scientific, ALAB, Poland). The RNA integrity and quality were checked in a Bioanalyzer 2100 (Agilent Technologies, Inc., Santa Clara, CA, USA). The resulting RNA integrity numbers were between 8.5 and 10 with an average of 9.2 (Agilent Technologies, Inc., Santa Clara, CA, USA). Each sample was diluted to the RNA concentration of 100 ng/μl, at the OD260/OD280 ratio of 1.8/2.0. From each RNA sample, 100 ng of RNA was taken for microarray experiments. The remaining amount of isolated RNA was used for RT-qPCR study.

Microarray Expression Analysis and Statistics

The Affimetrix procedure and methods of analyzes were described previously (19, 25–27). Total RNA (100 ng) from each sample was subjected to two rounds of sense cDNA amplification (Ambion® WT Expression Kit) (Ambion, TX, USA). The obtained cDNA was used for biotin labeling and fragmentation using AffymetrixGeneChip® WT Terminal Labeling and Hybridization kit (Affymetrix, Santa Clara, CA, USA). Biotin-labeled fragments of cDNA (5.5 μg) were hybridized to Affymetrix® Rat Gene 2.1 ST Array Strip (48°C/20 h). Then, microarrays were washed and stained according to the technical protocol, using Affymetrix GeneAtlas Fuidics Station. The array strips were scanned employing Imaging Station of GeneAtlas System. The preliminary analysis of the scanned chips was performed using AffymetrixGeneAtlasTM Operating Software. The quality of gene expression data was checked according to quality control criteria provided by the software. Obtained CEL files were imported into downstream data analysis.

All analyzes were performed using BioConductor software, based on the statistical R programming language. For background correction, normalization, and summation of raw data, the Robust Multiarray Averaging algorithm implemented in "affy" package of BioConductor was applied (28). Biological annotation was taken from BioConductor "oligo" package where annotated data frame object was merged with normalized data set, leading to a complete gene data table (29).

The selection criteria of a significantly changed gene expression were based on expression fold difference higher than abs. 2 and adjusted p value <0.05. The result of such a selection was presented as volcano plots, where total number of up- and down-regulated genes has been shown.

Data files were also deposited in the Gene Expression Omnibus (GEO) repository at the National Center for Biotechnology Information (http://www.ncbi.nlm.nih.gov/geo/) under the GEO accession number GEO: GSE93726.

Assignment of the Genes Regulated by Sex Hormones to Relevant Gene Ontology Terms

Sets of female and male genes regulated by sex hormones were also subjected to functional annotation clusterization using DAVID web-based bioinformatics tools (Database for Annotation, Visualization, and Integrated Discovery) (30). Gene symbols for up- or downregulated genes from each of the compared groups were loaded to DAVID by "RDAVIDWebService" BioConductor package (31). Functional annotation charts generated by DAVID with overrepresented gene annotations in gene ontology biological process database (BO BP FAT) were shown as box plot. Interested gene sets from DAVID functional annotation charts were also subjected to hierarchical clusterization algorithm and presented as a heatmaps. Such analyses were carried out separately for male and female data sets. Arbitrary signal intensities from selected genes were represented by colors (green—higher; red—lower expression value). Log2 signal intensity values for any single gene were resized to Row Z-score scale (from −1.5, the lowest expression, to +1.5, the highest expression for single gene). Additionally, gene names and calculated fold values were also shown.

Gene Set Enrichment Analysis (GSEA)

Gene Set Enrichment Analysis is a computational method used for testing *a priori* defined gene sets (GO terms, pathways) for association with one of the two compared biological groups. The method uses Kolmogorov–Smirnov (K-S) statistical test for identification of significantly enriched or depleted groups of genes (32). GSEA analysis has been conducted using GSEA Java Desktop Application from Broad Institute (http://software.broadinstitute.org/gsea/index.jsp). Normalized data from all of genes were transformed to an appropriate format and imported to application. Then, a predefined gene sets database named Hallmark was selected from Molecular Signatures Database (33). Genes belonging to the selected set were ranked according to the difference in their expression level using signal-to-noise ratio with 1,000 times permutation. By walking down the ranked list of genes, the enrichment score (ES) was calculated for each selected gene set. It was done by sum statistic when a gene was present in the gene set and decreasing it when it was not (34). ESs were normalized by their gene set size, and false positive finding were corrected by FDR.

QPCR

QPCR was performed by means of the Lightcycler 2.0 instrument (ROCHE) with the 4.05 software version. SYBR green detection system was applied as described earlier (19, 25–27, 35–37). Every 20 μl reaction mixtures contains 2 μl template cDNA (standard or control), 0.5 μM of specific primer, and a previously determined optimum $MgCl_2$ concentration (3.5 μM for each reaction). LightCyclerFastStart DNA Master SYBR Green I mix (ROCHE) was used. The real-time PCR program included 10 min denaturation step to activate the Taq DNA Polymerase, followed by a three-step amplification program: denaturation at 95°C for 10 s, annealing at 56°C for 5 s, and extension at 72°C for 10 s. Specificity of reaction products was checked by determination of melting points (0.1°C/s transition rate). Expression of studied genes was related to B2m, only in case of Hcrtr2 to PBGD.

The primers used were designed by Primer 3 software (Whitehead Institute for Biomedical Research, Cambridge, MA, USA) (**Table 1**). They were purchased from the Laboratory

TABLE 1 | Primers used for QPCR validation of selected genes.

cDNA	Genbank accession number	Primer	Primer sequence (5′–3′)	Position	PCR product size (bp)
Hcrtr2	NM_013074.1	S	GGCTTATCTCCAAATATTCCG	782–802	68
		A	CTCTGAACCACAGAAGAAGT	831–849	
AR	NM_012502.1	S	ATCATCTCTGTGCAAGTGCCC	3,634–3,654	162
		A	CCCATGCCAGAGAAGTAGTG	3,776–3,795	
ERa	NM_012689.1	S	ATGATGGGCTTATTGACCAAC	1,248–1,268	137
		A	AGGATCTCCAACCAGGCACA	1,365–1,384	
ERb	NM_012754.1	S	TCTGTGTGAAGGCCATGATC	1,474–1,493	237
		A	GCAGATGTTCCATGCCCTTG	1,691–1,710	
ERRa	NM_001008511.2	S	CTCTCTACCCAAACGCCTCT	334–353	234
		A	CGCACACCCTCCTTGAGCAT	548–567	
Mc2r	NM_001100491.1	S	GGACAAGGGGGGAGGCAGA	110–118	201
		A	TGGCACAACTACATCAGGAC	281–300	
Hmgcr	NM_013134.2	S	GACGCAACCTCTACATCCG	1,966–1,984	142
		A	TAGTTACCACTGACCGCCAGA	2,087–2,107	
B2m	NM_012512.2	S	CTTGCAGAGTTAAACACGTCA	316–336	70
		A	CTTGATTACATGTCTCGGTC	366–385	
PBGD	NM_013168.2	S	GAAAGACCCTGGAAACCTT	522–540	148
		A	AGCTCATCCAGCTTCCGTA	651–669	

Gene symbol, gene names, Genebank accession numbers, oligonucleotide sequences for sense and antisense primers, their position, and product size are shown.

of DNA Sequencing and Oligonucleotide Synthesis, Institute of Biochemistry and Biophysics, Polish Academy of Sciences, Warsaw.

Statistical Analysis

The applied statistical analyses of gene expression are parts of the softwares used. The RT-QPCR data, on the other hand, are expressed as the mean ± SE, and the statistical significance of the differences between the compared groups was estimated using the Student's *t*-test.

RESULTS

To study the modulatory effects of sex hormones on adrenal gland transcriptome profile, adult female and male rats were gonadectomized and replaced with estradiol or testosterone. The efficacy of the treatments has been demonstrated by seminal vesicles and uterine weights. As expected, weight of the examined organs decreased significantly after removal of gonads, whereas the weight of seminal vesicles and uteri were increased in the groups replaced with sex hormone [uterine weight (g): sham operated 0.42 ± 0.03, OVX 0.06 ± 0.01, OVX + estradiol replaced 0.37 ± 0.02; seminal vesicle weights: sham operated 0.41 ± 0.03, ORX 0.09 ± 0.01, ORX + testosterone replaced 0.85 ± 0.03; in each group $n = 6$; mean ± SE].

In these experimental conditions, ORX increases serum corticosterone concentrations, an effect reversed by testosterone replacement (Figure S1 in Supplementary Material). In the female, on the other hand, ovariectomy reduces serum corticosterone levels, while estradiol replacement restores corticosterone levels to the control values. In ORX rats, serum levels of the total cholesterol, LDL, and HDL were elevated, an effect reversed by testosterone replacement (Figure S2 in Supplementary Material). In OVX rats, serum levels of the total cholesterol, LDL, and HDL were higher and of triglyceride lower than in sham-operated animals. Estradiol supplementation restores these changes to the normal values.

Adrenals obtained from five rats from each group were used for whole transcriptome analysis using Afymetrix microarray method, where expression of approximately 30,000 genes was examined. General gene expression profiles resulting from the comparison of male and female controls with appropriate experimental groups are shown as volcano plots (**Figure 1**). The selection criteria of a significantly changed gene expression level was based on expression fold difference higher than abs. 2 and adjusted p value <0.05. Considering these assumptions, ORX vs. control male adrenal transcription profile comparisons revealed that 36 genes were expressed differentially (28 down- and 8 upregulated genes). In the next compared groups: ORX + T vs. control males, we revealed 93 differentially expressed genes (27 down- and 66 upregulated). The last comparison of ORX + T vs. ORX groups revealed 205 differentially expressed genes (65 down- and 140 upregulated). Similar comparisons performed between OVX vs. control females, OVX + E vs. control females and OVX + E vs. OVX revealed that 18 (0 down- and 18 upregulated), 30 (24 down- and 6 upregulated), and 193 (161 down- and 32 upregulated) genes are differentially expressed, respectively.

Correctness of presented study has been verified by detailed analysis of steroid-5-alpha-reductase alpha polypeptide 1 (Srd5a1) and hypocretin (orexin) receptor 2 (Hcrtr2) gene expression. Both, studied enzyme and receptor genes were earlier described as regulated by sex hormones. Profile of Srd5a1 gene expression was extracted from normalized microarray data set and presented on **Figure 2A**. Expression of Srd5a1 was significantly increased after gonadectomy (fold = 5.46, $p = 2.23\text{E-}05$ for male, and fold = 2.17, $p = 0.049$ for female, in relation to appropriate control groups) and reversed by sex hormone replacement (fold = −1.6, $p = 0.605$ for male and fold = −2.28, $p = 0.063$ for

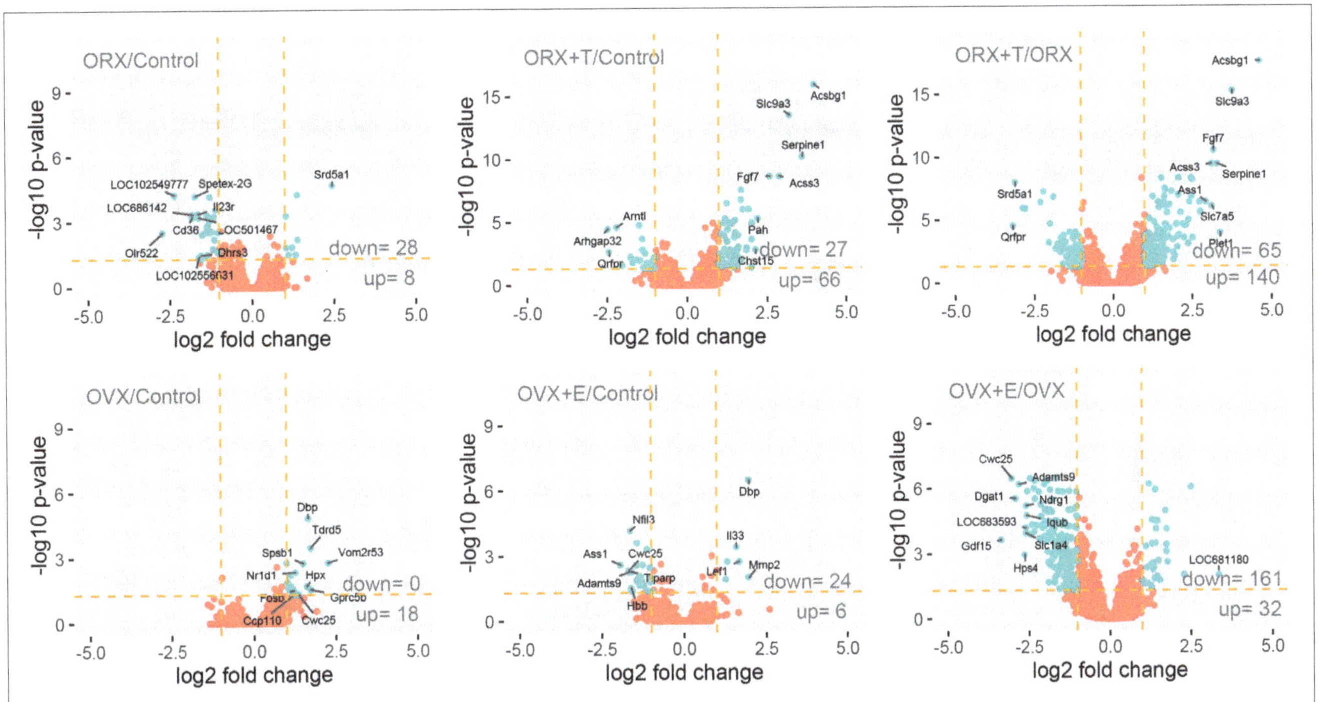

FIGURE 1 | Volcano plots showing the total gene expression profiles of adrenals of adult male and female control, gonadectomized and gonadal hormone replaced rats. Each dot represents mean expression ($n = 5$) of a single gene obtained from microarray normalized dataset. Orange dotted cutoff lines were established using the following parameters: fold > |2| and adjusted p value <0.05. Genes above cutoff are considered as differentially expressed and shown as blue dots. Total numbers of differentially expressed genes are written in the right bottom corner of the graph. Ten of the most regulated genes are described by their gene symbols.

female, in relation to control groups). As revealed by QPCR, also expression of Hcrtr2 is notably decreased in ORX and reversed by testosterone. On the contrary, in OVX rats expression of Hcrtr2 was elevated and again this effect was reversed by estradiol replacement (**Figure 2B**).

Differentially expressed gene sets were subsequently used for screening of their overrepresentation in some particular gene ontological groups. For this reason, gene symbols from all previously mentioned comparisons were loaded to DAVID searching system. Due to the small number of differentially expressed genes in ORX vs. control, OVX vs. control, and OVX + E vs. control, we did not obtain statistically significant GO groups in the abovementioned comparisons. Comparison between ORX + T vs. control males revealed two GO terms formed by differentially expressed genes: "small molecule biosynthetic process" and "lipid metabolic process" (**Figure 3A**). Genes from these GO terms were upregulated in ORX + T group in relation to male control. In the next comparison, 35 GO terms were formed from genes differentially expressed in ORX + T vs. ORX groups. Some of obtained GO groups have a general meaning, e.g., "response to organic substance," "response to chemical stimulus" but other seems to be more related to adrenal physiology, i.e., "response to steroid hormone" or "lipid metabolic process." All of presented GO terms were upregulated in ORX + T group in relation to ORX (**Figure 3B**). The last presented GO term graph demonstrates OVX + E vs. OVX groups comparisons, which delivered 24 GO terms. It is worth to notice that genes formed presented GO terms are downregulated in OVX + E vs. OVX group (**Figure 3C**). In this comparison, "lipid metabolic process" term was also statistically significant, and for this reason, genes belonging to this process in ORX + T vs. ORX as well as OVX + E vs. OVX were selected for hierarchical clusterization and presented as heatmap on **Figure 4**. To obtain the maps, 22 genes were selected from the "lipid metabolic process" in both male and female comparisons. All genes from male adrenals belonging to the "lipid metabolic process" are characterized by the highest expression levels in ORX + T group (green color) and the lowest in ORX group (red color). Expression of female genes has opposite profile. The highest gene expression levels are in OVX (green color) group, while the lowest in OVX + E (red color).

The above presented results were confirmed by another powerful bioinformatics tool that is the Gene Set Enrichment Analysis (GSEA). These analyzes were performed for: OXR/OXR + T and OVX/OVX + E experimental groups. After uploading of normalized expression level data from microarray to the software, we obtained a list of significantly represented terms from Hallmark database software. Ten of the most enrichment terms from each of the comparisons are presented on **Figure 5**. In accordance with DAVID and heatmap results, presented terms were enriched, it means that expressions of genes were higher in ORX + T (ORX + T/ORX) and OVX (OVX + E/OVX). The strongest enriched term in the comparison between ORX + T/ORX refers

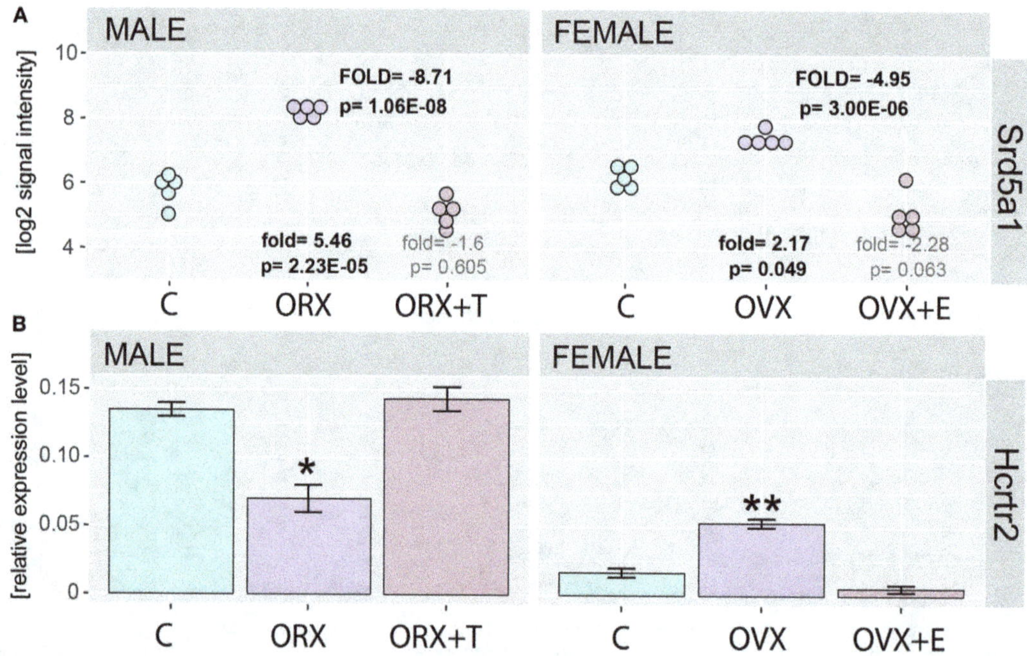

FIGURE 2 | Expression of Srd5a1 and Hcrtr2 genes in applied experimental model. (A) Expression values were extracted from microarray normalized data set and presented as log2 signal intensity scale. Fold and *p* values were calculated in relation to appropriate control groups (showed on bottom) or between gonadectomized [orchiectomy (ORX) or ovariectomy (OVX)] and gonadectomized + sex hormone replaced (ORX + T, OVX + E) groups (showed on the top "FOLD" in capitals). In each group, $n = 5$. *p* Value obtained from moderated *t* test with FDR correction (incorporated in the Limma package of the software). **(B)** QPCR assay of Hcrtr2 genes in adrenals of adult male and female control, gonadectomized and gonadal hormone replaced rats. Bars represent means ± SEM ($n = 5$). HPRT gene was used as reference for data normalization. Statistically significant differences in relation to control group (Student's *t*-test): $^{*}p < 0.05$; $^{**}p < 0.02$; $^{***}p < 0.01$; $^{****}p < 0.001$.

to "androgen response" while "TNFA signaling via NFKB" term was the strongest enriched in GSEA between OVX + E/OVX. Detailed results of those two terms are presented in **Figures 6** and **7**. List of the top 10 genes that strongly affect ES with their rank position are also shown.

One of the top enrichment term concerns the process strictly connected with adrenocortical steroidogenesis named "cholesterol homeostasis." Results of GSEA are presented in **Figure 8**. Genes belonging to "cholesterol homeostasis" hallmark term are highly enriched in ORX + T group in relation to ORX group. Opposite results were obtained in OVX/OVX + E comparison, where gene belonging to "cholesterol homeostasis" are enriched in OVX group, it means that the expressions are higher in OVX in relation to OVX + E. Obtained results from GSEA are in commitment with previously presented DAVID GO analysis. List of the top 10 genes with their rank position are also shown in these figures.

Regardless of experimental group, AR mRNA (androgen receptor) levels in rat adrenal are over 40 times higher than levels of estrogen receptors (**Figure 9**). As demonstrated by means of QPCR, expression levels of AR mRNA were not changed after OVX and OVX + E in relation to adrenals of control female rats. However, expression of AR was decreased after ORX and restored to control value after testosterone replacement. In both sexes, gonadectomy and sex hormone replacement did not change Esr1 and Esr2 gene expression. Expression of Esrra gene, on the other hand, was significantly elevated after OVX and restored to control level after estrogen replacement. Expression of Esrra in male adrenals was not changed in any experimental conditions. Expression of Mc2r was not significantly regulated in any experimental conditions in female adrenals, whereas it was lowered in gonadectomized males and elevated in testosterone-replaced animals. It is interesting to note that Hmgcr gene expression in the adrenal gland of male rats is significantly higher than in females. We also revealed that expression levels of this gene were affected neither by ORX nor testosterone replacement. On the other hand, ovariectomy resulted in a notable increase in Hmgcr gene expression levels, an effect reversed by estradiol replacement (**Figure 10**).

DISCUSSION

For many years, it is known that the multidirectional actions of androgen and estrogen lead to obvious sex differences in the structure and function of the adrenal cortex. As a result, in the adult female rat, adrenal cortex is larger and secretes more corticosterone than that of males (references in Section "Introduction"). It is commonly assumed that this effect depends on the stimulatory effect of estrogen on the HPA axis, while androgens have the opposite effect.

As revealed by global gene profiling method, distinct sex differences in the rat adrenal gland are accompanied by notable

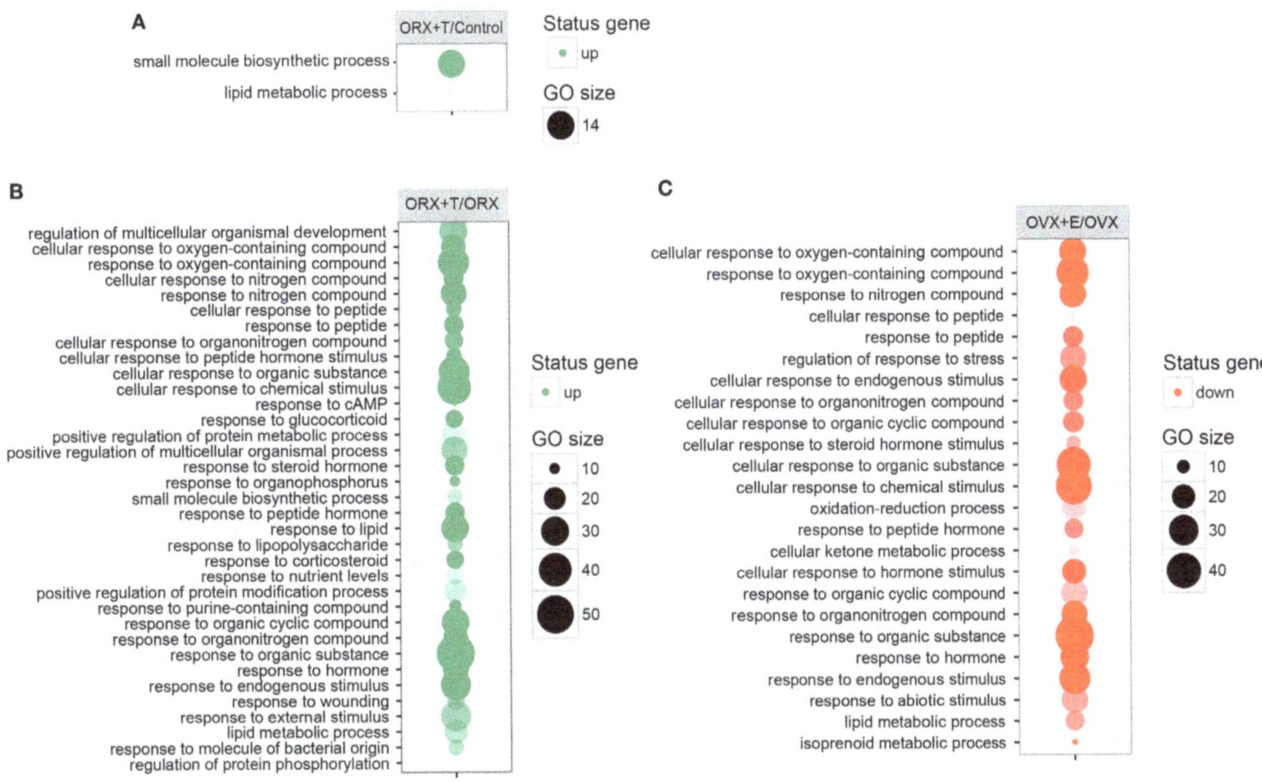

FIGURE 3 | Bubble plot of overrepresented gene set in DAVID GEOTERM BP FAT annotations database obtained from comparisons of expression profiles between: (A) male control/orchiectomy (ORX) + T, (B) ORX/ORX + T, (C) ovariectomy (OVX)/OVX + E. The graphs show only the GO groups above the established cutoff criteria (p with correction <0.01, minimal number of genes per group >5). The size of each bubble reflects the number of differentially expressed genes, assigned to the GO BP terms. Transparency of the bubbles displays p value (more transparent—closer to the border of $p = 0.01$).

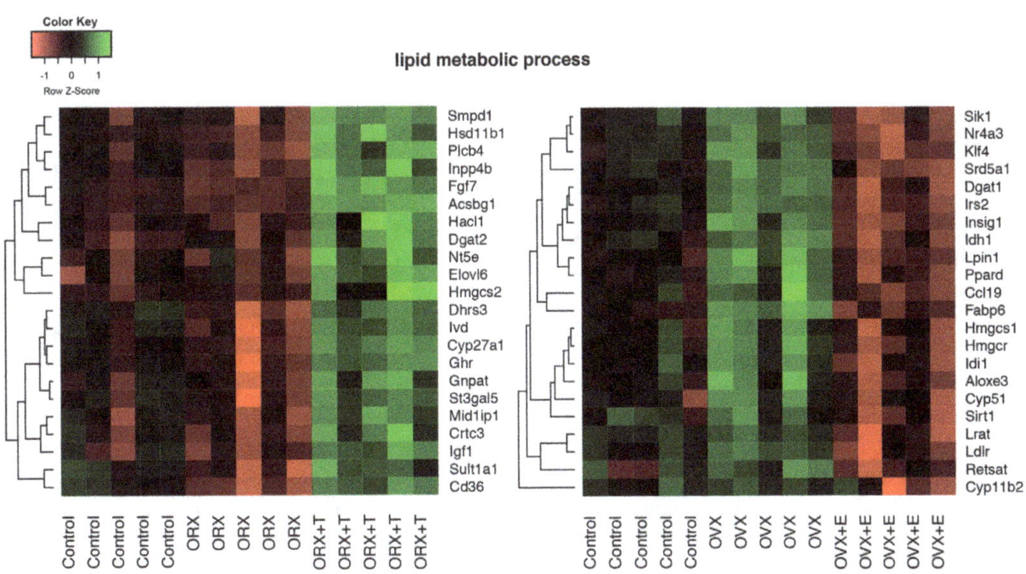

FIGURE 4 | Heat map graph of male and female adrenal gland genes regulated by sex hormones and belonging to "lipid metabolic process" GO BP term. Arbitrary signal intensity acquired from the microarray analysis is represented by colors (green—higher; red—lower expression). Log2 signal intensity values for any single gene were resized to Row Z-score scale (from −1.5, the lowest expression, to +1.5, the highest expression for single gene). Presented genes are described by their gene symbols. Genes were selected from David GO terms, obtained by comparison of orchiectomy (ORX)/ORX + T and ovariectomy (OVX)/OVX + E. For better data understanding, the control groups have also been shown; however, they were not included into comparisons.

GSEA result: ORX+T/ORX, enriched in ORX+T

HALLMARK GO TERM	SIZE	ES	NES	NOM.p.val	FDR.q.val	FWER.p.val
ANDROGEN RESPONSE	98	-0.58	-2.14	0.000	0.000	0.000
FATTY ACID METABOLISM	146	-0.50	-1.97	0.000	0.001	0.002
ADIPOGENESIS	193	-0.45	-1.83	0.000	0.006	0.015
XENOBIOTIC METABOLISM	192	-0.45	-1.82	0.000	0.004	0.015
ANGIOGENESIS	36	-0.59	-1.81	0.002	0.004	0.017
ESTROGEN RESPONSE EARLY	195	-0.44	-1.78	0.000	0.004	0.020
BILE ACID METABOLISM	112	-0.47	-1.78	0.002	0.003	0.020
UV RESPONSE DN	142	-0.44	-1.74	0.000	0.005	0.030
PROTEIN SECRETION	95	-0.46	-1.68	0.000	0.008	0.053
CHOLESTEROL HOMEOSTASIS	72	-0.47	-1.68	0.008	0.007	0.054

GSEA result: OVX+E/OVX, enriched in OVX

HALLMARK GO TERM	SIZE	ES	NES	NOM.p.val	FDR.q.val	FWER.p.val
TNFA SIGNALING VIA NFKB	200	0.72	3.00	0	0	0
CHOLESTEROL HOMEOSTASIS	72	0.76	2.72	0	0	0
MTORC1 SIGNALING	196	0.63	2.64	0	0	0
HYPOXIA	194	0.62	2.62	0	0	0
ANDROGEN RESPONSE	98	0.62	2.36	0	0	0
P53 PATHWAY	194	0.55	2.31	0	0	0
REACTIVE OXIGEN SPECIES PATHWAY	45	0.67	2.23	0	0	0
EPITHELIAL MESENCHYMAL TRANSITION	194	0.53	2.22	0	0	0
ESTROGEN RESPONSE LATE	191	0.53	2.21	0	0	0
UNFOLDED PROTEIN RESPONSE	112	0.57	2.20	0	0	0

FIGURE 5 | Ten of the highest enriched HALLMARK GO TERMS obtained from gene set enrichment analysis (GSEA) between orchiectomy (ORX)/ ORX + T and ovariectomy (OVX)/OVX + E groups. Size of the category (number of genes in the "TERM"), enrichment score (ES), normalized enrichment score (NES), *p* value (NOM.p.val), *q* value of FDR correction (FDR.q.val), and *p* corrected by FDR (FWER.p.val) are shown.

differences in expression levels of various groups of genes (19). We demonstrated that expression levels of genes involved in corticosteroid synthesis are higher and those regulating basal cell functions lower in adrenals of adult female rats. However, the control of adrenocortical gene expression by sex hormones is totally unknown. Regarding this, only one study presents data on global gene profiling in the adrenals of female intact and testosterone—administered mice (20). However, this experimental model is not a physiological one. To get information about the regulation by testosterone and estradiol of adrenal genes in male and female rats, we used the classic "remove and replace" experiments. As evidenced by changes in uterine and seminal vesicles weights, expected, gonadectomy-induced drop in the weight of these tissues was reversed by replacement with appropriate sex hormone.

In light of the above presented discussion on sex differences in adrenals of rats, one would expect the stimulatory effect of estradiol and the opposite effect of testosterone on the glands. To our surprise, global gene profiling analyses performed on adrenals of studied rats delivered rather unexpected results. It appeared that testosterone replacement mainly upregulates expression of adrenal genes while estradiol effect is opposite, large group of genes was downregulated. Regarding these results, the correctness of our experiments we tried to confirm by the more detailed studies of genes whose expression in a rat adrenal gland is known as dependent on testosterone or estradiol.

One of them is steroid-5-alpha-reductase alpha polypeptide 1 (Srd5a1). Expression of this gene and activity of the coded enzyme are notably elevated in ORX and OVX rats, changes prevented by testosterone or estradiol replacement, respectively (5, 38–43). Our microarray data are consistent with these findings. The second studied gene is orexin receptor 2 (Hcrtr2). Higher expression of Hcrtr2 in adrenals of the male rat in relation to female one as well as stimulatory effects of testosterone and inhibitory action of estradiol on this gene are well documented (19, 44–46). And again, our QPCR data are consistent with the earlier reports. Thus, obtained in the experiments performed, data on expression of specific genes in adrenals of rats of both sexes are consistent with earlier reports. In view of these, results still remains open while the global profile of gene expression regulated by sex hormones in the rat adrenal gland suggests prevalent inhibitory effect of estradiol and stimulatory effect of testosterone.

Higher expression in class:	ORX+T
Gene term:	HALLMARK_ANDROGEN_RESPONSE
Enrichment Score (ES)	-0.5787016
Normalized Enrichment Score (NES)	-2.1369805
Nominal p-value	0
FDR q-value	0
FWER p-Value	0

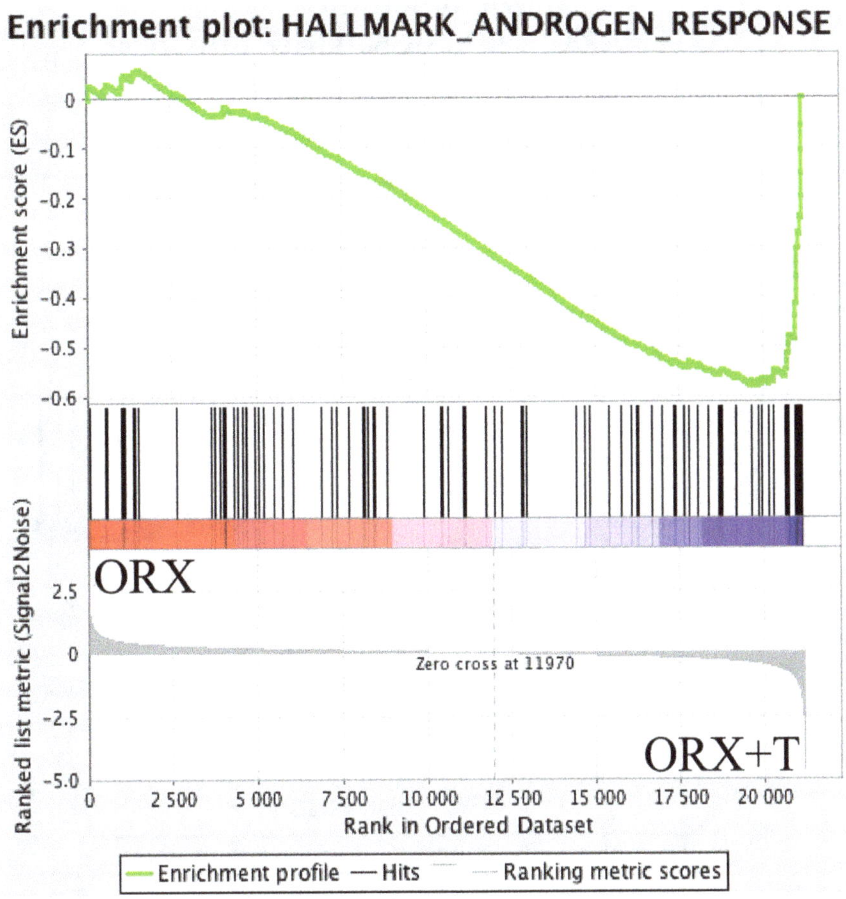

Gene symbol	Gene name	Rank in gene list
Gpd1l	glycerol-3-phosphate dehydrogenase 1-like	21224
Appbp2	amyloid beta precursor protein (cytoplasmic tail) binding protein 2	21203
Lifr	leukemia inhibitory factor receptor alpha	21195
Inpp4b	inositol polyphosphate-4-phosphatase, type II	21192
B4galt1	UDP-Gal:betaGlcNAc beta 1,4- galactosyltransferase, polypeptide 1	21180
Sepp1	selenoprotein P, plasma, 1	21129
Fkbp5	FK506 binding protein 5	21088
Dbi	diazepam binding inhibitor	21056
Hmgcr	3-hydroxy-3-methylglutaryl-CoA reductase	21055
Ankh	ANKH inorganic pyrophosphate transport regulator	21042

FIGURE 6 | **Summary results of gene set enrichment (GSEA) in HALLMARK_ANDROGEN_RESPONSE term.** Enrichment analysis was performed between orchiectomy (ORX) and ORX + T groups of male adrenal glands. Normalized enrichment score (NES) as well as *p* values are shown. Middle plot presents rank of each gene belonging to androgen response term with enrichment score (ES) peak values. Ten of the top relevant genes for enrichment calculation are shown in table with their symbol, names, and rank in gene list.

Higher expression in class:	OVX
Gene term:	HALLMARK_TNFA_SIGNALING_VIA_NFKB
Enrichment Score (ES)	0.71887577
Normalized Enrichment Score (NES)	2.998372
Nominal p-value	0
FDR q-value	0
FWER p-Value	0

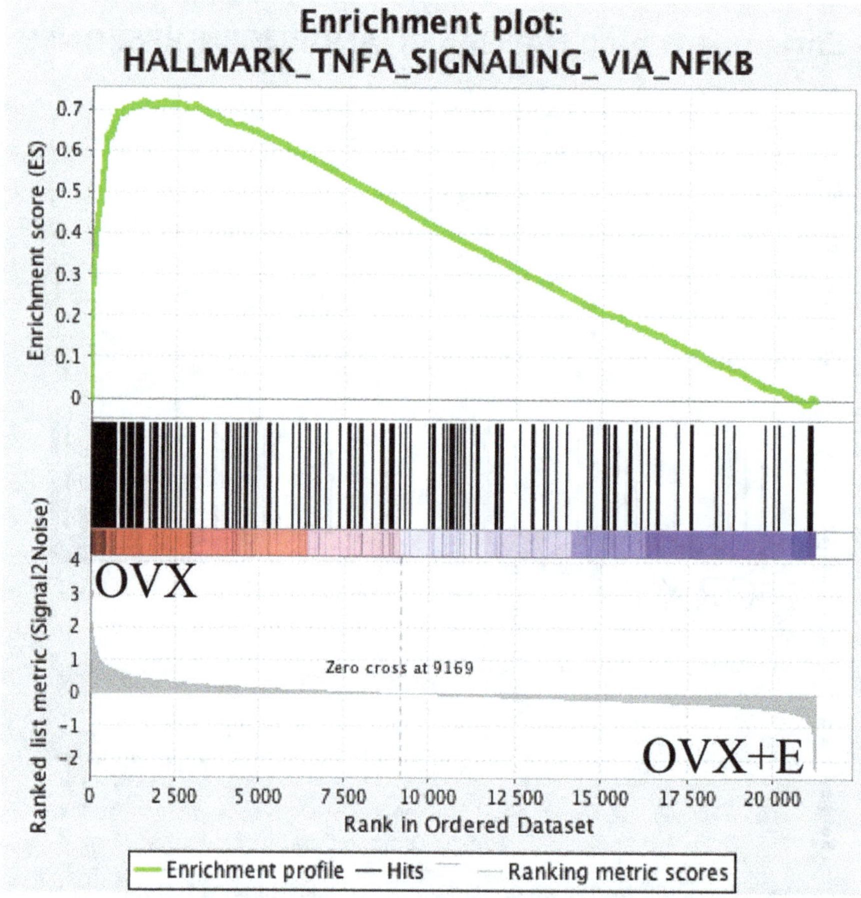

Gene symbol	Gene name	Rank in gene list
Tiparp	TCDD-inducible poly(ADP-ribose) polymerase	6
Spsb1	splA/ryanodine receptor domain and SOCS box containing 1	8
Klf4	Kruppel-like factor 4 (gut)	9
Nfil3	nuclear factor, interleukin 3 regulated	16
Nr4a2	nuclear receptor subfamily 4, group A, member 2	18
Sik1	salt-inducible kinase 1	27
Irs2	insulin receptor substrate 2	28
Nr4a3	nuclear receptor subfamily 4, group A, member 3	30
FosB	FBJ osteosarcoma oncogene B	35
Phlda1	pleckstrin homology-like domain, family A, member 1	38

FIGURE 7 | Summary results of gene set enrichment (GSEA) in HALLMARK_TNFA_SIGNALING_VIA_NFKB term. Enrichment analysis was performed between ovariectomy (OVX) and OVX + E groups of female adrenal glands. Normalized enrichment score (NES) as well as *p* values are shown. Middle plot presents rank of each gene belonging to Tnfa signaling via NFKB term with enrichment score (ES) peak values. Ten of the top relevant genes for enrichment calculation are shown in table with their symbol, names, and rank in gene list.

Higher expression in class:	ORX+T
Gene set:	HALLMARK_CHOLESTEROL_HOMEOSTASIS
Enrichment Score (ES)	-0.46569455
Normalized Enrichment Score (NES)	-1.6774724
Nominal p-value	0.007662835
FDR q-value	0.007083823
FWER p-Value	0.054

Higher expression in class:	OVX
Gene set:	HALLMARK_CHOLESTEROL_HOMEOSTASIS
Enrichment Score (ES)	0.7586827
Normalized Enrichment Score (NES)	2.7205517
Nominal p-value	0
FDR q-value	0
FWER p-Value	0

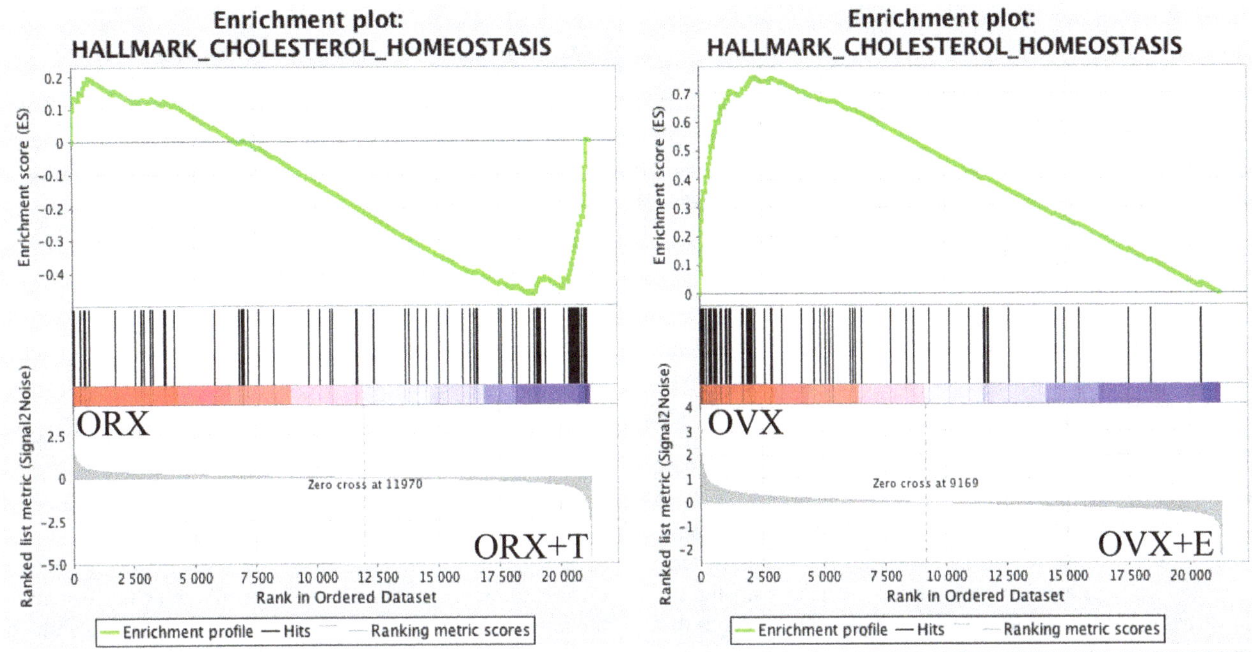

Gene symbol	Gene name	Rank in gene list
Acss2	acyl-CoA synthetase short-chain family member 2	21082
Lgals3	lectin, galactoside-binding, soluble, 3	21080
Hmgcr	3-hydroxy-3-methylglutaryl-CoA reductase	21055
Tm7sf2	transmembrane 7 superfamily member 2	21051
Scd	stearoyl-CoA desaturase (delta-9-desaturase)	21041
Ech1	enoyl CoA hydratase 1, peroxisomal	20979
Errfi1	ERBB receptor feedback inhibitor 1	20878
Stard4	StAR-related lipid transfer (START) domain containing 4	20789
Fdft1	farnesyl diphosphate farnesyl transferase 1	20748
Hmgcs1	3-hydroxy-3-methylglutaryl-CoA synthase 1 (soluble)	20694

Gene symbol	Gene name	Rank in gene list
Nfil3	nuclear factor, interleukin 3 regulated	16
Ldlr	low density lipoprotein receptor	67
Hmgcr	3-hydroxy-3-methylglutaryl-CoA reductase	74
Idi1	isopentenyl-diphosphate delta isomerase 1	79
Errfi1	ERBB receptor feedback inhibitor 1	83
Hmgcs1	3-hydroxy-3-methylglutaryl-CoA synthase 1 (soluble)	127
S100a11	S100 calcium binding protein A11	142
Mal2	mal, T-cell differentiation protein 2	176
Atf5	activating transcription factor 5	255
Atf3	activating transcription factor 3	282

FIGURE 8 | Summary results of gene set enrichment (GSEA) in HALLMARK_CHOLESTEROL_HOMEOSTASIS term. Enrichment analyses were done between gonadectomized and gonadectomized + sex hormone replaced groups, in both sexes. Normalized enrichment score (NES) as well as *p* values are shown. Middle plots present ranks of each gene belonging to cholesterol homeostasis term with enrichment score (ES) peak values. Ten of the top relevant genes for enrichment calculation from each sexes are shown in table with their symbol, names, and rank position.

To gain an insight into this problem, we performed numerous additional analyses of data delivered by Affymetrix microarray system. As demonstrated by Volcano plots, in adrenals of experimental rats, only small number of differentially expressed genes was found. Differentially expressed genes were further analyzed in order to get their representation in GO. This was accomplished by DAVID web-based bioinformatics tools. The highest numbers of GO terms were obtained in comparisons of ORX + T vs. ORX experimental groups (35 GO terms). In females, on the other hand, analogical comparison (OVX + E vs. OVX) delivered 24 GO terms. It is noteworthy to underline that testosterone replaced rat genes in obtained groups were upregulated, while those in estradiol-replaced ovariectomized animals were downregulated. One of these GO terms—"lipid metabolic process"—seems to be related to adrenal physiology. This term occurs in both, testosterone- or estradiol-replaced groups; however, in androgen-replaced rats, expression levels of genes included in this group are elevated, while in estrogen supplemented animals their expression is lowered.

Our results obtained by the DAVID web-based bioinformatic tools were confirmed by GSEA. GSEA revealed that in ORX + T group (in relation to ORX) genes belonging to the Hallmark GO terms "androgen response," "fatty acid metabolism," "adipogenesis," and "cholesterol homeostasis" are notably enriched.

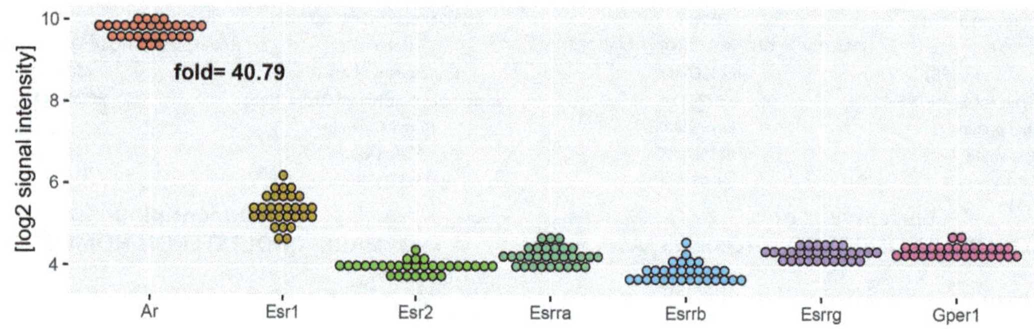

FIGURE 9 | Expression of androgen (Ar) and estrogen (Esr1, Esr2, Esrra, Esrrb, Esrrg, Gper) receptors in adrenal glands of studied rats (male and female control, gonadectomized and gonadal hormone replaced rats). Data obtained from Affymetrix® Rat Gene 2.1 ST Array. From microarray data sets, expression values of analyzed genes were extracted. Each dot on graph corresponds to single log2-transformed value of signal intensity from individual sample. Fold expression change was calculated from mean of Ar receptor gene and mean of all estrogen receptors.

Moreover, in OVX group (in relation to OVX + E), enriched genes are present, among others, within the following terms: "TNFA signaling via NFKB," "cholesterol homeostasis," and "androgen response." These data suggest that in adrenals of gonadectomized rats both, testosterone or estradiol replacement, potently affects genes involved in lipid and cholesterol metabolism, as well as intracellular pathways responsible for androgen response. Further GSEA analysis revealed that within the hallmark term "cholesterol homeostasis," in both, orchiectomized testosterone- and ovariectomized estradiol-replaced rats, among 10 genes that strongly affect ES Hmgcr is present.

There is some evidence that total lipid and cholesterol concentrations and contents in the rat adrenal gland are influenced by gonadal hormones. Lowered concentration of total lipid in adrenals of gonadectomized rats of both sexes was reported by Coleman et al. (47). Higher total lipid content, but not total lipid concentration in adrenals of female than male rats, has been reported by other group (48, 49). These studies demonstrated also higher concentrations and contents of total lipid in adrenals of orchiectomized testosterone replaced rats, while an opposite effects were observed in ovariectomized rats replaced with estradiol.

Although cholesterol is not a classical lipid, its physiological role in the adrenal cortex is often described in the aspects of the role of lipids. In contrast to lipids, numerous data are available on cholesterol and cholesterol esters in adrenals of intact male and female rats and on impact on them of sex hormones.

HMG-CoA reductase is the rate-limiting enzyme in cholesterol biosynthesis (50, 51). Administration of 17α-ethinylestradiol into aging male rats resulted in a notable stimulation of enzyme activity (52). Our results indicate that testosterone has no effect on the expression of Hmgcr gene; however, ovariectomy increases its expression, an effect reversed by estradiol replacement. Regarding these changes, it should be emphasized that HMG-CoA reductase is a highly regulated gene, among others by serum lipoprotein levels and intracellular cholesterol content (50, 53). Thus, it seems legitimate to suggest that observed in the present study changes in Hmgcr expression may be mediated by both, serum lipoprotein levels and adrenal cholesterol content. This assumption is supported by parallel changes in adrenal HMG-CoA reductase gene expression and serum HDL concentrations in studied female rats.

According to data reviewed in the earlier monographs, the majority of publications indicate a higher concentration of cholesterol (both, free or esterified) in the adrenal glands of adult female rats (5, 49). ORX increased cholesterol concentration in the gland, an effect reversed by testosterone replacement. Ovariectomy, on the other hand, either did not change or lowered the total cholesterol concentration in the rat adrenal gland. There is general agreement, on the other hand, that estrogens lower cholesterol content in adrenals of ovariectomized rats.

Free cholesterol, required for steroid hormone synthesis, is liberated from cholesterol esters by the action of ACTH-sensitive sterol ester hydrolase. The specific activity of this enzyme in adrenal homogenates is notably higher in male than female glands (54). Both, ORX and testosterone replacement had any effect on adrenal sterol ester hydrolase. Ovariectomy, on the other hand, resulted in an increase in activity of the enzyme, an effect reversed by estradiol replacement.

Thus, earlier data on the effects of testosterone and estradiol on adrenal lipids and enzymes involved in cholesterol metabolism in the rat are rather consistent with the transcriptome profile obtained in the respective experimental groups.

Also genes forming the hallmark GO term "androgen response" in rat adrenals are highly regulated by both, testosterone or estradiol replacement. In an aspect of this term in the present study, we analyzed the expression of the androgen receptor. Regardless of experimental group, AR mRNA levels in rat adrenal are over 40 times higher than levels of estrogen receptors, differences observed also by others (27, 55–59). We observed that expression of AR was decreased after ORX and restored to control value after testosterone replacement while no changes were observed after OVX and OVX + E. Our results are also consistent with the data on the sheep (60). Thus, our data did not confirm earlier reports on the effects of gonadectomy and sex hormone replacement on the levels of androgen- or estrogen-binding sites in the rat adrenals (56–58). Of estrogen receptor isoforms studied, only Esrra (estrogen

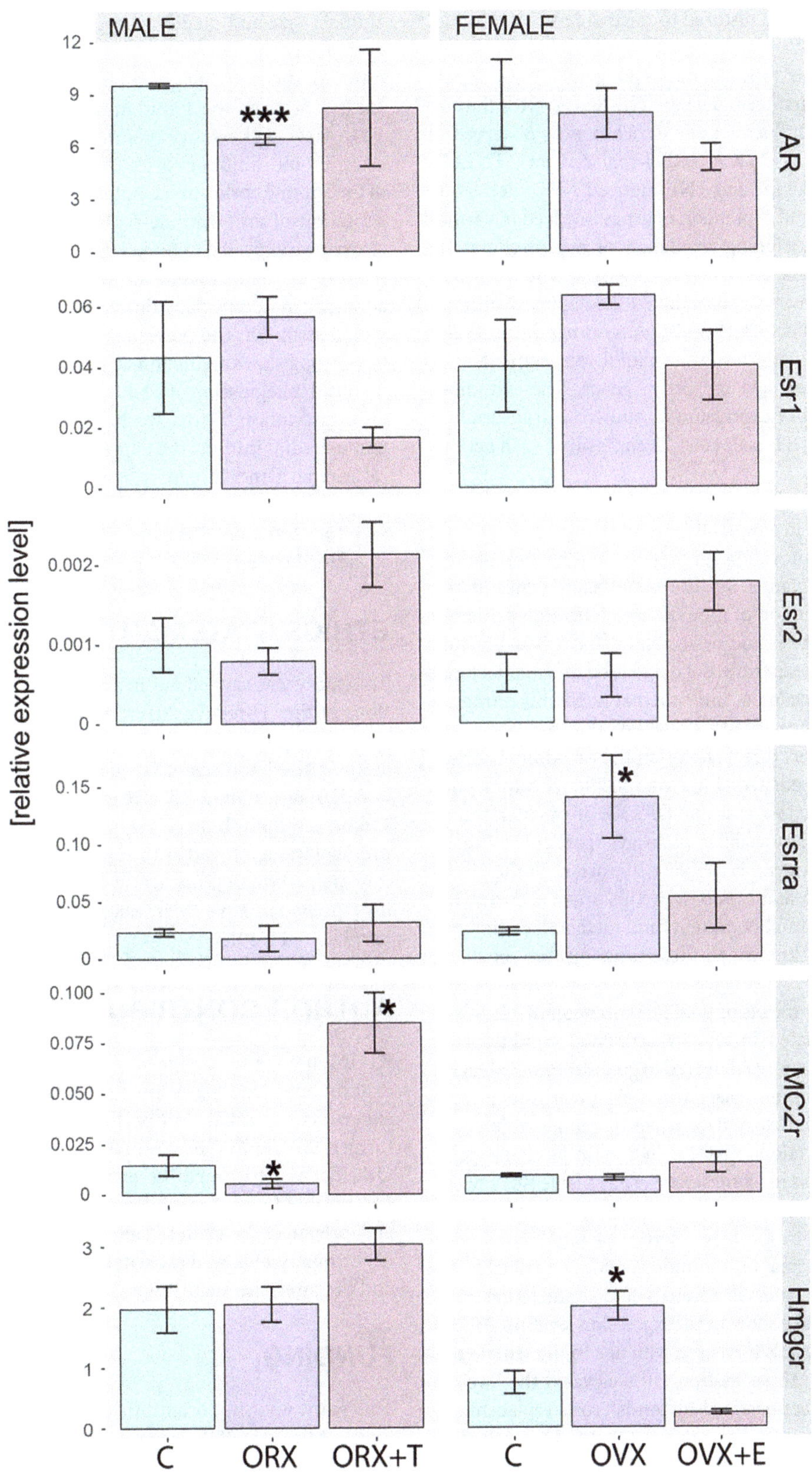

FIGURE 10 | QPCR assay of AR, Esr1, Esr2, Esrra, MC2r, and Hmgcr genes in adrenals of adult male and female control, gonadectomized and gonadal hormone replaced rats. Bars represent mean ± SEM ($n = 3$). All samples were amplified in triplicate, and HPRT gene was used as reference for data normalization. Statistically significant differences in relation to control group: $^{*}p < 0.05$; $^{***}p < 0.01$.

related receptor alpha, also known as NR3B1) is overexpressed in ovariectomized rats and restored to normal level by estradiol replacement.

In adrenals of female rats, hallmark GO term "TNFA signaling via NFKB" is the first term delivered by GSEA, with the size 200 (number of genes). Such a huge enrichment is observed in OVX rats, in relation to OVX estradiol-replaced rats. TNFA is a proinflammatory cytokine and TNF-induced NFKB activation induces transcription and expression of genes involved in various biological processes, including regulation of cell proliferation, differentiation, apoptosis, and immune response. The final steps of these signaling pathways are mediated through activation of nuclear transcription factors (61–63). Also other intracellular signaling pathways are affected by estradiol replacement, they predominantly downregulate respective genes. These findings may suggest inhibition of expression of numerous transcription factor genes in OVX + E female rats. Mechanism of such actions remains to be solved.

It is well documented that androgen and estrogen receptors are ubiquitously expressed in almost all tissues and organs. Therefore, *in vivo* experiments do not allow for precise identification of their action on the adrenal glands. Sex hormones exert a multidirectional effect on the function of the HPA axis, affecting primarily CRH and ACTH synthesis and/or secretion [for review, see Ref. (3–6, 64)]. Most of the experimental data based on gonadectomy and sex hormone replacement indicate that in the rat estrogens stimulate and androgens inhibit the HPA axis. However, sex hormones may also exert direct effects on the rat adrenal cortex. These effects may be mediated either via specific receptors, both nuclear and membrane (for example GPR30) or by interference with ACTH-sensitive intracellular pathways, particularly those associated with steroidogenesis (65–69). Important in the physiological control of HPA axis is also liver. This organ is critical for the regulation of CBG and lipoproteins and metabolizes circulating corticosteroids. As known, all these functions are regulated by sex hormones.

As demonstrated by means of QPCR, expression of Mc2r was not significantly regulated in any experimental conditions in female adrenals, whereas it was lowered in gonadectomized males and elevated in testosterone-replaced animals. In terms of gender differences, very contradictory data relate to gender differences in the content and secretion of ACTH by the rat pituitary gland and corticotrophin levels in blood serum are available [for review, see Malendowicz (5)]. The major part of these studies show a higher level of ACTH in the blood serum of rats treated with estrogen. Only scanty data, on the other hand, are available on expression of ACTH receptors in adrenals of male and female rats. Yoshimura et al. (70) have shown that expression levels of ACTH receptor mRNA in adrenals increased with age in the female rat, but not in the male. In these studies, ORX elevated the level of ACTH receptor, an effect reversed by testosterone replacement. In contrast, our experiments demonstrated that ORX resulted in lowering of Mc2r gene expression and testosterone replacement notable increased expression of this gene. It is difficult to explain these discrepancies, most likely they are the result of different experimental models and methods applied for determining the expression of a discussed gene [male rats aged 14 days (period of temporal decrease of adrenal ACTH responsiveness) vs. adult animals; size and quality of applied primers]. Our results, however, are consistent with the data on the sheep. In this species, estradiol did not change adrenal Mc2r expression, while higher Mc2r expression was found in testosterone-treated rams (60).

In view of the above literature data for stimulating effects of estradiol and inhibitory of testosterone on the growth and function of the adrenal cortex of rat, obtained results of the analysis of transcriptome of sex hormone-replaced rats are surprising. Contrary to what we expected to find, it appeared that testosterone replacement resulted in a potent stimulation of expression of numerous adrenal genes, especially those involved in lipids and cholesterol metabolism. On the other hand, estradiol replacement resulted in a strong downregulation of numerous genes, especially those involved in regulation of TNFA signaling via NFKB pathways and on transcription factors synthesis. Obtained results may suggest that estradiol inhibits the expression of corepressor genes in the rat adrenal gland. It seems possible that this mechanism of action may lead to an increase in both the adrenal gland growth and secretory function. The physiological relevance of these findings await further research.

ETHICS STATEMENT

This study was carried out in accordance with the recommendations of the "Directive 2010/63/EU of the European Parliament and of the Council of 22 September 2010 on the protection of animals used for scientific purposes." as stated in the Polish law "Ustawa z dnia 15 stycznia 2015 r. o ochronie zwierzat wykorzystywanych do celów naukowych lub edukacyjnych." The protocol was approved by the Local Ethics Committee for Animal Research (Poznan, Poland) (in Polish: Lokalna Komisja Etyczna ds. Doświadczeń na zwierzętach w Poznaniu), permission number: LKE—11/2015.

AUTHOR CONTRIBUTIONS

KJ invented and designed the experiments, performed the experiments, and performed microarrays; PC performed the experiments, QPCR; MS performed the experiments and performed QPCR; MT performed the experiments and performed QPCR; PM performed the experiments and performed QPCR; LM invented and designed the experiments, analyzed the data, and prepared the manuscript; MR invented and designed the experiments, analyzed the data, prepared graphical presentation, and prepared the manuscript.

FUNDING

This work was supported by "Diamond Grant" program of the Polish Ministry of Science and Higher Education No. 0171/DIA/2015/44 (to KJ).

SUPPLEMENTARY MATERIAL

FIGURE S1 | Serum corticosterone concentrations in adult male and female control, gonadectomized and gonadal hormone replaced rats.

Bars represent mean ± SEM. Each circle represents an individual value. Statistically significant differences in relation to control or gonadectomized group: $^*p < 0.05$; $^{**}p < 0.02$; $^{***}p < 0.01$; $^{****}p < 0.001$.

FIGURE S2 | Serum total cholesterol, LDL, HDL, and triglyceride concentrations in adult male and female control, gonadectomized and gonadal hormone-replaced rats. Bars represent mean ± SEM. Each circle represents an individual value. Statistically significant differences in relation to control or gonadectomized group: $^*p < 0.05$; $^{**}p < 0.02$; $^{***}p < 0.01$; $^{****}p < 0.001$.

TABLE S1 | List off all regulated genes in adrenals of adult male and female control, gonadectomized and gonadal hormone replaced rats. Their fold change, *p* values, and their localization to chromosomes.

REFERENCES

1. Bachmann R. *Handbuch der Mikroskopischen Anatomie des Menschen*. Berlin, Göttingen, Heidelberg: Springer (1954).
2. Kitay JI. Effects of estrogen and androgen on the adrenal cortex of the rat. In: McKerns KW, editor. *Functions of the Adrenal Cortex*. Vol. 2. Amsterdam: North Holland Publishing Corpany (1968). p. 775–811.
3. Kime D, Vinson GP, Major P, Kilpatrick R. Adrenal-gonad relationship. In: McKerns KW, editor. *Functions of the Adrenal Cortex*. Vol. 3. London: Academic Press (1979). p. 183–347.
4. Handa RJ, Weiser MJ. Gonadal steroid hormones and the hypothalamo-pituitary-adrenal axis. *Front Neuroendocrinol* (2014) 35:197–220. doi:10.1016/j.yfrne.2013.11.001
5. Malendowicz LK. *Cytophysiology of the Mammalian Adrenal Cortex as Related to Sex, Gonadectomy and Gonadal Hormones*. Poznan: PTPN Press (1994).
6. Goel N, Workman JL, Lee TT, Innala L, Viau V. Sex differences in the HPA axis. *Compr Physiol* (2014) 4:1121–55. doi:10.1002/cphy.c130054
7. Green MR, McCormick CM. Sex and stress steroids in adolescence: gonadal regulation of the hypothalamic-pituitary-adrenal axis in the rat. *Gen Comp Endocrinol* (2016) 234:110–6. doi:10.1016/j.ygcen.2016.02.004
8. Gala RR, Westphal U. Corticosteroid-binding globulin in the rat: studies on the sex difference. *Endocrinology* (1965) 77:841–51. doi:10.1210/endo-77-5-841
9. Rosner W. The functions of corticosteroid-binding globulin and sex hormone-binding globulin: recent advances. *Endocr Rev* (1990) 11:80–91. doi:10.1210/edrv-11-1-80
10. Mattos GE, Heinzmann JM, Norkowski S, Helbling JC, Minni AM, Moisan MP, et al. Corticosteroid-binding globulin contributes to the neuroendocrine phenotype of mice selected for extremes in stress reactivity. *J Endocrinol* (2013) 219:217–29. doi:10.1530/JOE-13-0255
11. Meyer EJ, Nenke MA, Rankin W, Lewis JG, Torpy DJ. Corticosteroid-binding globulin: a review of basic and clinical advances. *Horm Metab Res* (2016) 48:359–71. doi:10.1055/s-0042-108071
12. Herbst AL, Yates FE, Glenister DW, Urquhart J. Variations in hepatic inactivation of corticosterone with changes in food intake: an explanation of impaired corticosteroid metabolism following noxious stimuli. *Endocrinology* (1960) 67:222–38. doi:10.1210/endo-67-2-222
13. Kitay JI. Sex differences in adrenal cortical secretion in the rat. *Endocrinology* (1961) 68:818–24. doi:10.1210/endo-68-5-818
14. Glenister DW, Yates FE. Sex difference in the rate of disappearance of corticosterone-4-C14 from plasma of intact rats: further evidence for the influence of hepatic Delta4-steroid hydrogenase activity on adrenal cortical function. *Endocrinology* (1961) 68:747–58. doi:10.1210/endo-68-5-747
15. Seal US, Doe RP. Vertebrate distribution of corticosteroid-binding globulin and some endocrine effects on concentration. *Steroids* (1965) 41:827–41. doi:10.1016/0039-128X(65)90174-1
16. Kitay JI. Effects of estradiol on pituitary-adrenal function in male and female rats. *Endocrinology* (1963) 72:947–54. doi:10.1210/endo-72-6-947
17. Labrie F. *Interactions hormonales et rôle de la transcortine dans l'ajustement de l'activité hypophysosurrénalienne [These Doctorate Sciences]*. Quebec: Universite Laval (1967).
18. Kamoun A. Activité cortico-surrénale au cours de la gestation, de la lactation et du développement pre- et postnatal chez le rat. *J Physiol* (1970) 65:5–32.
19. Trejter M, Hochol A, Tyczewska M, Ziolkowska A, Jopek K, Szyszka M, et al. Sex-related gene expression profiles in the adrenal cortex in the mature rat: microarray analysis with emphasis on genes involved in steroidogenesis. *Int J Mol Med* (2015) 35:702–14. doi:10.3892/ijmm.2015.2064
20. El Wakil A, Mari B, Barhanin J, Lalli E. Genomic analysis of sexual dimorphism of gene expression in the mouse adrenal gland. *Horm Metab Res* (2013) 45:870–3. doi:10.1055/s-0033-1349881
21. Cagen LM, Baer PG. Effects of gonadectomy and steroid treatment on renal prostaglandin 9-ketoreductase activity in the rat. *Life Sci* (1987) 40:95–100. doi:10.1016/0024-3205(87)90257-8
22. Longhurst PA, Kauer J, Leggett RE, Levin RM. The influence of ovariectomy and estradiol replacement on urinary bladder function in rats. *J Urol* (1992) 148:915–9.
23. Udagawa K, Ogawa T, Watanabe T, Tamura Y, Kita K, Kubota Y. Testosterone administration promotes regeneration of chemically impaired spermatogenesis in rats. *Int J Urol* (2006) 13:1103–8. doi:10.1111/j.1442-2042.2006.01484.x
24. Schulte-Beerbühl M, Nieschlag E. Comparison of testosterone, dihydrotestosterone, luteinizing hormone, and follicle-stimulating hormone in serum after injection of testosterone enanthate of testosterone cypionate. *Fertil Steril* (1980) 33:201–3. doi:10.1016/S0015-0282(16)44543-7
25. Tyczewska M, Rucinski M, Trejter M, Ziolkowska A, Szyszka M, Malendowicz LK. Angiogenesis in the course of enucleation-induced adrenal regeneration – expression of selected genes and proteins involved in development of capillaries. *Peptides* (2012) 38:404–13. doi:10.1016/j.peptides.2012.09.025
26. Tyczewska M, Rucinski M, Ziolkowska A, Szyszka M, Trejter M, Hochol-Molenda A, et al. Enucleation-induced rat adrenal gland regeneration: expression profile of selected genes involved in control of adrenocortical cell proliferation. *Int J Endocrinol* (2014) 2014:130359. doi:10.1155/2014/130359
27. Trejter M, Jopek K, Celichowski P, Tyczewska M, Malendowicz LK, Rucinski M. Expression of estrogen, estrogen related and androgen receptors in adrenal cortex of intact adult male and female rats. *Folia Histochem Cytobiol* (2015) 53:133–44. doi:10.5603/FHC.a2015.0012
28. Gautier L, Cope L, Bolstad BM, Irizarry RA. affy – analysis of Affymetrix GeneChip data at the probe level. *Bioinformatics* (2004) 20:307–15. doi:10.1093/bioinformatics/btg405
29. Carvalho BS, Irizarry RA. A framework for oligonucleotide microarray preprocessing. *Bioinformatics* (2010) 26:2363–7. doi:10.1093/bioinformatics/btq431
30. Huang da W, Sherman BT, Lempicki RA. Systematic and integrative analysis of large gene lists using DAVID bioinformatics resources. *Nat Protoc* (2009) 4:44–57. doi:10.1038/nprot.2008.211
31. Fresno C, Fernandez EA. RDAVIDWebService: a versatile R interface to DAVID. *Bioinformatics* (2013) 29:2810–1. doi:10.1093/bioinformatics/btt487
32. Damian D, Gorfine M. Statistical concerns about the GSEA procedure. *Nat Genet* (2004) 36:663; author reply 663. doi:10.1038/ng0704-663a
33. Liberzon A, Birger C, Thorvaldsdottir H, Ghandi M, Mesirov JP, Tamayo P. The Molecular Signatures Database (MSigDB) hallmark gene set collection. *Cell Syst* (2015) 1:417–25. doi:10.1016/j.cels.2015.12.004
34. Subramanian A, Tamayo P, Mootha VK, Mukherjee S, Ebert BL, Gillette MA, et al. Gene set enrichment analysis: a knowledge-based approach for interpreting genome-wide expression profiles. *Proc Natl Acad Sci U S A* (2005) 102:15545–50. doi:10.1073/pnas.0506580102
35. Rucinski M, Ziolkowska A, Szyszka M, Hochol A, Malendowicz LK. Evidence suggesting that ghrelin *O*-acyl transferase inhibitor acts at the hypothalamus to inhibit hypothalamo-pituitary-adrenocortical axis function in the rat. *Peptides* (2012) 35:149–59. doi:10.1016/j.peptides.2012.04.007
36. Trejter M, Hochol A, Tyczewska M, Ziolkowska A, Jopek K, Szyszka M, et al. Visinin-like peptide 1 in adrenal gland of the rat. Gene expression

and its hormonal control. *Peptides* (2015) 63:22–9. doi:10.1016/j.peptides.2014.10.017

37. Szyszka M, Paschke L, Tyczewska M, Rucinski M, Grabowska P, Malendowicz LK. Lack of expression of preproorexin and orexin receptors genes in human normal and prostate cancer cell lines. *Folia Histochem Cytobiol* (2015) 53:333–41. doi:10.5603/fhc.a2015.0035
38. Kitay JI, Coyne MD, Swygert NH. Adrenal 5 alpha-reductase activity in the rat: effects of gonadectomy: some cofactor and substrate requirements. *Proc Soc Exp Biol Med* (1971) 137:229–32. doi:10.3181/00379727-137-35550
39. Colby HD, Kitay JI. Effects of gonadal hormones on adrenal steroid metabolism in vitro. *Steroids* (1972) 20:143–57. doi:10.1016/0039-128X(72)90066-9
40. Malendowicz LK. Sex differences in adrenocortical structure and function. III. The effects of postpubertal gonadectomy and gonadal hormone replacement on adrenal cholesterol sidechain cleavage activity and on steroids biosynthesis by rat adrenal homogenates. *Endokrinologie* (1976) 67:26–35.
41. Malendowicz LK, Fichna P. Sex differences in adrenocortical structure and function. IV. Effects of postpubertal gonadectomy and sex hormones on adrenal steroid 5alpha-reductase activity in the rat. *Endokrinologie* (1978) 72:36–42.
42. Lephart ED, Simpson ER, Trzeciak WH. Rat adrenal 5 alpha-reductase mRNA content and enzyme activity are sex hormone dependent. *J Mol Endocrinol* (1991) 6:163–70. doi:10.1677/jme.0.0060163
43. Yokoi H, Tsuruo Y, Ishimura K. Steroid 5alpha-reductase type 1 immunolocalized in the rat peripheral nervous system and paraganglia. *Histochem J* (1998) 30:731–9. doi:10.1023/A:1003482512567
44. Johren O, Neidert SJ, Kummer M, Dendorfer A, Dominiak P. Prepro-orexin and orexin receptor mRNAs are differentially expressed in peripheral tissues of male and female rats. *Endocrinology* (2001) 142:3324–31. doi:10.1210/en.142.8.3324
45. Johren O, Bruggemann N, Dendorfer A, Dominiak P. Gonadal steroids differentially regulate the messenger ribonucleic acid expression of pituitary orexin type 1 receptors and adrenal orexin type 2 receptors. *Endocrinology* (2003) 144:1219–25. doi:10.1210/en.2002-0030
46. Johren O, Bruggemann N, Dominiak P. Orexins (hypocretins) and adrenal function. *Horm Metab Res* (2004) 36:370–5. doi:10.1055/s-2004-814569
47. Coleman RD, Chen YM, Alfinslater RB. Cholesterol metabolism in gonadectomized rats. *Circ Res* (1958) 6:172–7. doi:10.1161/01.RES.6.2.172
48. Malendowicz LK, Mlynarczyk W. Sex differences in adrenocortical structure and function. X. Lipid and corticosterone in the rat adrenal as affected by gonadectomy and testosterone or estradiol replacement. *Endokrinologie* (1982) 79:292–300.
49. Duda T, Waliszewska A, Trzeciak WH, Malendowicz LK. Sex differences in adrenocortical structure and function. XX. The effects of gonadectomy and testosterone or estradiol replacement on cholesterol content and distribution in the gland. *J Steroid Biochem* (1985) 23:577–81. doi:10.1016/0022-4731(85)90007-X
50. Goldstein JL, Brown MS. Regulation of the mevalonate pathway. *Nature* (1990) 343:425–30. doi:10.1038/343425a0
51. Brown MS, Goldstein JL. Lipoprotein receptors: therapeutic implications. *J Hypertens* (1990) 8(Suppl):S33–5; discussion S35–6. doi:10.1097/00004872-199003001-00007
52. Popplewell PY, Azhar S. Effects of aging on cholesterol content and cholesterol-metabolizing enzymes in the rat adrenal gland. *Endocrinology* (1987) 121:64–73. doi:10.1210/endo-121-1-64
53. Friesen JA, Rodwell VW. The 3-hydroxy-3-methylglutaryl coenzyme-A (HMG-CoA) reductases. *Genome Biol* (2004) 5:248. doi:10.1186/gb-2004-5-11-248
54. Trzeciak WH, Malendowicz LK. Sex differences in adrenocortical structure and function. VII. Adrenal sterol ester hydrolase activity in the rat and its dependence on gonadal hormones. *Horm Metab Res* (1981) 13:519–22. doi:10.1055/s-2007-1019321
55. Muller RE, Wotiz HH. Estrogen-binding protein in mouse and rat adrenal glands. *J Biol Chem* (1978) 253:740–5.
56. Calandra RS, Naess O, Purvis K, Attramadal A, Djoseland O, Hansson V. Oestrogen receptors in the rat adrenal gland. *J Steroid Biochem* (1978) 9:957–62. doi:10.1016/0022-4731(78)90057-2
57. Calandra RS, Purvis K, Naess O, Attramadal A, Djoseland O, Hansson V. Androgen receptors in the rat adrenal gland. *J Steroid Biochem* (1978) 9:1009–15. doi:10.1016/0022-4731(78)90057-2
58. Calandra RS, Luthy I, Finocchiaro L, Terrab RC. Influence of sex and gonadectomy on sex steroid receptors in rat adrenal gland. *J Steroid Biochem* (1980) 13:1331–5. doi:10.1016/0022-4731(80)90094-1
59. Bentvelsen FM, McPhaul MJ, Wilson CM, Wilson JD, George FW. Regulation of immunoreactive androgen receptor in the adrenal gland of the adult rat. *Endocrinology* (1996) 137:2659–63. doi:10.1210/en.137.7.2659
60. van Lier E, Carriquiry M, Meikle A. Sex steroid modulation of cortisol secretion in sheep. *Animal* (2014) 8:960–7. doi:10.1017/S1751731114000780
61. Schutze S, Wiegmann K, Machleidt T, Kronke M. TNF-induced activation of NF-kappa B. *Immunobiology* (1995) 193:193–203. doi:10.1016/S0171-2985(11)80543-7
62. Aggarwal BB. Signalling pathways of the TNF superfamily: a double-edged sword. *Nat Rev Immunol* (2003) 3:745–56. doi:10.1038/nri1184
63. Wajant H, Pfizenmaier K, Scheurich P. Tumor necrosis factor signaling. *Cell Death Differ* (2003) 10:45–65. doi:10.1038/sj.cdd.4401189
64. Lesniewska B, Miskowiak B, Nowak M, Malendowicz LK. Sex differences in adrenocortical structure and function. XXVII. The effect of ether stress on ACTH and corticosterone in intact, gonadectomized, and testosterone- or estradiol-replaced rats. *Res Exp Med (Berl)* (1990) 190:95–103. doi:10.1007/PL00020011
65. Provencher PH, Tremblay Y, Belanger A. Effects of C19 steroids on adrenal steroidogenic enzyme activities and their mRNA levels in guinea-pig fasciculata-glomerulosa cells in primary culture. *J Endocrinol* (1992) 132:269–76. doi:10.1677/joe.0.1320269
66. Nowak KW, Neri G, Nussdorfer GG, Malendowicz LK. Effects of sex hormones on the steroidogenic activity of dispersed adrenocortical cells of the rat adrenal cortex. *Life Sci* (1995) 57:833–7. doi:10.1016/0024-3205(95)02015-B
67. Rossi R, Zatelli MC, Valentini A, Cavazzini P, Fallo F, del Senno L, et al. Evidence for androgen receptor gene expression and growth inhibitory effect of dihydrotestosterone on human adrenocortical cells. *J Endocrinol* (1998) 159:373–80. doi:10.1677/joe.0.1590373
68. Yanes LL, Romero DG. Dihydrotestosterone stimulates aldosterone secretion by H295R human adrenocortical cells. *Mol Cell Endocrinol* (2009) 303:50–6. doi:10.1016/j.mce.2008.12.020
69. Caroccia B, Seccia TM, Campos AG, Gioco F, Kuppusamy M, Ceolotto G, et al. GPER-1 and estrogen receptor-beta ligands modulate aldosterone synthesis. *Endocrinology* (2014) 155:4296–304. doi:10.1210/en.2014-1416
70. Yoshimura S, Sakamoto S, Kudo H, Sassa S, Kumai A, Okamoto R. Sex-differences in adrenocortical responsiveness during development in rats. *Steroids* (2003) 68:439–45. doi:10.1016/S0039-128X(03)00045-X

5

Phase-Dependent Shifting of the Adrenal Clock by Acute Stress-Induced ACTH

William C. Engeland, J. Marina Yoder, Carley A. Karsten and Paulo Kofuji*

Department of Neuroscience, University of Minnesota, Minneapolis, MN, USA

***Correspondence:**
William C. Engeland
engel002@.umn.edu

The adrenal cortex has a molecular clock that generates circadian rhythms in glucocorticoid production, yet it is unclear how the clock responds to acute stress. We hypothesized that stress-induced ACTH provides a signal that phase shifts the adrenal clock. To assess whether acute stress phase shifts the adrenal clock *in vivo* in a phase-dependent manner, mPER2:LUC mice on a 12:12-h light:dark cycle underwent restraint stress for 15 min or no stress at zeitgeber time (ZT) 2 (early subjective day) or at ZT16 (early subjective night). Adrenal explants from mice stressed at ZT2 showed mPER2:LUC rhythms that were phase-advanced by ~2 h, whereas adrenals from mice stressed at ZT16 showed rhythms that were phase-delayed by ~2 h. The biphasic response was also observed in mice injected subcutaneously either with saline or with ACTH at ZT2 or ZT16. Blockade of the ACTH response with the glucocorticoid, dexamethasone, prevented restraint stress-induced phase shifts in the mPER2:LUC rhythm both at ZT2 and at ZT16. The finding that acute stress results in a phase-dependent shift in the adrenal mPER2:LUC rhythm that can be blocked by dexamethasone indicates that stress-induced effectors, including ACTH, act to phase shift the adrenal clock rhythm.

Keywords: adrenal clock, acute stress, restraint stress, dexamethasone, ACTH, circadian, mPER2:LUC

INTRODUCTION

The suprachiasmatic nucleus (SCN) is responsible for generating circadian rhythms in mammals (1). The molecular clock that underlies SCN rhythmicity is found in most mammalian cells (2), providing a peripheral clock mechanism that subserves tissue-specific functional rhythms (3). A fundamental question is how peripheral clocks are entrained to light and to other environmental signals (4). The adrenal cortex expresses a clock that can control the corticosterone rhythm by inducing rhythmic expression of the clock-controlled gene, steroidogenic acute regulatory (StAR) protein (5). Knockdown of the adrenal clock results in a corticosterone rhythm with reduced amplitude under constant dark, yet the rhythm is maintained under light–dark (LD) conditions (5). These results argue for redundancy in controlling corticosterone rhythms, with both clock-dependent and clock-independent mechanisms.

Our results using the mPER2:LUC mouse have shown that the adrenal clock can be reset *in vitro* by ACTH in a phase-dependent manner (6). The *in vitro* experiments showed that ACTH produced a phase delay when administered at a circadian time analogous to subjective night, but no phase shift at the circadian time representing subjective day. To examine whether stress is capable of phase-shifting the adrenal clock *in vivo*, we examined the adrenal clock in mPER2:LUC mice after exposure to chronic subordinate stress (7). The chronic subordinate stress model consisted of a brief period

(10 min or less) of daily physical contact between subordinate and dominant mice at early subjective day [zeitgeber time (ZT) 3] followed by cohabitation for the remainder of the 24-h period. We found that a single exposure to subordination stress produced a phase advance in the adrenal mPER2:LUC rhythm that was maintained after 14 days of chronic subordinate stress. However, it is unclear (1) whether the effect of acute stress on the adrenal clock is dependent on the phase of the circadian rhythm and (2) whether the phase shift depends on the release of ACTH. Using acute stress to activate the hypothalamic–pituitary–adrenal (HPA) axis in mPER2:LUC mice, experiments were done to determine whether stress shifts the phase of the adrenal clock in a phase-dependent fashion and whether the adrenal response occurs after blockade of ACTH release.

MATERIALS AND METHODS

Animals

Homozygous male mPER2:LUC mice (8) (3–6 months old) bred in-house were housed on a 12:12-h LD cycle (lights on at 0600 hours). Animals were maintained and cared for in accordance with the NIH Guide for the Care and Use of Laboratory Animals. Experimental procedures were approved by the University of Minnesota Animal Care and Use Committee.

Bioluminescence

Animals were killed by decapitation 3.5–4.0 h before lights out (at ZT 8–8.5). Adrenals were rapidly excised and placed in cold Hank's balanced salt solution. Cleaned and hemisected adrenals were placed on Millicell organotypic inserts (PICMORG50, 30 mm hydrophilic PTFE membrane, 0.4 μm pore size) in a 35 mm Petri dish with 1.5 ml of warmed culture media (Dulbecco's Modified Eagle media w/o Phenol Red) supplemented with luciferin and penicillin/streptomycin, as described previously (6, 8). Dishes were sealed with circular glass coverslips and silicon grease. Cultures were maintained at 36°C, and bioluminescence was measured using photomultiplier tubes in an Actimetrics Lumicycle.

Experiments

Experiment 1a

Male mPER2:LUC mice (n = 7/group) housed under a 12:12 L:D cycle underwent a 15-min restraint stress or no stress at ZT2. Mice were restrained by being placed in 50 ml conical tubes (Fisher Scientific, cat. # 05-539-13) with air holes drilled in tube bottoms to permit respiration. Mice were returned to their home cages following restraint and killed by decapitation at ZT8. Adrenals were processed for monitoring rhythms in bioluminescence.

Experiment 1b

Male mPER2:LUC mice (n = 6/group) housed under a 12:12 L:D cycle underwent a 15-min restraint stress or no stress at ZT16; at ZT16 all procedures were performed under dim red light. Mice were returned to their home cages following restraint and killed by decapitation on the next day at ZT8. Adrenals were processed for monitoring rhythms in bioluminescence.

Experiment 2a

Male mPER2:LUC mice (n = 5–6/group) housed under a 12:12 L:D cycle were injected with saline (100 μl sc; vehicle for ACTH) or ACTH (0.3 μg/100 μl sc) or underwent no stress at ZT2. Mice were returned to their home cages following injection and killed by decapitation at ZT8. Adrenals were processed for monitoring rhythms in bioluminescence.

Experiment 2b

Male mPER2:LUC mice (n = 5/group) housed under a 12:12 L:D cycle were injected with saline (100 μl sc; vehicle for ACTH) or ACTH (0.3 μg/100 μl sc) or no stress at ZT16 under dim red light. Mice were returned to their home cages following restraint and killed by decapitation on the next day at ZT8. Adrenals were processed for monitoring rhythms in bioluminescence.

Experiment 3

Male mPER2:LUC mice (n = 4–5/group) were pretreated with dexamethasone [Dexamethasone phosphate (Bimeda Inc.); 250 μg/kg BW sc] or needle puncture only as a control at ZT14 and underwent restraint stress for 15 min or no stress at ZT16. Mice were decapitated immediately following restraint, and trunk blood was collected for hormone assay. Plasma ACTH and corticosterone were measured by RIA, as described previously (9).

Experiment 4a

Male mPER2:LUC mice (n = 4–5/group) were pretreated with dexamethasone (250 μg/kg BW sc) or needle puncture at ZT1 and underwent restraint stress for 15 min or no stress at ZT3. For experiment 4, the dexamethasone treatment was given at ZT1, instead of ZT0, to avoid manipulation of mice at light onset. To maintain a 2-h exposure to dexamethasone before stress, acute restraint was initiated at ZT3. Mice were returned to their home cages following restraint and killed by decapitation at ZT8. Adrenals were processed for monitoring rhythms in bioluminescence.

Experiment 4b

Male mPER2:LUC mice (n = 4–5/group) were pretreated with dexamethasone (250 μg/kg BW sc) or needle puncture at ZT14 and underwent restraint stress for 15 min or no stress at ZT16. Mice were returned to their home cages following restraint and killed by decapitation the next day at ZT8. Adrenals were processed for monitoring rhythms in bioluminescence.

Data Analysis

Data from the first day of recording were omitted from analysis due to transient bioluminescent activity (10). The remaining data were smoothed and detrended using a 2- and 24-h running average, baseline subtracted, and fit to a damped sine wave using Lumicycle Analysis software (Actimetrics). Only tissue showing rhythms with a goodness of fit >85% were accepted. To assess changes in the adrenal clock rhythm induced by *in vivo* manipulations, phase was determined from the peak measured on the second day of incubation, and period was calculated using data from two cycles spanning the second and third days of incubation.

Statistical Analysis

Data are presented as means ± SEM. Statistical differences were determined using one-way ANOVA (using Dunnett's correction for *post hoc* analysis), two-way ANOVA (using Bonferroni's correction for *post hoc* analysis), or unpaired Student's *t*-test, where appropriate, using Prism software (GraphPad). Differences were considered significant if $p < 0.05$.

RESULTS

A schematic showing the time line of treatments for each experiment as shown in **Figure 1**. Experiment 1 was done to determine if acute restraint stress results in a phase-dependent shift in the adrenal clock rhythm. Representative examples of mPER2:LUC bioluminescent activity are shown for adrenals collected from non-stressed mice and mice exposed to a 15-min restraint stress at ZT2 (**Figure 2A**) or at ZT16 (**Figure 2B**). Adrenals from mice that underwent a 15-min restraint stress at ZT2 showed a phase advance in the mPER2:LUC rhythm compared with adrenals from non-stressed (control) mice (**Figure 3A**), whereas adrenal rhythms from mice that were stressed at ZT16 showed a phase delay compared with controls (**Figure 3B**). Acute restraint stress had no effect on the period of the rhythm at ZT2 (CTRL: 23.25 ± 0.11; RESTRAINT: 23.32 ± 0.23) or at ZT16 (CTRL: 23.37 ± 0.08; RESTRAINT: 22.78 ± 0.23).

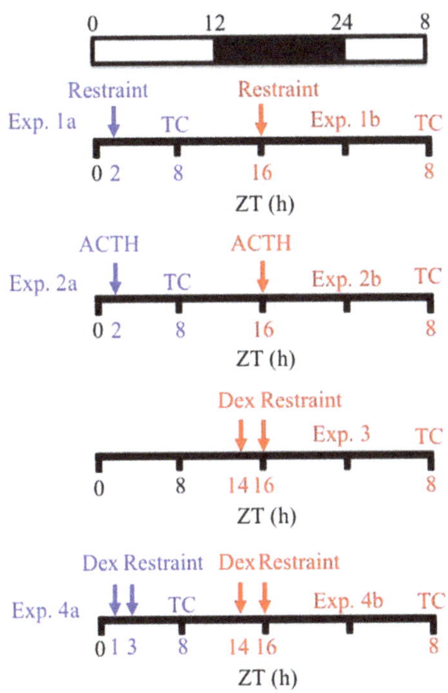

FIGURE 1 | Schematic showing the time-line for each experiment relative to zeitgeber time (ZT). Mice were on a 12:12-h LD cycle (0600:1800 hours) with lights on at ZT0 and lights off at ZT12. Experimental manipulations were done in early subjective day (denoted by blue font) or early subjective night (denoted by red font). Dex, dexamethasone; TC, time of tissue collection.

Two approaches were used to examine whether stress-induced ACTH contributed to stress-induced phase-dependent shifts in the adrenal mPER2:LUC rhythm. In experiment 2, mice were injected with a supramaximal dose of ACTH [100 μl, 3.0 μg/kg BW; Ref. (9)] and compared with mice injected with saline (100 μl) or no injection (Control) at ZT2 or ZT16. Adrenals from mice injected with saline at ZT2 showed a phase advance in the mPER2:LUC rhythm compared with adrenals from Control mice (**Figure 4A**), whereas rhythms from adrenals from mice injected with saline or ACTH at ZT16 showed a phase delay compared with Control mice (**Figure 4B**). No differences were observed between saline and ACTH at ZT2 or ZT16, indicating that the handling and injection stress was sufficient to shift the adrenal mPER2:LUC rhythm in a phase-dependent fashion. Neither injection of saline nor ACTH had an effect on the period of the rhythm at ZT2 (CTRL: 23.60 ± 0.18; saline: 23.58 ± 0.23; ACTH: 22.88 ± 0.49) or at ZT16 (CTRL: 22.12 ± 0.10; saline: 22.48 ± 0.28; ACTH: 22.32 ± 0.25).

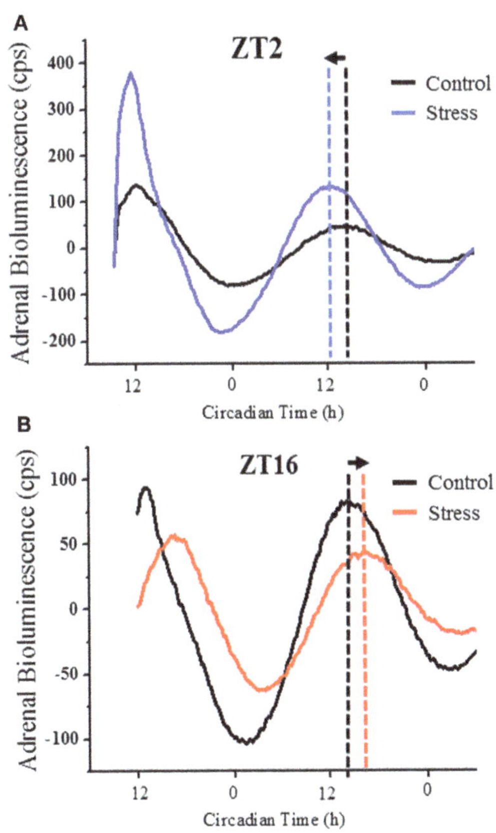

FIGURE 2 | Representative experiment showing the mPER2:LUC rhythm after detrending and baseline subtraction; adrenal explants were collected from control mice (black line) and mice exposed to acute (15 min) restraint stress at ZT2 (blue line) (A) or at ZT16 (red line) (B). The peak in adrenal PER2 bioluminescence is phase-advanced by ~2 h following restraint stress at ZT2 **(A)** and phase-delayed by ~2 h following restraint stress at ZT16 **(B)**. The vertical dashed lines identify the time of the peak phase in the mPER2:LUC rhythm. Adrenal bioluminescence is reported as counts per second (cps).

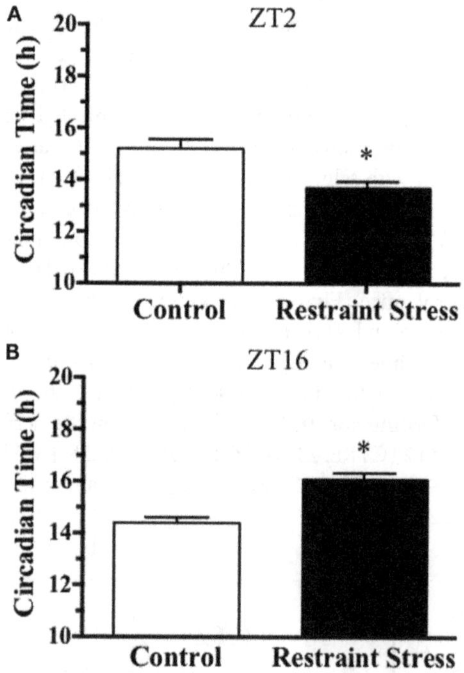

FIGURE 3 | Effect of acute (15 min) restraint stress at ZT2 (A) and at ZT16 (B) on the peak phase of the *in vitro* adrenal mPER2:LUC rhythm. Values represent means ± SEM (n = 6–7/group). Based on unpaired Student's *t*-test, $^*p < 0.05$ vs. Control at ZT2 and ZT16.

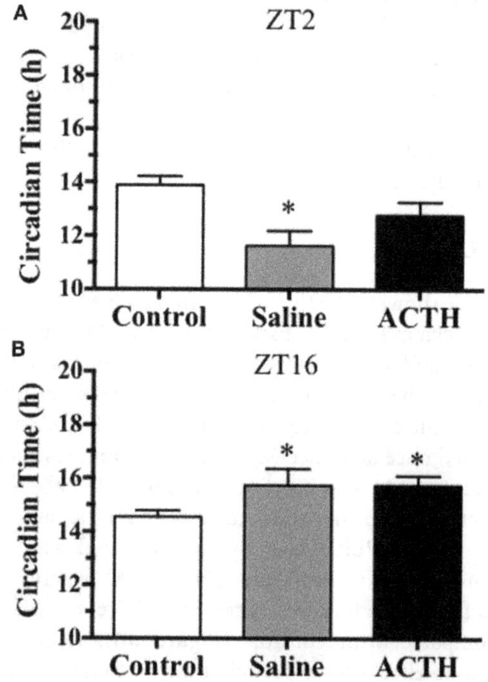

FIGURE 4 | Effect of injection of ACTH or saline or no treatment (Control) at ZT2 (A) and at ZT16 (B) on the peak phase of the *in vitro* adrenal mPER2:LUC rhythm. Values represent means ± SEM (n = 5–6/group). Based on one-way ANOVA (using Dunnett's correction for *post hoc* analysis), $^*p < 0.05$ vs. Control at ZT2 and ZT16.

To further examine a possible role for stress-induced ACTH in the phase-dependent shift of the mPER2:LUC rhythm, dexamethasone was used to block ACTH release induced by restraint stress. In experiment 3, mice were pretreated with dexamethasone 2 h before undergoing restraint stress at ZT16. Plasma ACTH and corticosterone increased at 15 min after restraint in mice that were not treated with dexamethasone. In contrast, dexamethasone pretreatment blocked the plasma ACTH and corticosterone response to restraint (**Figure 5**). In experiment 4, dexamethasone was used to block ACTH 2 h prior to restraint at ZT3 or at ZT16, and adrenals were collected to measure changes in the mPER2:LUC rhythm *in vitro*. Results showed that dexamethasone prevented both the phase advance in the mPER2:LUC rhythm induced by restraint stress at ZT3 (**Figure 6A**) and the phase delay induced by restraint stress at ZT16 (**Figure 6B**), suggesting that increased ACTH induced by restraint stress contributes to the phase-dependent shift in the mPER2:LUC rhythm. Although the period of the mPER2:LUC rhythm was not affected by restraint stress in the absence of dexamethasone, the period was lengthened in adrenals from mice that underwent dexamethasone treatment followed by stress at ZT3 (**Figure 7A**) and ZT16 (**Figure 7B**).

DISCUSSION

Experiments were done to determine whether acute stress shifts the phase of the adrenal clock in a phase-dependent manner and whether the adrenal response is dependent on stress-induced release of ACTH. The present results show that a single 15-min restraint stress at ZT2 produced an ~2-h phase advance in the mPER2:LUC rhythm. In marked contrast, the same manipulation performed at ZT16 produced an ~2-h phase delay. To examine whether increased ACTH was responsible for the phase-dependent shift, we injected ACTH at ZT2 or at ZT16 to mimic restraint stress-induced ACTH. Injection stress was sufficient to phase shift the adrenal mPER2:LUC rhythm in a phase-dependent manner, yet responses to ACTH injection were comparable to saline injection. To assess a possible role for ACTH more clearly, mice were treated with dexamethasone to inhibit restraint stress-induced ACTH; results showed that dexamethasone blocked the phase-dependent shift in the mPER2:LUC rhythm. Taken together, these experiments show that acute stress is capable of producing a biphasic shift in the adrenal mPER2:LUC rhythm that can be blocked by dexamethasone, suggesting that ACTH is a necessary component in stress-induced alterations in adrenal clock timing.

Our previous work showed that a single exposure to subordination stress at early subjective day (ZT3) followed by cohabitation for the remainder of the day produced an ~2-h phase advance in the adrenal mPER2:LUC rhythm in male mice (7). By using a single acute restraint or injection stress, the present experiments were designed to allow more precise control of the timing of stress exposure. Similar to the response to single subordination stress, acute restraint or injection stress at early subjective day (ZT2–3) phase-advanced the adrenal mPER2:LUC rhythm. In

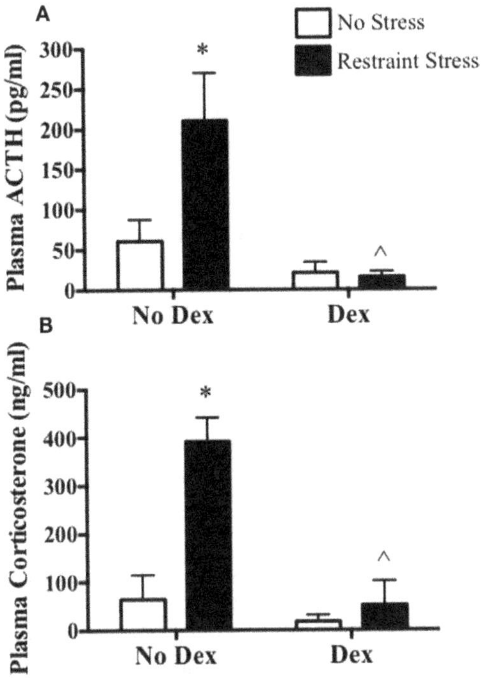

FIGURE 5 | Effect of dexamethasone blockade on restraint stress-induced plasma ACTH (A) and corticosterone (B) at ZT16 in mPER2:LUC mice. Values represent means ± SEM (n = 4–5/group). Based on two-way ANOVA (using Bonferroni's correction for *post hoc* analysis), $^{*}p < 0.05$ vs. No Dex-No Stress and $^{\wedge}p < 0.05$ vs. No Dex-Stress.

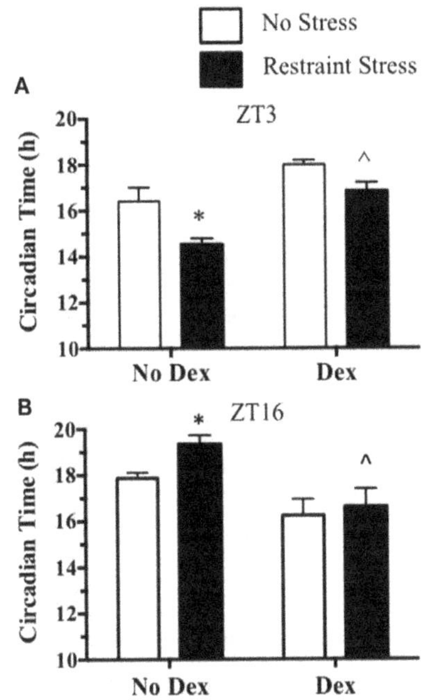

FIGURE 6 | Effect of dexamethasone treatment before restraint stress at ZT3 (A) or at ZT16 (B) on the peak phase of the *in vitro* adrenal mPER2:LUC rhythm. Values represent means ± SEM (n = 4–5/group). Based on two-way ANOVA (using Bonferroni's correction for *post hoc* analysis), $^{*}p < 0.05$ vs. No Dex-No Stress and $^{\wedge}p < 0.05$ vs. No Dex-Stress at ZT3 and ZT16.

addition, when acute stress was applied at early subjective night (ZT16), the adrenal mPER2:LUC rhythm was phase-delayed (**Figures 3** and **4**). Others have examined whether repeated stress results in a phase-dependent effect on the adrenal mPER2:LUC rhythm (11). A 2-h exposure to subordination stress in early subjective day for 3 weeks resulted in a phase advance in the adrenal rhythm, but repeated subordination stress in early subjective night did not produce a phase shift in the adrenal rhythm. The effect of repeated stress at early subjective day confirmed our previous work showing that the phase advance in the adrenal mPER2:LUC rhythm was maintained after chronic (14-day) subordination stress, indicating that changes in the timing of the adrenal clock did not habituate to chronic stress applied at ZT3 (7). Since exposure to a single acute stressor, but not repeated exposure to stress, results in a biphasic effect on the adrenal mPER2:LUC rhythm, it is possible that the phase delay produced by acute stress in early subjective night habituates to repeated exposure to stress. Additional experiments are required to test this possibility.

The observation that acute restraint stress shifts the phase of the adrenal mPER2:LUC rhythm led to experiments assessing whether ACTH contributed to the response. This possibility was based in part on our previous study showing that ACTH *in vitro* induced a phase shift of adrenal mPER2:LUC rhythm (6). The 2-h phase delay of the mPER2:LUC rhythm following acute restraint stress during the dark period (ZT16) parallels the phase-dependent delay produced by ACTH *in vitro*. In contrast, the phase advances in the mPER2:LUC rhythm observed after restraint stress during the light period (ZT2) was not mimicked by ACTH *in vitro* (6). By injecting ACTH *in vivo*, experiments were done to assess the effect of ACTH directly on the phase-dependent response. Results showed that ACTH injection was comparable to saline injection in changing the phase of the adrenal mPER2:LUC rhythm, suggesting that injection stress alone was sufficient for producing a phase-dependent shift (**Figure 4**). To examine whether ACTH responses to acute stress were required for the phase shift, mice were treated with dexamethasone, a synthetic glucocorticoid, to block ACTH secretion. This approach takes advantage of the known effect of dexamethasone to act at the anterior pituitary as a negative feedback signal to inhibit ACTH release (12). Pretreatment with a low dose (250 μg/kg) of dexamethasone, similar to the dose used to block stress-induced ACTH in rats (9, 13), effectively blocked both restraint stress-induced plasma ACTH and corticosterone (**Figure 5**). In addition, dexamethasone pretreatment prevented both the phase advance produced by restraint stress at ZT3 and the phase delay produced by restraint stress at ZT16 (**Figure 6**). These findings show that acute stress shifts the phase of the adrenal clock rhythm *in vivo* and suggest that the response results at least in part from increased plasma ACTH.

Activation of glucocorticoid receptors by dexamethasone can entrain other peripheral clocks (14, 15). Thus, in addition to ACTH blockade, it is possible that the activation of glucocorticoid receptors in the adrenal (16) could be involved in

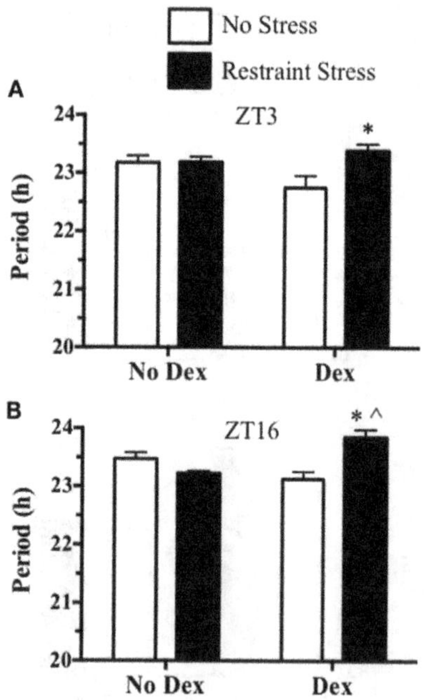

FIGURE 7 | Effect of dexamethasone treatment before restraint stress at ZT3 (A) or at ZT16 (B) on the period of the *in vitro* adrenal mPER2:LUC rhythm. Values represent means ± SEM (n = 4–5/group). Based on two-way ANOVA (using Bonferroni's correction for *post hoc* analysis), *p < 0.05 vs. Dex-No Stress and ^p < 0.05 vs. No Dex-Stress at ZT3 and ZT16.

phase-dependent changes in the adrenal mPER2:LUC rhythm. Although the high doses (10 mg/kg) of dexamethasone result in phase-dependent shifts in the body temperature rhythm, lower doses like those used in the present study have no effect (17). By evaluating the effects of dexamethasone alone on the adrenal mPER2:LUC rhythm, we were unable to find differences in peak phases between non-stress groups treated with or without dexamethasone (**Figure 6**). However, whereas changes in the period were not observed after stress or dexamethasone alone, dexamethasone combined with stress at ZT3 and ZT16 prolonged the period of the mPER2:LUC rhythm (**Figure 7**). Additional experiments are necessary to determine whether the mechanism for period lengthening includes activation of adrenal glucocorticoid receptors.

In non-photic entrainment, SCN-controlled rhythms, such as locomotor activity, shift in response to acute arousal (18). Non-photic entrainment by arousal is more prevalent during subjective day (19) and is characterized by a phase advance (20). Since we observed a phase advance in the adrenal mPER2:LUC rhythm following stress at ZT2, it is possible that the adrenal response is dependent on a change in SCN activity. Although we did not assess SCN mPER2:LUC activity, others have shown that repeated subordination stress at ZT1–3 does not affect the phase of the SCN clock gene rhythm (11). Moreover, acute subordinate stress during subjective night in rats does not shift the phase of activity or temperature rhythms, reflections of SCN activity, suggesting that acute stress during the active period acts independently of the SCN (19, 21). Since mice were housed under a 12:12-h LD cycle in the present study, it is likely that photic entrainment predominates in maintaining the phase of the SCN clock over stress-related stimuli. The biphasic stress-induced phase shifts of the adrenal clock may not result from non-photic entrainment of the SCN but instead may represent a direct phase-dependent response of the adrenal clock to stress.

The mechanism for a phase-dependent response of the adrenal clock rhythm to stress is unclear. The ability to block the phase-resetting induced by stress with dexamethasone implicates ACTH. Since the magnitude of the ACTH response to stress differs diurnally (22), exposure to different levels of ACTH may contribute to phase dependency. However, our *in vitro* data showed that the phase response was not dependent on the magnitude of the ACTH stimulus, since high concentrations of ACTH administered at early CTs were ineffective in phase-shifting the mPER2:LUC rhythm (6). It is likely that factors, in addition to ACTH, play a role. Since increases in adrenal sympathetic activity synergize with ACTH to increase adrenal steroidogenic responses (23) and also increase adrenal Per expression (24), sympathetic neural input may be involved in altering timing of the adrenal clock. The adrenal cortex includes sympathetic innervation by vasoactive intestinal peptide (VIP)-ergic fibers (25). Corticosterone rhythms are dampened in constitutive VIP knockout (26, 27) and in VIP receptor knockout mice (28, 29), supporting the possibility that stress-induced VIPergic activity could complement ACTH in phase-shifting the adrenal clock. As shown for light-induced phase shifts of the SCN clock (30), phase-shifting of the adrenal clock may result from stress-induced increases in adrenal PER that vary with the time of stress to differentially change PER negative feedback on the molecular clock. Additional studies are required to assess this possibility.

The present results show that acute stress produces a shift in the adrenal clock gene rhythm that is phase-dependent. The physiological importance of this observation stems in large part from the role of the adrenal clock in regulating glucocorticoid secretion. Rhythms in plasma glucocorticoids are paralleled by rhythms in adrenal sensitivity to ACTH (9, 22, 31), and the adrenal clock is thought to control rhythmic steroidogenesis by gating sensitivity to ACTH (32). Since the adrenal clock controls circadian rhythms in glucocorticoid production (5), it will be important to determine whether acute stress also shifts the phase of the plasma glucocorticoid rhythm in a phase-dependent manner. Since glucocorticoid rhythms entrain other peripheral clocks (14, 33), altered glucocorticoid rhythms produced by stress-induced phase shifts could have effects on metabolic, hemodynamic, and cognitive function.

AUTHOR CONTRIBUTIONS

WE designed the experiments, assisted in performing the experiments, analyzed the results, wrote the initial draft of the manuscript, and completed the final edited version of the manuscript. JY and CK assisted in designing and performing the experiments, analyzing the results, and editing the manuscript. PK assisted in designing the experiments, performing the experiments, and editing the manuscript.

ACKNOWLEDGMENTS

The authors thank Sofiya Hupalo, Shubhendru Mishra, and Logan Massman, undergraduate students, who provided technical assistance.

FUNDING

This work was supported in part by NSF grant IOS1025119, NIH grant RO3NS094419, the Wallin Discovery Fund, and a grant-in-aid from the University of Minnesota.

REFERENCES

1. Mohawk JA, Green CB, Takahashi JS. Central and peripheral circadian clocks in mammals. *Annu Rev Neurosci* (2012) 35:445–62. doi:10.1146/annurev-neuro-060909-153128
2. Dibner C, Schibler U, Albrecht U. The mammalian circadian timing system: organization and coordination of central and peripheral clocks. *Annu Rev Physiol* (2010) 72:517–49. doi:10.1146/annurev-physiol-021909-135821
3. Sahar S, Sassone-Corsi P. Regulation of metabolism: the circadian clock dictates the time. *Trends Endocrinol Metab* (2012) 23:1–8. doi:10.1016/j.tem.2011.10.005
4. Mahoney CE, Brewer D, Costello MK, Brewer JM, Bittman EL. Lateralization of the central circadian pacemaker output: a test of neural control of peripheral oscillator phase. *Am J Physiol Regul Integr Comp Physiol* (2010) 299:R751–61. doi:10.1152/ajpregu.00746.2009
5. Son GH, Chung S, Choe HK, Kim H-D, Baik S-M, Lee H, et al. Adrenal peripheral clock controls the autonomous circadian rhythm of glucocorticoid by causing rhythmic steroid production. *Proc Natl Acad Sci U S A* (2008) 105:20970–5. doi:10.1073/pnas.0806962106
6. Yoder JM, Brandeland M, Engeland WC. Phase-dependent resetting of the adrenal clock by ACTH in vitro. *Am J Physiol Regul Integr Comp Physiol* (2014) 306:387–93. doi:10.1152/ajpregu.00519.2013
7. Razzoli M, Karsten C, Yoder JM, Bartolomucci A, Engeland WC. Chronic subordination stress phase advances adrenal and anterior pituitary clock gene rhythms. *Am J Physiol Regul Integr Comp Physiol* (2014) 307:R198–205. doi:10.1152/ajpregu.00101.2014
8. Yoo SH, Yamazaki S, Lowrey PL, Shimomura K, Ko CH, Buhr ED, et al. PERIOD2::LUCIFERASE real-time reporting of circadian dynamics reveals persistent circadian oscillations in mouse peripheral tissues. *Proc Natl Acad Sci U S A* (2004) 101:5339–46. doi:10.1073/pnas.0308709101
9. Ulrich-Lai YM, Arnhold MM, Engeland WC. Adrenal splanchnic innervation contributes to the diurnal rhythm of plasma corticosterone in rats by modulating adrenal sensitivity to ACTH. *Am J Physiol Regul Integr Comp Physiol* (2006) 290:R1128–35. doi:10.1152/ajpregu.00042.2003
10. Davidson AJ, Castanon-Cervantes O, Leise TL, Molyneux PC, Harrington ME. Visualizing jet lag in the mouse suprachiasmatic nucleus and peripheral circadian timing system. *Eur J Neurosci* (2009) 29:171–80. doi:10.1111/j.1460-9568.2008.06534.x
11. Bartlang MS, Savelyev SA, Johansson AS, Reber SO, Helfrich-Förster C, Lundkvist GB. Repeated psychosocial stress at night, but not day, affects the central molecular clock. *Chronobiol Int* (2014) 31(9):996–1007. doi:10.3109/07420528.2014.940085
12. Bradbury MJ, Akana SF, Dallman MF. Roles of type I and II corticosteroid receptors in regulation of basal activity in the hypothalamo-pituitary-adrenal axis during the diurnal trough and the peak: evidence for a nonadditive effect of combined receptor occupation. *Endocrinology* (1994) 134:1286–96. doi:10.1210/endo.134.3.8119168
13. Engeland WC, Shinsako J, Winget CM, Vernikos-Danellis J, Dallman MF. Circadian patterns of stress-induced ACTH secretion are modified by corticosterone response. *Endocrinology* (1977) 100:138–47. doi:10.1210/endo-100-1-138
14. Balsalobre A, Brown SA, Marcacci L, Tronche F, Kellendonk C, Reichardt HM, et al. Resetting of circadian time in peripheral tissues by glucocorticoid signaling. *Science* (2000) 289:2344–7. doi:10.1126/science.289.5488.2344
15. So AY, Bernal TU, Pillsbury ML, Yamamoto KR, Feldman BJ. Glucocorticoid regulation of the circadian clock modulates glucose homeostasis. *Proc Natl Acad Sci U S A* (2009) 106:17582–7. doi:10.1073/pnas.0909733106
16. Gummow BM, Scheys JO, Cancelli VR, Hammer GD. Reciprocal regulation of a glucocorticoid receptor-steroidogenic factor-1 transcription complex on the Dax-1 promoter by glucocorticoids and adrenocorticotropic hormone in the adrenal cortex. *Mol Endocrinol* (2006) 20:11–23. doi:10.1210/me.2005-0461
17. Horseman ND, Ehret CF. Glucocorticosteroid injection is a circadian zeitgeber in the laboratory rat. *Am J Physiol* (1982) 243:R373–8.
18. Maywood ES, Mrosovsky N. A molecular explanation of interactions between photic and non-photic circadian clock-resetting stimuli. *Brain Res Gene Expr Patterns* (2001) 1:27–31. doi:10.1016/S1567-133X(01)00005-9
19. Mistlberger RE, Antle MC, Webb IC, Jones M, Weinberg J, Pollock MS. Circadian clock resetting by arousal in Syrian hamsters: the role of stress and activity. *Am J Physiol Regul Integr Comp Physiol* (2003) 285:R917–25. doi:10.1152/ajpregu.00222.2003
20. Maywood ES, Mrosovsky N, Field MD, Hastings MH. Rapid down-regulation of mammalian period genes during behavioral resetting of the circadian clock. *Proc Natl Acad Sci U S A* (1999) 96:15211–6. doi:10.1073/pnas.96.26.15211
21. Meerlo P, Hoofdakker RH, Koolhaas JM, Daan S. Stress-induced changes in circadian rhythms of body temperature and activity in rats are not caused by pacemaker changes. *J Biol Rhythms* (1997) 12:80–92. doi:10.1177/074873049701200109
22. Dallman MF, Engeland WC, Rose JC, Wilkinson CW, Shinsako J, Siedenburg F. Nycthemeral rhythm in adrenal responsiveness to ACTH. *Am J Physiol* (1978) 235:R210–8.
23. Ulrich-Lai YM, Engeland WC. Adrenal splanchnic innervation modulates adrenal cortical responses to dehydration stress in rats. *Neuroendocrinology* (2002) 76:79–92. doi:10.1159/000064426
24. Ishida A, Mutoh T, Ueyama T, Bando H, Masubuchi S, Nakahara D, et al. Light activates the adrenal gland: timing of gene expression and glucocorticoid release. *Cell Metab* (2005) 2:297–307. doi:10.1016/j.cmet.2005.09.009
25. Kondo H, Kuramoto H, Fujita T. An immuno-electron-microscopic study of the localization of VIP-like immunoreactivity in the adrenal gland of the rat. *Cell Tissue Res* (1986) 245:531–8. doi:10.1007/BF00218554
26. Loh DH, Abad C, Colwell CS, Waschek JA. Vasoactive intestinal peptide is critical for circadian regulation of glucocorticoids. *Neuroendocrinology* (2008) 88:246–55. doi:10.1159/000140676
27. Loh DH, Dragich JM, Kudo T, Schroeder AM, Nakamura TJ, Waschek JA, et al. Effects of vasoactive intestinal peptide genotype on circadian gene expression in the suprachiasmatic nucleus and peripheral organs. *J Biol Rhythms* (2011) 26:200–9. doi:10.1177/0748730411401740
28. Sheward WJ, Maywood ES, French KL, Horn JM, Hastings MH, Seckl JR, et al. Entrainment to feeding but not to light: circadian phenotype of VPAC2 receptor-null mice. *J Neurosci* (2007) 27:4351–8. doi:10.1523/JNEUROSCI.4843-06.2007
29. Fahrenkrug J, Georg B, Hannibal J, Jørgensen HL. Altered rhythm of adrenal clock genes, StAR and serum corticosterone in VIP receptor 2-deficient mice. *J Mol Neurosci* (2012) 48:584–96. doi:10.1007/s12031-012-9804-7
30. Yan L, Silver R. Resetting the brain clock: time course and localization of mPER1 and mPER2 protein expression in suprachiasmatic nuclei during phase shifts. *Eur J Neurosci* (2004) 19:1105–9. doi:10.1111/j.1460-9568.2004.03189.x
31. Kaneko M, Hiroshige T, Shinsako J, Dallman MF. Diurnal changes in amplification of hormone rhythms in the adrenocortical system. *Am J Physiol* (1980) 239:R309–16.
32. Oster H, Damerow S, Kiessling S, Jakubcakova V, Abraham D, Tian J, et al. The circadian rhythm of glucocorticoids is regulated by a gating mechanism residing in the adrenal cortical clock. *Cell Metab* (2006) 4:163–73. doi:10.1016/j.cmet.2006.07.002

6

ACTH Antagonists

Adrian John Clark[1], Rachel Forfar[2], Mashal Hussain[1], Jeff Jerman[2], Ed McIver[2], Debra Taylor[2] and Li Chan[1]*

[1] Centre for Endocrinology, William Harvey Research Institute, Queen Mary University of London, London, UK, [2] Centre for Therapeutics Discovery, MRC Technology, Stevenage, UK

Correspondence:
Adrian John Clark
a.j.clark@qmul.ac.uk

Adrenocorticotropin (ACTH) acts via a highly selective receptor that is a member of the melanocortin receptor subfamily of type 1 G protein-coupled receptors. The ACTH receptor, also known as the melanocortin 2 receptor (MC2R), is unusual in that it is absolutely dependent on a small accessory protein, melanocortin receptor accessory protein (MRAP) for cell surface expression and function. ACTH is the only known naturally occurring agonist for this receptor. This lack of redundancy and high degree of ligand specificity suggests that antagonism of this receptor could provide a useful therapeutic aid and a potential investigational tool. Clinical situations in which this could be useful include (1) Cushing's disease and ectopic ACTH syndrome – especially while preparing for definitive treatment of a causative tumor, or in refractory cases, or (2) congenital adrenal hyperplasia – as an adjunct to glucocorticoid replacement. A case for antagonism in other clinical situations in which there is ACTH excess can also be made. In this article, we will explore the scientific and clinical case for an ACTH antagonist, and will review the evidence for existing and recently described peptides and modified peptides in this role.

Keywords: adrenocorticotropin hormone, receptor antagonism, Cushing's syndrome, congenital adrenal hyperplasia, high throughput screening, G protein-coupled receptor, receptor modelling, peptide hormone antagonists

INTRODUCTION

The impact of receptor antagonism on modern medicine cannot be understated. Classical examples include the β-blockers in the treatment of hypertension and cardiovascular disease (1) and histamine H2 antagonism in the treatment of gastric hyperacidity (2). Even in the field of endocrinology, receptor antagonism of steroid hormones [e.g., tamoxifen (3), eplerenone (4), and flutamide (5)] and some peptide hormones [e.g., pegvisomant (6) and conivaptan (7)] has had major life-changing impact. The pituitary–adrenal axis is one endocrine axis that when disrupted can be associated with a wide range of pathologies, and yet, despite the fact that it comprises several unique and thus highly targetable components, receptor antagonism has received little attention as a therapeutic approach.

In this article, we will examine the possible benefits of development of an effective antagonist to a key component of this axis, the peptide hormone adrenocorticotropin (ACTH). The disorders in which clinical benefit might be attained will be considered. We will then consider the nature of the target – ACTH and the ACTH receptor complex, and certain unique features before discussing the history of ACTH antagonist research, ending with a description of the current state-of-the art. Initially, a brief description of the pituitary–adrenal axis and its key components is necessary.

THE PITUITARY–ADRENAL AXIS

The corticotroph cells of the anterior pituitary gland are responsible for synthesis and secretion of the 39 residue peptide, ACTH (8). ACTH is derived from a larger precursor protein, pro-opiomelanocortin (POMC), by the action of a specific pro-hormone convertase enzyme (PC1 or PCSK1) (9). In other tissues – for example, the hypothalamus – this precursor is processed differently to produce α-MSH instead of ACTH (10). ACTH is synthesized and secreted by the pituitary in response to tonic control from the hypothalamus – principally in the form of two peptide hormones – corticotrophin-releasing hormone (CRH) and vasopressin (AVP), which in turn are regulated by multiple higher factors including stress (11).

Adrenocorticotropin has a short half-life in the circulation (12) and acts on a highly specific G protein-coupled receptor expressed almost uniquely in the adrenal cortex (13). This receptor, the MC2R is one of five members of the melanocortin receptor family – see **Table 1**. ACTH can activate all five of these receptors, although at physiological circulating levels, the sensitivity of the other receptors is such that they are not activated. Importantly, the naturally occurring agonists for these other receptors – α-MSH, γ-MSH, and possibly β-MSH – have no affinity for the MC2R (14, 15). Thus the MC2R is a highly sensitive and highly specific receptor for ACTH with a major, essential function of stimulating the fasciculata cells of the adrenal cortex to synthesize and secrete glucocorticoid. In addition, ACTH can stimulate zona glomerulosa cells to secrete mineralocorticoid and zona reticularis cells to secrete adrenal androgens.

Glucocorticoid (cortisol in man and most other species, corticosterone in rodents), secreted by the adrenal gland exert a plethora of physiological actions on virtually every cell in the organism. These actions are the result of interaction with the widely expressed glucocorticoid receptor – a nuclear hormone receptor. Glucocorticoid may also activate a second related receptor – the mineralocorticoid receptor – which is less widely expressed. However, the action of the 11 β-hydroxysteroid dehydrogenase type 2 enzyme inactivates glucocorticoid in mineralocorticoid receptor expressing tissues under normal circumstances leaving these receptors responsive to aldosterone (16). From an endocrine perspective, a key role of glucocorticoid is to feedback negatively on the pituitary and hypothalamus to inhibit ACTH secretion (17).

From this brief description, it can be seen that in theory, the MC2R should provide a perfect substrate for receptor targeting. This is a receptor with, effectively, a single function, expressed in a highly tissue-restricted way and activated by a single, highly specific agonist. The question is – if it were possible to design the perfect antagonist – what clinical role might it play?

DISORDERS OF THE PITUITARY–ADRENAL AXIS

Disorders of this axis are, fortunately, uncommon and can be subdivided into disorders of hormone deficiency and excess. Glucocorticoid deficiency seems unlikely to benefit from MC2R antagonism, but in certain specific circumstances, there could be a valuable role for this therapeutic option as discussed later.

Glucocorticoid Excess

Glucocorticoid excess may result from primary adrenal disease – typically an adrenal adenoma or carcinoma – and is independent of ACTH. Indeed ACTH is normally suppressed by the actions of the negative feedback loop. More often, cortisol excess or Cushing's syndrome is the result of a pituitary adenoma secreting excess ACTH – known as Cushing's Disease – or less commonly a non-pituitary tumor that "ectopically" secretes ACTH. This group of disorders might theoretically provide a suitable target for an MC2R antagonist.

Cushing's Disease

Corticotroph adenomas are small, usually slow growing, benign tumors that normally come to clinical attention as a result of the effects of glucocorticoid excess, rather than because of the physical effects of an expanding tumor. Typically, Cushing's syndrome may take many years to develop. Consequently the diagnosis of the disorder and exclusion of other causes of Cushing's syndrome is a significant challenge. Once a diagnosis is conclusively made, the optimal treatment is surgical removal of the tumor – ideally preserving the remaining pituitary function. Surgery for Cushing's disease requires extensive experience and skill and is normally undertaken in specialist centers (18).

In some patients, the metabolic consequences of their untreated glucocorticoid excess are so significant that there would be risks in immediately proceeding to complex or prolonged surgery. The glucocorticoid synthesis blockers metyrapone and/or ketoconazole are frequently used in this situation to reduce steroid production (see **Figure 1**), and most patients tolerate and respond to this treatment reasonably well (19–21). However, an MC2R antagonist could be equally effective in this situation.

TABLE 1 | A summary of the main features of each of the melanocortin receptors in the human.

	Major sites of expression	Ligand preference	Function	Effect of deletion	Comments
MC1R	Melanocytes	α-MSH > ACTH > γ-MSH	Pigmentation of hair and skin	Red hair, pale skin	Agouti antagonizes
MC2R	Adrenal cortex	ACTH	Steroidogenesis adrenal growth	Adrenal failure	Absolute dependency on MRAP
MC3R	Brain, spinal cord	γ-MSH > α-MSH = ACTH	Complex, inhibits POMC neurones	Obesity	
MC4R	Brain, spinal cord	α-MSH > ACTH > γ-MSH	Appetite regulation	Obesity	Enhanced action with MRAP2 AGRP is natural antagonist
MC5R	Multiple tissues	α-MSH > ACTH > γ-MSH	Exocrine gland function	Defective water repulsion	

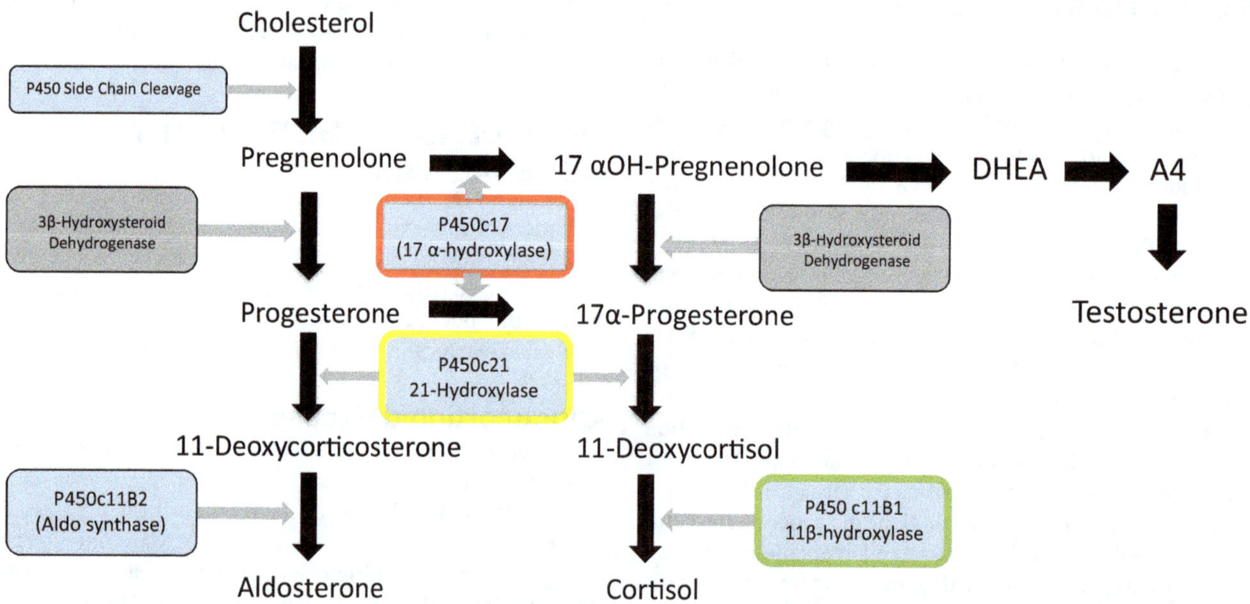

FIGURE 1 | Major steroid synthetic pathways in the human showing the three main end products – cortisol, testosterone and aldosterone, the key intermediates, and the main enzymes. 21-Hydroxylase deficiency (enzyme highlighted in yellow) is the major cause of congenital adrenal hyperplasia. It can be seen that deficiency or inhibition will result in cortisol and aldosterone deficiency and androgen excess. Inhibition of 17 α-hydroxylase (highlighted in red) by abiraterone in contrast will lead to cortisol and testosterone deficiency and overproduction of aldosterone. Metyrapone inhibits 11 β-hydroxylase (highlighted in green) and this may lead to an overproduction of adrenal androgens. The p450 inhibitor, ketoconazole will impair the action of all these enzymes and other P450 enzymes (shown in blue) and thus will not result in overproduction of steroid.

Following surgery, the glucocorticoid excess will come under rapid control in a minority of patients. More frequently, there will be a reduction in steroid over-secretion that may tail off over several weeks. In other cases, it may be necessary to re-explore the pituitary surgically, and this may result in pituitary clearance with a loss of other pituitary hormones (18). Control of glucocorticoid excess during this interim period will often necessitate the use of metyrapone and/or ketoconazole.

If further surgical measures are unsuccessful, endocrinologists may turn to the somatostatin receptor 5 agonist, pasireotide, which directly targets the corticotroph adenoma and provides partial or complete control of Cushing's in a proportion of cases (22). Other second-line options in this situation include pituitary radiotherapy or adrenalectomy. The former may take several years to normalize the glucocorticoid excess, necessitating metyrapone and/or ketoconazole during this time. An MC2R antagonist could be a possible alternative.

While glucocorticoid synthesis inhibitors are usually effective and reasonably well tolerated in these situations, there are some potential disadvantages to their prolonged use. Metyrapone blocks the 11β-hydroxylase enzyme, required for the last step of cortisol synthesis from 11-deoxycortisol. Consequently, as shown in **Figure 1**, steroid precursors are channeled through the androgen pathways resulting in increased secretion of adrenal androgens. In women, this may induce hirsutism and in pre-pubertal children both virilization and early puberty (23, 24). Ketoconazole, a cytochrome P450 inhibitor, inhibits several steps of steroidogenesis and does not usually cause androgen excess. However, complications include potential rare but serious hepatotoxicity and multiple drug interactions. Consequently, although these treatments are effective and inexpensive, there could be a place for a highly specific MC2R antagonist in the management of Cushing's disease.

Ectopic ACTH Syndrome

The mechanisms of ectopic ACTH syndrome are essentially the same as those of Cushing's disease except that the underlying tumor is outside the pituitary gland. These rare tumors are often small carcinoid tumors that may occur anywhere in the lungs and gastrointestinal tract. Improvements in imaging over the last 10–20 years together with intravenous sampling for ACTH have made identification of the primary source far simpler. Once identified, and if surgical removal of the underlying tumor is possible, then this can be curative. As with Cushing's disease, it may be helpful to use a cortisol synthesis blocking drug while waiting for definitive treatment (18) and in cases where definitive treatment is not possible. Hence, for the same reasons described above, an MC2R antagonist may have a place in the clinical management of such conditions.

Small cell lung cancer makes up about 20% of all lung cancer is a highly malignant neuroendocrine tumor of poor prognosis. This tumor is frequently associated with ectopic ACTH secretion, and the development of Cushing's syndrome in this disease may obviously worsen prognosis. Thus there may also be value in using an ACTH antagonist in this clinical situation.

Glucocorticoid Deficiency

The second group of disorders in which there may be an place for antagonizing ACTH action are those in which the physiological negative feedback of cortisol is reduced or lost, leading to a compensatory increase in ACTH secretion. In this situation, it is the stimulation of non-glucocorticoid adrenal steroidogenesis by ACTH, which requires control.

Congenital Adrenal Hyperplasia

The most prominent example of such a situation is that of congenital adrenal hyperplasia, caused in the majority of cases by mutations in both alleles of the *CYP21* gene encoding the 21-hydroxylase enzyme necessary for the penultimate step of cortisol synthesis (**Figure 1**) (25, 26). This is one of the commonest human autosomal recessive disorders occurring in about 1 in 15,000 live births. Reduced glucocorticoid feedback results in ACTH stimulation of adrenal androgen production. As a consequence, affected female children are likely to be virilized or have ambiguous genitalia at presentation. Life-long treatment with glucocorticoids will restore any cortisol deficiency and suppress ACTH secretion and subsequent androgen production (27). However, achieving the optimal dose and timings of hydrocortisone replacement to avoid the adverse effects of excessive glucocorticoid on growth and metabolism while maintaining adequate androgen suppression is challenging, resulting in poor health outcomes (28). Availability of an easily administered ACTH antagonist would be likely to facilitate treatment, allowing a "block and replace" approach in which the physician could focus on treatment of glucocorticoid replacement alone rather than androgen suppression.

Prostate Cancer Treatment

The use of the drug Abiratarone in the treatment of prostate cancer induces a form of acquired adrenal hyperplasia. Abiratarone is a potent inhibitor of the 17 α-hydroxylase and 17,20 lyase enzymes in the adrenal and is used to very effectively reduce the production of adrenal androgens in castration-resistant prostate cancer, with valuable benefits to prostate cancer treatment (29). Examination of adrenal steroid synthetic pathways (**Figure 1**) demonstrates that this inhibition is likely to channel steroid synthesis toward deoxycorticosterone synthesis and aldosterone production, leading to mineralocorticoid excess and glucocorticoid deficiency. The latter requires glucocorticoid replacement, but the fluid overload, hypertension, and hypokalemia resulting from aldosterone excess require treatment with a mineralocorticoid antagonist such as eplerenone (30). Use of an ACTH antagonist together with a replacement dose of hydrocortisone may be a preferred approach in this situation.

Investigation of Endocrine Disease

A further potential use of an ACTH antagonist is in the investigation of adrenal disorders. One of the key questions in the investigation of Cushing's syndrome is whether the cortisol excess is ACTH dependent. A number of tests have been used to determine this including the dexamethasone suppression test and the CRH stimulation test, combined with measurements of plasma ACTH and imaging studies. Hypoglycemic stress tests and metyrapone tests may also be required in complex cases (31). It is conceivable that the use of a single dose ACTH antagonist test could provide a simple and clear solution to this question, although it is more likely that its use in combination with other investigations would be required in most cases.

THE TARGET

As discussed in the Section "Introduction," the receptor for ACTH presents a remarkably attractive target for pharmacological manipulation. It is highly specific for a single peptide agonist – ACTH [1–39], and has no affinity or response to any other naturally occurring agonist. It is expressed in functional quantities only in the adrenal cortex, and thus the possibility of unwanted off-target effects of an antagonist is unlikely.

The key component of the ACTH receptor complex is the seven transmembrane domain MC2R – perhaps surprisingly, the smallest of all the G protein-coupled receptor (GPCR) family at only 289 residues in length (32). The MC2R cannot function alone as an ACTH receptor, which led to many difficulties in its characterization after initial cloning (33). The discovery that deficiency of a small, single transmembrane domain protein caused a clinical syndrome essentially identical to that caused by MC2R deficiency led to the identification of the melanocortin 2 receptor accessory protein (MRAP) as the MC2R co-receptor (34, 35).

Melanocortin receptor accessory protein is a highly unusual protein in that it naturally exists as an antiparallel homodimer and seems to be necessary for trafficking and cell surface expression of the MC2R, as well as binding of ACTH and hence signal transduction (36, 37). In common, with many other GPCRs, MC2R has the potential to homodimerise and the evidence suggests that it exists as a homodimer with two MRAP molecules, in an antiparallel homodimer formation, associated with each MC2R component (38) (**Figure 2**).

The nature of the ligand, ACTH is important in understanding receptor function (**Figure 3A**). The strongly conserved N-terminal 24 residues of ACTH are almost as efficient as the 39 residue naturally occurring peptide in activating this receptor. Further truncation of ACTH from the C-terminus is associated with gradual loss of activity until removal of the four basic residues (Lys–Lys–Arg–Arg) in positions 15–18, which inactivates this peptide at the ACTH receptor (39, 40). The first 13 residues are however active at all the other melanocortin receptors and thus it seems that this "tetrabasic" region acts as a "key" to unlock the MC2R–MRAP complex.

The evidence suggests that once the receptor is "unlocked," the N-terminal region is an effective agonist for the receptor. As with all the melanocortin receptors, the His–Phe–Arg–Trp sequence (or HFRW sequence using the single letter amino acid code) at positions 6–9 and to some extent those residues flanking this induce the conformational changes required to activate the receptor. This HFRW sequence is fundamental to activation of all the melanocortin receptors and can be considered the "message" region of the peptide (40, 43, 44). Interestingly, a naturally occurring human mutation of Arg 8 in the HFRW sequence results in biologically inactive ACTH (45). The most N-terminal region (Ser–Tyr–Ser) has been reported to potentiate the action of the HFRW sequence (46).

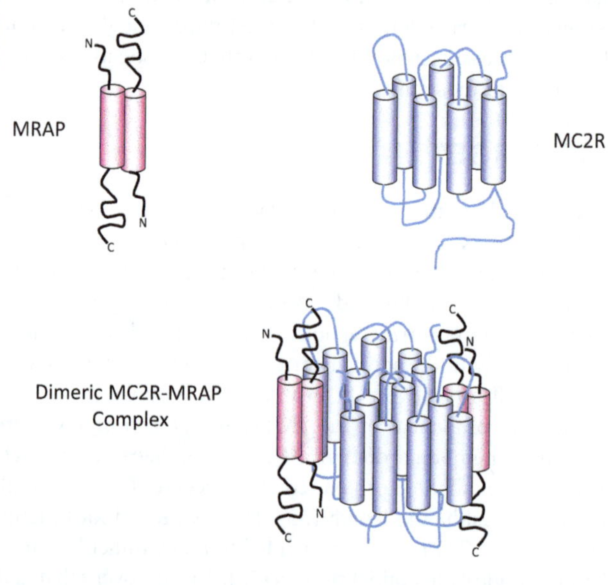

FIGURE 2 | Diagrammatic representation of the components of the ACTH receptor complex. MRAP (pink) exists as an antiparallel homodimer with one short N-terminus and one longer C-terminus on either side of the plasma membrane. The cylindrical components represent the α-helical transmembrane domains. MC2R (blue) contains seven transmembrane domains (blue cylinders) with an N-terminal extracellular domain and a C-terminal intracellular domain. Evidence suggests that one MRAP homodimer associates with one MC2R molecule and that MC2R probably exist as homodimers as shown in the lower panel, or possibly as higher order multimers.

Great strides have been made in recent years in understanding the three dimensional nature of GPCRs, based around a growing number of receptor crystal structures. No melanocortin receptor crystal structure has yet been reported, but increasingly sophisticated modeling exercises combined with receptor mutagenesis and substitution studies are providing information on how ligands interact with their receptor.

Pogozheva et al. studied the MC4R-binding site for NDP-MSH (a highly potent analog of α-MSH) and two small molecule agonists using a combination of alanine scanning mutagenesis of the receptor followed by functional analysis and *in silico* modeling. They concluded that the HFRW sequence of NDP-MSH was required to form a β-hairpin-like structure so that the phenyl ring of Phe 7 interacts with the indole ring of Trp 9 (**Figure 3B**). This allows interaction between His 6 of NDP-MSH and Glu 100 in transmembrane domain 2 (TM2) of MC4R, and Arg 8 of NDP-MSH and Asp 115 and 119 inTM3 of MC4R. The interacting aromatic residues of this sequence, Phe 7 and Trp 9 interact with the aromatic Phe at positions 261 and His 264 of MC4R in TM6 (41).

A relatively similar picture of NDP-MSH binding to the MC5R was constructed by Yang and colleagues using site-directed mutagenesis and structural modeling. They also suggested that Asp 115 and 119 in TMD 3 interact with Arg 8 of the HFRW sequence and that Phe 195 (in TMD 5) and Phe 254 (TMD 6) interact with Phe 7 and Trp 9 of HFRW. All of these residues are conserved in the MC2R (and other melanocortin receptors), and it seems highly likely that these interactions are critical in determining the HFRW binding and activation of this receptor (42). Indeed, naturally occurring homozygous mutations of Asp 103 and 107 in MC2R, the equivalent conserved Asp residues in this receptor, lead to ACTH resistance/Familial Glucocorticoid Deficiency (47). This arrangement is shown in **Figure 3C**.

Using a receptor chimera approach in which regions of the MC4R were substituted into the MC2R, Fridmanis et al. suggested that one of the MRAP molecules binds to MC2R in the region of transmembrane domains 4 and 5 to create a binding pocket for the tetrabasic "address" sequence in ACTH. Following this interaction, a conformational shift in the receptor transmembrane domains takes place, which permits the formation of the HFRW-binding pocket (14). Although this remains speculative, it is an attractive hypothesis. It is notable that Malik et al. have shown that it is the N-terminal region of the MRAP molecule that is required on the extracellular surface of the cell for ACTH binding (48). Clearly complete understanding of this complex area will ultimately require determination of a crystal structure of the MC2R–MRAP–ACTH complex.

APPROACHES TO ANTAGONIZING ACTH

Given the extensive knowledge of the interaction of ACTH with its receptor gained over about 50 years one might anticipate that it would be a relatively straightforward matter to design an ACTH-like peptide with antagonist properties. The first attempts to do this resulted in peptides that retained the tetrabasic address region, but lacked the HFRW message sequence. This led to the development of ACTH [11–24] (49, 50) as a potential receptor antagonist. Li et al. isolated a naturally occurring peptide, ACTH [8–39], from human pituitary, which they showed to have ACTH antagonistic effects *in vitro*, and they called this corticotrophin-inhibiting peptide (CIP) (51). However, the data with each of these potential antagonists has been confusing with discrepant results for steroidogenesis and cAMP generation in some cases. For example, Szalay demonstrated that ACTH [11–24] stimulated steroidogenesis in dispersed zona glomerulosa and zona fasciculata cells (52), and Goverde and Smals (53) demonstrated some steroidogenesis with this peptide.

More recently, Kovalitskaia et al. investigated the binding of a wide range of ACTH fragments derived from an ACTH [11–24] parent peptide. They reported that the ACTH [15–18] tetrabasic fragment alone was an effective competitor for ACTH [11–24] in ligand-binding assays, and that it also failed to stimulate cAMP generation in adrenocortical membranes (54). Its use in competition with ACTH in cAMP generation or steroidogenesis has not been reported.

The consensus from most researchers seems to be that ACTH [11–24] is not an effective ACTH antagonist. This may be because the interaction between the tetrabasic region of ACTH converts the MC2R into a "primed receptor with an unoccupied HFRW-binding site, which may then be activated by the natural agonist." Hoffman therefore used a different approach and developed an analog in which the Trp residue at position 9 of the HFRW message sequence was substituted with Phe or *N*-methyl Trp,

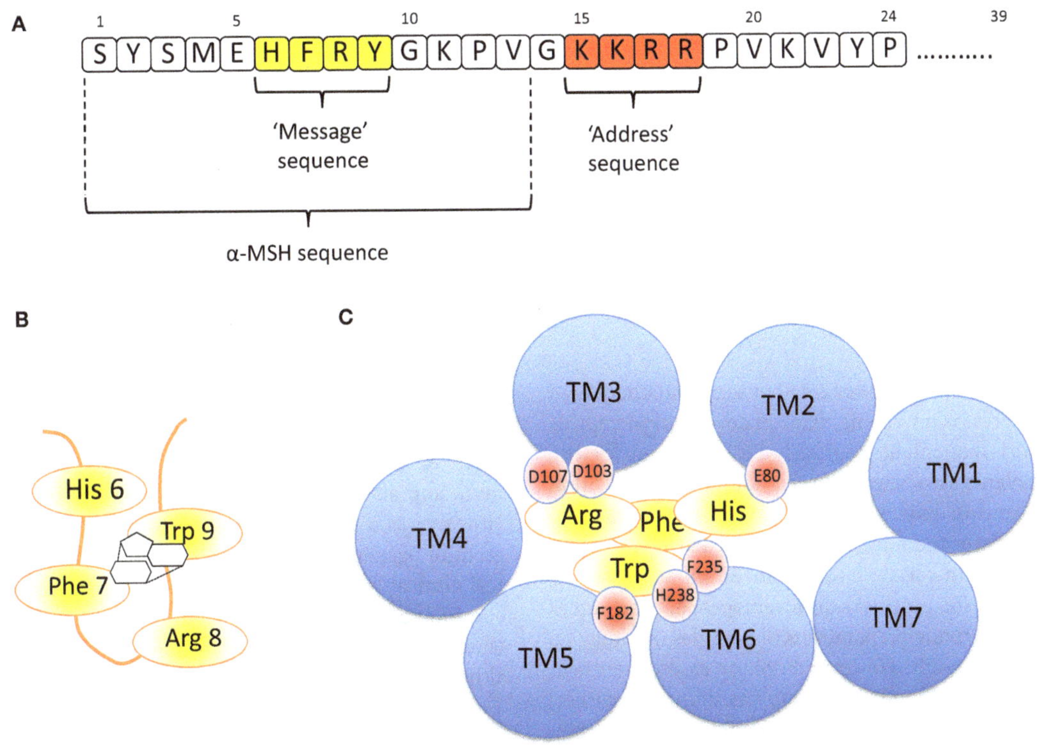

FIGURE 3 | **(A)** Amino acid sequence of ACTH [1-24] using the single letter amino acid code. Note – the naturally occurring peptide is 39 residues in length. The key functional domains are the "message" sequence (yellow), which is required for activation of all the melanocortin receptors, and the "address" sequence (red), which enables only ACTH to activate the MC2R. α-MSH is equivalent to the first 13 residues of ACTH. **(B)** The "message" sequence folds into a β-hairpin loop in which the aromatic amino acids Phe 7 and Trp 9 interact with each other *via* their phenyl and indole rings, respectively, as shown. **(C)** If the MC2R is viewed from above, each of the transmembrane domains is seen as a blue circle (labeled TM1, TM2, etc). By extrapolation from modeling data from the MC4R (41) and from the MC5R (42), it seems likely that His 6 of ACTH interacts with E80 in TM2 of the MC2R, and Arg 8 interacts with D103 and 107 (of MC2R). Phe 7 and Trp 9 interact with multiple residues including F182, F235, and H238 of MC2R.

and showed inhibition of ACTH stimulated cAMP generation on bovine adrenal membranes (55).

Liang et al. has described a number of peptide analogs of ACTH based on alanine and histidine substitutions around the HFRW region and in the spacing between this and the tetrabasic region (56). In this work, they described the marked reduction in MC2R activation observed with some of these peptides and, in a US patent filed the preceeding year, they reported potent ACTH antagonism with an ACTH [15–24] decapeptide (57).

In all of the above studies, the actions on adrenal tissues, slices, cells, or membranes have been studied, but little or no data on the selectivity of these peptide antagonists for the MC2R, or even melanocortin receptors in general have been obtained. It is usually highly desirable that any receptor active drug used therapeutically is selective for its target receptor and lacks off-target effects. The functions of the other melanocortin receptors and the effects of antagonizing or deleting them are summarized in **Table 1**, and it can be seen that a non-selective agent could induce a number of unwanted effects.

Bouw and colleagues reported an approach in which ACTH peptides that retain the intact tetrabasic region were substituted at various positions in the HFRW sequence and in some cases were cyclized in order to enhance stability. HEK293 cells stably expressing human MC2R and MRAP were used, and cAMP production was measured with a luminescence assay. Several peptides exhibited significant antagonist actions among which GPS1573 – a variant of ACTH [7–18] with an N-terminal nor leucine – proline sequence and D-Phe and DD-Trp (in place of the L-Phe and L-Trp) in the HFRW sequence, and a cyclized variant of this – GPS1574 were most potent (IC50s of 66 ± 23 nM and 260 ± 1 nM, respectively). These peptides retain some antagonist effect on the MC3R, MC4R and MC5R at approximately an order of magnitude less than that on the MC2R (58).

In work published in this issue, Nensey et al. report the actions of these same analogs on rat adrenal cells and show inhibitory effects in which the dose responses to ACTH [1–39] were shifted to the right by one log order or more. They also conducted *in vivo* experiments in young rats but were unable to show inhibition of the ACTH response even at 400-fold molar excess of antagonist in the case of GPS1573. GPS1574 was partially inhibitory at 30 min after ACTH injection (59).

In a recent study, presented in abstract form, researchers from Ipsen Bioscience Inc. reported the development of an ACTH-related peptide, IRC-274. This peptide was shown to inhibit ACTH binding to the human MC2R and MRAP expressed in HEK 293 cells with an IC50 of 3 nM (60). cAMP generation in response to ACTH in this same model is inhibited with an IC50 of 38 nM. Using an *in vivo* hypophysectomized rat model in which ACTH is infused by osmotic minipump, significant inhibition of corticosterone production was observed. Using a second model in which mouse AtT20 pituitary corticotroph tumor cells were implanted into athymic nude mice, inhibition of corticosterone was again observed until the implanted tumors outgrew the inhibitory action of IRC-274. Interestingly, this antagonist exhibits a high degree of selectivity for the MC2R and has no significant actions on other melanocortin receptors. The sequence and structure of this peptide have not been revealed.

ALTERNATIVE APPROACHES

Small Molecules

From the above, it seems that after a rather long and chequered history some progress is now being made in developing a peptide ACTH antagonist that might ultimately be developed for use *in vivo*. The problems associated with peptide-based medication are well-known and include a short half-life in the circulation, the need to administer them by injection and the risk of inducing immunogenicity. In certain circumstances, the benefits of a peptide outweigh these potential disadvantages, and advances are being made in deriving preparations of peptides that may be taken orally or intranasally. However in many cases, there will be a need for a reliable long-term therapy as discussed earlier. Under these circumstances, it would be desirable to have an orally active agent, which would most likely be a small (non-peptide) molecule. Substantial efforts have been made to develop small molecules as agonists of the MC4 receptor with some limited success (61). With this objective in mind, we have undertaken a high throughput screen of about 200,000 small molecules using a cell-line expressing the human MC2R and MRAP, and this may provide a promising approach if a molecule with sufficient potency and selectivity can be identified.

Antibody-Based Approaches

Humanized monoclonal antibodies directed against key signaling molecules have proven to provide effective therapeutic solutions in inflammatory diseases and cancer. This approach has been used to target ACTH and the pituitary–adrenal axis by a number of investigators and one pharmaceutical company aims to begin human studies in the near future (62). While such antibodies may not necessarily provide a long-term therapeutic solution, they seem likely to have potential in shorter-term therapeutic situations, such as around the time of pituitary surgery for Cushing's disease.

Corticostatins

Solomon and colleagues identified a novel lung and neutrophil peptide belonging to the defensin class of highly cationic antimicrobial peptides. They showed this peptide exhibited a number of functions including inhibition of ACTH binding and corticosterone secretion and named this corticostatin (63). It is also known as defensin α-4. These functions appear to be relatively non-specific, and little work has been published on this in recent years. We are not aware that this action of corticostatin has been explored for therapeutic purposes.

SUMMARY

We have reviewed the case for the development of an ACTH antagonist for therapeutic purposes. The conditions in which there is a potential clinical indication are relatively uncommon, and alternative therapies are well described in each case. However as a refinement to existing therapies or for the treatment of particularly difficult or complex cases, there would be a real clinical benefit. We have not considered a number of more common conditions, such as depressive illness or septic shock in which there might ultimately be a role for an ACTH antagonist, although these have been considered elsewhere (64).

The evidence suggests that progress is being made on more than one front in developing an antagonist. This has been delayed for many years by the absence of "clean" systems in which to test candidate peptides and compounds, owing to the problems in expressing the MC2R. This should no longer be a problem as a result of the identification of MRAP that enables cell surface expression of the MC2R. As a result there does seem to be a growing interest in this area and the next decade may witness exciting developments.

AUTHOR CONTRIBUTIONS

This work is part of the result of a 5-year project. Over this time, all authors have contributed information, ideas, and data to the work. The manuscript was primarily written by AC, with comment and editing from the other authors.

FUNDING

LC is supported by an MRC/Academy of Medical Sciences Clinician Scientist Fellowship (G0802796) and MH by a MRC CASE studentship (MR/J006394/1).

REFERENCES

1. Lorimer AR, Dunn FG, Jones JV, Lawrie TD. Beta-adrenoreceptor blockade in hypertension. *Am J Med* (1976) 60:877–85. doi:10.1016/0002-9343(76)90908-6
2. Siepler JK, Campagna KD, Donahue PE, Bombeck CT. H2 receptor antagonists. *Am J Hosp Pharm* (1978) 35:141–5.
3. Osborne CK. Tamoxifen in the treatment of breast cancer. *N Engl J Med* (1998) 339:1609–18. doi:10.1056/NEJM199811263392207
4. Seferovic PM, Pelliccia F, Zivkovic I, Ristic A, Lalic N, Seferovic J, et al. Mineralocorticoid receptor antagonists, a class beyond spironolactone – focus on the special pharmacologic properties of eplerenone. *Int J Cardiol* (2015) 200:3–7. doi:10.1016/j.ijcard.2015.02.096
5. Singh SM, Gauthier S, Labrie F. Androgen receptor antagonists (antiandrogens): structure-activity relationships. *Curr Med Chem* (2000) 7:211–47. doi:10.2174/0929867003375371
6. Capatina C, Wass JA. 60 years of neuroendocrinology: acromegaly. *J Endocrinol* (2015) 226:T141–60. doi:10.1530/JOE-15-0109
7. Peri A. Clinical review: the use of vaptans in clinical endocrinology. *J Clin Endocrinol Metab* (2013) 2013(98):1321–32. doi:10.1210/jc.2012-4082
8. Clark AJ. 60 years of POMC: the proopiomelanocortin gene: discovery, deletion and disease. *J Mol Endocrinol* (2016) 56(4):T27–37. doi:10.1530/JME-15-0268
9. Chretien M, Mbikay M. 60 years of POMC: from the prohormone theory to proopiomelanocortin and to proprotein convertases (PCSK1 to PCSK9). *J Mol Endocrinol* (2016) 56(4):T49–62. doi:10.1530/JME-15-0261

10. Lowry P. 60 years of POMC: purification and biological characterisation of melanotrophins and corticotrophins. *J Mol Endocrinol* (2016) 56(4):T1–12. doi:10.1530/JME-15-0260
11. Lim CT, Grossman A, Khoo B. Normal physiology of ACTH and GH release in the hypothalamus and anterior pituitary in man. In: De Groot LJ, Beck-Peccoz P, Chrousos G, Dungan K, Grossman A, Hershman JM, et al., editors. *Endotext [Internet]*. South Dartmouth, MA: MDText.com, Inc. (2014).
12. Schöneshöfer M, Goverde HJ. Corticotropin in human plasma. General considerations. *Surv Immunol Res* (1984) 3:55–63.
13. Ramachandrappa S, Gorrigan RJ, Clark AJ, Chan LF. The melanocortin receptors and their accessory proteins. *Front Endocrinol (Lausanne)* (2013) 4:9. doi:10.3389/fendo.2013.00009
14. Fridmanis D, Petrovska R, Kalnina I, Slaidina M, Peculis R, Schiöth HB, et al. Identification of domains responsible for specific membrane transport and ligand specificity of the ACTH receptor (MC2R). *Mol Cell Endocrinol* (2010) 321:175–83. doi:10.1016/j.mce.2010.02.032
15. Veo K, Reinick C, Liang L, Moser E, Angleson JK, Dores RM. Observations on the ligand selectivity of the melanocortin 2 receptor. *Gen Comp Endocrinol* (2011) 172:3–9. doi:10.1016/j.ygcen.2011.04.006
16. Draper N, Stewart PM. 11beta-hydroxysteroid dehydrogenase and the pre-receptor regulation of corticosteroid hormone action. *J Endocrinol* (2005) 186:251–71. doi:10.1677/joe.1.06019
17. Keller-Wood M. Hypothalamic-pituitary – adrenal axis-feedback control. *Compr Physiol* (2015) 5:1161–82. doi:10.1002/cphy.c140065
18. Biller BM, Grossman AB, Stewart PM, Melmed S, Bertagna X, Bertherat J, et al. Treatment of adrenocorticotropin-dependent Cushing's syndrome: a consensus statement. *J Clin Endocrinol Metab* (2008) 93:2454–62. doi:10.1210/jc.2007-2734
19. Beardwell CG, Adamson AR, Shalet SM. Prolonged remission in florid Cushing's syndrome following metyrapone treatment. *Clin Endocrinol (Oxf)* (1981) 14:485–92. doi:10.1111/j.1365-2265.1981.tb00638.x
20. Boscaro M, Sonino N, Rampazzo A, Mantero F. Response of pituitary-adrenal axis to corticotrophin releasing hormone in patients with Cushing's disease before and after ketoconazole treatment. *Clin Endocrinol (Oxf)* (1987) 27:461–7. doi:10.1111/j.1365-2265.1987.tb01174.x
21. Sonino N. The use of ketoconazole as an inhibitor of steroid production. *N Engl J Med* (1987) 317:812–8. doi:10.1056/NEJM198709243171307
22. Colao A, Petersenn S, Newell-Price J, Findling JW, Gu F, Maldonado M, et al. A 12-month phase 3 study of pasireotide in Cushing's disease. *N Engl J Med* (2012) 366:914–24. doi:10.1056/NEJMoa1105743
23. Verhelst JA, Trainer PJ, Howlett TA, Perry L, Rees LH, Grossman AB, et al. Short and long-term responses to metyrapone in the medical management of 91 patients with Cushing's syndrome. *Clin Endocrinol (Oxf)* (1991) 35:169–78. doi:10.1111/j.1365-2265.1991.tb03517.x
24. Juszczak A, Ertorer ME, Grossman A. The therapy of Cushing's disease in adults and children: an update. *Horm Metab Res* (2013) 45:109–17. doi:10.1055/s-0032-1330009
25. Miller WL. Clinical review 54: genetics, diagnosis, and management of 21-hydroxylase deficiency. *J Clin Endocrinol Metab* (1994) 78:241–6. doi:10.1210/jc.78.2.241
26. Nimkarn S, Lin-Su K, New MI. Steroid 21 hydroxylase deficiency congenital adrenal hyperplasia. *Endocrinol Metab Clin North Am* (2009) 38:699–718. doi:10.1016/j.ecl.2009.08.001
27. Joint LWPES/ESPE CAH Working Group. Consensus statement on 21-hydroxylase deficiency from the Lawson Wilkins Pediatric Endocrine Society and the European Society for Paediatric Endocrinology. *J Clin Endocrinol Metab* (2002) 87:4048–53. doi:10.1210/jc.2002-020611
28. Han TS, Conway GS, Willis DS, Krone N, Rees DA, Stimson RH, et al. Relationship between final height and health outcomes in adults with congenital adrenal hyperplasia: United Kingdom congenital adrenal hyperplasia adult study executive (CaHASE). *J Clin Endocrinol Metab* (2014) 99:E1547–55. doi:10.1210/jc.2014-1486
29. Ryan CJ, Smith MR, Fizazi K, Saad F, Mulders PF, Sternberg CN, et al. Abiraterone acetate plus prednisone versus placebo plus prednisone in chemotherapy-naive men with metastatic castration-resistant prostate cancer (COU-AA-302): final overall survival analysis of a randomised, double-blind, placebo-controlled phase 3 study. *Lancet Oncol* (2015) 16:152–60. doi:10.1016/S1470-2045(14)71205-7
30. Attard G, Reid AH, Auchus RJ, Hughes BA, Cassidy AM, Thompson E, et al. Clinical and biochemical consequences of CYP17A1 inhibition with abiraterone given with and without exogenous glucocorticoids in castrate men with advanced prostate cancer. *J Clin Endocrinol Metab* (2012) 97:507–16. doi:10.1210/jc.2011-2189
31. Kola B, Grossman AB. Dynamic testing in Cushing's syndrome. *Pituitary* (2008) 11:155–62. doi:10.1007/s11102-007-0079-x
32. Mountjoy KG, Robbins LS, Mortrud MT, Cone RD. The cloning of a family of genes that encode the melanocortin receptors. *Science* (1992) 257:1248–51. doi:10.1126/science.1325670
33. Noon LA, Franklin JM, King PJ, Goulding NJ, Hunyady L, Clark AJ. Failed export of the adrenocorticotrophin receptor from the endoplasmic reticulum in non-adrenal cells: evidence in support of a requirement for a specific adrenal accessory factor. *J Endocrinol* (2002) 174:17–25. doi:10.1677/joe.0.1740017
34. Metherell LA, Chapple JP, Cooray S, David A, Becker C, Rüschendorf F, et al. Mutations in MRAP, encoding a new interacting partner of the ACTH receptor, cause familial glucocorticoid deficiency type 2. *Nat Genet* (2005) 37:166–70. doi:10.1038/ng1501
35. Webb TR, Clark AJ. Minireview: the melanocortin 2 receptor accessory proteins. *Mol Endocrinol* (2010) 24:475–84. doi:10.1210/me.2009-0283
36. Sebag JA, Hinkle PM. Melanocortin-2 receptor accessory protein MRAP forms antiparallel homodimers. *Proc Natl Acad Sci U S A* (2007) 104:20244–9. doi:10.1073/pnas.0708916105
37. Cooray SN, Almiro, Do Vale I, Leung KY, Webb TR, Chapple JP, et al. The melanocortin 2 receptor accessory protein exists as a homodimer and is essential for the function of the melanocortin 2 receptor in the mouse y1 cell line. *Endocrinology* (2008) 149:1935–41. doi:10.1210/en.2007-1463
38. Cooray SN, Chung TT, Mazhar K, Szidonya L, Clark AJ. Bioluminescence resonance energy transfer reveals the adrenocorticotropin (ACTH)-induced conformational change of the activated ACTH receptor complex in living cells. *Endocrinology* (2011) 152:495–502. doi:10.1210/en.2010-1053
39. Schwyzer R. Chemistry and metabolic action of nonsteroid hormones. *Ann Rev Biochem* (1964) 33:259–86. doi:10.1146/annurev.bi.33.070164.001355
40. Schwyzer R. ACTH: a short introductory review. *Ann N Y Acad Sci* (1977) 297:3–26. doi:10.1111/j.1749-6632.1977.tb41843.x
41. Pogozheva ID, Chai BX, Lomize AL, Fong TM, Weinberg DH, Nargund RP, et al. Interactions of human melanocortin 4 receptor with nonpeptide and peptide agonists. *Biochemistry* (2005) 44:11329–41. doi:10.1021/bi0501840
42. Yang Y, Mishra VK, Chen M, Duffee E, Dimmitt R, Harmon CM. Molecular characterization of human melanocortin-5 receptor ligand-receptor interaction. *Biochemistry* (2013) 52:1737–45. doi:10.1021/bi3013593
43. Hofmann K. Chemistry and function of polypeptide hormones. *Annu Rev Biochem* (1962) 31:213–46. doi:10.1146/annurev.bi.31.070162.001241
44. Eberle A, Schwyzer R. Hormone-receptor interactions. Demonstration of two message sequences (active sites) in alpha-melanotropin. *Helv Chim Acta* (1975) 58:1528–35. doi:10.1002/hlca.19750580604
45. Samuels ME, Gallo-Payet N, Pinard S, Hasselmann C, Magne F, Patry L. Bioinactive ACTH causing glucocorticoid deficiency. *Clin Endocrinol Metab* (2013) 98:736–42. doi:10.1210/jc.2012-3199
46. Schwyzer R. Structure and function in neuropeptides. *Proc R Soc Lond B Biol Sci* (1980) 210:5–20. doi:10.1098/rspb.1980.0115
47. Chung TT, Webb TR, Chan LF, Cooray SN, Metherell LA, King PJ, et al. The majority of adrenocorticotropin receptor (melanocortin 2 receptor) mutations found in familial glucocorticoid deficiency type 1 lead to defective trafficking of the receptor to the cell surface. *J Clin Endocrinol Metab* (2008) 93:4948–54. doi:10.1210/jc.2008-1744
48. Malik S, Dolan TM, Maben ZJ, Hinkle PM. Adrenocorticotropic hormone (ACTH) responses require actions of the melanocortin-2 receptor accessory protein on the extracellular surface of the plasma membrane. *J Biol Chem* (2015) 290:27972–85. doi:10.1074/jbc.M115.668491
49. Seelig S, Sayers G, Schwyzer R, Schiller P. Isolated adrenal cells: ACTH(11-24), a competitive antagonist of ACTH(1-39) and ACTH(1-10). *FEBS Lett* (1971) 19:232–4. doi:10.1016/0014-5793(71)80521-5
50. Seelig S, Sayers G. Isolated adrenal cortex cells: ACTH agonists, partial agonists, antagonists; cyclic AMP and corticosterone production. *Arch Biochem Biophys* (1973) 154:230–9. doi:10.1016/0003-9861(73)90053-2
51. Li CH, Chung D, Yamashiro D, Lee CY. Isolation, characterization, and synthesis of a corticotropin-inhibiting peptide from human pituitary glands. *Proc Natl Acad Sci U S A* (1978) 75:4306–9. doi:10.1073/pnas.75.9.4306

52. Szalay KS, De Wied D, Stark E. Effects of ACTH-(11-24) on the corticosteroid production of isolated adrenocortical cells. *J Steroid Biochem* (1989) 32:259–62. doi:10.1016/0022-4731(89)90261-6
53. Goverde HJ, Smals AG. The anomalous effect of some ACTH-fragments missing the amino acid sequence 1-10 on the corticosteroidogenesis in purified isolated rat adrenal cells. *FEBS Lett* (1984) 173:23–6. doi:10.1016/0014-5793(84)81009-1
54. Kovalitskaia IA, Kolobov AA, Kampe-Nemm EA, Iurovskií VV, Sadovnikov VB, Lipkin VM, et al. Synthetic peptide KKRR corresponding to the human ACTH fragment 15-18 is an antagonist of the ACTH receptor. *Bioorg Khim* (2008) 34:29–35.
55. Hofmann K, Montibeller JA, Finn FM. ACTH antagonists. *Proc Natl Acad Sci U S A* (1974) 71:80–3. doi:10.1073/pnas.71.1.80
56. Liang L, Angleson JK, Dores RM. Using the human melanocortin-2 receptor as a model for analyzing hormone/receptor interactions between a mammalian MC2 receptor and ACTH(1-24). *Gen Comp Endocrinol* (2013) 181: 203–10. doi:10.1016/j.ygcen.2012.11.011
57. Dores RM. *ACTH Antagonist Peptides*. US Patent application US 2012/0309696 A1 (2012).
58. Bouw E, Huisman M, Neggers SJ, Themmen AP, van der Lely AJ, Delhanty PJ. Development of potent selective competitive-antagonists of the melanocortin type 2 receptor. *Mol Cell Endocrinol* (2014) 394:99–104. doi:10.1016/j.mce.2014.07.003
59. Nensey NK, Bodager J, Gehrand AL, Raff H. Effect of novel melanocortin type 2 receptor antagonists on the corticosterone response to ACTH in the neonatal rat adrenal gland in vivo and in vitro. *Front Endocrinol (Lausanne).* (2016) 7:23. doi:10.3389/fendo.2016.00023
60. Halem HA, Ufret M, Jewett I, Mattei A, Bastille A, Beech J, et al. In vivo suppression of corticosterone in rodent models of Cushing's disease with a selective, peptide MC2 receptor antagonist. *Abstract presented to the Endocrine Society Annual Meeting*, Boston (2016).
61. Fani L, Bak S, Delhanty P, van Rossum EF, van den Akker EL. The melanocortin-4 receptor as target for obesity treatment: a systematic review of emerging pharmacological therapeutic options. *Int J Obes (Lond)* (2014) 38:163–9. doi:10.1038/ijo.2013.80
62. Feldhaus AL, Anderson K, Dutzar B, Ojala E, McNeill PD, Fan P, et al. A novel anti-ACTH antibody (ALD1613) neutralizes ACTH activity and reduced glucocorticoids in rats and nonhuman primates. *Abstract presented to the Endocrine Society Annual Meeting*, Boston (2016).
63. Zhu QZ, Hu J, Mulay S, Esch F, Shimasaki S, Solomon S. Isolation and structure of corticostatin peptides from rabbit fetal and adult lung. *Proc Natl Acad Sci U S A* (1988) 85:592–6. doi:10.1073/pnas.85.2.592
64. Clark AJ, Metherell LA. Mechanisms of disease: the adrenocorticotropin receptor and disease. *Nat Clin Pract Endocrinol Metab* (2006) 2:282–90. doi:10.1038/ncpendmet0165

7

ACTH Receptor (MC2R) Specificity: What Do We Know About Underlying Molecular Mechanisms?

Davids Fridmanis, Ance Roga and Janis Klovins*

Latvian Biomedical Research and Study Centre, Riga, Latvia

***Correspondence:**
Davids Fridmanis
davids@biomed.lu.lv

Coincidentally, the release of this Research Topic in Frontiers in Endocrinology takes place 25 years after the discovery of the adrenocorticotropic hormone receptor (ACTHR) by Mountjoy and colleagues. In subsequent years, following the discovery of other types of mammalian melanocortin receptors (MCRs), ACTHR also became known as melanocortin type 2 receptor (MC2R). At present, five types of MCRs have been reported, all of which share significant sequence similarity at the amino acid level, and all of which specifically bind melanocortins (MCs)—a group of biologically active peptides generated by proteolysis of the proopiomelanocortin precursor. All MCs share an identical -H-F-R-W- pharmacophore sequence. α-Melanocyte-stimulating hormone (α-MSH) and adrenocorticotropic hormone (ACTH) are the most extensively studied MCs and are derived from the same region. Essentially, α-MSH is formed from the first 13 amino acid residues of ACTH. ACTHR is unique among MCRs because it binds one sole ligand—ACTH, which makes it a very attractive research object for molecular pharmacologists. However, much research has failed, and functional studies of this receptor are lagging behind other MCRs. The reason for these difficulties has already been outlined by Mountjoy and colleagues in their publication on ACTHR coding sequence discovery where the Cloudman S91 melanoma cell line was used for receptor expression because it was a "more sensitive assay system." Subsequent work showed that ACTHR could be successfully expressed only in endogenous MCR-expressing cell lines, since in other cell lines it is retained within the endoplasmic reticulum. The resolution of this methodological problem came in 2005 with the discovery of melanocortin receptor accessory protein, which is required for the formation of functionally active ACTHR. The decade that followed this discovery was filled with exciting research that provided insight into the molecular mechanisms underlying the action of ACTHR. The purpose of this review is to summarize the advances in this fascinating research field.

Keywords: MC2R, ACTHR, specificity, mutation, mutagenesis, site directed

INTRODUCTION

Adrenocorticotropic hormone (ACTH), discovered in 1933 (1), is the primary regulator of aldosterone and corticosterone/cortisol production in mammalian adrenal glands (2–5). It is secreted into the circulating blood stream by corticotropic cells in the anterior pituitary (6) in response to short- and/or long-term stress (7). Due to its chemical structure, biological activity, and origin,

ACTH is classified as a member of the peptide hormone group named melanocortins (MCs), which in addition to ACTH also comprises α-, β-, γ- and δ-melanocyte-stimulating hormones (MSHs), of which the latter is only found within cartilaginous fish (8). All MCs are formed through tissue- and site-specific proteolysis of the propeptide proopiomelanocortin (POMC; **Figure 1**) (7, 9), and all share the –M–X–H–F–R–W– consensus sequence (**Figure 2**), which is the main determinant of their biological activity (8, 10). Experimental data suggest that this core sequence adopts a β-turn secondary structure in most MCs that is generally essential for ligand binding (11). The exception to this rule is γ-MSH, but since it is not directly relevant to the main subject of this article, the reasons underlying this difference are not discussed [for details on molecular mechanisms underlying the action of this peptide see Ref. (12)]. α-MSH and ACTH are overlapping peptides since the aa sequence of the former is identical to the first 13 aa of the latter, because the former is the result of proteolytic cleavage of the latter (**Figure 1**). Following their discovery and aa sequence determination (1, 13–19), there was an ongoing discussion about the melanotropic activity of ACTH and the possible adrenocorticotropic activity of α-MSH (13, 20). However, the latter of these was soon dismissed following overwhelming evidence from *ex vivo* assays that suggested ACTH-derived peptides, which lack the basic –K–K–R–R– motif (**Figure 2**), have minimal effect on steroid production [(21, 22); reviewed in Ref. (23–25)]. Detailed mutational research performed a few decades later extended this motif by including a C-terminal proline, since the replacement of this residue with alanine or tryptophan significantly decreased the potency of the peptide (26). A similar alanine scanning mutagenesis experimental approach was also used to investigate the properties of the ACTH region, which is located between the –M–X–H–F–R–W– and –K–K–R–R–P– motifs (**Figure 2**). The results demonstrated that although replacement of one or two residues had no effect on receptor activation, substitution of all five residues (–G–K–P–V–G–) resulted in dramatic decrease in response sensitivity. Thus, it was concluded that the secondary structure of this motif is of paramount importance because it properly orients the other two motifs in relation to each other so that they can properly fit into the receptor-binding pocket(s) (27). This highly condensed introduction to ACTH, the ligand of ACTHR that is the main subject of this review, barely skims the enormous amount of knowledge acquired for mammalian and other lineages (6, 8, 10, 28–37). However, although having a detailed understanding of the functional properties of the ligand is very import because the interaction of both elements results in the physiological effect, reviewing the ligand in detail is beyond the scope of this article. We believe the core information provided here will be sufficient for interpretation of the research on the molecular mechanisms underlying the action of the adrenocorticotropic hormone receptor (ACTHR).

Although the main subunit of the receptor was discovered in 1992 (38) and the functional receptor was obtained in 2005 (39), research on the structure and function of the mammalian ACTHR dates back as far as 1954, when the aa sequence of ACTH was determined (14–18), or perhaps even to 1933, when

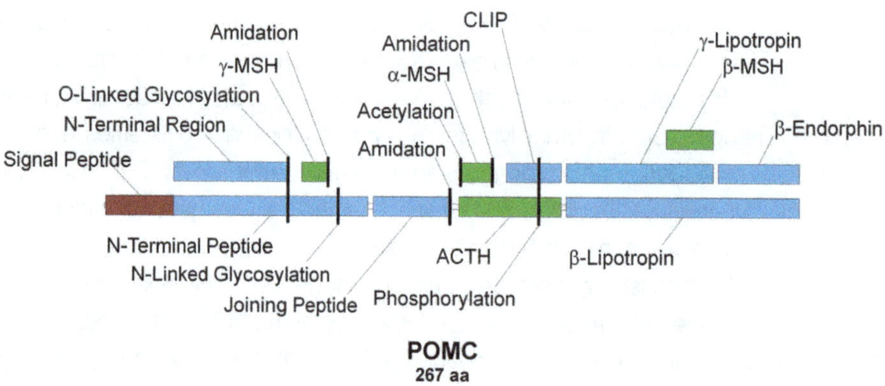

FIGURE 1 | Schematic representation of the proopiomelanocortin precursor, the products of its proteolysis, and known posttranslational modifications. Melanocortins are colored green, signal peptide is colored red, and other peptides are colored blue. Posttranslational modification sites are marked with vertical black lines.

ACTH H_2N-SYSMEHFRWGKPVG*KKRRP*VKVYPNGAEDESAEAFPLEF-COOH

α-MSH HOOC-SYSMEHFRWGKPV-NH_2

β-MSH H_2N-AEKKDEGPYRMEHFRWGSPPKD-COOH

γ-MSH H_2N-YVMGHFRWDRFG-NH_2

FIGURE 2 | Sequence alignment of melanocortin (MC) peptides. All MCs share the conserved –M–X–H–F–R–W– motif, which serves as the pharmacophore for receptor binding (8, 10). The –K–K–R–R–P– motif within adrenocorticotropic hormone (ACTH) is considered the second pharmacophore and is required for successful activation of adrenocorticotropic hormone receptor (26).

the hormone itself was discovered (1). Although to some readers this statement might seem exaggerated, *ex vivo* research on the physiological effects of ACTH was performed on tissue samples containing endogenously expressed ACTHR from these dates. Thus, a large amount of knowledge was accumulated well before the discovery of the receptor itself, and some of these early studies revealed that the receptor was also present in murine fat cells (40–42) and in addition to increasing corticosteroid production (1, 43), activation of the ACTHR is accompanied by the activation of phosphorylases (44, 45), an increase in cyclic adenosine 3′,5′-monophosphate (cAMP) concentration (46–50), and subsequently desensitization (51). Research performed in the 1980s also revealed that stimulation with ACTH increases the number of ACTH-binding sites at adrenal cell membranes (52) and promotes calcium influx (53–56). The information gained during these studies was extensive, and it provided researchers with clues on the nature of the ACTHR and accelerated research in related areas.

At the beginning of the 1990s, a significant number of G-protein coupled receptors (GPCRs) were already identified, all of which share the typical seven transmembrane (TM) domain core structure with the N-terminus located on the exterior of the cell. These receptors were shown to activate intracellular signaling pathways through coupling to the α-subunit of heterotrimeric G-proteins (Gα) that comprise also β and γ subunits. At the time, it was already known that there are several types of G-proteins that induce distinct intracellular responses (57). The most notable of these from the perspective of melanocortin receptors (MCRs) and the ACTHR were those coupling to the $G\alpha_s$ subunit that activates adenylyl cyclase, which in turn increases the intracellular concentration of cAMP. This knowledge was consistent with the observed ACTH-induced intracellular responses, which indicated that MCRs are members of this structurally conserved GPCR family.

The coding sequences of receptors that specifically bind ACTH were first reported in 1992 by two research groups, one led by Cone, and the other led by Wikberg (38, 58). Although both groups employed similar methodology (degenerate primer PCR followed by northern blot screening of melanoma cDNA libraries), the first group identified two receptor-encoding genes, and the second group identified one such gene. This discrepancy could partially be explained by the source of the PCR template, since Cone's group used cDNAs from melanoma cells, while Wikberg's group used genomic DNA. Subsequent pharmacological characterization of receptors and post-publication sequence comparison revealed that both groups discovered the same MCR, which is highly expressed within melanocytes and specifically binds all MCs (ACTH, α-, β- and γ-MSH), and was thus designated the MSH receptor (MSHR) (38, 58). In addition to MC1R, Cone's group also discovered a receptor sharing significant aa sequence identity with MSHR (~39%), yet it proved to be difficult to characterize *in vitro*. Functional expression of this protein was achieved only in an endogenous MCR-expressing Cloudman S91 melanoma cell line, and unlike MSHR, this receptor was found to be expressed in adrenal tissue and activated only by ACTH and was hence named the ACTHR (38). In the following 2 years, three additional MC-binding receptors were uncovered—two by Yamada's group (59, 60) and one by both the Wikberg's and Yamada's groups (61, 62). Due to this simultaneous discovery, there was some ambiguity in the nomenclature of these novel MCRs, but the scientific community soon came to agreement and named them using Yamada's nomenclature as the MC type 3 receptor (MC3R), MC4R, and MC5R. Evaluation of the pharmacological properties of these novel receptors revealed that, like previously characterized homologs, they all coupled with $G\alpha_s$ [it was later discovered that the exception to this rule is MC3R, which is also able to interact with the $G\alpha_{q/11}$ subunit (63)]. However, from a ligand selectivity and *in vitro* expression perspective, they are more akin to MSHR since they are activated by all four MCs and successfully expressed in non-melanoma cells. Since these new receptors also shared significant aa sequence identity with previously discovered homologs (all MCRs share 39–61% sequence identity), their nomenclature was reviewed and, as a result, MSHR became synonymous with MC1R, and ACTHR with MC2R. To avoid any further confusion, in this article, we use ACTHR throughout, since this name better describes the unique functional properties, while the HGNC approved name of MC2R is a better descriptor of its evolutionary origin.

Considered together, the results on MCR expression and ligand selectivity highlighted the unique nature of each receptor because all displayed distinct pharmacological and tissue distribution profiles (**Table 1**). From this perspective, MC3R and ACTHR are the most specialized MCRs, because MC3R is the only receptor in this family that effectively binds γ-MSH and, as mentioned above, ACTHR specifically binds only ACTH (64). The molecular mechanisms underlying the ability of MC3R to effectively bind γ-MSH were soon uncovered (12, 65) following the expression of this receptor in a variety of mammalian cell lines. However, the mechanisms underlying the ACTHR ligand selectivity remained concealed for more than a decade due to the unusual expression selectivity of this receptor.

Although the period following the determination of the DNA sequence encoding the ACTHR was marked by very few molecular studies, this knowledge did facilitate functional and genetic research, which confirmed expression in the *zona reticularis* and *zona fasciculata* of the adrenal cortex, where its activation upregulates its own mRNA production (66). ACTHR mRNA was also found to be present in murine adipocytes (67–69) [where

TABLE 1 | Ligand selectivity and expression profiles of melanocortin receptors.

Receptor	Potency of ligands	Site of expression
MC1R	α-MSH = ACTH > β-MSH > γ-MSH	Melanocytes
ACTHR	ACTH	Adrenal cortex, adipocytes
MC3R	α-MSH = β-MSH = γ-MSH = ACTH	Hypothalamus, limbic system, placenta, digestive tract
MC4R	α-MSH = ACTH > β-MSH > γ-MSH	Hypothalamus, limbic system, cerebrum, brain stem
MC5R	α-MSH > ACTH > β-MSH > γ-MSH	Muscles, liver, spleen, lungs, brain, adipocytes

it affects lipolysis (67, 70) as well as leptin (71) and interleukin 6 production (69)], skin (72–74), pituitary (75), rat sympathetic ganglia (76), fetal and neonatal mouse testis (77, 78), human endometrium (79), human erythroblasts (80), and human osteoblasts (81, 82). The concept of receptor desensitization was not forgotten and was investigated in detail, and findings were somewhat contentious, but all agreed that receptor phosphorylation by various kinases (GPCR kinase and protein kinases A and C) is essential for desensitization and subsequent internalization *via* clathrin-coated pits (83–87).

There are several disorders associated with aberrant ACTH action. Familial glucocorticoid deficiency (FDG), which is also known as familial glucocorticoid insufficiency, hereditary adrenocortical unresponsiveness to ACTH, and familial Addison's disease, is a rare, early onset, autosomal recessive disorder characterized by low or undetectable plasma cortisol levels, normal mineralocorticoid levels, excess plasma ACTH, and hypoplasia of adrenal cortex *zona fasciculata* and *zona reticularis*. Typical physical symptoms include frequent hypoglycemia and/or infective episodes accompanied by excessive skin pigmentation. This disease was described in detail for the first time by Shepard in 1959 (88), and other studies soon followed (89–96). All reports highlighted an unusual resistance to ACTH in patients and a positive response to glucocorticosteroid treatment. Nevertheless, until 1993, when the first mutations within *ACTHR* coding sequence were discovered (97), the genetic cause of this disorder remained unknown. From this pivotal moment, the number of reports involving sequencing of *ACTHR*, which is located on the small arm of chromosome 18 (18p11.21-pter) (98), increased significantly (99–101) and facilitated accumulation of some structural information that is reviewed in a separate chapter. However, although this information did provide some clear links between genetic cause and physiological effect, surprisingly, mutations within *ACTHR* were the cause of FGD in only 25% of cases, indicating additional ACTHR-related factors. In the aftermath of these initial genetic discoveries, the disorder caused by a faulty *ACTHR* gene was designated as FDG type I, while disorders of unknown cause were designated FDG type II (100, 102–104).

As the incoming information from genetic studies was in a good agreement with the difficulties in expressing ACTHR, interest remained intense and molecular research continued. The first breakthrough was achieved in 1995 when Schimmer and colleagues revealed that ACTH-resistant Y6 and OS3 cell lines derived a decade earlier from the Y1 adrenal cell line (105) completely failed to express ACTHR (106). This provided for the first time a platform for sensitive and unbiased ACTHR characterization (107–109). An important study using one of these cell lines was performed by Noon and colleagues who expressed an ACTHR-green fluorescent protein (GFP) fusion protein and observed that the receptor is retained within the endoplasmic reticulum (ER) of CHO cells, but successfully reached the cell membrane in Y6 cells. Thus, they concluded that adrenal cells produce some kind of ACTHR accessory factor that overcomes receptor trafficking arrest (110).

The discovery of this accessory factor was reported in 2005 by Metherell and colleagues (39) who performed SNP array genotyping on an FGD type 2 family to map the causal mutation to chromosome 21 locus 21q22.1, which spanned 30 known or predicted genes at the time. Subsequent *in silico* and mRNA expression analyses revealed that one of these genes, a predicted small single TM domain protein encoding a six exon gene named "chromosome 21 open reading frame 61 (C21orf61)," was expressed in adrenals and carried a mutation within the third intron donor splice site. *In vitro* co-expression of this protein with ACTHR-GFP in CHO and SK-N-SH cells confirmed that the receptor successfully reached the cell membrane and was functionally active. Based on these results, the newly identified protein was renamed the melanocortin receptor accessory protein (MRAP). Following the confirmation of its functional purpose, Matherell and colleagues performed an in-depth analysis of the gene and its expression profile. They discovered two isoforms of MRAP resulting from alternative splicing: MRAP-α and MRAP-β. The 172 aa MRAP-α is the product of the first five exons, while the 102 aa MRAP-β is formed from the third, fourth, and sixth exons. Since the "Start" codon is located within the third exon, both isoforms have identical N-termini and TM domains, but distinct C-termini. Analysis of protein expression patterns revealed that both proteins are differentially expressed in various tissues. Simultaneous expression was observed in the adrenals, testis, breast, ovary, adipocytes, skin, and jejunum. MRAP-α is also expressed in the thyroid, lymph nodes, ileum, liver, stomach, and pituitary, while MRAP-β is only expressed in the brain (39). It was later revealed that mutations in *MRAP* account for another 20–25% of FGD cases, thus it was established that there are additional causal factors for this disease that distinguish FGD type 2 and FGD type 3, the later referring to cases of unknown genetic cause (111).

As would be expected, the discovery of MRAP stimulated research aimed at uncovering the molecular mechanisms of ACTHR action. However, it also initiated an additional line of research aimed at investigating MRAP itself. These studies demonstrated that ACTHR is differentially affected by MRAP isoforms, with MRAP-α providing higher sensitivity to ACTH, whereas higher cAMP response and membrane trafficking occur during co-expression with MRAP-β (112). Detailed investigations on the actions of the accessory proteins revealed a unique feature; in the cell, MRAP is present as a highly stable, SDS-resistant, antiparallel homodimer in which the C-terminus of one monomer is on the cytoplasmic side of the cell membrane, while the C-terminus of the other is on the extracellular side of the cell membrane (113, 114). A few years later, the same dimer topology was also observed in another membrane protein sharing 39% aa sequence identity with MRAP that was also able to facilitate ACTHR trafficking to the cell membrane, and this evolutionary related protein was therefore named MRAP2 (115). There was, however, one major difference between MRAP1 (the name was accordingly updated) and MRAP2; when co-expressed with MRAP2, ACTHR was located on the surface of the cell, but stimulation with ACTH induced the cAMP response with 1000-fold lower potency than when co-expressed with MRAP1 (116). This observation indicated that MRAP1 is more than a mere "deliverer" and is instead an essential functional component of ACTHR (115). Indeed, it was soon discovered that the N-terminal region comprising residues 18–21 (–L–D–Y–L–) is essential for

ACTHR ligand recognition (117). Its substitution with alanine residues resulted in an MRAP2-like protein that promoted only the trafficking of receptors to the plasma membrane. Alignment of both MRAPs revealed that this is the exact region missing from the MRAP2 sequence, and its insertion using site-directed mutagenesis allowed MRAP2 to form a functionally active ACTHR (117, 118). Further mutagenesis of various MRAP1 regions also revealed that the N-terminal side of TM region, formed from residues 31–37 (-L-K-A-N-K-H-S-), is required for MRAP1 to form an antiparallel dimer, since its removal resulted in the formation of a protein with the N-terminus always oriented on the extracellular side of the cell membrane (117). Additional aa replacement experiments showed that the TM domain of MRAP1 provides specific coupling to ACTHR, although the nature of this interaction remains unclear (117, 118). It should be noted that this review only considers MRAP1 in relation to ACTHR, but the functions of this protein extend beyond formation of functionally active ACTHR (115, 119–123).

The latest development in the field of ACTHR research regards the dimerization of the receptor itself. It has been known for a long time that various GPCRs form homo- and heterodimers and that dimerization is essential for the formation of functionally active receptors and implementation of their physiological effects (124–126). Therefore, the discovery of MCR homo- and heterodimerization was not surprising (127). However, initial difficulties with expression prevented such experiments on ACTHR, but this changed in 2011 when Cooray and colleagues performed bioluminescence resonance energy transfer analysis on functionally active ACTHR (the ACTHR and MRAP1 complex) which revealed that, just like other GPCRs, ACTHR formed dimers. Furthermore, only when each ACTHR subunit was accompanied by an MRAP1 dimer was a functionally active ACTHR formed, hence the realization that a hetero-hexameric structure is required for full activity (**Figure 3**) (128).

Finally, we would like to highlight the important contribution made by *ACTHR* knock-out mice. Phenotypic data from these animals were in a very good agreement with observations by medical practitioners on the effects of ACTHR deficiencies in humans. *ACTHR* knock-out mice therefore provided an experimental system for investigating the complexity of ACTHR action in mammals (129–134), but these studies are too voluminous and are beyond the immediate scope of this article.

MCs AND MCRs

More targeted research aimed at understanding the molecular mechanisms that underlie the action of MCRs was undertaken soon after their discovery. The majority of these studies focused on MC1R or MC4R, as they were either considered the best representatives, or the pharmacologically most relevant MCRs. Some research was also carried out on MC3R and MC5R, but due to expression difficulties, targeted studies on ACTHR were not performed until after 2000. Nevertheless, despite being highly specific, ACTHR is a member of the MCRs family and thus general MCR ligand-binding mechanisms are relevant and likely to apply.

Among the first to explore these mechanisms through active intervention were Frandberg and colleagues who performed PCR-based site-directed mutagenesis, a novel method at that time, to substitute selected aa residues with alanine to evaluate

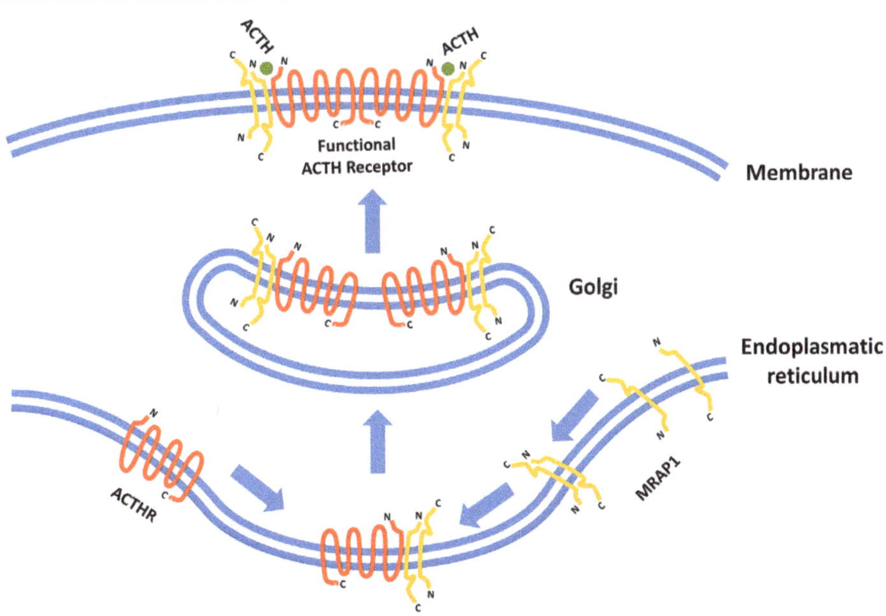

FIGURE 3 | Formation of functionally active adrenocorticotropic hormone receptor (ACTHR). The functional form of ACTHR is a hetero-hexameric structure formed from two molecules of ACTHR and four molecules of MRAP1. The antiparallel dimer of MRAP1 is formed within the endoplasmic reticulum, where it couples to one molecule of ACTHR. Afterward, this complex is transported to the Golgi where it "dimerizes," thus forming the hetero-hexameric functional ACTHR (128). Symbols representing ACTHR and MRAP1 were selected to highlight the protein secondary structure. The depicted intermolecular interactions are therefore general and do not reflect the actual situation in detail.

the role of four human MC1R aa residues (D^{117}, H^{260}, F^{179}, and H^{209}) in ligand recognition and receptor activation. The selection criteria for these residues were the location within the TM domains, the presence of reactive groups, and sequence conservation between known MCRs. The employment of the last two criteria was somewhat traditional, since reactive groups are necessary for molecular interactions, whereas the degree of conservation indicates structural and/or functional importance of residue. However, the first criterion was unusual because known binding pockets for the majority of receptors were on their surface. MCRs were the smallest known GPCRs, and they bind relatively large peptide ligands, thus it was predicted that their binding pocket would be located between the helices. The results of these experiments revealed that two residues of the four (D^{117} and H^{260}) were essential for binding of α-, β- and γ-MSH peptides, while their substitution had no effect on coupling with artificial ligand NDP-MSH ([Nle^4,D-Phe^7]-α-MSH). This demonstrated not only the importance of these residues but also the principle that different ligands may interact with different regions of the binding pocket (135).

Researchers employed a more sophisticated approach in one subsequent study; instead of creating a large number of receptors by mutating conserved residues, they generated a three-dimensional molecular model of human MC1R based on the cryo-electron microscopy structure of bacteriorhodopsin and the electron density footprint of bovine rhodopsin and docked several natural and synthetic ligands. The results suggested the cavity of MC1R consists of two distinct acidic- and aromatic-binding pockets. According to this model, the acidic pocket is formed from E^{94} (TM2), D^{117} (TM3), and D^{121} (TM3), while the aromatic pocket is formed from F^{175} (TM4), F^{179} (TM4), F^{195} (TM5), F^{196} (TM5), F^{257} (TM6), Y^{182} (TM4), and/or Y^{183} (TM4). Being acidic, the first pocket interacts with basic R residues and to some extent H residues in the MC consensus motif -M-X-H-F-R-W-, while the second pocket interacts with aromatic F and W residues of the same motif (136). In the following years, this research group rigorously tested this model with various point mutations, different native and synthetic ligands, and even through conversion to MC4R. Their results confirmed that residues in the predicted acidic pocket were of paramount importance for ligand binding and do indeed interact predominantly with R residue from the -M-X-H-F-R-W- motif. Data on the aromatic-binding pocket were harder to interpret because considerable alterations in ligand binding were achieved only when multiple mutations were introduced at the same time, suggesting each individual residue plays a small part, and the loss of one may be compensated by the others. However, this conclusion was not supported by an acidic pocket eradication experiment in which all three pocket-forming residues were replaced with alanines. The resulting receptor was functionally inactive yet able to bind α-MSH with modest affinity, indicating other potentially more important ligand-binding elements within the aromatic pocket. Thus, the repertoire of mutated aromatic residues was extended, and W^{254} (TM6), Phe^{257} (TM6), and H^{260} (TM6) were recognized as crucial elements of this ligand-binding pocket (137–139). In the following years, this type of research was performed on all five MCRs, which highlighted the uniqueness of the individual receptor-binding pockets by identifying the aa residues responsible for differential ligand recognition. However, all studies agreed that the six previously mentioned aa residues (**Figure 4**) form the "backbone" of the MCR-binding pocket, while the residues surrounding these act as binding pocket "modifiers" [(65, 140–143); reviewed in Ref. (144–147)].

An interesting attempt to redesign the three-dimensional model of MC4R was undertaken by Pogozheva et al. (149) and Chai et al. (150). Unlike previous groups, these researchers employed data from functional analysis of receptors with point mutations and also used the crystal structure of bovine rhodopsin which had been recently determined (150). In addition, to test the validity of their model, they also performed docking of various native and artificial ligands. According to their model, the binding pocket of MC4R is a large elongated cavity formed by L^{44}, V^{46}, F^{51}, E^{100}, I^{103}, I^{104}, D^{122}, I^{125}, D^{126}, I^{129}, C^{130}, L^{133}, F^{184}, S^{188}, S^{190}, V^{193}, C^{196}, M^{200}, W^{258}, F^{261}, H^{264}, L^{265}, Y^{268}, M^{281}, F^{284}, L^{288}, and M^{292}. This cavity contains several acidic and multiple aromatic residues located in groups on opposing sides thus forming the predicted-binding pockets with "backbone" MC-binding residues (**Figures 4** and **5**). Although hypothetical, this model clearly demonstrates that a significant amount of space is required to incorporate the relatively large β-turn structure of MCs (148), and a similar situation would be expected with all MCRs (links to models are available at http://www.uniprot.org/uniprot/P32245).

In the following years, a number of groups generated 3D models of various MCRs, and each explored MCR-specific themes, whether mutation-induced structural changes or differences in ligand recognition. However, the majority of these models are unavailable for download, and we were therefore unable to assess their intramolecular and intermolecular interactions in detail. For this reason, we used the model generated by Pogozheva et al. (148) and Chai et al. (149) as a reference in our following analysis.

NATURALLY OCCURRING MUTATIONS

Historically, the first source that provided information on the molecular mechanisms underlining the action of ACTHR were genetic studies on FGD—a rare autosomal recessive disorder that, as mentioned in Section "Introduction," can be caused by defects in the *ACTHR* gene. From a genetic standpoint, all these alterations can be subdivided in three groups: mutations within regulatory sequences, mutations that result in severely truncated proteins (frameshift mutations or mutations that introduce STOP codons), and mutations that alter a single aa residue. Since the first two groups, from perspective of this article, are uninformative, they are not reviewed in detail [for reports on this subject see Ref. (107, 151–160)]. However, the third group has provided the scientific community with some valuable knowledge.

The first report on a missense mutation within FGD patients was published by Clark and colleagues soon after the discovery of the ACTHR coding sequence (97). The mutation was located within the extracellular part of the TM2 domain and resulted in substitution of S^{74} with I (**Figure 6**). Subsequent functional characterization of the mutated receptor confirmed that its ability to induce cAMP (107, 161, 162), bind ACTH (107), and even reach the cellular surface (despite being able to couple to

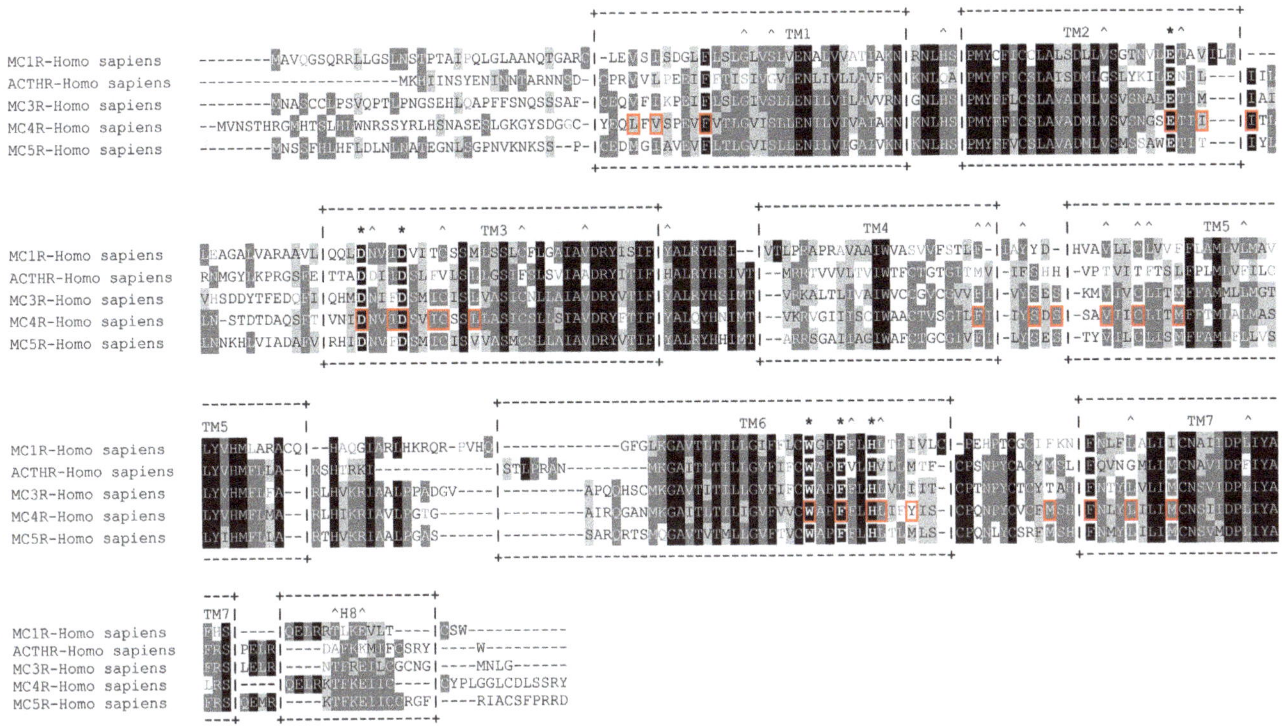

FIGURE 4 | Amino acid sequence alignment of human melanocortin receptors (MCRs). +--+ and vertical dashes mark transmembrane domain boundaries, acquired from GPCRdb (http://gpcrdb.org/). *Indicates residues that form the "backbone" of the MCR-binding pocket. ^Indicates residues that are unique to adrenocorticotropic hormone receptor (ACTHR). Red boxes indicate amino acid residues that, according to the model created by Pogozheva et al. (148) and Chai et al. (149), form the ligand-binding cavity of MC4R.

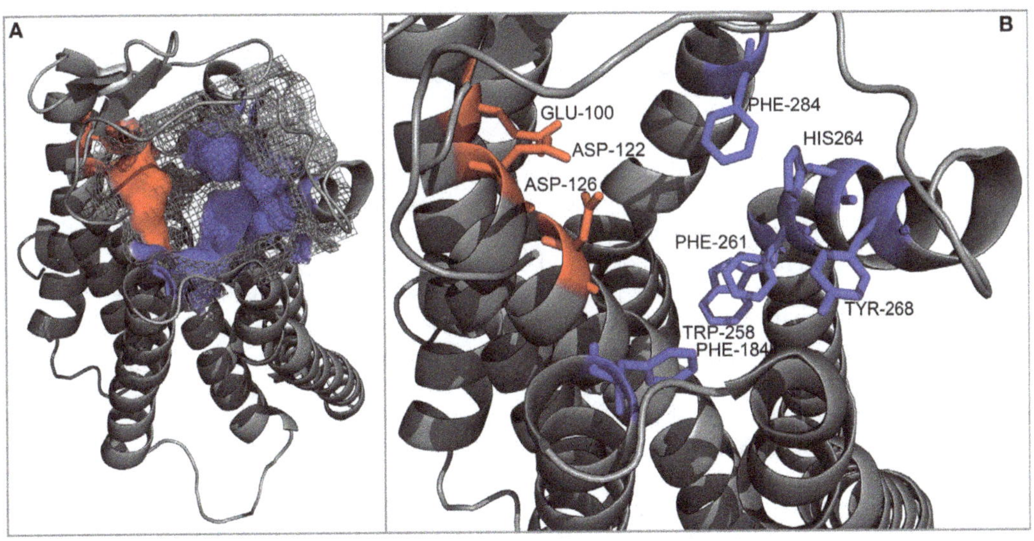

FIGURE 5 | Cartoon representation of the backbone of the MC4R model created by Pogozheva et al. (148) and Chai et al. (149). (A) View from the side and top on the surface of the ligand-binding cavity that contains several acidic (red) and multiple aromatic residues (blue) located in groups at opposite sides of the cavity and forming acidic- and aromatic-binding pockets, respectively. **(B)** Close-up view of the binding cavity without the surface layer.

MRAP1) (156) was severely reduced in comparison to wild-type (WT) ACTHR. As expected, the discovery of this mutation was soon followed by others, and at present 35 different coding sequence alleles have been associated with adrenocortical disorders (detailed information on these mutations is summarized in **Table 2; Figure 6**).

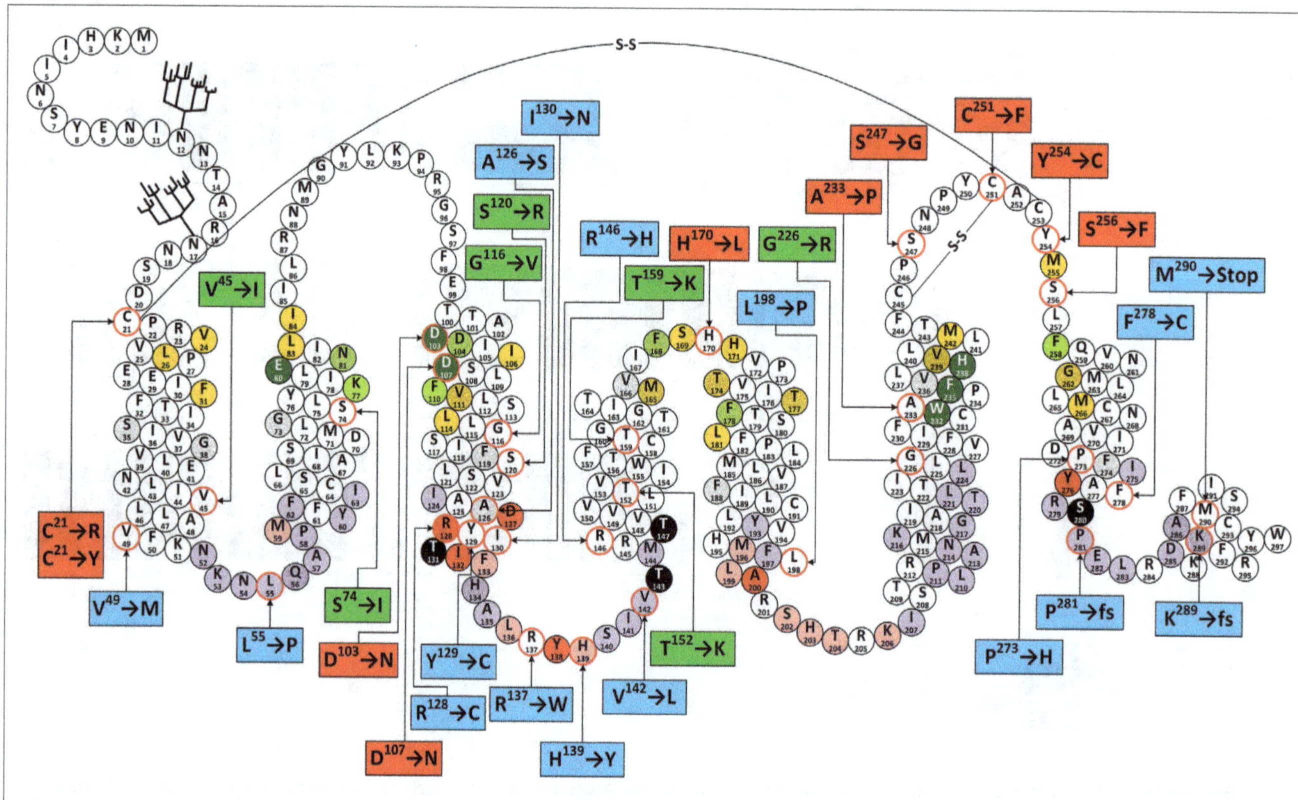

FIGURE 6 | Snake-like plot of adrenocorticotropic hormone receptor (ACTHR). Forked structures represent glycosylation. –S–S– represents disulfide bonds. Circles with a red outline represent naturally occurring missense mutations (labels enclose information on the resulting residue replacement). Red labels indicate residues located on the extracellular part of the receptor. Green labels indicate residues located within the central part of transmembrane domains. Blue labels indicate residues located within the intracellular part of receptor. Dark green circles represent residues that form the backbone of the melanocortin receptor (MCR)-binding pocket. Orange circles represent residues equivalent to those forming the ligand-binding cavity of MC4R based on the model created by Pogozheva et al. (148) and Chai et al. (149). Light green circles represent residues that Yang et al. (146) identified as important for ligand recognition. Circles shaded in red, pink, and light purple represent residues equivalent to those that, according to the ADRB2 model (163), directly interact with Gα, are involved in Gα coupling-related intramolecular interactions, and that form the surface of the Gα-binding cavity, respectively. Circles shaded in black represent S/T residues that are crucial for ACTHR expression and functional regulation. Circles with angled cross-hatching represent residues that are unique to ACTHR (yet conserved in other MCRs).

From a functional point of view, these mutations can be divided into three groups: (1) those located within the intracellular part of the receptor (**Table 2**; blue labels in **Figure 6**) that are most likely to affect G-protein interactions; (2) those located on the extracellular part of the receptor (**Table 2**; red labels in **Figure 6**) that are most likely to affect receptor–ligand interactions; (3) those located within the central regions of TM domains (**Table 2**; green labels in **Figure 6**) that are most likely to affect the overall conformation of the receptor. Despite the fact that this division is quite general, it is in good agreement with data from modeling of the MCR-binding pocket (148) and also the crystal structure of the β_2 adrenergic receptor–G_s protein complex (163).

The majority of extracellular mutations altered either the previously mentioned "backbone" MC-binding residues (dark green in **Figure 6**), as is the case for D^{103} and D^{107}, or residues that are adjacent to other MC ligand cavity-forming residues (orange in **Figure 6**). According to the model, MC4R-S^{259} (ACTHR-A^{233}) and the conserved MC4R-P^{260} (ACTHR-P^{234}) are located between aromatic-binding pocket-forming residues MC4R-W^{258} (ACTHR-W^{232}) and MC4R-F^{261} (ACTHR-F^{235}) (**Figures 4** and **6**). The presence of conserved P within the TM domain is rather unusual, since due to its chemical structure it is unable to participate in the formation of an α-helix, and when present it introduces a "kink"-like structure that is often employed for the proper positioning of surrounding reactive aa residues. Indeed, this appears to be exactly the case for MC4R-P^{260} (ACTHR-P^{234}), and it is logical to presume that additional proline located adjacent to this conserved one, as is the case of ACTHR-A^{233} → P, would not only disrupt the binding pocket but also alter the overall conformation of the receptor to the extent that it is recognized as misfolded and retained within intracellular compartments and ultimately degraded.

According to both the model and other experimental data, there are two structure-stabilizing disulfide bonds within the extracellular region of MCRs (148, 183, 184). It is presumed that in the case of ACTHR these are formed between C^{245} and C^{251}, and between C^{21} and C^{253} (**Figure 6**). Both the MC4R model and predictions using the NetTurnP 1.0 server (185) indicate that the bond between this first pair of residues "locks" the conserved –P–Q–N–P–Y– motif of extracellular loop (EL) 3 into a β-turn-like structure, thus exposing its N and Y residues to the entrance of the binding pocket, and this also limits the physical distance

TABLE 2 | Amino acid residue replacements of naturally occurring *ACTHR* gene missense mutations and their effects on receptor function.

Mutation	Binding	Cyclic adenosine 3′,5′-monophosphate (cAMP)	Basal cAMP activity	Membrane trafficking	Reference
$_{EC}C^{21} \rightarrow R$	↓		↔		(164, 165)
$_{EC}C^{21} \rightarrow Y$					(166)
$_{TM}V^{45} \rightarrow I$	↔	↔			(159)
$_{IC}V^{49} \rightarrow M$					(153)
$_{IC}L^{55} \rightarrow P$				↓	(156)
$_{TM}S^{74} \rightarrow I$	↓	↓		↓	(97, 107, 108, 156–158, 161, 162)
$_{EC}D^{103} \rightarrow N$	↓	↓	↑	↔	(107, 156, 167–170)
$_{EC}D^{107} \rightarrow N$	↓	↓		↔	(156, 159, 171–173)
$_{TM}G^{116} \rightarrow V$		↓		↓	(156, 174)
$_{TM}S^{120} \rightarrow R$				↓	(151, 156)
$_{IC}A^{126} \rightarrow S$		↓			(160)
$_{IC}R^{128} \rightarrow C$	↓	↓		↔	(107, 156, 158)
$_{IC}Y^{129} \rightarrow C$		↓		↓	(156, 175)
$_{IC}I^{130} \rightarrow N$				↓	(156, 176)
$_{IC}R^{137} \rightarrow W$		↓		↓	(108, 156)
$_{IC}H^{139} \rightarrow Y$				↓	(156, 176)
$_{IC}V^{142} \rightarrow L$		↓			(167–169)
$_{IC}R^{146} \rightarrow H$	↓	↓	↑	↓	(107, 156–158, 166, 177)
$_{TM}T^{152} \rightarrow K$				↓	(156, 178)
$_{TM}T^{159} \rightarrow K$	↓	↓	↑	↓	(107, 156, 179)
$_{EC}H^{170} \rightarrow L$		↓		↔	(156)
$_{IC}L^{198} \rightarrow P$				↓	(156, 176)
$_{TM}G^{226} \rightarrow R$				↓	(156)
$_{EC}A^{233} \rightarrow P$		↓		↓	(156, 168, 169)
$_{EC}S^{247} \rightarrow G$	↓		↔		(164, 165)
$_{EC}C^{251} \rightarrow F$		↓		↓	(156, 159, 171, 172)
$_{EC}Y^{254} \rightarrow C$		↓		↓	(108, 156, 180, 181)
$_{EC}S^{256} \rightarrow F$				↓	(156)
$_{IC}P^{273} \rightarrow H$		↓		↓	(156, 162)
$_{IC}F^{278} \rightarrow C$	↔	↔	↑	↔	(109, 175)
$_{IC}P^{281} \rightarrow fs$					(173)
$_{IC}K^{289} \rightarrow fs$				↓	(182)
$_{IC}M^{290} \rightarrow Stop$				↓	(182)
$_{EC}C^{21} \rightarrow R$ + $_{EC}S^{247} \rightarrow G$			↑		(164)
$_{IC}Y^{129} \rightarrow C$ + $_{IC}F^{278} \rightarrow C$		↓		↓	(175)

EC, located within the extracellular part; IC, located within the intracellular part; TM, located within the central part of the TM domain; fs, frameshift; ↔, functional properties were unaffected; ↑, functional properties were improved; ↓, functional properties were hampered; empty field, no data available.

between TM6 and TM7. Although data on the role of "locked" aa residues in MCR ligand recognition is ambiguous, the disruption of this disulfide bond ($C^{251} \rightarrow F$) apparently prevents proper receptor folding and results in intracellular retention. From this perspective, it is hard to explain the negative effect of the $S^{247} \rightarrow G$ mutation, because according to model, the side chain of the residue homologous to ACTHR-S^{247} in MC4R is located on the exterior surface of the receptor and thus cannot be involved in ligand recognition. Perhaps the function of this β-turn-like structure is to serve as a physical barrier that restricts the movement of the ligand while it occupies the cavity, or as a physical support that keeps the cavity entrance open. Thus, replacement of S^{274} with most other residues would not have any effect, but replacement with the highly flexible G allows it to adopt an alternative conformation that does not provide the necessary physical support. The disulfide bond between C^{21} and C^{253} connects TM1 and TM7 domains and locks the TM domain bundle in a "closed" conformation, which reduces flexibility and the number of available conformations. This effect appears to be crucial for formation of a functionally active receptor, as the disruption of this bond by $C^{21} \rightarrow R$ or $C^{21} \rightarrow Y$ mutations resulted in receptors incapable of binding ACTH. One possible explanation is probably connected to fact that the surface of the MCR ligand-binding cavity is predominantly formed from the TM domains. Another mutation that falls within the disulfide bond category is $Y^{254} \rightarrow C$, since it introduces an additional C residue within the EL3 region that could interfere with the formation of one or other of the previously mentioned disulfide bonds. Therefore, unsurprisingly, the $Y^{254} \rightarrow C$ mutant was intracellularly retained, similar to the $C^{251} \rightarrow F$ mutant.

The effects of the last two extracellular mutations ($S^{256} \rightarrow F$ and $H^{170} \rightarrow L$) are harder to explain. Alignment of MCR coding sequences reveals that residue S^{256} is somewhat conserved (present in three out of five human MCRs), while the model suggests that the side chain of MC4R-S^{282} (ACTHR-S^{256}) is oriented toward the external surface of the receptor and thus cannot directly interact with the ligand. However, it is located adjacent to MC4R-M^{281} (ACTHR-M^{255}) that lines the binding cavity, and in close proximity to the disulfide bond forming MC4R-C^{279} (ACTHR-C^{253}). Thus, replacement of the small, polar, and hydrophilic S with a bulky, non-polar, and hydrophobic F could affect these functionally important residues by misfolding the extracellular region, resulting in the retention of the receptor in the interior of the cell. The mechanisms of this effect may vary; for example, to minimize contact with water molecules, the side chain of F could reorient from the exterior surface to the internal cavity of the receptor, or as predicted by TMpred software (186), increase the length of TM7 by introducing an additional turn so that it is embedded within the lipid bilayer of the membrane.

Although difficult to explain, the $H^{170} \rightarrow L$ variant is perhaps the most interesting mutation of on the extracellular side of ACTHR because it is located within EL2, which is the shortest of the three loops. In most MCRs, this region is well conserved and formed from one acidic residue (E or D) and a number of hydrophilic and/or polar residues (**Figure 4**), but within ACTHR there are two basic H and one hydrophilic S residue. The conservation of acidic residues and the participation of both flanking residues in the formation of the binding cavity of MC4R are indicative of a functional purpose. Perhaps it works as "bait" for basic residues on the MC pharmacophore to recruit/direct ligand to the cavity entrance. Alternatively, it could interact with the basic -K–K–R–R–P- motif of ACTH, thus modulating its receptor activation ability. Determination of the true purpose clearly requires additional research. Nevertheless, such speculation is at least partially untrue in the case of ACTHR because the basic H^{170} is in the exact position occupied by an acidic residue in other MCRs, yet the loss of functional activity observed by Clark's group (156) shows that it is still important. Peculiarly, the Clark group also observed that $H^{170} \rightarrow L$, $D^{103} \rightarrow N$, $D^{107} \rightarrow N$, and $R^{128} \rightarrow C$ were the only 4 out of 22 functionally hampered receptors that were effectively transported to the cell membrane. Unifying the other three mutations was their location and functional purpose, since all are located deep within the cavities of ACTHR, and all participate in ligand–receptor or receptor–G-protein interactions. Thus, it can be presumed that these substitutions altered only the internal surface and not the overall structure of ACTHR. In light of this knowledge, it is tempting to speculate that $H^{170} \rightarrow L$ could have similar effects. However, being located on the edge of a binding cavity, this residue cannot participate in interactions with the MC consensus pharmacophore and must instead interact with either the second ACTH pharmacophore (-K–K–R–R–P–) or with MRAP1.

According to the MC4R model, mutations in the central part of the TM domains are located either on the external surface of ACTHR and thus in contact with the lipid bilayer ($S^{74} \rightarrow I$ $T^{152} \rightarrow K$, $T^{159} \rightarrow K$, and $G^{226} \rightarrow R$) or buried within the tightly packed core of the TM bundle ($S^{120} \rightarrow R$ and $G^{116} \rightarrow V$). Therefore, it was not surprising that all native residues were small and/or hydrophobic, and mutated residues were hydrophilic ($S^{120} \rightarrow R$, $T^{152} \rightarrow K$, $T^{159} \rightarrow K$, and $G^{226} \rightarrow R$) or significantly larger than native residues ($S^{74} \rightarrow I$ and $G^{116} \rightarrow V$). The mechanisms underlying the changes in receptor activity for all these substitutions thus appear to be very simple. In the case of hydrophobic → hydrophilic alterations, the introduced residue would likely induce a rotational shift of the TM domain to minimize exposure to the hydrophobic environment, while for small → large alterations, the surrounding structure would have to shift to accommodate the larger residue. Either type of rearrangement would likely result in misfolding and/or altered functional cavities.

Analogous to mutations located on the extracellular side of receptor, those on the intracellular side likely affect receptor–G-protein interactions. The crystal structure of the β_2 adrenergic receptor–Gs protein complex identified a number of receptor residues that are involved in interactions between both partners (163). Although the β_2 adrenergic receptor (ADRB2) and ACTHR are relatively distantly related (~26% sequence identity), they both couple with the $G\alpha_s$ subunit, thus the ACTHR surface that interacts with Gα should be similarly folded to that of ADRB2 (**Figure 6**). For this very reason, we based our subsequent analysis described in the next paragraphs on this receptor–ligand complex crystal structure (PDB ID: 3SN6).

Given that there are a significantly larger number of GPCR subtypes than G-protein subtypes, the correct folding of the intracellular parts of receptors is presumably rigorously monitored and misfolded molecules intracellularly retained and degraded. Indeed, this was observed by the Clark group (156) who characterized a number of intracellular mutations located within ACTHR regions that either directly interact with $G\alpha_s$ ($R^{128} \rightarrow C$) or are homologous to residues that form the surface of ADRB2 $G\alpha_s$ coupling cavity ($L^{55} \rightarrow P$, $H^{139} \rightarrow Y$, $V^{142} \rightarrow L$, $P^{281} \rightarrow fs$, and $K^{289} \rightarrow fs$). The effect of $R^{128} \rightarrow C$ can be easily explained because it is located within the highly conserved rhodopsin GPCR family –D–R–Y– motif, which is involved in signal transduction. The retention of $L^{55} \rightarrow P$, $H^{139} \rightarrow Y$, and $V^{142} \rightarrow L$ is most probably caused by relevant changes in the properties of the residues. Mutation to P often restricts the backbone of the polypeptide chain and prevents the adoption of its native conformation, while the replacement of more hydrophilic H and V to more hydrophobic Y and L generally causes local structural rearrangements because the introduced residues tend to get buried deeper within the protein or lipid bilayer to minimize contact with water molecules. In the case of V^{142}, these local rearrangements and the increased size of the hydrophobic side chain could possibly affect phosphorylation of the adjacent T^{143} because the homologous position (T^{157}) within MC1R is critical for receptor functional activity (86, 187, 188). Peculiar, however, were the P^{281} and K^{289} frameshifts and the $M^{290} \rightarrow$ Stop mutation affecting located within the small C-terminal intracellular α-helix (often referred as H8). Since neither structural data nor experimental results have illuminated the role of this region in signal transduction *via* G-protein binding, the retention caused by its loss seems interesting. Several research groups have undertaken efforts to uncover the purpose of this structural element, but results are ambiguous (189–191). Its primary role could be to properly orient the GPCR within the plasma membrane, so that it can be effectively accessed by both ligand and G-protein.

Results from mutations located outside the binding cavity are harder to interpret, yet some appear relatively straightforward. Substitution of $Y^{129} \rightarrow C$, located within the previously mentioned –D–R–Y– motif, can be interpreted based on the ADRB2 structure, which suggests this particular residue is oriented toward the exterior of the molecule, and a role in signal transduction has been demonstrated in other MCRs (192). The $A^{126} \rightarrow S$ and $I^{130} \rightarrow N$ replacements involve changes from hydrophobic to hydrophilic residues. In both cases, the side chains of native residues are predicted to be located on the surface of the receptor and oriented toward the lipid bilayer; therefore, these replacements most probably induce some structural rearrangements so that the mutated residues have limited interaction with the hydrophobic environment of the membrane. The opposite is likely true of $R^{137} \rightarrow W$, in which the hydrophilic R is replaced with the hydrophobic W. R^{137} (ADRB2-K^{140}) is located between Y^{138} (ADRB2-Y^{141}), and L^{136} (ADRB2-F^{139}), and the first of these two residues interacts with D in the –D–R–Y– motif that orients the second residue toward the hydrophobic pocket of the G-protein. It appears the purpose of the basic R^{137} is to serve as a kind of a "lever" that keeps this otherwise hydrophobic region at the surface of the cell membrane. Its replacement would likely cause this region to adopt a different conformation and possibly "sink" deeper in to the membrane. As already mentioned, replacements involving P are often associated with large changes in the protein backbone, and this appears to be the case for $P^{273} \rightarrow H$ and $L^{198} \rightarrow P$. P^{273} (ADRB2-P^{323}) is one of the most highly conserved residues within rhodopsin GPCRs, where it introduces a kink in TM7 that allows the highly conserved Y^{276} (ADRB2-Y^{326}) to interact with $G\alpha_s$. Introduction of H at this position would likely disrupt the native conformation. The opposite is true of L^{198} which is located at the base of TM5 and followed by IL3, which plays a crucial role in receptor–G-protein interactions. Introduction of P and an associated α-helical kink would alter the orientation of the entire loop, resulting in a misfolded receptor with hampered signal transduction ability.

Of all the intracellular mutations, the effects of $V^{49} \rightarrow M$ and $R^{146} \rightarrow H$ are hardest to interpret, because in both cases the native residue is replaced with a residue that has similar properties. Nevertheless, closer examination involving analysis of the ADRB2 structure can shed light on the underlying mechanisms. Replacement of $V^{49} \rightarrow M$ involves only a change in size and the introduction of a sulfur atom. V^{49} (ADRB2-I^{58}) is located on the surface at the base of TM1 and being hydrophobic, it does not protrude outwards but is instead oriented along the surface of the ACTHR molecule toward the TM2 domain and the receptor interior. V is a small residue compared with M, therefore the size difference could account for the observed effects. However, in ADRB2, the same position is occupied by I, which is also larger than V, yet this receptor has high activity, indicating that the introduction of a sulfur atom cannot be excluded. Interestingly, both sulfur-containing residues (C and M) and H are able to bind metal ions, and if several similar residues are present in a given location, they may simultaneously bind single metal ion to form a bridge-like structure. According to the crystal structure of ADRB2, the base of both TM1 and TM2 is located in close proximity, and there is an additional M^{59} at the base of the TM2 domain in ACTHR that may be sufficiently close to form a metal-binding site with the mutated M^{49} ($V^{49} \rightarrow M$). Based on the structural similarity with ADRB2, this second M^{59} (ADRB2-T^{68}) is likely located within the functionally important region that interacts with the previously mentioned Y^{138} (ADRB2-Y^{141}) and D^{127} (ADRB2-D^{130}) from the –D–R–Y– motif, hence the formation of this putative metal bridge-like structure could alter the ability of the receptor to activate the G-protein. Although this theory seems highly speculative, in our previous studies, we successfully introduced similar albeit artificial metal-binding sites into the structure of MC4R (147).

The $R^{146} \rightarrow H$ replacement involves residues that both are basic, suggesting the observed decrease in receptor's ability to bind ligand, induce functional response and reach cellular surface is due to size differences, aromatic interactions, or the ability to bind metal ions rather than the loss of a reactive group. R^{146} (ADRB2-K^{149}) is located on the surface of the receptor at the base of the TM4 domain. Being hydrophilic, this residue is oriented toward the surface of the molecule, thus structural alterations due to size differences are unlikely to affect receptor function. Coincidentally, as with the TM1 domain, the base of this domain is also located in close proximity to the TM2 domain. Therefore, the formation of a M^{59}–H^{146} metal-binding pocket that alters the conformation of the intracellular region is also plausible. Additionally, within the TM2 domain, approximately one α-helical turn above M^{59} is located F^{62} (ADRB2-F^{71}), which is conserved in rhodopsin GPCRs. The side chain of this residue is oriented toward the TM4 domain, suggesting that abnormal aromatic interactions could prohibit ACTHR from adopting its native conformation in a similar way to that proposed for the putative metal-binding pockets described above.

In addition to mutations that hamper receptor activity, the intracellular part of ACTHR includes two constitutive activity mutations $F^{278} \rightarrow C$ and the double mutation $C^{21} \rightarrow R + S^{247} \rightarrow G$. The first of these mutations was discovered in a patient with ACTH-independent Cushing's syndrome, a disease typically caused by excess ACTH. Functional analysis revealed that this mutated receptor was effectively transported to the cell surface and displayed functional activity parameters that were comparable with WT ACTHR. The only difference was the elevated basal activity. Further research revealed that this effect was due to deficient receptor desensitization, and site-directed mutation of the phosphorylation site in the $S^{280} \rightarrow A$ variant resulted in a receptor with similar properties (109). The authors of this article concluded that the $F^{278} \rightarrow C$ mutation somehow masks the presence of the phosphorylation site. However, the mechanism of this masking is still unknown and hard to interpret. Some years later, a patient was identified that in addition to $F^{278} \rightarrow C$ also carried an inactivating $Y^{129} \rightarrow C$ mutation (as described in previous paragraphs). As a result, this double mutant receptor was intracellularly retained.

Although considered to be rare, this $C^{21} \rightarrow R + S^{247} \rightarrow G$ double mutant was identified in another ACTH hypersensitivity patient (164). However, unlike in the previous patient, this mutant displayed only basal activity, and cAMP accumulation was not observed upon stimulation with ACTH. Expressed separately, both mutations generated functionally inactive receptors (as described in previous paragraphs), thus the authors speculated that within the double mutant these residues are located in close proximity and are required to maintain the receptor in an activated conformation.

Taken together, the knowledge gained from naturally occurring mutations is in good agreement with the findings of Pogozheva et al. (148), the MC4R-binding pocket model, and the crystal structure of the β_2 adrenergic receptor–Gs protein complex of Rasmussen et al. (163). Thus, both models appear to be useful for evaluation of the effects caused by single residue mutations.

SITE-DIRECTED MUTAGENESIS

Although analysis of naturally occurring mutations has provided us with a significant amount of functional data, the nature of this type of research can be somewhat random and unfocused. Thus, in order to pursue a broader knowledge on ACTHR specificity and the underlying molecular mechanisms, several research groups employed site-directed mutagenesis and subsequent functional characterization of mutated ACTHRs. Due to the difficulties to express functionally active ACTHR (193), majority of such studies were performed only after the characterization of Y6 and OS3 adrenal cell lines (106) and/or discovery of MRAP1 (39).

One of the first to perform systematic mutagenesis of ACTHR was Yang and colleagues who had already performed similar analyses on other MCRs (138, 139, 142). They introduced 16 point mutations within various ACTHR regions to assess their functional role in ligand binding and receptor activation. The repertoire of mutations covered both residues that were known to alter the activity of MC1-3R, and residues that, according to sequence alignment, were unique to ACTHR. The results of these analyses are summarized in **Table 3** (146). In Section "Discussion," the authors concluded that the general organization of the ACTHR ligand-binding cavity is similar to that of other MCRs, as it also consists of acidic- and aromatic-binding pockets formed by the same "backbone" residues (E^{80}, D^{103}, D^{107}, F^{235}, and H^{238}). However, there are also significant differences. Compared with other MCRs, the role of D^{103} in ligand binding and receptor activation is significantly diminished, as its alteration caused only a 2.8-fold decrease in ACTH (1–24) affinity and a 7.3-fold decrease in potency. The role of this residue appears to be compensated by the adjacent D^{104} that is unique to ACTHR, since replacement of this residue had a greater effect (10.2-fold and 18.3-fold decrease, respectively). A number of aromatic residues unique to ACTHR were also tested, and their replacement with alanine had a significant (F^{168}) or even tremendous (F^{110} and F^{178}) effect on ligand binding and receptor activation. This led to speculation that the binding cavity of ACTHR could be "broader" than that of other MCRs and could accommodate additional ligand residues that would interact with some of the identified functionally relevant unique residues (146). However, work based on the MC4R-binding pocket model (148) partially counters this speculation, because homologous positions of these high effect aromatic residues (F^{110} and F^{178}) were located in close proximity to aromatic residues of the MC consensus pharmacophore (F^{235} and W^{232}, respectively), thus indicating their role in ligand binding and receptor activation. Nevertheless, this "broader" binding cavity remained possible because homologous position of the basic ACTHR-K^{77} within MC4R model resides within the densely packed and hydrophobic TM domain bundle region adjacent to the acidic D^{103}. Being charged and larger than N (in MC1, MC3, and MC4R) or S (in MC5R), this residue could conceivably thread through this region toward the surface of the binding cavity and interact with D^{103} to alter (broaden) the cavity. In light of the previously discussed naturally occurring $H^{170} \rightarrow L$ mutation is was particularly interesting to test F^{168} which, like H^{170}, is located within EL2 at the entrance to the binding cavity, and, like H^{170}, it affects ligand binding, although apparently to a lesser extent. This provided further evidence of the role of this region in receptor functional activity.

Although very informative, this work by Yang and colleagues was not their first involving ACTHR. In their preceding study (published only a few months earlier), they used chimeric MC4/ACTHR receptors to probe TM domain residues of MC4R that are responsible for the high affinity for the synthetic ligand NDP-MSH (195). Due to the high ligand recognition specificity, they

TABLE 3 | Site-directed mutants of adrenocorticotropic hormone receptor (ACTHR) and their effects on receptor function.

Mutation	Binding (×wtACTHR)	Cyclic adenosine 3′,5′-monophosphate (×wtACTHR)	Membrane trafficking (×wtACTHR)	Rate of internalization (% of initial rate)	Reference
$D^{70} \rightarrow A$	X	X	X		(146)
$^{*}K^{77} \rightarrow A$	$K_i = 4.5×\uparrow$	$EC_{50} = 7.8×\uparrow$	$1.4×\downarrow$		
$E^{80} \rightarrow A$	$K_i = 11.6×\uparrow$	$EC_{50} = 9.8×\uparrow$	$1.3×\downarrow$		
$^{*}N^{81} \rightarrow A$	$K_i = 1.8×\uparrow$	$EC_{50} = 2.4×\uparrow$	$1.1×\downarrow$		
$D^{103} \rightarrow N$	$K_i = 2.8×\uparrow$	$EC_{50} = 7.3×\uparrow$	$1.5×\downarrow$		
$^{*}D^{104} \rightarrow N$	$K_i = 10.2×\uparrow$	$EC_{50} = 18.3×\uparrow$	$1.3×\downarrow$		
$D^{107} \rightarrow N$	$K_i > 178.6×\uparrow$	$EC_{50} > 1250.0×\uparrow$	$1.5×\downarrow$		
$^{*}F^{110} \rightarrow A$	$K_i > 116.3×\uparrow$	$EC_{50} > 208.3×\uparrow$	$1.5×\downarrow$		
$^{*}T^{164} \rightarrow A$	$K_i = 1.2×\downarrow$	$EC_{50} = 1.3×\downarrow$	$1.1×\downarrow$		
$^{*}F^{168} \rightarrow A$	$K_i = 25.3×\uparrow$	$EC_{50} = 68.3×\uparrow$	$1.8×\downarrow$		
$^{*}F^{178} \rightarrow A$	$K_i > 178.6×\uparrow$	$EC_{50} > 1250.0×\uparrow$	$1.5×\downarrow$		
$F^{235} \rightarrow A$	$K_i = 17.5×\uparrow$	$EC_{50} = 270.0×\uparrow$	$1.2×\downarrow$		
$H^{238} \rightarrow A$	$K_i > 178.6×\uparrow$	$EC_{50} > 1250.0×\uparrow$	$1.4×\downarrow$		
$^{*}F^{244} \rightarrow A$	$K_i = 1×\leftrightarrow$	$EC_{50} = 1.1×\uparrow$	$1.1×\downarrow$		
$F^{258} \rightarrow A$	$K_i = 13.9×\uparrow$	$EC_{50} = 233.8×\uparrow$	$1.3×\downarrow$		
$D^{272} \rightarrow A$	X	X	X		
$N^{12}N^{13} \rightarrow QQ$		$EC_{50} = \sim 1.4×\uparrow$	$\leftrightarrow$		(194)
$N^{17}N^{18} \rightarrow QQ$		$EC_{50} = \sim 2.1×\uparrow$	$\leftrightarrow$		
$N^{12}N^{13}N^{17}N^{18} \rightarrow QQQQ$		$EC_{50} = \sim 4.5×\uparrow$	$\sim 3.2×\downarrow$		
wtACTHR		$R_{max} = 1×\leftrightarrow$	$1×\leftrightarrow$	33.1	(86)
$T^{131} \rightarrow A$		$R_{max} = 1.1×\downarrow$	$1.27×\uparrow$	<0.1	
$T^{131} \rightarrow D$		$R_{max} = 4.5×\downarrow$	$1.3×\uparrow$	<0.1	
$S^{140} \rightarrow A$		$R_{max} = 1.1×\downarrow$	$1.1×\downarrow$	25.5	
$S^{140} \rightarrow D$		$R_{max} = 1.2×\downarrow$	$1.25×\uparrow$	43.2	
$T^{143} \rightarrow A$		$R_{max} = 33.3×\downarrow$	$100×\downarrow$	22.2	
$T^{143} \rightarrow D$		$R_{max} = 1×\leftrightarrow$	$3.1×\downarrow$	16.3	
$T^{143} \rightarrow S$		$R_{max} = 1.1×\uparrow$	$2.3×\downarrow$	27.7	
$T^{143} \rightarrow G$		X	$11.1×\downarrow$	X	
$T^{143} \rightarrow K$		$R_{max} = 2.9×\downarrow$	$12.5×\downarrow$	X	
$T^{147} \rightarrow A$		$R_{max} = 1.2×\uparrow$	$1.2×\uparrow$	23.6	
$T^{147} \rightarrow D$		$R_{max} = > 100×\downarrow$	$>100×\downarrow$	<0.1	
$S^{202} \rightarrow A$		$R_{max} = 1×\leftrightarrow$	$1.5×\uparrow$	40.6	
$S^{202} \rightarrow D$		$R_{max} = 1.1×\uparrow$	$1.1×\downarrow$	60.7	
$S^{204} \rightarrow A$		$R_{max} = 1.2×\uparrow$	$1×\leftrightarrow$	18.8	
$S^{204} \rightarrow D$		$R_{max} = 1×\leftrightarrow$	$1.5×\downarrow$	39.4	
$S^{208} \rightarrow A$		$R_{max} = 1.1×\uparrow$	$1.1×\downarrow$	22.6	
$S^{208} \rightarrow D$		$R_{max} = 1.1×\downarrow$	$1.1×\downarrow$	56.7	
$T^{209} \rightarrow A$		$R_{max} = 1.1×\uparrow$	$1×\leftrightarrow$	32.4	
$T^{209} \rightarrow D$		$R_{max} = 1.1×\downarrow$	$1.2×\downarrow$	20.1	
$S^{280} \rightarrow A$		$R_{max} = 1×\leftrightarrow$	$1.4×\downarrow$	50.8	
$S^{280} \rightarrow D$		$R_{max} = 1.5×\downarrow$	$1.1×\downarrow$	<0.1	
$S^{294} \rightarrow A$		$R_{max} = 1×\leftrightarrow$	$1.3×\downarrow$	36.4	
$S^{294} \rightarrow D$		$R_{max} = 1.4×\downarrow$	$1.3×\downarrow$	49.0	
$N^{12}N^{13}N^{17}N^{18} \rightarrow QQQQ$		$R_{max} = 1.2×\downarrow$	$3.0×\downarrow$	80.5	

×, fold difference compared with wtACTHR; ↔, value unaffected; ↑, value increased; ↓, value decreased; X, not determined; empty field, no data available.

intended to use the TM domains of ACTHR for loss of function studies, and in order to localize the alterations and simplify data interpretation, they replaced only one TM domain (TM2, TM3, TM4, TM5, or TM6) at a time without disruption of adjacent intracellular or ELs. The results revealed that in majority of cases these replacements had little or no effect on receptor surface expression, NDP-MSH recognition or receptor activation efficiency. The exception was the replacement of TM3 (hMC4R/TM3 hMC2R); although this receptor was transported to the cell surface, it displayed significantly reduced ligand affinity and potency (a 12.7-fold and 40-fold decrease, respectively; Table S1 in Supplementary Material). Therefore, the authors concluded that non-conserved residues in this region determine the ability of MC4R to effectively bind NDP-MSH (195). However, based on the above knowledge, we believe that these observations are more likely due to peculiarities of ligand recognition within ACTHR rather than MC4R, in particular binding pocket disturbance caused by the presence of an additional acidic (D^{104}) residue, and also possibly the aromatic F^{110} residue (195).

The successful application of a chimeric receptor strategy for various MCRs has been reported on multiple occasions (195–198). Since this initial work number of groups including our own group has used this platform for functional research on ACTHR (199–202). However, since the results of these studies are to a degree speculative, and because different analytical methods were employed, the findings are quite difficult to summarize and so are reviewed in chronological order.

Although many groups were working in parallel, we were the first group to publish in this area. During the initial stages of our research (199), we were more interested in exploring the structural elements that determine the selectivity of ACTHR membrane expression rather than its ligand recognition selectivity. Therefore, since it was already known that posttranslational modification of the N-terminus affected the membrane transport of cell-surface glycoproteins, in our first set of chimeric receptors, we substituted this region in both ACTHR and MC4R. The results partially confirmed our hypothesis; the membrane expression of MC4R with the ACTHR N-terminus (Ch1 in Table S1 in Supplementary Material) was significantly reduced compared with wt MC4R. The results also demonstrated that the N-terminus is not the only region of ACTHR that facilitates its intracellular retention, because ACTHR with the N-terminus of MC4R (Ch2 in Table S1 in Supplementary Material) was not trafficked to the cell membrane. Thus, to explore further, we created additional sets of chimeric receptors by replacing ACTHR TM domains with corresponding regions of MC4R in various combinations (Ch3–Ch15 in Table S1 in Supplementary Material). Subsequent evaluation of the membrane transportation efficiency revealed that retention occurred only when both TM3 and TM4 from ACTHR were present simultaneously, suggesting this region, or elements of this region, is responsible for intracellular retention. In addition to membrane transportation, we also carried out binding and cAMP response analyses. Although, due to their sensitivity, the initial purpose of these assays was to enable the detection of low-level membrane trafficking, the results also identified regions that determine ACTHR ligand-binding specificity. MC4R-based chimeric receptors were able to bind ligands when TM4–5 and TM6–7 were replaced with the corresponding parts of ACTHR, but binding was not observed when both regions were replaced simultaneously. Thus, we speculated that there must be some kind of interaction between these two elements, which disrupts the conformation required for formation of the MC consensus pharmacophore (M–X–H–F–R–W) binding pocket (199).

A year after publication of our report, Hinkle and colleagues reported on employment of remarkably similar strategy (201). Indeed, several of the chimeric receptors were identical in spite of being independently created. However, they employed distinct methods for characterization of the chimeric receptor properties (i.e., measurement of surface transport and activation efficiency), and they also evaluated the effects of co-expression with MRAP1. As in our study, the chimeric receptors were generated in sets. The first set included ACTHR-based chimeric receptors with a variety of TM domains replaced to corresponding regions from MC4R (2C1–2C6 in Table S1 in Supplementary Material), while the second set mirrored these so that the same TM domains within MC4R were replaced with the corresponding regions from ACTHR (4C1–4C6 in Table S1 in Supplementary Material). Functional analysis confirmed that co-expression with MRAP1 promoted the cell-surface trafficking of ACTHR-based chimeric receptors, but this was decreased with MC4R-based receptors. However, the ACTHR-based receptor with only the N-terminus, TM1 domain, and IL1 replaced to the corresponding regions of MC4R (2C1 in Table S1 in Supplementary Material) was an exception, since it was located on the cell surface even in the absence of MRAP1, but despite its successful transportation it was functionally inactive. To investigate this further, Hinkle and colleagues created an additional set of chimeric receptors (C2C1a, C2C1b, and C2C1c in Table S1 in Supplementary Material), and subsequent evaluation of their properties narrowed the region responsible for intracellular retention to TM1 alone, because the corresponding receptor variant (C2C1b in Table S1 in Supplementary Material) was both effectively transported to the cell plasma membrane, and functionally active in the presence of MRAP1. Functional analysis of receptors from the main set also revealed another surprising discovery; when co-expressed with MRAP1, ACTHR-based chimeric receptor with TM2, EL1, and TM3 replaced to the corresponding regions of MC4R (2C2 in Table S1 in Supplementary Material) was able to induce intracellular response upon stimulation with both NDP-MSH and ACTH and also displayed substantial constitutive activity. Since both of these traits are known to be characteristic of MC4R, the authors attempted to pinpoint the responsible region by undertaking the creation of another set of C2C2 derivative chimeric receptors (C2C2a, C2C2b, C2C2c, and C2C2d in Table S1 in Supplementary Material), but functional data showed that none shared the properties of the parental chimeric or wt receptors. Based on this and other studies, Hinkle and colleagues proposed that a more likely explanation for these observations was the general misfolding of ACTHR that, without the assistance of MRAP1, is unable to pass the rigorous quality control system in the ER and is subsequently degraded. Regarding our article, the authors simply remarked that although they did not study exactly the same chimeras, but according to their data introduction of the TM2–TM3 or TM4–TM5 regions of ACTHR receptor had little effect on MC4R surface expression (201).

Based on confidence in our own results and given that the action of ACTHR remained largely unexplained, we decided to further investigate the matter. In our following study (200), we generated additional sets of ACTHR-based chimerical receptors. Given our previously proposed hypothesis that the N-terminus and TM3–TM5 region of ACTHR was important for receptor transportation and ligand recognition specificity, we replaced various elements of these regions with the corresponding elements of MC4R (Ch16–Ch22 in Table S1 in Supplementary Material). Similarly to the Hinkle group, we tested all receptors for their ability to reach the cell plasma membrane and induce intracellular cAMP responses upon stimulation with ACTH and α-MSH during both standalone expression and co-expression with MRAP. The results were somewhat unexpected because they indicated that the integrity of the extracellular part of receptor and not the separate TM domains was of paramount importance for the formation of ACTHR-specific and MRAP1-dependent arrest signal. Although initially these observations seemed to conflict with the conclusions of our former publication, in-depth reanalysis of data from both studies revealed a good agreement. In most cases, when the N-terminus, EL1 and EL2 of ACTHR were present the chimera was retained, but when two of the three elements were present, transport of the chimera to the membrane was hampered (Table S1 in Supplementary Material). Intrigued by this finding, we decided to verify and investigate it in more detail by making smaller (two to five aa) replacements within the TM3–TM5 region of Ch2, a chimera from our previous study, which is essentially ACTHR with the N-terminus of MC4R (Table S1 in Supplementary Material). While performing the same analyses as carried out on previous sets of receptors, we observed that in most cases these replacements increased the membrane export efficiency during standalone expression, but replacement of residues located within the central part of TM3 and the intracellular part of TM4 had no effect (Ch24, Ch27, and Ch28 in Figure S1 in Supplementary Material). Co-expression with MRAP1 revealed a whole spectrum of effects, including receptors that were unaffected by MRAP1 and still retained (Ch28 in Figure S1 in Supplementary Material), receptors unaffected by MRAP1 and still effectively transported to the membrane (Ch26, Ch32, and Ch35 in Figure S1 in Supplementary Material), receptors with improved transportation efficiency comparable with ACTHR (Ch24, Ch27, Ch30, Ch31, and Ch34 in Figure S1 in Supplementary Material), and receptors with decreased transportation efficiency comparable to MC4R (Ch23, Ch25, Ch29, and Ch33 in Figure S1 in Supplementary Material). As observed with large-scale replacements, these results were unexpected because we believed we finally understood ACTHR specificity. Nevertheless, like Hinkle and colleagues, we came to the conclusion that the overall structure of ACTHR must be somewhat attuned for misfolding as changes within various regions could avert this effect. Thus, we speculated that similarly to bovine rhodopsin, the extracellular part of ACTHR might form a lid-like structure over the ligand-binding pocket (**Figure 7**), but rather than being permanent like in rhodopsin, it must be able to undergo MRAP1- and -K-K-R-R-P- pharmacophore-induced conformational changes that result in opening of the -M-X-H-F-R-W- binding cavity. In addition, this lid-like structure could also serve as an arrest signal, since being located on the surface of the cell membrane, it is readily accessible to components of the ER quality control system. However, it also appeared that the correct formation of this structure requires a precise alignment of the TM domains, as even the slightest changes were able to disrupt its formation. Although this study, like the previous one, mainly focused on identification of mechanisms underlying the ACTHR membrane transportation

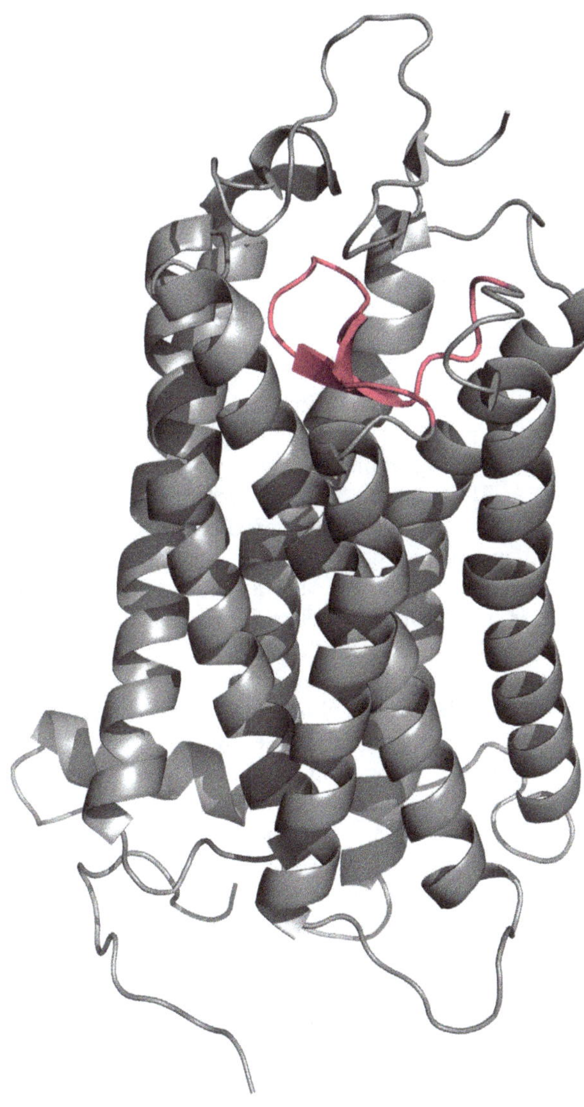

FIGURE 7 | Cartoon representation of the crystal structure of bovine rhodopsin (150). EL2 (magenta) forms a lid-like structure over the ligand-binding pocket that prevents any external molecular interference with the covalently bound ligand.

specificity, we were also able to gain some insight regarding structures that determine its ligand recognition specificity. Since all chimeric receptors created during this study were ACTHR based, it was not surprising that the majority of them were able to induce cAMP responses only when co-expressed with MRAP1 and stimulated with ACTH; therefore, the most interesting in this respect were the functionally inactive Ch24 and Ch31 (Figure S1 in Supplementary Material). The functional inactivity of Ch24 was rather easy to explain, since all affected residues were located in close proximity to residues known to form the –M–X–H–F–R–W– acidic-binding pocket. However, residues replaced within Ch31 were far more interesting because they are located within EL2 that forms the edge of the binding cavity, as described above regarding the naturally occurring $H^{170} \rightarrow L$ mutation. Since none of the adjacent alterations displayed a similar effect, and because selected residues were substituted with corresponding ones from MC4R, we concluded that this region must be either involved in the formation of the –K–K–R–R– binding pocket or functional interaction between ACTHR and MRAP1 that mediates receptor activation. In an attempt to explain this observation, we also compared the properties of the original and substituted residues, which showed that H^{170} and H^{171} (substituted with D and S, respectively) were the most plausible candidates for residues with a functional role because their replacement had the most significant effect on properties of this region, and due to its potential positive charge, propensity for hydrogen-bonding, and aromatic nature, histidine is often a functionally important residue (200).

The latest in a series of publications on chimeric ACTH/MC4 receptors was published by Yang and colleagues (202). This study assessed the binding affinity and potency of the synthetic ligand [D-Phe7]ACTH(1–24) on chimera receptors that were very similar to those described in their previous report in 2007 (195) (Table S1 in Supplementary Material). Their main conclusion was also very similar to their former conclusion that TM3 of ACTHR is critical for ligand selectivity and potency. Therefore, due to their lack of novelty, these results are not reviewed in detail, although there is one aspect that must be mentioned. In this article, the authors also described the creation of five ACTHR-based receptors with single TM domain substitutions to corresponding regions of MC4R (TM2, TM3, TM4, TM5, or TM6; Table S1 in Supplementary Material). In the experimental procedures section, the authors indicated that expression of chimeric receptors was performed in both OS3 and HEK cell lines, the former of which is known to support functional expression of ACTHR. However, during the experiments, they observed that all ACTHR-based chimeric receptors were transported to the cell surface at very low levels, and they therefore failed to assess their ligand-binding affinity and potency (202). Although co-expression with MRAP1 in HEK293 or CHO cell lines and the OS3 cell line may not be directly comparable, in our view, these results are somewhat contrary to the observation made by us and the Hinkle group that most ACTHR-based chimeras co-expressed of with MRAP1 were able to reach the cell membrane and many were functionally active.

Interpreting the results of studies using ACTH/MC4 chimera receptors can be difficult and even controversial. We believe this is due to using a small-scale approach such as few chimeric receptors with single domain replacements to investigate large-scale problems such as the molecular structure and intermolecular interactions of ACTHR (i.e., overinterpretation of results acquired using the reductionist approach). This could be compared with observing the construction of a building through small holes in the fence that surrounds it. Since each group generates their own hypotheses and is only able to generate and test a limited number of mutant receptors, they see only a small part of the "bigger picture" and thus were viewing the problems from a different perspective. Nevertheless, in spite of these differences, we have attempted to summarize the disparate results in Table S1 in Supplementary Material, and, to our surprise, data obtained by different groups are generally in good agreement. Of course, some seemingly identical receptors displayed very different properties in the hands of different research groups, and differences in the expression systems may account for the apparent discrepancies (for example, Ch5 or Ch6 in our study and 2C6 or 4C4 in the Hinkle group). However, the overall general agreement allowed us to draw some summative conclusions. Firstly, it appears there is no single domain that is responsible for ACTHR intracellular retention, but rather the general structure of ACTHR may be somewhat misfolded and coupling with MRAP1 is required to either correct or mask this. Secondly, the results indicated that the role of the extracellular and possibly even the intracellular parts of ACTHR had been underestimated, because in multiple cases the substitution of even a single loop or terminus was crucial on determining receptor localization and the ability to induce an intracellular response.

While ourselves and others were working on large-scale replacements and searching for domains and regions that determine the membrane transportation and ligand recognition specificity of ACTHR, a group led by Gallo-Payet was taking a more focused approach on ACTHR glycosylation (194) and phosphorylation (86) and their effects on receptor functionality. These simple, elegant studies are reviewed below, again in chronological order.

It has been known for quite some time that glycosylation of cell-surface proteins is often required for their successful transport to the plasma membrane (203, 204). In the case of GPCRs, however, the effects of glycosylation are wider and range from being important for correct receptor folding and maturation, to having no apparent function (205–208). Prediction of potential glycosylation sites within ACTHR using such online tools as NetNGlyc 1.0 Server[1] or GlycoEP[2] identifies two glycosylation sites within the N-terminus of the receptor: $N^{12}N^{13}T^{14}$ and $N^{17}N^{18}S^{19}$ (**Figure 6**). Since this aspect of ACTHR functionality had not been previously researched in detail, Roy et al. (194) employed site-directed mutagenesis to eliminate these sites and performed functional expression and characterization of the resultant mutated ACTHRs within the HEK293/FRT cell line to evaluate the role of glycosylation. Upon first reading, the results of this study seemed rather confusing, as the authors observed that during standalone expression abolishment of one

[1]http://www.cbs.dtu.dk/services/NetNGlyc/.

[2]http://www.imtech.res.in/raghava/glycoep/.

glycosylation site had a moderate effect on the surface transportation of ACTHR, while abolishment of both significantly reduced it. In addition, co-expression with MRAP1 (α, β, or C-terminally truncated) resulted in the effective rescue of surface expression for mutants with only one valid glycosylation site, and moderate rescue for mutants with no glycosylation sites (**Table 3**). The confusing part, of course, was the presence of ACTHR at the cell membrane in the absence MRAP. However, this was later explained by the discovery that this cell line actually expresses low levels of MRAP2 that promotes ACTHR membrane transportation. Although at the first glance the selection of this expression system might seem unfortunate, it actually allowed the researchers to observe the effects of glycosylation in detail because, due to overexpression and MRAP1 rescue effects, the employment of any other MRAP2-less cell line most probably would not have allowed them to distinguish between unhampered and moderately hampered transportation efficiency. The causal reason for the endogenous expression of this accessory protein could be related to the source of the particular human embryonic kidney cell line. Based on MRAP2 expression data available at "The Human Protein Atlas"[3] (209, 210), adult kidney tissue expresses this protein at low levels. Although the same database suggests the parent (HEK293) cell line does not express this protein, it is plausible that this cell line is prone to triggering expression during later passages, hence its use in ACTHR surface expression studies should be carefully considered. In addition to cell-surface transportation measurements, the authors also performed receptor activation experiments, and all mutated receptors were functionally active, but there was a tendency for EC_{50} values to increase with the number of mutated glycosylation sites, thus it was concluded that N-glycosylation of ACTHR is not critical but does have a slight influence on receptor activity (**Table 3**) (194).

Another type of posttranslational modification that often plays a major role in protein functionality is phosphorylation. In the case of GPCRs, it is usually associated with receptor desensitization and internalization, and it is performed by a group of serine/threonine protein kinases known as G-protein-coupled receptor kinases (211–215). Since this aspect of ACTHR action was not previously researched in detail, Roy and coworkers (86) introduced point mutations that altered all S and T residues located within the intracellular part of the receptor to the non-phosphorylatable residue A, or to the negatively charged D that can mimic phosphorylation. Additionally, T^{143} was also mutated to S, G, and K because, as already mentioned above, the homologous position (T^{157}) within MC1R is critical for receptor export to the plasma membrane and thus functional activity (86, 187, 188). Detailed activation, surface expression, and receptor internalization analyses both standalone and during co-expression with MRAP1β in the HEK293/FRT cell line generated a large number of results, the most relevant of which (in the context of this review) are presented in **Table 3**. The authors initially evaluated the internalization of WT ACTHR and established that ligand binding is a necessary prerequisite for ACTHR internalization. Additionally, MRAP1 was internalized along with ACTHR, further confirming that a functional receptor is formed following the formation of ACTHR and MRAP1 complex. They also revealed that stimulation with low concentrations of ACTH (<0.3 nM) did not induce any apparent internalization, and ~28% of internalized receptor molecules were recycled back to the cell surface. Having established a baseline and confirmed the necessity of further investigations on the role of intracellular S/T residues, Roy et al. (86) carried out similar analyses on all mutated receptors, and the results showed that $T^{143} \rightarrow A$ and $T^{147} \rightarrow D$ replacements disrupted transportation to the cell surface and abolished the ability to respond to stimulation with ACTH, while the internalization of receptors carrying mutations $T^{131} \rightarrow A$, $T^{131} \rightarrow D$, and $S^{280} \rightarrow D$ was essentially undetectable. Thus, it was concluded that these four residues (T^{131}, T^{143}, T^{147}, and S^{280}) are crucial for ACTHR expression and functional regulation (86).

CONCLUSION

Data presented in this review are rather voluminous and reflect the heterogeneity of available information and applied research methodology. However, despite the difficulties, we hope that condensing this large body of work has proved useful and shall provide some novel insight. At the beginning of this article, we implied that functional ACTHR was discovered only in 2005 by Metherell et al. (39), while 1992 marks the discovery of the main subunit (38). This statement is clearly at odds with the currently used nomenclature, and the name ACTHR is even more at odds (the HGNC accepted name is MC2R). But, through this review, we have come to the conclusion that using term "receptor" is inappropriate because without MRAP1 ACTHR/MC2R does not bind to its ligand. Thus, while in this article we have ignored this, we propose that the name ACTHR should not be abandoned entirely but rather used to describe the molecular complex that specifically binds only ACTH (ACTHR-2 × MRAP1).

AUTHOR CONTRIBUTIONS

Preparation of this article was a joint effort of all authors. DF was coordinating the process of manuscript preparation.

ACKNOWLEDGMENTS

The authors are grateful to Helgi B. Schioth for supporting us throughout our research on ACTHR (MC2R). Preparation of this article was supported by the Latvian Council of Science grant 364/2012.

[3] http://www.proteinatlas.org/.

REFERENCES

1. Collip JB, Anderson E, Thomson DL. The adrenotropic hormone of the anterior pituitary lobe. *Lancet* (1933) 222:347–8. doi:10.1016/S0140-6736(00)44463-6
2. Gallo-Payet N, Payet MD. Mechanism of action of ACTH: beyond cAMP. *Microsc Res Tech* (2003) 61:275–87. doi:10.1002/jemt.10337
3. Saffran M, Grad B, Bayliss MJ. Production of corticoids by rat adrenals in vitro. *Endocrinology* (1952) 50:639–43. doi:10.1210/endo-50-6-639
4. Saffran M, Bayliss MJ. In vitro bioassay of corticotrophin. *Endocrinology* (1953) 52:140–8. doi:10.1210/endo-52-2-140
5. Haynes R, Savard K, Dorfman RI. The action of adrenocorticotropic hormone on beef adrenal slices. *J Biol Chem* (1954) 207:925–38.
6. Vale W, Spiess J, Rivier C, Rivier J. Characterization of a 41-residue ovine hypothalamic peptide that stimulates secretion of corticotropin and beta-endorphin. *Science* (1981) 213:1394–7. doi:10.1126/science.6267699
7. Cawley NX, Li Z, Loh YP. 60 YEARS OF POMC: biosynthesis, trafficking and secretion of pro-opiomelanocortin-derived peptides. *J Mol Endocrinol* (2016) 56(4):T77–97. doi:10.1530/JME-15-0323
8. Metz JR, Peters JJ, Flik G. Molecular biology and physiology of the melanocortin system in fish: a review. *Gen Comp Endocrinol* (2006) 148:150–62. doi:10.1016/j.ygcen.2006.03.001
9. Nakanishi S, Inoue A, Kita T, Nakamura M, Chang AC, Cohen SN, et al. Nucleotide sequence of cloned cDNA for bovine corticotropin-beta-lipotropin precursor. *Nature* (1979) 278:423–7. doi:10.1038/278423a0
10. Sahm UG, Olivier GW, Branch SK, Moss SH, Pouton CW. Synthesis and biological evaluation of alpha-MSH analogues substituted with alanine. *Peptides* (1994) 15:1297–302. doi:10.1016/0196-9781(94)90157-0
11. Haslach EM, Schaub JW, Haskell-Luevano C. Beta-turn secondary structure and melanocortin ligands. *Bioorg Med Chem* (2009) 17:952–8. doi:10.1016/j.bmc.2008.02.090
12. Adan RA, Gispen WH. Melanocortins and the brain: from effects via receptors to drug targets. *Eur J Pharmacol* (2000) 405:13–24. doi:10.1016/S0014-2999(00)00537-9
13. Lerner AB, Lee TH. Isolation of homogeneous melanocyte stimulating hormone from hog pituitary gland. *J Am Chem Soc* (1955) 77:1066–7. doi:10.1021/ja01609a098
14. Bell PH. Purification and structure of β-corticotropin. *J Am Chem Soc* (1954) 76:5565–7. doi:10.1021/ja01650a094
15. Li CH, Geschwind II, Cole RD, Raacke ID, Harris JI, Dixon JS. Amino-acid sequence of alpha-corticotropin. *Nature* (1955) 176:687–9. doi:10.1038/176687a0
16. Shepherd RG, Willson SD, Howard KS, Bell PH, Davies DS, Davis SB, et al. Studies with corticotropin. III. Determination of the structure of β-corticotropin1and its active degradation products. *J Am Chem Soc* (1956) 78:5067–76. doi:10.1021/ja01600a067
17. Li CH, Dixon JS, Chung D. The structure of bovine corticotropin1,2. *J Am Chem Soc* (1958) 80:2587–8. doi:10.1021/ja01543a061
18. Lee TH, Lerner AB, Buettner-Janusch V. On the structure of human corticotropin (adrenocorticotropic hormone). *J Biol Chem* (1961) 236:2970–4.
19. Harris JI, Lerner AB. Amino-acid sequence of the alpha-melanocyte-stimulating hormone. *Nature* (1957) 179:1346–7. doi:10.1038/1791346a0
20. Steelman SL, Guillemin R. Adrenocorticotropic activity of alpha melanocyte stimulating hormone (alpha-MSH). *Proc Soc Exp Biol Med* (1959) 101:600–1. doi:10.3181/00379727-101-25031
21. Schwyzer R, Schiller P, Seelig S, Sayers G. Isolated adrenal cells: log dose response curves for steroidogenesis induced by ACTH(1-24), ACTH(1-10), ACTH(4-10) and ACTH(5-10). *FEBS Lett* (1971) 19:229–31.
22. Seelig S, Sayers G, Schwyzer R, Schiller P. Isolated adrenal cells: ACTH(11-24), a competitive antagonist of ACTH(1-39) and ACTH(1-10). *FEBS Lett* (1971) 19:232–4. doi:10.1016/0014-5793(71)80521-5
23. Schwyzer R. ACTH: a short introductory review. *Ann N Y Acad Sci* (1977) 297:3–26. doi:10.1111/j.1749-6632.1977.tb41843.x
24. Otsuka H, Inouye K. Structure-activity relationships of adrenocorticotropin. *Pharmacol Ther B* (1975) 1:501–27.
25. Dores RM. Adrenocorticotropic hormone, melanocyte-stimulating hormone, and the melanocortin receptors: revisiting the work of Robert Schwyzer: a thirty-year retrospective. *Ann N Y Acad Sci* (2009) 1163:93–100. doi:10.1111/j.1749-6632.2009.04434.x
26. Costa JL, Bui S, Reed P, Dores RM, Brennan MB, Hochgeschwender U. Mutational analysis of evolutionarily conserved ACTH residues. *Gen Comp Endocrinol* (2004) 136:12–6. doi:10.1016/j.ygcen.2003.11.005
27. Liang L, Angleson JK, Dores RM. Using the human melanocortin-2 receptor as a model for analyzing hormone/receptor interactions between a mammalian MC2 receptor and ACTH(1-24). *Gen Comp Endocrinol* (2013) 181:203–10. doi:10.1016/j.ygcen.2012.11.011
28. Samuels ME, Gallo-Payet N, Pinard S, Hasselmann C, Magne F, Patry L, et al. Bioinactive ACTH causing glucocorticoid deficiency. *J Clin Endocrinol Metab* (2013) 98:736–42. doi:10.1210/jc.2012-3199
29. Lowry P. 60 YEARS OF POMC: purification and biological characterisation of melanotrophins and corticotrophins. *J Mol Endocrinol* (2016) 56:T1–12. doi:10.1530/JME-15-0260
30. Dores RM, Liang L, Davis P, Thomas AL, Petko B. 60 YEARS OF POMC: Melanocortin receptors: evolution of ligand selectivity for melanocortin peptides. *J Mol Endocrinol* (2016) 56:T119–33. doi:10.1530/JME-15-0292
31. Orth DN, Nicholson WE. Different molecular forms of Acth. *Ann N Y Acad Sci* (1977) 297:27–48. doi:10.1111/j.1749-6632.1977.tb41844.x
32. Chan JS, Lu CL, Seidah NG, Chretien M. Corticotropin releasing factor (CRF): effects on the release of pro-opiomelanocortin (POMC)-related peptides by human anterior pituitary cells in vitro. *Endocrinology* (1982) 111:1388–90. doi:10.1210/endo-111-4-1388
33. Medzihradszky K. Synthesis of human ACTH and its biologically active fragments. In: Katsoyannis PG, editor. *The Chemistry of Polypeptides: Essays in Honor of Dr. Leonidas Zervas*. Boston, MA: Springer (1973). p. 259–78.
34. Goverde HJ, Pesman GJ, Smals AG. Major contribution of the basic amino acid lysine at position 11 to the bioactivity of ACTH in purified isolated rat adrenocortical cells. *Biochem Biophys Res Commun* (1993) 190:1060–5. doi:10.1006/bbrc.1993.1156
35. Gallo-Payet N. 60 YEARS OF POMC: Adrenal and extra-adrenal functions of ACTH. *J Mol Endocrinol* (2016) 56:T135–56. doi:10.1530/JME-15-0257
36. Dores RM. Observations on the evolution of the melanocortin receptor gene family: distinctive features of the melanocortin-2 receptor. *Front Neurosci* (2013) 7:28. doi:10.3389/fnins.2013.00028
37. Clark AJ. 60 YEARS OF POMC: the proopiomelanocortin gene: discovery, deletion and disease. *J Mol Endocrinol* (2016) 56:T27–37. doi:10.1530/JME-15-0268
38. Mountjoy KG, Robbins LS, Mortrud MT, Cone RD. The cloning of a family of genes that encode the melanocortin receptors. *Science* (1992) 257:1248–51. doi:10.1126/science.1325670
39. Metherell LA, Chapple JP, Cooray S, David A, Becker C, Ruschendorf F, et al. Mutations in MRAP, encoding a new interacting partner of the ACTH receptor, cause familial glucocorticoid deficiency type 2. *Nat Genet* (2005) 37:166–70. doi:10.1038/ng1501
40. Rodbell M. Metabolism of isolated fat cells. I. Effects of hormones on glucose metabolism and lipolysis. *J Biol Chem* (1964) 239:375–80.
41. Rodbell M. Metabolism of isolated fat cells. V. Preparation of "ghosts" and their properties; adenyl cyclase and other enzymes. *J Biol Chem* (1967) 242:5744–50.
42. Oelofsen W, Ramachandran J. Studies of corticotropin receptors on rat adipocytes. *Arch Biochem Biophys* (1983) 225:414–21. doi:10.1016/0003-9861(83)90048-6
43. Simpson ER, Waterman MR. Regulation of the synthesis of steroidogenic enzymes in adrenal cortical cells by ACTH. *Annu Rev Physiol* (1988) 50:427–40. doi:10.1146/annurev.ph.50.030188.002235
44. Haynes RC Jr, Berthet L. Studies on the mechanism of action of the adrenocorticotropic hormone. *J Biol Chem* (1957) 225:115–24.
45. Haynes RC Jr. The activation of adrenal phosphorylase by the adrenocorticotropic hormone. *J Biol Chem* (1958) 233:1220–2.
46. Grahame-Smith DG, Butcher RW, Ney RL, Sutherland EW. Adenosine 3′,5′-monophosphate as the intracellular mediator of the action of adrenocorticotropic hormone on the adrenal cortex. *J Biol Chem* (1967) 242:5535–41.
47. Taunton OD, Roth J, Pastan I. ACTH stimulation of adenyl cyclase in adrenal homogenates. *Biochem Biophys Res Commun* (1967) 29:1–7. doi:10.1016/0006-291X(67)90531-1

48. Taunton OD, Roth J, Pastan I. Studies on the adrenocorticotropic hormone-activated adenyl cyclase of a functional adrenal tumor. *J Biol Chem* (1969) 244:247–53.
49. Lefkowitz RJ, Roth J, Pricer W, Pastan I. ACTH receptors in the adrenal: specific binding of ACTH-125I and its relation to adenyl cyclase. *Proc Natl Acad Sci U S A* (1970) 65:745–52. doi:10.1073/pnas.65.3.745
50. Haynes RC Jr, Koritz SB, Peron FG. Influence of adenosine 3′,5′-monophosphate on corticoid production by rat adrenal glands. *J Biol Chem* (1959) 234:1421–3.
51. Morera AM, Cathiard AM, Saez JM. ACTH-induced refractoriness in cultured adrenal cell line (Y1). *Biochem Biophys Res Commun* (1978) 83:1553–60. doi:10.1016/0006-291X(78)91398-0
52. Penhoat A, Jaillard C, Saez JM. Corticotropin positively regulates its own receptors and cAMP response in cultured bovine adrenal cells. *Proc Natl Acad Sci U S A* (1989) 86:4978–81. doi:10.1073/pnas.86.13.4978
53. Kojima I, Kojima K, Rasmussen H. Role of calcium and cAMP in the action of adrenocorticotropin on aldosterone secretion. *J Biol Chem* (1985) 260:4248–56.
54. Durroux T, Gallo-Payet N, Payet MD. Effects of adrenocorticotropin on action potential and calcium currents in cultured rat and bovine glomerulosa cells. *Endocrinology* (1991) 129:2139–47. doi:10.1210/endo-129-4-2139
55. Yamazaki T, Kimoto T, Higuchi K, Ohta Y, Kawato S, Kominami S. Calcium ion as a second messenger for o-nitrophenylsulfenyl-adrenocorticotropin (NPS-ACTH) and ACTH in bovine adrenal steroidogenesis. *Endocrinology* (1998) 139:4765–71. doi:10.1210/endo.139.12.6338
56. Enyeart JJ, Mlinar B, Enyeart JA. T-type Ca2+ channels are required for adrenocorticotropin-stimulated cortisol production by bovine adrenal zona fasciculata cells. *Mol Endocrinol* (1993) 7:1031–40. doi:10.1210/mend.7.8.8232302
57. Probst WC, Snyder LA, Schuster DI, Brosius J, Sealfon SC. Sequence alignment of the G-protein coupled receptor superfamily. *DNA Cell Biol* (1992) 11:1–20. doi:10.1089/dna.1992.11.1
58. Chhajlani V, Wikberg JE. Molecular cloning and expression of the human melanocyte stimulating hormone receptor cDNA. *FEBS Lett* (1992) 309:417–20. doi:10.1016/0014-5793(92)80820-7
59. Gantz I, Konda Y, Tashiro T, Shimoto Y, Miwa H, Munzert G, et al. Molecular cloning of a novel melanocortin receptor. *J Biol Chem* (1993) 268:8246–50.
60. Gantz I, Miwa H, Konda Y, Shimoto Y, Tashiro T, Watson SJ, et al. Molecular cloning, expression, and gene localization of a fourth melanocortin receptor. *J Biol Chem* (1993) 268:15174–9.
61. Chhajlani V, Muceniece R, Wikberg JE. Molecular cloning of a novel human melanocortin receptor. *Biochem Biophys Res Commun* (1993) 195:866–73. doi:10.1006/bbrc.1993.2125
62. Gantz I, Shimoto Y, Konda Y, Miwa H, Dickinson CJ, Yamada T. Molecular cloning, expression, and characterization of a fifth melanocortin receptor. *Biochem Biophys Res Commun* (1994) 200:1214–20. doi:10.1006/bbrc.1994.1580
63. Konda Y, Gantz I, DelValle J, Shimoto Y, Miwa H, Yamada T. Interaction of dual intracellular signaling pathways activated by the melanocortin-3 receptor. *J Biol Chem* (1994) 269:13162–6.
64. Gantz I, Fong TM. The melanocortin system. *Am J Physiol Endocrinol Metab* (2003) 284:E468–74. doi:10.1152/ajpendo.00434.2002
65. Oosterom J, Nijenhuis WA, Schaaper WM, Slootstra J, Meloen RH, Gispen WH, et al. Conformation of the core sequence in melanocortin peptides directs selectivity for the melanocortin MC3 and MC4 receptors. *J Biol Chem* (1999) 274:16853–60. doi:10.1074/jbc.274.24.16853
66. Mountjoy KG, Bird IM, Rainey WE, Cone RD. ACTH induces up-regulation of ACTH receptor mRNA in mouse and human adrenocortical cell lines. *Mol Cell Endocrinol* (1994) 99:R17–20. doi:10.1016/0303-7207(94)90160-0
67. Boston BA, Cone RD. Characterization of melanocortin receptor subtype expression in murine adipose tissues and in the 3T3-L1 cell line. *Endocrinology* (1996) 137:2043–50. doi:10.1210/endo.137.5.8612546
68. Kubo M, Shimizu C, Kijima H, Nagai S, Koike T. Alternate promoter and 5′-untranslated exon usage of the mouse adrenocorticotropin receptor gene in adipose tissue. *Endocr J* (2004) 51:25–30. doi:10.1507/endocrj.51.25
69. Jun DJ, Na KY, Kim W, Kwak D, Kwon EJ, Yoon JH, et al. Melanocortins induce interleukin 6 gene expression and secretion through melanocortin receptors 2 and 5 in 3T3-L1 adipocytes. *J Mol Endocrinol* (2010) 44:225–36. doi:10.1677/JME-09-0161
70. Boston BA. The role of melanocortins in adipocyte function. *Ann N Y Acad Sci* (1999) 885:75–84. doi:10.1111/j.1749-6632.1999.tb08666.x
71. Norman D, Isidori AM, Frajese V, Caprio M, Chew SL, Grossman AB, et al. ACTH and alpha-MSH inhibit leptin expression and secretion in 3T3-L1 adipocytes: model for a central-peripheral melanocortin-leptin pathway. *Mol Cell Endocrinol* (2003) 200:99–109. doi:10.1016/S0303-7207(02)00410-0
72. Slominski A, Ermak G, Mihm M. ACTH receptor, CYP11A1, CYP17 and CYP21A2 genes are expressed in skin. *J Clin Endocrinol Metab* (1996) 81:2746–9. doi:10.1210/jc.81.7.2746
73. Park HJ, Kim HJ, Lee JY, Cho BK, Gallo RL, Cho DH. Adrenocorticotropin hormone stimulates interleukin-18 expression in human HaCaT keratinocytes. *J Invest Dermatol* (2007) 127:1210–6. doi:10.1038/sj.jid.5700703
74. Cirillo N, Prime SS. Keratinocytes synthesize and activate cortisol. *J Cell Biochem* (2011) 112:1499–505. doi:10.1002/jcb.23081
75. Morris DG, Kola B, Borboli N, Kaltsas GA, Gueorguiev M, McNicol AM, et al. Identification of adrenocorticotropin receptor messenger ribonucleic acid in the human pituitary and its loss of expression in pituitary adenomas. *J Clin Endocrinol Metab* (2003) 88:6080–7. doi:10.1210/jc.2002-022048
76. Nankova BB, Kvetnansky R, Sabban EL. Adrenocorticotropic hormone (MC-2) receptor mRNA is expressed in rat sympathetic ganglia and up-regulated by stress. *Neurosci Lett* (2003) 344:149–52. doi:10.1016/S0304-3940(03)00361-6
77. O'Shaughnessy PJ, Fleming LM, Jackson G, Hochgeschwender U, Reed P, Baker PJ. Adrenocorticotropic hormone directly stimulates testosterone production by the fetal and neonatal mouse testis. *Endocrinology* (2003) 144:3279–84. doi:10.1210/en.2003-0277
78. Johnston H, King PJ, O'Shaughnessy PJ. Effects of ACTH and expression of the melanocortin-2 receptor in the neonatal mouse testis. *Reproduction* (2007) 133:1181–7. doi:10.1530/REP-06-0359
79. Lantang AM, Innes BA, Gan EH, Pearce SH, Lash GE. Expression of melanocortin receptors in human endometrium. *Hum Reprod* (2015) 30:2404–10. doi:10.1093/humrep/dev188
80. Simamura E, Arikawa T, Ikeda T, Shimada H, Shoji H, Masuta H, et al. Melanocortins contribute to sequential differentiation and enucleation of human erythroblasts via melanocortin receptors 1, 2 and 5. *PLoS One* (2015) 10:e0123232. doi:10.1371/journal.pone.0123232
81. Zhong Q, Sridhar S, Ruan L, Ding KH, Xie D, Insogna K, et al. Multiple melanocortin receptors are expressed in bone cells. *Bone* (2005) 36:820–31. doi:10.1016/j.bone.2005.01.020
82. Bohm M, Grassel S. Role of proopiomelanocortin-derived peptides and their receptors in the osteoarticular system: from basic to translational research. *Endocr Rev* (2012) 33:623–51. doi:10.1210/er.2011-1016
83. Baig AH, Swords FM, Szaszak M, King PJ, Hunyady L, Clark AJ. Agonist activated adrenocorticotropin receptor internalizes via a clathrin-mediated G protein receptor kinase dependent mechanism. *Endocr Res* (2002) 28:281–9. doi:10.1081/ERC-120016798
84. Clark AJ, Baig AH, Noon L, Swords FM, Hunyady L, King PJ. Expression, desensitization, and internalization of the ACTH receptor (MC2R). *Ann N Y Acad Sci* (2003) 994:111–7. doi:10.1111/j.1749-6632.2003.tb03169.x
85. Kilianova Z, Basora N, Kilian P, Payet MD, Gallo-Payet N. Human melanocortin receptor 2 expression and functionality: effects of protein kinase A and protein kinase C on desensitization and internalization. *Endocrinology* (2006) 147:2325–37. doi:10.1210/en.2005-0991
86. Roy S, Roy SJ, Pinard S, Taillefer LD, Rached M, Parent JL, et al. Mechanisms of melanocortin-2 receptor (MC2R) internalization and recycling in human embryonic kidney (hek) cells: identification of Key Ser/Thr (S/T) amino acids. *Mol Endocrinol* (2011) 25:1961–77. doi:10.1210/me.2011-0018
87. Baig AH, Swords FM, Noon LA, King PJ, Hunyady L, Clark AJ. Desensitization of the Y1 cell adrenocorticotropin receptor: evidence for a restricted heterologous mechanism implying a role for receptor-effector complexes. *J Biol Chem* (2001) 276:44792–7. doi:10.1074/jbc.M108572200
88. Shepard TH, Landing BH, Mason DG. Familial Addison's disease; case reports of two sisters with corticoid deficiency unassociated with hypoaldosteronism. *AMA J Dis Child* (1959) 97:154–62. doi:10.1001/archpedi.1959.02070010156002
89. Migeon CJ, Kenny EM, Kowarski A, Snipes CA, Spaulding JS, Finkelstein JW, et al. The syndrome of congenital adrenocortical unresponsiveness to ACTH. Report of six cases. *Pediatr Res* (1968) 2:501–13.

90. Franks RC, Nance WE. Hereditary adrenocortical unresponsiveness to ACTH. *Pediatrics* (1970) 45:43–8.
91. Moshang T Jr, Rosenfield RL, Bongiovanni AM, Parks JS, Amrhein JA. Familial glucocorticoid insufficiency. *J Pediatr* (1973) 82:821–6. doi:10.1016/S0022-3476(73)80073-3
92. Thistlethwaite D, Darling JA, Fraser R, Mason PA, Rees LH, Harkness RA. Familial glucocorticoid deficiency. Studies of diagnosis and pathogenesis. *Arch Dis Child* (1975) 50:291–7. doi:10.1136/adc.50.4.291
93. Stempfel RS Jr, Engel FL. A congenital, familial syndrome of adrenocortical insufficiency without hypoaldosteronism. *J Pediatr* (1960) 57:443–51. doi:10.1016/S0022-3476(60)80252-1
94. Williams HE, Freeman M. Primary familial Addison's disease. *J Paediatr Child Health* (1965) 1:93–7. doi:10.1111/j.1440-1754.1965.tb02588.x
95. Kelch RP, Kaplan SL, Biglieri EG, Daniels GH, Epstein CJ, Grumbach MM. Hereditary adrenocortical unresponsiveness to adrenocorticotropic hormone. *J Pediatr* (1972) 81:726–36. doi:10.1016/S0022-3476(72)80093-3
96. Kershnar AK, Roe TF, Kogut MD. Adrenocorticotropic hormone unresponsiveness: report of a girl with excessive growth and review of 16 reported cases. *J Pediatr* (1972) 80:610–9. doi:10.1016/S0022-3476(72)80058-1
97. Clark AJ, McLoughlin L, Grossman A. Familial glucocorticoid deficiency associated with point mutation in the adrenocorticotropin receptor. *Lancet* (1993) 341:461–2. doi:10.1016/0140-6736(93)90208-X
98. Vamvakopoulos NC, Rojas K, Overhauser J, Durkin AS, Nierman WC, Chrousos GP. Mapping the human melanocortin 2 receptor (adrenocorticotropic hormone receptor; ACTHR) gene (MC2R) to the small arm of chromosome 18 (18p11.21-pter). *Genomics* (1993) 18:454–5. doi:10.1006/geno.1993.1499
99. Clark AJ, Weber A. Adrenocorticotropin insensitivity syndromes. *Endocr Rev* (1998) 19:828–43. doi:10.1210/edrv.19.6.0351
100. Cooray SN, Chan L, Metherell L, Storr H, Clark AJ. Adrenocorticotropin resistance syndromes. *Endocr Dev* (2008) 13:99–116. doi:10.1159/000134828
101. Meimaridou E, Hughes CR, Kowalczyk J, Guasti L, Chapple JP, King PJ, et al. Familial glucocorticoid deficiency: new genes and mechanisms. *Mol Cell Endocrinol* (2013) 371:195–200. doi:10.1016/j.mce.2012.12.010
102. Weber A, Clark AJ. Mutations of the ACTH receptor gene are only one cause of familial glucocorticoid deficiency. *Hum Mol Genet* (1994) 3:585–8. doi:10.1093/hmg/3.4.585
103. Naville D, Weber A, Genin E, Durand P, Clark AJ, Begeot M. Exclusion of the adrenocorticotropin (ACTH) receptor (MC2R) locus in some families with ACTH resistance but no mutations of the MC2R coding sequence (familial glucocorticoid deficiency type 2). *J Clin Endocrinol Metab* (1998) 83:3592–6. doi:10.1210/jcem.83.10.5166
104. Genin E, Huebner A, Jaillard C, Faure A, Halaby G, Saka N, et al. Linkage of one gene for familial glucocorticoid deficiency type 2 (FGD2) to chromosome 8q and further evidence of heterogeneity. *Hum Genet* (2002) 111:428–34. doi:10.1007/s00439-002-0806-3
105. Watt VM, Schimmer BP. Association of a 68,000-dalton protein with adrenocorticotropin-sensitive adenylate cyclase activity in Y1 adrenocortical tumor cells. *J Biol Chem* (1981) 256:11365–71.
106. Schimmer BP, Kwan WK, Tsao J, Qiu R. Adrenocorticotropin-resistant mutants of the Y1 adrenal cell line fail to express the adrenocorticotropin receptor. *J Cell Physiol* (1995) 163:164–71. doi:10.1002/jcp.1041630119
107. Elias LL, Huebner A, Pullinger GD, Mirtella A, Clark AJ. Functional characterization of naturally occurring mutations of the human adrenocorticotropin receptor: poor correlation of phenotype and genotype. *J Clin Endocrinol Metab* (1999) 84:2766–70. doi:10.1210/jcem.84.8.5924
108. Fluck CE, Martens JW, Conte FA, Miller WL. Clinical, genetic, and functional characterization of adrenocorticotropin receptor mutations using a novel receptor assay. *J Clin Endocrinol Metab* (2002) 87:4318–23. doi:10.1210/jc.2002-020501
109. Swords FM, Baig A, Malchoff DM, Malchoff CD, Thorner MO, King PJ, et al. Impaired desensitization of a mutant adrenocorticotropin receptor associated with apparent constitutive activity. *Mol Endocrinol* (2002) 16:2746–53. doi:10.1210/me.2002-0099
110. Noon LA, Franklin JM, King PJ, Goulding NJ, Hunyady L, Clark AJ. Failed export of the adrenocorticotrophin receptor from the endoplasmic reticulum in non-adrenal cells: evidence in support of a requirement for a specific adrenal accessory factor. *J Endocrinol* (2002) 174:17–25. doi:10.1677/joe.0.1740017
111. Chan LF, Clark AJ, Metherell LA. Familial glucocorticoid deficiency: advances in the molecular understanding of ACTH action. *Horm Res* (2008) 69:75–82. doi:10.1159/000111810
112. Roy S, Rached M, Gallo-Payet N. Differential regulation of the human adrenocorticotropin receptor [melanocortin-2 receptor (MC2R)] by human MC2R accessory protein isoforms alpha and beta in isogenic human embryonic kidney 293 cells. *Mol Endocrinol* (2007) 21:1656–69. doi:10.1210/me.2007-0041
113. Sebag JA, Hinkle PM. Melanocortin-2 receptor accessory protein MRAP forms antiparallel homodimers. *Proc Natl Acad Sci U S A* (2007) 104:20244–9. doi:10.1073/pnas.0708916105
114. Cooray SN, Almiro Do Vale I, Leung KY, Webb TR, Chapple JP, Egertova M, et al. The melanocortin 2 receptor accessory protein exists as a homodimer and is essential for the function of the melanocortin 2 receptor in the mouse y1 cell line. *Endocrinology* (2008) 149:1935–41. doi:10.1210/en.2007-1463
115. Chan LF, Webb TR, Chung TT, Meimaridou E, Cooray SN, Guasti L, et al. MRAP and MRAP2 are bidirectional regulators of the melanocortin receptor family. *Proc Natl Acad Sci U S A* (2009) 106:6146–51. doi:10.1073/pnas.0809918106
116. Gorrigan RJ, Guasti L, King P, Clark AJ, Chan LF. Localisation of the melanocortin-2-receptor and its accessory proteins in the developing and adult adrenal gland. *J Mol Endocrinol* (2011) 46:227–32. doi:10.1530/JME-11-0011
117. Sebag JA, Hinkle PM. Regions of melanocortin 2 (MC2) receptor accessory protein necessary for dual topology and MC2 receptor trafficking and signaling. *J Biol Chem* (2009) 284:610–8. doi:10.1074/jbc.M804413200
118. Webb TR, Chan L, Cooray SN, Cheetham ME, Chapple JP, Clark AJ. Distinct melanocortin 2 receptor accessory protein domains are required for melanocortin 2 receptor interaction and promotion of receptor trafficking. *Endocrinology* (2009) 150:720–6. doi:10.1210/en.2008-0941
119. Hinkle PM, Sebag JA. Structure and function of the melanocortin2 receptor accessory protein (MRAP). *Mol Cell Endocrinol* (2009) 300:25–31. doi:10.1016/j.mce.2008.10.041
120. Webb TR, Clark AJ. Minireview: the melanocortin 2 receptor accessory proteins. *Mol Endocrinol* (2010) 24:475–84. doi:10.1210/me.2009-0283
121. Jackson DS, Ramachandrappa S, Clark AJ, Chan LF. Melanocortin receptor accessory proteins in adrenal disease and obesity. *Front Neurosci* (2015) 9:213. doi:10.3389/fnins.2015.00213
122. Ramachandrappa S, Gorrigan RJ, Clark AJ, Chan LF. The melanocortin receptors and their accessory proteins. *Front Endocrinol* (2013) 4:9. doi:10.3389/fendo.2013.00009
123. Dores RM, Garcia Y. Views on the co-evolution of the melanocortin-2 receptor, MRAPs, and the hypothalamus/pituitary/adrenal-interrenal axis. *Mol Cell Endocrinol* (2015) 408:12–22. doi:10.1016/j.mce.2014.12.022
124. Angers S, Salahpour A, Bouvier M. Biochemical and biophysical demonstration of GPCR oligomerization in mammalian cells. *Life Sci* (2001) 68:2243–50. doi:10.1016/S0024-3205(01)01012-8
125. Devi LA. Heterodimerization of G-protein-coupled receptors: pharmacology, signaling and trafficking. *Trends Pharmacol Sci* (2001) 22:532–7. doi:10.1016/S0165-6147(00)01799-5
126. Hebert TE, Bouvier M. Structural and functional aspects of G protein-coupled receptor oligomerization. *Biochem Cell Biol* (1998) 76:1–11. doi:10.1139/o98-012
127. Mandrika I, Petrovska R, Wikberg J. Melanocortin receptors form constitutive homo- and heterodimers. *Biochem Biophys Res Commun* (2005) 326:349–54. doi:10.1016/j.bbrc.2004.11.036
128. Cooray SN, Chung TT, Mazhar K, Szidonya L, Clark AJ. Bioluminescence resonance energy transfer reveals the adrenocorticotropin (ACTH)-induced conformational change of the activated ACTH receptor complex in living cells. *Endocrinology* (2011) 152:495–502. doi:10.1210/en.2010-1053
129. Chida D, Sato T, Sato Y, Kubo M, Yoda T, Suzuki H, et al. Characterization of mice deficient in melanocortin 2 receptor on a B6/Balbc mix background. *Mol Cell Endocrinol* (2009) 300:32–6. doi:10.1016/j.mce.2008.10.027
130. Matsuwaki T, Nishihara M, Sato T, Yoda T, Iwakura Y, Chida D. Functional hypothalamic amenorrhea due to increased CRH tone in melanocortin

receptor 2-deficient mice. *Endocrinology* (2010) 151:5489–96. doi:10.1210/en.2010-0687

131. Sato Y, Suzuki H, Sato T, Suda T, Yoda T, Iwakura Y, et al. The role of endogenous glucocorticoids in lymphocyte development in melanocortin receptor 2-deficient mice. *Biochem Biophys Res Commun* (2010) 403:253–7. doi:10.1016/j.bbrc.2010.11.002
132. Chida D, Miyoshi K, Sato T, Yoda T, Kikusui T, Iwakura Y. The role of glucocorticoids in pregnancy, parturition, lactation, and nurturing in melanocortin receptor 2-deficient mice. *Endocrinology* (2011) 152:1652–60. doi:10.1210/en.2010-0935
133. Kameda H, Miyoshi H, Shimizu C, Nagai S, Nakamura A, Kondo T, et al. Expression and regulation of neuromedin B in pituitary corticotrophs of male melanocortin 2 receptor-deficient mice. *Endocrinology* (2014) 155:2492–9. doi:10.1210/en.2013-2077
134. Chida D, Nakagawa S, Nagai S, Sagara H, Katsumata H, Imaki T, et al. Melanocortin 2 receptor is required for adrenal gland development, steroidogenesis, and neonatal gluconeogenesis. *Proc Natl Acad Sci U S A* (2007) 104:18205–10. doi:10.1073/pnas.0706953104
135. Frandberg PA, Muceniece R, Prusis P, Wikberg J, Chhajlani V. Evidence for alternate points of attachment for alpha-MSH and its stereoisomer [Nle4, D-Phe7]-alpha-MSH at the melanocortin-1 receptor. *Biochem Biophys Res Commun* (1994) 202:1266–71. doi:10.1006/bbrc.1994.2067
136. Haskell-Luevano C, Sawyer TK, Trumpp-Kallmeyer S, Bikker JA, Humblet C, Gantz I, et al. Three-dimensional molecular models of the hMC1R melanocortin receptor: complexes with melanotropin peptide agonists. *Drug Des Discov* (1996) 14:197–211.
137. Haskell-Luevano C, Hendrata S, North C, Sawyer TK, Hadley ME, Hruby VJ, et al. Discovery of prototype peptidomimetic agonists at the human melanocortin receptors MC1R and MC4R. *J Med Chem* (1997) 40:2133–9. doi:10.1021/jm960840h
138. Yang Y, Dickinson C, Haskell-Luevano C, Gantz I. Molecular basis for the interaction of [Nle4,D-Phe7]melanocyte stimulating hormone with the human melanocortin-1 receptor. *J Biol Chem* (1997) 272:23000–10. doi:10.1074/jbc.272.37.23000
139. Yang YK, Fong TM, Dickinson CJ, Mao C, Li JY, Tota MR, et al. Molecular determinants of ligand binding to the human melanocortin-4 receptor. *Biochemistry* (2000) 39:14900–11. doi:10.1021/bi001684q
140. Haskell-Luevano C, Cone RD, Monck EK, Wan YP. Structure activity studies of the melanocortin-4 receptor by in vitro mutagenesis: identification of agouti-related protein (AGRP), melanocortin agonist and synthetic peptide antagonist interaction determinants. *Biochemistry* (2001) 40:6164–79. doi:10.1021/bi010025q
141. Nickolls SA, Cismowski MI, Wang X, Wolff M, Conlon PJ, Maki RA. Molecular determinants of melanocortin 4 receptor ligand binding and MC4/MC3 receptor selectivity. *J Pharmacol Exp Ther* (2003) 304:1217–27. doi:10.1124/jpet.102.044974
142. Chen M, Aprahamian CJ, Celik A, Georgeson KE, Garvey WT, Harmon CM, et al. Molecular characterization of human melanocortin-3 receptor ligand-receptor interaction. *Biochemistry* (2006) 45:1128–37. doi:10.1021/bi0521792
143. Ignatovica V, Petrovska R, Fridmanis D, Klovins J. Expression of human melanocortin 4 receptor in *Saccharomyces cerevisiae*. *Cent Eur J Biol* (2011) 6:167–75. doi:10.2478/s11535-011-0002-3
144. Yang Y. Structure, function and regulation of the melanocortin receptors. *Eur J Pharmacol* (2011) 660:125–30. doi:10.1016/j.ejphar.2010.12.020
145. Yang Y, Mishra VK, Chen M, Duffee E, Dimmitt R, Harmon CM. Molecular characterization of human melanocortin-5 receptor ligand-receptor interaction. *Biochemistry* (2013) 52:1737–45. doi:10.1021/bi3013593
146. Chen M, Aprahamian CJ, Kesterson RA, Harmon CM, Yang Y. Molecular identification of the human melanocortin-2 receptor responsible for ligand binding and signaling. *Biochemistry* (2007) 46:11389–97. doi:10.1021/bi700125e
147. Lagerstrom MC, Klovins J, Fredriksson R, Fridmanis D, Haitina T, Ling MK, et al. High affinity agonistic metal ion binding sites within the melanocortin 4 receptor illustrate conformational change of transmembrane region 3. *J Biol Chem* (2003) 278:51521–6. doi:10.1074/jbc.M307683200
148. Pogozheva ID, Chai BX, Lomize AL, Fong TM, Weinberg DH, Nargund RP, et al. Interactions of human melanocortin 4 receptor with nonpeptide and peptide agonists. *Biochemistry* (2005) 44:11329–41. doi:10.1021/bi0501840
149. Chai BX, Pogozheva ID, Lai YM, Li JY, Neubig RR, Mosberg HI, et al. Receptor-antagonist interactions in the complexes of agouti and agouti-related protein with human melanocortin 1 and 4 receptors. *Biochemistry* (2005) 44:3418–31. doi:10.1021/bi0478704
150. Palczewski K, Kumasaka T, Hori T, Behnke CA, Motoshima H, Fox BA, et al. Crystal structure of rhodopsin: a G protein-coupled receptor. *Science* (2000) 289:739–45. doi:10.1126/science.289.5480.739
151. Tsigos C, Arai K, Hung W, Chrousos GP. Hereditary isolated glucocorticoid deficiency is associated with abnormalities of the adrenocorticotropin receptor gene. *J Clin Invest* (1993) 92:2458–61. doi:10.1172/JCI116853
152. Tsiotra PC, Koukourava A, Kaltezioti V, Geffner ME, Naville D, Begeot M, et al. Compound heterozygosity of a frameshift mutation in the coding region and a single base substitution in the promoter of the ACTH receptor gene in a family with isolated glucocorticoid deficiency. *J Pediatr Endocrinol Metab* (2006) 19:1157–66. doi:10.1515/JPEM.2006.19.9.1157
153. Mazur A, Koehler K, Schuelke M, Skunde M, Ostanski M, Huebner A. Familial glucocorticoid deficiency type 1 due to a novel compound heterozygous MC2R mutation. *Horm Res* (2008) 69:363–8. doi:10.1159/000117393
154. Chan LF, Metherell LA, Krude H, Ball C, O'Riordan SM, Costigan C, et al. Homozygous nonsense and frameshift mutations of the ACTH receptor in children with familial glucocorticoid deficiency (FGD) are not associated with long-term mineralocorticoid deficiency. *Clin Endocrinol (Oxf)* (2009) 71:171–5. doi:10.1111/j.1365-2265.2008.03511.x
155. al Kandari HM, Katsumata N, al Alwan I, al Balwi M, Rasoul MS. Familial glucocorticoid deficiency in five Arab kindreds with homozygous point mutations of the ACTH receptor (MC2R): genotype and phenotype correlations. *Horm Res Paediatr* (2011) 76:165–71. doi:10.1159/000328035
156. Chung TT, Webb TR, Chan LF, Cooray SN, Metherell LA, King PJ, et al. The majority of adrenocorticotropin receptor (melanocortin 2 receptor) mutations found in familial glucocorticoid deficiency type 1 lead to defective trafficking of the receptor to the cell surface. *J Clin Endocrinol Metab* (2008) 93:4948–54. doi:10.1210/jc.2008-1744
157. Lin L, Hindmarsh PC, Metherell LA, Alzyoud M, Al-Ali M, Brain CE, et al. Severe loss-of-function mutations in the adrenocorticotropin receptor (ACTHR, MC2R) can be found in patients diagnosed with salt-losing adrenal hypoplasia. *Clin Endocrinol (Oxf)* (2007) 66:205–10. doi:10.1111/j.1365-2265.2006.02709.x
158. Weber A, Toppari J, Harvey RD, Klann RC, Shaw NJ, Ricker AT, et al. Adrenocorticotropin receptor gene mutations in familial glucocorticoid deficiency: relationships with clinical features in four families. *J Clin Endocrinol Metab* (1995) 80:65–71. doi:10.1210/jc.80.1.65
159. Naville D, Barjhoux L, Jaillard C, Faury D, Despert F, Esteva B, et al. Demonstration by transfection studies that mutations in the adrenocorticotropin receptor gene are one cause of the hereditary syndrome of glucocorticoid deficiency. *J Clin Endocrinol Metab* (1996) 81:1442–8. doi:10.1210/jc.81.4.1442
160. Artigas RA, Gonzalez A, Riquelme E, Carvajal CA, Cattani A, Martinez-Aguayo A, et al. A novel adrenocorticotropin receptor mutation alters its structure and function, causing familial glucocorticoid deficiency. *J Clin Endocrinol Metab* (2008) 93:3097–105. doi:10.1210/jc.2008-0048
161. Weber A, Kapas S, Hinson J, Grant DB, Grossman A, Clark AJ. Functional characterization of the cloned human ACTH receptor: impaired responsiveness of a mutant receptor in familial glucocorticoid deficiency. *Biochem Biophys Res Commun* (1993) 197:172–8. doi:10.1006/bbrc.1993.2456
162. Wu SM, Stratakis CA, Chan CH, Hallermeier KM, Bourdony CJ, Rennert OM, et al. Genetic heterogeneity of adrenocorticotropin (ACTH) resistance syndromes: identification of a novel mutation of the ACTH receptor gene in hereditary glucocorticoid deficiency. *Mol Genet Metab* (1998) 64:256–65. doi:10.1006/mgme.1998.2724
163. Rasmussen SG, DeVree BT, Zou Y, Kruse AC, Chung KY, Kobilka TS, et al. Crystal structure of the beta2 adrenergic receptor-Gs protein complex. *Nature* (2011) 477:549–55. doi:10.1038/nature10361
164. Swords FM, Noon LA, King PJ, Clark AJ. Constitutive activation of the human ACTH receptor resulting from a synergistic interaction between

two naturally occurring missense mutations in the MC2R gene. *Mol Cell Endocrinol* (2004) 213:149–54. doi:10.1016/j.mce.2003.10.052

165. Hiroi N, Yakushiji F, Shimojo M, Watanabe S, Sugano S, Yamaguchi N, et al. Human ACTH hypersensitivity syndrome associated with abnormalities of the ACTH receptor gene. *Clin Endocrinol (Oxf)* (1998) 48:129–34. doi:10.1046/j.1365-2265.1998.3971187.x
166. Matsuura H, Shiohara M, Yamano M, Kurata K, Arai F, Koike K. Novel compound heterozygous mutation of the MC2R gene in a patient with familial glucocorticoid deficiency. *J Pediatr Endocrinol Metab* (2006) 19:1167–70. doi:10.1515/JPEM.2006.19.9.1167
167. Berberoglu M, Aycan Z, Ocal G, Begeot M, Naville D, Akar N, et al. Syndrome of congenital adrenocortical unresponsiveness to ACTH. Report of six patients. *J Pediatr Endocrinol Metab* (2001) 14:1113–8. doi:10.1515/jpem-2001-0807
168. Penhoat A, Naville D, El Mourabit H, Buronfosse A, Durand P, Begeot M. Functional expression of the human ACTH receptor gene. *Endocr Res* (2000) 26:549–57. doi:10.3109/07435800009048569
169. Penhoat A, Naville D, El Mourabit H, Buronfosse A, Berberoglu M, Ocal G, et al. Functional relationships between three novel homozygous mutations in the ACTH receptor gene and familial glucocorticoid deficiency. *J Mol Med* (2002) 80:406–11. doi:10.1007/s00109-002-0333-7
170. Kim CJ, Woo YJ, Kim GH, Yoo HW. Familial glucocorticoid deficiency with a point mutation in the ACTH receptor: a case report. *J Korean Med Sci* (2009) 24:979–81. doi:10.3346/jkms.2009.24.5.979
171. Naville D, Penhoat A, Barjhoux L, Jaillard C, Fontanay S, Saez J, et al. Characterization of the human ACTH receptor gene and in vitro expression. *Endocr Res* (1996) 22:337–48. doi:10.1080/07435809609043716
172. Naville D, Barjhoux L, Jaillard C, Saez JM, Durand P, Begeot M. Stable expression of normal and mutant human ACTH receptor: study of ACTH binding and coupling to adenylate cyclase. *Mol Cell Endocrinol* (1997) 129:83–90. doi:10.1016/S0303-7207(97)04043-4
173. Delmas O, Marrec C, Caietta E, Simonin G, Morel Y, Girard N, et al. [Uncommon neonatal case of hypoglycemia: ACTH resistance syndrome]. *Arch Pediatr* (2014) 21:1353–8. doi:10.1016/j.arcped.2014.09.010
174. Collares CV, Antunes-Rodrigues J, Moreira AC, Franca SN, Pereira LA, Soares MM, et al. Heterogeneity in the molecular basis of ACTH resistance syndrome. *Eur J Endocrinol* (2008) 159:61–8. doi:10.1530/EJE-08-0079
175. Chan LF, Chung TT, Massoud AF, Metherell LA, Clark AJ. Functional consequence of a novel Y129C mutation in a patient with two contradictory melanocortin-2-receptor mutations. *Eur J Endocrinol* (2009) 160:705–10. doi:10.1530/EJE-08-0636
176. Naville D, Penhoat A, Bégeot M. Syndromes de résistance à l'ACTH. *Ann Endocrinol* (2000) 61:428–39. doi:AE-11-2000-61-5-00034266-101019-ART5
177. Slavotinek AM, Hurst JA, Dunger D, Wilkie AO. ACTH receptor mutation in a girl with familial glucocorticoid deficiency. *Clin Genet* (1998) 53:57–62. doi:10.1111/j.1399-0004.1998.tb02583.x
178. Turan S, Hughes C, Atay Z, Guran T, Haliloglu B, Clark AJ, et al. An atypical case of familial glucocorticoid deficiency without pigmentation caused by coexistent homozygous mutations in MC2R (T152K) and MC1R (R160W). *J Clin Endocrinol Metab* (2012) 97:E771–4. doi:10.1210/jc.2011-2414
179. Habeb AM, Hughes CR, Al-Arabi R, Al-Muhamadi A, Clark AJ, Metherell LA. Familial glucocorticoid deficiency: a diagnostic challenge during acute illness. *Eur J Pediatr* (2013) 172:1407–10. doi:10.1007/s00431-013-2044-1
180. Tsigos C, Arai K, Latronico AC, DiGeorge AM, Rapaport R, Chrousos GP. A novel mutation of the adrenocorticotropin receptor (ACTH-R) gene in a family with the syndrome of isolated glucocorticoid deficiency, but no ACTH-R abnormalities in two families with the triple A syndrome. *J Clin Endocrinol Metab* (1995) 80:2186–9. doi:10.1210/jcem.80.7.7608277
181. Francescato G, Salvatoni A, Persani L, Agosti M. A rare genetic disorder causing persistent severe neonatal hypoglycaemia the diagnostic workup. *BMJ Case Rep* (2012) 2012:bcr0320125979. doi:10.1136/bcr-03-2012-5979
182. Hirsch A, Meimaridou E, Fernandez-Cancio M, Pandey AV, Clemente M, Audi L, et al. Loss of the C terminus of melanocortin receptor 2 (MC2R) results in impaired cell surface expression and ACTH insensitivity. *J Clin Endocrinol Metab* (2011) 96:E65–72. doi:10.1210/jc.2010-1056
183. Yang Y, Chen M, Kesterson RA Jr, Harmon CM. Structural insights into the role of the ACTH receptor cysteine residues on receptor function. *Am J Physiol Regul Integr Comp Physiol* (2007) 293:R1120–6. doi:10.1152/ajpregu.00240.2007
184. Frändberg P-A, Doufexis M, Kapas S, Chhajlani V. Cysteine residues are involved in structure and function of melanocortin 1 receptor: substitution of a cysteine residue in transmembrane segment two converts an agonist to antagonist. *Biochem Biophys Res Commun* (2001) 281:851–7. doi:10.1006/bbrc.2001.4429
185. Petersen B, Lundegaard C, Petersen TN. NetTurnP – neural network prediction of beta-turns by use of evolutionary information and predicted protein sequence features. *PLoS One* (2010) 5:e15079. doi:10.1371/journal.pone.0015079
186. Hofmann K, Stoffel W. TMbase – a database of membrane spanning proteins segments. *Biol Chem Hoppe-Seyler* (1993) 374:166.
187. Sanchez-Laorden BL, Jimenez-Cervantes C, Garcia-Borron JC. Regulation of human melanocortin 1 receptor signaling and trafficking by Thr-308 and Ser-316 and its alteration in variant alleles associated with red hair and skin cancer. *J Biol Chem* (2007) 282:3241–51. doi:10.1074/jbc.M606865200
188. Sanchez-Laorden BL, Herraiz C, Valencia JC, Hearing VJ, Jimenez-Cervantes C, Garcia-Borron JC. Aberrant trafficking of human melanocortin 1 receptor variants associated with red hair and skin cancer: steady-state retention of mutant forms in the proximal golgi. *J Cell Physiol* (2009) 220:640–54. doi:10.1002/jcp.21804
189. Aratake Y, Okuno T, Matsunobu T, Saeki K, Takayanagi R, Furuya S, et al. Helix 8 of leukotriene B4 receptor 1 inhibits ligand-induced internalization. *FASEB J* (2012) 26:4068–78. doi:10.1096/fj.12-212050
190. Bruno A, Costantino G, de Fabritiis G, Pastor M, Selent J. Membrane-sensitive conformational states of helix 8 in the metabotropic Glu2 receptor, a class C GPCR. *PLoS One* (2012) 7:e42023. doi:10.1371/journal.pone.0042023
191. Sensoy O, Weinstein H. A mechanistic role of Helix 8 in GPCRs: computational modeling of the dopamine D2 receptor interaction with the GIPC1-PDZ-domain. *Biochim Biophys Acta* (2015) 1848:976–83. doi:10.1016/j.bbamem.2014.12.002
192. Huang H, Tao YX. Functions of the DRY motif and intracellular loop 2 of human melanocortin 3 receptor. *J Mol Endocrinol* (2014) 53:319–30. doi:10.1530/JME-14-0184
193. Schioth HB, Chhajlani V, Muceniece R, Klusa V, Wikberg JE. Major pharmacological distinction of the ACTH receptor from other melanocortin receptors. *Life Sci* (1996) 59:797–801. doi:10.1016/0024-3205(96)00370-0
194. Roy S, Perron B, Gallo-Payet N. Role of asparagine-linked glycosylation in cell surface expression and function of the human adrenocorticotropin receptor (melanocortin 2 receptor) in 293/FRT cells. *Endocrinology* (2010) 151:660–70. doi:10.1210/en.2009-0826
195. Chen M, Cai M, Aprahamian CJ, Georgeson KE, Hruby V, Harmon CM, et al. Contribution of the conserved amino acids of the melanocortin-4 receptor in [corrected] [Nle4,D-Phe7]-alpha-melanocyte-stimulating [corrected] hormone binding and signaling. *J Biol Chem* (2007) 282:21712–9. doi:10.1074/jbc.M702285200
196. Kim CS, Lee SH, Kim RY, Kim BJ, Li SZ, Lee IH, et al. Identification of domains directing specificity of coupling to G-proteins for the melanocortin MC3 and MC4 receptors. *J Biol Chem* (2002) 277:31310–7. doi:10.1074/jbc.M112085200
197. Muceniece R, Mutule I, Mutulis F, Prusis P, Szardenings M, Wikberg JE. Detection of regions in the MC1 receptor of importance for the selectivity of the MC1 receptor super-selective MS04/MS05 peptides. *Biochim Biophys Acta* (2001) 1544:278–82. doi:10.1016/S0167-4838(00)00227-2
198. Schioth HB, Yook P, Muceniece R, Wikberg JE, Szardenings M. Chimeric melanocortin MC1 and MC3 receptors: identification of domains participating in binding of melanocyte-stimulating hormone peptides. *Mol Pharmacol* (1998) 54:154–61.
199. Fridmanis D, Petrovska R, Kalnina I, Slaidina M, Peculis R, Schioth HB, et al. Identification of domains responsible for specific membrane transport and ligand specificity of the ACTH receptor (MC2R). *Mol Cell Endocrinol* (2010) 321:175–83. doi:10.1016/j.mce.2010.02.032
200. Fridmanis D, Petrovska R, Pjanova D, Schioth HB, Klovins J. Replacement of short segments within transmembrane domains of MC2R disrupts retention signal. *J Mol Endocrinol* (2014) 53:201–15. doi:10.1530/JME-14-0169
201. Hinkle PM, Serasinghe MN, Jakabowski A, Sebag JA, Wilson KR, Haskell-Luevano C. Use of chimeric melanocortin-2 and -4 receptors to identify regions responsible for ligand specificity and dependence on melanocortin 2 receptor accessory protein. *Eur J Pharmacol* (2011) 660:94–102. doi:10.1016/j.ejphar.2010.10.113

202. Yang Y, Mishra V, Crasto CJ, Chen M, Dimmitt R, Harmon CM. Third transmembrane domain of the adrenocorticotropic receptor is critical for ligand selectivity and potency. *J Biol Chem* (2015) 290:7685–92. doi:10.1074/jbc.M114.596122
203. Petrecca K, Atanasiu R, Akhavan A, Shrier A. N-linked glycosylation sites determine HERG channel surface membrane expression. *J Physiol* (1999) 515(Pt 1):41–8. doi:10.1111/j.1469-7793.1999.041ad.x
204. Gut A, Kappeler F, Hyka N, Balda MS, Hauri HP, Matter K. Carbohydrate-mediated Golgi to cell surface transport and apical targeting of membrane proteins. *EMBO J* (1998) 17:1919–29. doi:10.1093/emboj/17.7.1919
205. Duvernay MT, Filipeanu CM, Wu G. The regulatory mechanisms of export trafficking of G protein-coupled receptors. *Cell Signal* (2005) 17:1457–65. doi:10.1016/j.cellsig.2005.05.020
206. Boer U, Neuschafer-Rube F, Moller U, Puschel GP. Requirement of N-glycosylation of the prostaglandin E2 receptor EP3beta for correct sorting to the plasma membrane but not for correct folding. *Biochem J* (2000) 350(Pt 3):839–47. doi:10.1042/bj3500839
207. Davis D, Liu X, Segaloff DL. Identification of the sites of N-linked glycosylation on the follicle-stimulating hormone (FSH) receptor and assessment of their role in FSH receptor function. *Mol Endocrinol* (1995) 9:159–70. doi:10.1210/me.9.2.159
208. Michineau S, Muller L, Pizard A, Alhenc-Gelas F, Rajerison RM. N-linked glycosylation of the human bradykinin B2 receptor is required for optimal cell-surface expression and coupling. *Biol Chem* (2004) 385:49–57. doi:10.1515/BC.2004.007
209. Uhlen M, Fagerberg L, Hallstrom BM, Lindskog C, Oksvold P, Mardinoglu A, et al. Proteomics. Tissue-based map of the human proteome. *Science* (2015) 347:1260419. doi:10.1126/science.1260419
210. Uhlen M, Oksvold P, Fagerberg L, Lundberg E, Jonasson K, Forsberg M, et al. Towards a knowledge-based Human Protein Atlas. *Nat Biotechnol* (2010) 28:1248–50. doi:10.1038/nbt1210-1248
211. Gurevich EV, Gainetdinov RR, Gurevich VV. G protein-coupled receptor kinases as regulators of dopamine receptor functions. *Pharmacol Res* (2016) 111:1–16. doi:10.1016/j.phrs.2016.05.010
212. Packiriswamy N, Parameswaran N. G-protein-coupled receptor kinases in inflammation and disease. *Genes Immun* (2015) 16:367–77. doi:10.1038/gene.2015.26
213. Park JY, Lee SY, Kim HR, Seo MD, Chung KY. Structural mechanism of GPCR-arrestin interaction: recent breakthroughs. *Arch Pharm Res* (2016) 39:293–301. doi:10.1007/s12272-016-0712-1
214. Prihandoko R, Bradley SJ, Tobin AB, Butcher AJ. Determination of GPCR phosphorylation status: establishing a phosphorylation barcode. *Curr Protoc Pharmacol* (2015) 69:2.13.1–26. doi:10.1002/0471141755.ph0213s69
215. Gurevich EV, Tesmer JJ, Mushegian A, Gurevich VV. G protein-coupled receptor kinases: more than just kinases and not only for GPCRs. *Pharmacol Ther* (2012) 133:40–69. doi:10.1016/j.pharmthera.2011.08.001

8

Hypothesis and Theory: Revisiting Views on the Co-evolution of the Melanocortin Receptors and the Accessory Proteins, MRAP1 and MRAP2

*Robert M. Dores**

Department of Biological Sciences, University of Denver, Denver, CO, USA

***Correspondence:**
Robert M. Dores
rdores@du.edu

The evolution of the melanocortin receptors (MCRs) is closely associated with the evolution of the melanocortin-2 receptor accessory proteins (MRAPs). Recent annotation of the elephant shark genome project revealed the sequence of a putative MRAP1 ortholog. The presence of this sequence in the genome of a cartilaginous fish raises the possibility that the *mrap1* and *mrap2* genes in the genomes of gnathostome vertebrates were the result of the chordate 2R genome duplication event. The presence of a putative MRAP1 ortholog in a cartilaginous fish genome is perplexing. Recent studies on melanocortin-2 receptor (MC2R) in the genomes of the elephant shark and the Japanese stingray indicate that these MC2R orthologs can be functionally expressed in CHO cells without co-expression of an exogenous *mrap1* cDNA. The novel ligand selectivity of these cartilaginous fish MC2R orthologs is discussed. Finally, the origin of the *mc2r* and *mc5r* genes is reevaluated. The distinctive primary sequence conservation of MC2R and MC5R is discussed in light of the physiological roles of these two MCR paralogs.

Keywords: melanocortin receptors, MRAP1, MRAP2, MC2R, MC5R, evolution

INTRODUCTION

In many respects, the features of the melanocortin receptor (MCR) gene family (i.e., *mc1r, mc2r, mc3r, mc4r, mc5r*) are rather straightforward. These G Protein-coupled receptors are only found in chordates (1), and the proliferation of paralogous genes in this family has been influenced by the two genome duplication events that occurred during the early evolution of the chordates (2–4). In addition, these receptors appear to be predominately coupled to a cAMP/PKA pathway at their respective target cells (5). Finally, all of the MCRs are activated by one or more of the melanocortin-related peptides (i.e., ACTH, α-MSH, β-MSH, γ-MSH, or δ-MSH), which are derived from the precursor protein, POMC in gnathostomes (6), and the precursors POM or POC in lampreys (7).

There are also features of this gene family that are somewhat unique. For example, some of the MCRs interact with the accessory proteins melanocortin-2 receptor accessory protein (MRAP)1 and MRAP2 (8, 9), and these interactions can affect receptor trafficking and activation. In addition, for teleosts and tetrapods, the MC2R paralog has exclusive ligand selectivity for ACTH as compared to the more permissive ligand selectivity of the other MCR paralogs for ACTH and the MSH-sized ligands (10). Finally, while it is assumed that two genome duplications should yield four paralogous genes, there are five paralogous genes present in this family. Hence, the origin of the fifth gene and the physiological significance of the fifth gene are another issue that will be revisited.

PHYLOGENY AND PROPOSED EVOLUTION OF THE MRAPs

Following the initial cloning of the five MCRs, pharmacology studies for each receptor were done in heterologous non-adrenal cortex-derived mammalian cell lines with one exception – MC2R (6). Mountjoy et al. (11) found that in order to examine the ligand selectivity of human MC2R, the receptor cDNA needed to be expressed in Cloudman S91 melanoma cells; a cell line that endogenously expresses the *Mc1r* gene. Subsequent studies would show that mammalian MC2R orthologs could be functionally expressed in cell lines derived from adrenal cortex cells, but not in non-adrenal mammalian cell lines (12–15). These observations contributed to the discovery of the accessory protein, MRAP (16).

Melanocortin-2 receptor accessory protein is a single chain polypeptide with one membrane-spanning domain. This transmembrane (TM) protein forms a homodimer at the endoplasmic reticulum in which the two monomers are oriented in an anti-parallel manner [reverse topology; for reviews, see Ref. (8, 9)]. In the human genome, there are two paralogous *MRAP* genes, *MRAP* or *MRAP1* (16), and *MRAP2* (17). For this discussion, "*mrap*" will be used to refer to the ancestral accessory protein gene, and *mrap1* and *mrap2* will be used to designate the two paralogous members of the gene family. As a reference for the discussion that will follow, **Table 1** summarizes the observations from Chan et al. (17) with respect to the effects of human MRAP1α and human MRAP2 on the activation and trafficking of the five human MCRs.

The salient features of the MRAPs are illustrated by mouse MRAP1 and MRAP2 (**Figure 1**). For MRAP1, the LKANKH motif is required for reverse topology (18), and the corresponding reverse topology motif in mouse MRAP2 is LKAHKY, [(8); **Figure 1**]. Reverse topology motifs are also apparent in the chicken and zebrafish MRAP1 and MRAP2 orthologs (**Figure 1**).

The TM domain of mouse Mrap1 is required for the trafficking of MC2R to the plasma membrane (18), and the corresponding sequence in mouse Mrap2 (**Figure 1**) has 43% amino acid sequence identity with the TM domain of mouse Mrap1. Among the MRAP1 orthologs presented in **Figure 1**, the amino acid sequence identity between mouse Mrap1 and chicken MRAP1, and mouse Mrap1 and zebrafish MRAP1 is 74 and 48%, respectively. This level of sequence identity is apparently adequate since both chicken MC2R (19) and zebrafish MC2R (20) can be activated when co-expressed in heterologous mammalian cells with their respective MRAP1 ortholog. It is interesting that the amino acid sequence identity for the TM region of the MRAP2 orthologs presented in **Figure 1** is 74%. Since MRAP2 is expressed in brain and adrenal cortex cells, there appears to be selection pressure to maintain the TM sequences of MRAP2 orthologs. The physiological roles of the MRAP2 orthologs will be discussed later in this section.

Given the preceding comments on primary sequence similarity, the most striking difference between mouse Mrap1 and Mrap2 is the activation motif present in Mrap1 that is conspicuously absent in Mrap2 (**Figure 1**). As a result, although MC2R will move to the plasma membrane in the presence of MRAP2, activation of the receptor following an ACTH-binding event is barely detectable at concentrations of ACTH of 10^{-8}M or less (8, 9, 21). Conversely, in the presence of MRAP1, the activation of MC2R is robust following an ACTH-binding event [(16); **Table 1**]. It would appear then, that when a mammalian MC2R ortholog is expressed alone, the receptor miss-folds, and is non-functional (22). When co-expressed with MRAP1, MC2R assumes an active conformation, and the MC2R/MRAP1 complex can be activated by ACTH. Interaction with an MRAP1 paralog to achieve functional expression is a strict requirement for teleost and tetrapod MC2R orthologs (20, 23).

Sebag and Hinkle (18) found that if the activation motif (LDYI) in the N-terminal domain of mouse Mrap1 (**Figure 1**) was replaced with alanine residues, the activation of MC2R was blocked. Furthermore, a single alanine substitution of the Y residue in the mouse Mrap1 LDYI motif resulted in a 50% drop in activation. Note that similar activation motifs are present in the N-terminal domains of the chicken and zebrafish MRAP1

TABLE 1 | Summary of the interactions between human melanocortin receptors and human MRAP1α and human MRAP2.

	MRAP1α		MRAP2	
	Trafficking	**Activation**	**Trafficking**	**Activation**
MC1R	Not required	Not required	Not required	Lowers
MC2R	Facilitates	Required	Facilitates	Required
MC3R	Not required	Lowers	Not required	Lowers
MC4R	Restricts	Lowers	Restricts	Lowers
MC5R	Restricts	Lowers	Restricts	Lowers

Chan et al. (17) expressed individual human melanocortin receptors in CHO cells either in the presence or absence of either human MRAP1α or human MRAP2, and measured either trafficking to the plasma membrane or activation with human ACTH (1–39) (MC2R; single dose 10^{-6}M) or NDP-MSH (MC1R, MC3R, MC4R, MC5R: single dose 10^{-9}M). For the trafficking experiments, "not required" indicates that co-expression with an MRAP had no negative or positive effect on trafficking to the plasma membrane relative to CHO cells transfected with only the melanocortin receptor. "Facilitates" indicates that the receptor did not translocate to the plasma membrane in the absence of the MRAP. "Restricts" indicates that there was a decline in trafficking to the plasma membrane when the receptor was co-expressed with an MRAP. For activation experiments, "not required" indicates that co-expression with an MRAP had no negative or positive effect on activation relative to CHO cells transfected with only the melanocortin receptor. "Requires" indicates that the receptor could not be activated when expressed alone in CHO cells. "Lowers" indicates that there was a statistically significant drop in activation when the receptor was co-expressed with an MRAP.

```
MRAP1
   [--------------------N-Terminal------------------][----------TM----------]
es M-ADVEAFTNSSEDLRLNHSNSEYRFEYEYY-EYE--VDVSFEGLQVNKYSIVAFFWVGLAVFMIHQVHIIPE
zf M-------KNSS----------EYVWGYEYYYDYVDPVLVNASTLKYSRYSIVLIFWMILAAFIGFFFLILSL
c  M-------ANRT-------NSSEYFWSYEYYWDYIDPIPVDGRKLKVNKYSIVIAFWVGLAAFVMFLFLILLY
m  M-------ANGT-------DASVPLTSYEYYLDYIDLIPVDEKKLKANKHSIVIALWLSLATFVVLLFLILLY

                                Activation      Reverse          Trafficking
                                  Motif     Topology Motif          Motif
MRAP2
m  M-EMSAQRLASNRTSPQSPSNSDYTWEYEYY----EIGPVSFEGLKAHKYSIVIGFWVGLAVFVIFMFFVLTL
c  M---SALRLISNRTSQQALSNSDYTWEYEYY----EYGPVSFEGLKAHKYSIVIGFWVGLAVFVIFMFFVLTL
zf MPRMSENNPVVNKTTHHPGFNNDYTWGYEYY----DYGPVSFEGLKAHRYSIVIGFWVGLAVFVIFMFFVLTL
es M---SENNPVVNKTTHHPGFNNDYTWGYEYY----DYGPVSFEGLKAHRYSIVIGFWVGLVVFVIFMFFVLTL
lp      LNGSERASARTPGSNRSKEYYWDFEYY----DYEPISFEGLRAHRYSIVIGFWVGIASFVLFMFFILVM

MRAP1
   [----------------------C-Terminal-------------------------]
es RPQSLLDNTILLPGGVNP
zf ISHSGQLPRGPRVKKSGLPLMKGYASSQ
c  MSRSGSNPVKQVVVRNRVEESSSNSEQPHGDNLSSPFPDPVAPGTPSCLPDHSGIHGSI
m  MSWSGSPQMRHSPQPQPICSWTHSFNLPLCLRRASLQTTEEPGRRAGTDQWLTQQSPS

MRAP2
m  LTKTGAPHQDNAESSERRFRMNSFVSDFGKPLESDKVFSRQGNEESRSLFHCYINEVEH..............
c  LTKTGAPHQENTESSEKRFRMNSFVADFGRPLESERVFSRQIAEESRSLFHFCINEVEH..............
zf LTKTGAPHPEAAEPYEKRMRLTSCADGLGRQRETDGRTGLSRPLLEESRSLFHCYINEE..............
es LTKTGAPHQENVDLPAKQHRMNGFSVGYPMLQKPDKAFVHRVSEESRSLFHCYVNEVGH..............
lp LVRSGV
```

FIGURE 1 | Amino acid sequence alignment of MRAP1 and MRAP2 paralogs. The amino acid sequences of mouse (m) MRAP1 (NP_084120.1), zebrafish (z) MRAP1 (XP001342923.2), chicken (c) MRAP1 (XR_001470382) elephant shark (es) MRAP1 (XM_007903550.1), mouse (m) MRAP2 (XP_006511239.1), chicken (c) MRAP2 (XP_015140201), zebrafish (zf) MRAP2a (XP_001342923.4), elephant shark (es) MRAP2 (XP_007906624.1), and lamprey (lp) MRAP2 (FAA00710.1) were aligned to the sequences of mouse MRAP1 and mouse MRAP2, respectively. Note that only a partial sequence for lamprey (*Petromyzon marinus*) MRAP2 has been reported (1). In addition, only the partial C-terminal sequences for the MRAP2 orthologs are presented. Predicted N-linked glycosylation sites are underlined. Note that there are two potential N-linked glycosylation sites in the putative elephant shark MRAP1 amino acid sequence. The amino acids in the activation motif for mouse MRAP1 are highlighted in red. Conserved amino acid positions in the proposed activation motifs of the chicken, zebrafish, elephant shark MRAP1 orthologs are also highlighted in red. The amino acids in the reverse topology motif of mouse MRAP1 were highlighted in green. Conserved amino acid positions in the reverse topology motif of chicken, zebrafish, elephant shark, mouse, and lamprey MRAP1 and MRAP2 sequences, respectively, were also highlighted in green. Finally, the amino acids in the transmembrane domain of mouse MRAP1 are highlighted in blue, and the conserved amino acid positions in the chicken, zebrafish, elephant shark, mouse and lamprey MRAP1 and MRAP2 sequences, respectively, were also highlighted in blue.

orthologs (**Figure 1**). In addition, a recent study indicated that alanine substitution of the DY residues in the YDYV motif of zebrafish MRAP1 blocks activation of MC2R (24).

While it appears that the direct interaction of mammalian MRAP2 orthologs with mammalian MC2R orthologs might be pharmacological rather physiological [**Table 1**; (8, 9, 21)], there are cells such as mouse adipocytes (25) and embryonic mouse adrenal cortex cells (26) that co-express Mrap2 as well as Mc2r and Mc5r. Sebag and Hinkle (27) found that when human MC5R and mouse Mrap2 were co-expressed in CHO cells, the trafficking of human MC5R to the plasma membrane decreased. The implication of these experiments was that by decreasing the number of MC5 receptors on the plasma membrane, Mrap2 would make the target cells more selective for stimulation by ACTH, rather than α-MSH. Since, MC2R and MC5R are co-expressed in chicken adrenal cortex cells (28), frog interrenal tissue (23), and rainbow trout interrenal tissue (29), an interaction between MC5R and MRAP2 could have physiological implications for non-mammalian vertebrates as well. Hence, an evaluation of the pharmacological interactions of MC5R and MRAP2 orthologs with respect to trafficking to the plasma membrane and ligand selectivity in these species is warranted.

When considering a physiological role for MRAP2, a promising area of study has been the interaction between MRAP2 and MC4R in the modulation of feeding behavior by neurons in the hypothalamus (30). In both zebrafish (31) and mice (32), endogenous MRAP2 orthologs appear to play roles in the ligand sensitivity of the MC4 receptor. For example, Asai et al. (32) observed that when mouse Mc4r and Mrap2 are co-expressed in HEK-293 cells, Mc4R has a higher sensitivity for α-MSH; an outcome that would decrease feeding activity *in vivo*. Conversely, in mice in which the *Mrap2* gene was selectivity deleted from neurons in the hypothalamus, the result was an obese phenotype. While the implications of these results are intriguing from a biomedical perspective, it appears that for mammals there may be species specific difference in the regulation of MC4R. For example, Kay et al. (33) observed that co-expression of human MC4R and human MRAP2 in HEK-293 cells had no effect on ligand sensitivity. However, a shift in ligand sensitivity was observed when human MC4R was co-expressed with human MRAPα. Clearly, studies are needed on other tetrapods (i.e., amphibians, reptiles, and birds) are needed to determine the role that MRAP2 may play in modulating the ligand selectivity of MC4R in the regulation of feeding behavior in these organisms.

A more complex mechanism for the role of MRAP2 in regulating feeding behavior has been observed for the zebrafish (31, 34). As a result of a teleost-specific genome duplication [3R event; (35)], two paralogs of the *mrap2* gene (*mrap2a* and *mrap2b*) are present in the zebrafish genome (20). Furthermore, the expression of these paralogs appears to be developmentally regulated. Sebag et al. (31) report that during the larval stage of development, MRAP2a lowers the ligand sensitivity of zebrafish MC4R (as measured by *V*max), and as a result the animal eats more; an outcome that would favor growth. During larval development, the expression levels of the zebrafish *mrap2b* gene are low. Conversely in the adult stage, zebrafish *mrapb* gene expression is elevated, and zebrafish *mrapa* gene expression declines. Sebag et al. (31) also report that co-expression of zebrafish MC2R and zebrafish MRAP2 in HEK-293 cells increases the sensitivity of zebrafish MC4R for α-MSH. These results are interpreted as giving the adult zebrafish fine control over food consumption; a trait that would be considered adaptive (31). Hence, it would appear that zebrafish MRAPb is functioning in a manner analogous to mouse Mrap2 (32). However, Aguilleiro et al. (34) observed that co-expression of zebrafish MC4R and zebrafish MRAP2a in HEK-293 cells resulted in a higher sensitivity of the zebrafish MC4R for ACTH as compared to α-MSH. The latter study proposes that ACTH may be playing a role in the control of feeding behavior, and that role can be influenced by the expression levels of zebrafish MRAP2a. In the later study, the *in vitro* effect of zebrafish MRAP2b on zebrafish MC4R ligand selectivity was not apparent. Finally, zebrafish MRAP2a had no negative or positive effect on the trafficking of zebrafish MC4R to the plasma membrane (31, 34); whereas zebrafish MRAP2b appeared to increase the surface expression of zebrafish MC4R (31). Hence, there appears to be species-specific differences in way the MC4R orthologs respond to interaction with MRAP2 (See **Table 1**) That said, at the molecular level it is not clear which domain(s) of MRAP2 (MRAP2a or MRAP2b) are making contact with MC4R to alter ligand selectivity. The possibility of an "activation motif" in MRAP2 orthologs, analogous to the activation motif in MRAP1 orthologs, has not been investigated.

In terms of the evolution of the MRAP gene family, an earlier review concluded that MRAP2 was the ancestral "MRAP" (1). This conclusion was based on the apparent absence of MRAP1 orthologs in the genomes of a cartilaginous fish (*Callorhinchus milii*, the elephant shark) and the lamprey (*Petromyzon marinus*), and the presence of MRAP2 orthologs in both these species. In this scenario, the duplication of the ancestral *mrap* gene may have occurred in the bony fishes following the divergence of the ancestral cartilaginous fishes and the ancestral bony fishes (36) over 420 million years ago. However, recent annotation of the elephant shark genome project[1] revealed a cDNA (accession number: XM_007903550.1) that Blast analysis[2] has identified as an MRAP1 ortholog. The deduced amino acid sequence of the putative elephant shark MRAP1 ortholog is presented in **Figure 1**. The putative elephant shark MRAP1 has a reverse topology motif (LQVNKY), and the TM region has 39% amino acid sequence identity with the mouse MRAP1 TM region. The C-terminal domain of the putative elephant shark MRAP1 is very short relative to the other MRAP1 orthologs. However, Sebag and Hinkle (18) have shown that the C-terminal of mouse MRAP1 is not required for either trafficking or activation of mammalian MC2R orthologs. The N-terminal domain of the putative elephant shark MRAP1 is nearly 43% longer than the other MRAP1 orthologs in **Figure 1**. By inserting gaps, it was possible to align these sequences and identify a putative activation motif (EYE) in the putative elephant shark MRAP1. The presence of the Y residue in this domain is particularly interesting, given the importance of this residue for mammalian and teleost MRAP1 orthologs (18, 24).

From a phylogenetic/evolutionary perspective, the detection of the putative cartilaginous fish MRAP1 ortholog fills a gap. The elephant shark is in Subclass Holocephali (Class Chondrichithyes), and it is very probable that *mrap1* orthologs are present in the genomes of members of Subclass Elasmobranchii (i.e., sharks and rays). Hence, *mrap1* and *mrap2* paralogs may have been present in the genome of the ancestral gnathostomes (**Figure 2**). Given these assumptions, the evolution of the *mrap* gene family may have involved the following scenario. In the ancestral agnathan vertebrates that underwent the 2R genome duplication event, the ancestral *mrap* gene would have been duplicated to yield the *mrap1* and *mrap2* genes, and these paralogous genes presumably would have been distributed on separate chromosomes. Currently, *mrap1* and *mrap2* genes have been found on separate chromosomes in the various gnathostome genome databases where chromosomes maps are available.[3] Among extant 2R

[1] http://esharkgenome.imcb.a-star.edu.sg
[2] https://blast.ncbi.nlm.nih.gov/Blast.cgi
[3] http://ensemble.org

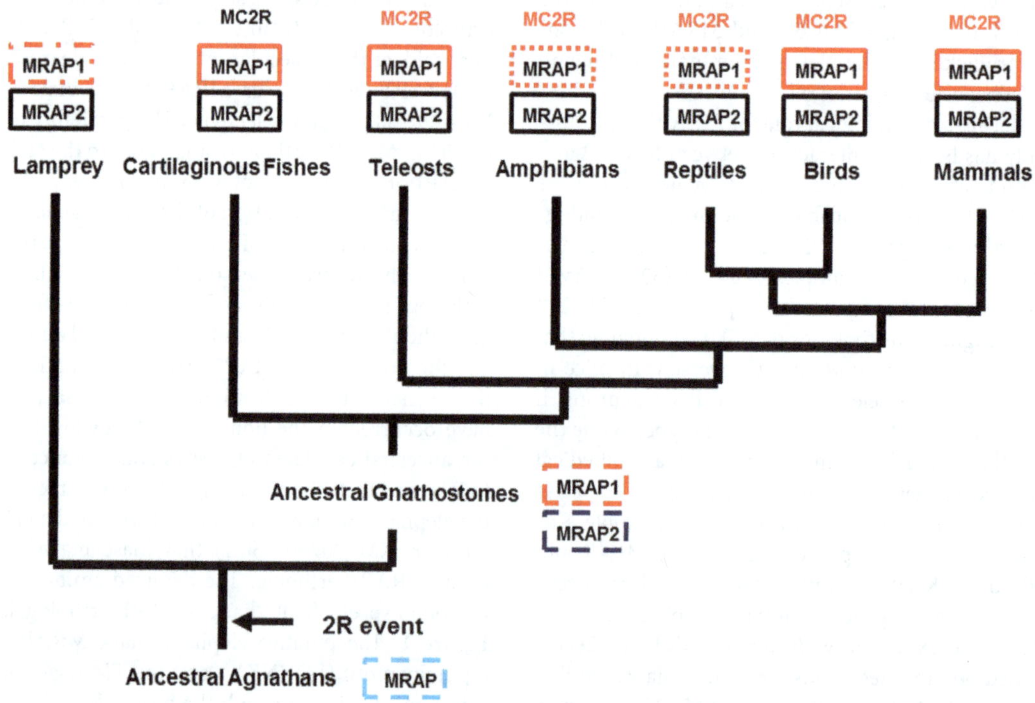

FIGURE 2 | Proposed evolution for the MRAP Gene Family. The evolutionary tree presented in this figure assumes that there was an ancestral *mrap* (MRAP) gene in the genome of ancestral agnathans. Following the 2R genome duplication event, two paralogous mrap genes emerged (MRAP1 and MRAP2) and are present in the genomes of many extant 2R chordates. A solid black box indicates that the gene has been reported in the respective taxa. A box with a dashed line border indicates a gene that is predicted, but has not been detected (i.e., lamprey MRAP1) or the organism is extinct (e.g., ancestral agnathans, ancestral in gnathostomes). A box with a dotted border indicates a taxonomic group in which MRAP1 is required for the functional expression of MC2R, but a MRAP1 sequence has not been identified in the genome of a representative from that taxonomic group.

vertebrates (**Figure 2**), an *mrap1* ortholog has not been detected in the current version of the lamprey genome project[4] (**Figure 2**). Whether the absence of this ortholog represents the incomplete state of the lamprey genome project, or a secondary loss of the ortholog cannot be determined at this time. In addition, *mrap1* orthologs have not been detected in the genomes of either the frog, *Xenopus tropicalis* or the reptile, *Anolis carolinensis*. However, the MC2R orthologs for both species requires co-expression with a tetrapod MRAP1 ortholog for functional expression in CHO cells (21, 37). It would appear that either the *X. tropicalis* and *A. carolinensis* genome projects are not complete, or some other accessory protein is utilized in these species.

From a pharmacological perspective, the presence of the putative elephant shark MRAP1 ortholog is perplexing. An earlier study had shown that the elephant shark MC2R ortholog could be functionally expressed in CHO cells in the absence of co-transfection of an exogenous *mrap1* cDNA (38). Elephant shark MC2R could be stimulated in a dose-dependent manner by either human ACTH (1–24) or by dogfish (*Squalus acanthias*) ACTH (1–25). More recently, a MC2R cDNA cloned from the genome of the stingray, *Dasyatis akajei*, was also functionally expressed in CHO cells in the absence of co-transfection of an exogenous *mrap1* cDNA (39). The stingray MC2R ortholog also could be stimulated by stingray ACTH (1–24) and stingray Des-Acetyl-α-MSH. Hence, there are several issues with respective to the putative elephant shark MRAP1 that need to be resolved. It will be important to determine whether the elephant shark *mrap1* mRNA is expressed in the same cells as elephant shark *mcr* mRNAs. In addition, pharmacological studies are needed to determine whether co-expression of cartilaginous fish MCR orthologs with the putative elephant shark MRAP1 ortholog have any effect on either trafficking of the MCR orthologs to the plasma membrane or sensitivity to melanocortin ligands.

LIGAND SELECTIVITY OF MC2R ORTHOLOGS

Several studies have shown that the MC2R orthologs of teleosts and tetrapods (**Figure 2**) require co-expression with a corresponding MRAP1 ortholog. Perhaps as a result of this interaction, and the intrinsic tertiary features of these MC2R orthologs, all of these receptors can only be activated by ACTH, and not by any MSH-sized ligand (19–21, 37, 40). Nearly 40 years ago, analog studies on mammalian ACTH sequences revealed the dual importance of the $H^6F^7R^8W^9$ motif and the $K^{15}K^{16}R^{17}R^{18}$ (tetrabasic) motif in ACTH for the activation of the "ACTH" (MC2R) receptor on mammalian adrenal cortex cells (41). These same features are required for the activation of MC2R on the interrenal and

[4]http://www.ensembl.org/Petromyzon_marinus/Info/Index

adrenal cortex cells of non-mammalian tetrapods and teleosts as well (42). Although, teleost and tetrapod α-MSH sequences have the $H^6F^7R^8W^9$ motif, these ligands lack the tetrabasic motif, and as a result are incapable of activating either teleost or tetrapod MC2R orthologs. By contrast, the teleost and tetrapod MC1R, MC3R, MC4R, and MC5R paralogs can be activated by either ACTH or the MSH-sized polypeptides derived from POMC with varying potencies (10, 42, 43). It would appear that teleost and tetrapod MCR paralogs all have an HFRW-binding site, and MC2R orthologs have an addition R/KKRR-binding site. These generalizations apply for the ligand selectivity properties of the MCRs of cartilaginous fishes (class Chondrichthyes) with one notable exception.

Studies on the ligand selectivity of dogfish, *Squalus acanthias* (order Squaliformes, subclass Elasmobranchii), MC3R, MC4R, and MC5R paralogs (44–46), and the MC1R, MC3R, MC4R, and MC5R paralogs of the stingray, *D. akajei* [order Rajiformes, subclass Elasmobranchii; (39)] found that these MCR paralogs could be activated by either ACTH or MSH-sized ligands in a manner analogous to the corresponding MCR paralogs in teleosts or tetrapods. Hence, these paralogs have an HFRW-binding site. However, the MC2R ortholog of the stingray, *D. akajei*, and the MC2R ortholog from the elephant shark, *C. milii* (order Chimaeriformes, subclass Holocephali) could also be activated by either ACTH or MSH-sized ligands (38, 39), and as noted in Phylogeny and Proposed Evolution of the MRAPs, both of these MC2R orthologs could be functionally expressed in CHO cells without co-expression of an exogenous *mrap1* cDNA. The two cartilaginous fish MC2R orthologs, from different subclasses of the cartilaginous fishes, have ligand selectivity properties more similar to MC4R paralogs, and most likely have only a HFRW-binding pocket. This apparent feature for the cartilaginous fishes MC2R orthologs would be quite distinct from teleost and tetrapod MC2R orthologs. Whether the ligand selectivity properties

```
                              N-TERMINAL                          [----------TM1----------]  IC1
hMC2R M----------------------------------------KHIINSYENINNTARNNSDCPRVVLPEEIFFTISIVGVLENLIVLLAVFKNKNLQA  97
zMC2R M----------------------------------------------NPSAESPSSIHTDCAEVQVPGQVFLVIAVASLSENLLVIVAVIKNKNLHS
sMC2R MPDMMIPGYGTLLDSNGILPMPPDATISPHSHPTISPWLPYGTEVVIDTINQTNMNATEECSQIEIPTEVYLILGLVSLLENLLVVIAVLKNKKLHF
eMC2R M----------------------------SGADTSASPWLANVTTAVMNTSGFMNGSGGICRQLEIPLEVYLILGGVGMLENLLVIIAVVNNRNLHS
sMC4R M---------------------------------------DLSYTRGPADTTQNRNQSVSGFTGANILHSNGSSSGCNEQLWILVVAAIVKNKNLHS

      [----------TM2---------]       EC1        [---------TM3----------]      IC2      [---------
hMC2R PMYFFICSLAISDMLGSLYKILENILIILRNMGYLKPRGSFETTADDIIDSLFVLSLLGSIFSLSVIAADRYITIFHALRYHSIVTMRRTVVVLTVI 194
zMC2R PMYCFICNLAVFNTISSFSKALENILLLFKDAGRLNSRGPFELKIDDIMDSLLCMCFLGSIFSILAIAVDRYISIFHALRYHMLMTMRRVLIILFTI
sMC2R PMYFFICSLAVSDILLCLSKAWEAFTISLVNNHEDLFTQTFLLSLDNVFDTLICISFLASIFNLAAITTDRYISIFHCLRYHNIMTGKRVAFAIAGI
eMC2R PMYLFICSLAMADMLVSVGKASEAVIIFLDQNSHLL-TETLIDHLDYLFDSLICISLIASILSLGAIATDRYLTIFHALRYHQIMTVKRAALIISAL
sMC4R PMYFFICSLAVADMLISVSNAWETITIAMLKSRHLLAQDKLIKSIDNVFDSVICSSLLASICSLLAVAVDRYITIFYALRYHNIMTVRRALTVIAGI
                            *                       *    *  **  *

      ----TM4-----]  EC2  [-------TM5---------]            IC3           [----------TM6----------]
hMC2R WTFCTGTGITMVIFSHHVPTVITFTSLFPLMLVFILCLYVHMFLLARSH-------TRKISTLPRANMKGAITLTILLGVFIFCWAPFVLHVLLMTF 291
zMC2R WVLCGTSGALMVGFFEAATVKIFFIVLFFTALLLILLLYVHMFLLARHHANRIASMPGAQAQHRKSGLRGALTLTILIGVFVACWAPFSLHLLIMMI
sMC2R WVFCTATGILMINFHNSQGIISFYIIFFLLSVVLIVSLYIYMFLLAQMH-ARKIRILPGHTAHQGINFKGAFTVTVLLGVFIFCWAPLSLHFILFLL
eMC2R WTFCTFSGSFIIKFNRKNAFPGSLITMYFTTLFVIVSLYVYMFLLARRH-AQCIRSLPGQRVHQGTSLKGAITLTILLGIFIICWAPFFLHLILVLA
sMC4R WAVCIGSGILFIIYSESTTAVICLIAMFFAMLAIMASLYVHMFMLARLHLKRIAALPSSGAICQAANMKGAITLTILLGVFVVCWAPFFLHLILMIS
                                                                                            *   *   *

          EC3     [-------TM7-----------]      C-TERMINAL
hMC2R CPSNPYCACYMSLFQVNGMLIMCNAVIDPFIYAFRSPELRDAFKKMIFCSRYW
zMC2R CPENPYCECYRSLFQLHVVLLVSHAVIDPAIYAFRSVELRNTYKKMLLSSASRICKRCA
sMC2R CPSDPYCACFMSLFQIDLIFIMCHSIIDPLIYAFRDPELSNTFKKMMFCHKKQWYFHASPSFLNI                              353
eMC2R CPSNPYCTCYMSLFQVDLILIMCNSIIDPLIFAFRSPELRNTFKKMCICFNKQLY
sMC4R CPRNPYCICFMSHFNMYLILILCNSIIDPLIYAFRSQEMRKTFKEIICCYSLRGSCDLLSNINTH
                     *  *
```

A) Overall % Amino acid Identity for all five sequences - 33%

B) Sequence identity by region

	% Amino Acid Identity		% Amino Acid Identity
N-TERMINAL	2	EC2	11
TM1	35	TM5	33
IC1	83	IC3	24
TM2	46	TM6	76
EC1	5	EC3	57
TM3	58	TM7	55
IC2	81	C-TERMINAL	39
TM4	22		

FIGURE 3 | Amino Acid Alignment of MC2R Orthologs. The amino acid sequences of human (h) MC2R (NP_ 001278840.1), zebrafish (z) MC2R (XP_00518229.1) stingray (s) MC2R (LC108747), elephant shark (e) MC2R (FAA704.1), stingray (s) MC4R (LC108749) were aligned, and amino acid positions in which four of the five sequences were identical are marked in red. The position of critical amino acids in the HFRW-binding site of MC4R orthologs (47) are marked with a star. The overall percent primary sequence identify **(A)** and the percent identity within each domain **(B)** are presented.

of the cartilaginous fishes MC2R orthologs are an ancestral trait or a derived trait unique to the cartilaginous fishes is not clear at this time.

In any event, there should be distinct sites within the teleost/tetrapod MC2R orthologs and the cartilaginous fishes MC2R orthologs that can account for the ligand selectivity properties of these receptors. In this regard, a comparison of MC2R orthologs with an MC4R paralog my reveal these potential sites. As shown in **Figure 3**, the human, zebrafish, elephant shark, and stingray MC2R amino acid sequences could be aligned to the stingray MC4R sequence by inserting a minimum of two gaps. The positions of critical residues in TM2, TM3, TM6, and TM7 that correspond to the HFRW-binding site for a MC4R ortholog (47) are marked with a star. For the teleost and tetrapod MC2R orthologs, six of these sites are conserved, and for the cartilaginous fishes MC2R orthologs eight of these positions are conserved. Overall only 33% of the positions in this alignment are identical in at least four of the five sequences, however, there are very clear regions of primary sequence identity, which serve as markers for MCR-related sequences. The highly conserved regions (sequence identify greater than 50%) include: IC1, TM3, IC2, TM6, EC3, and TM7. Moderately conserved regions (sequence identity greater than 35%) include: TM1, TM2, and the C-terminal domain. The highest primary sequence divergence (<15%) was observed for the N-terminal domain, EC1, and EC2.

Previous studies used chimeric proteins of human MC2R and human MC4R to analyze the functions of these regions. For example, Fridmanis et al. (48) observed that replacing the N-terminal domain of human MC4R with the N-terminal domain of human MC2R inhibited trafficking of the chimeric MC4R protein to the plasma membrane. However, since the N-terminal of stingray MC4R is nearly the same length as the human MC2R domain (**Figure 3**), and the stingray receptor could be functionally expressed in CHO cells (39), length alone may not be a factor in influencing trafficking to the plasma membrane. Hinkle et al. (49) observed that exchanging the TM2/EC1/TM3 region of human MC2R with the corresponding region of human MC4R resulted in a chimeric MC2R protein that could be activated by either ACTH or NDP-MSH. Presumably making a similar chimeric protein for human MC2R, but using the TM2/EC1/TM3 region of either elephant shark or stingray MC2R should yield the same outcome. Finally, Fridmanis et al. (48) observed that substitution of the TM4 and TM5 domains in human MC2R affected ACTH activation, and this region of human MC2R may be the KKRR-binding site. In support of the later conclusion, studies on naturally occurring mutations in the TM4/EC2/TM5 domain of human MC2R, and alanine substitution experiments point to the TM4/EC2/TM5 region as playing an important role in the activation of human MC2R [for review see Ref. (50)]. It would now seem advantageous to extend the chimeric protein paradigm to the cartilaginous fishes MC2R orthologs to determine whether exchanging the TM2/EC1/TM3 and TM4/EC2/TM5 domains of teleost/tetrapod MC2R orthologs with the corresponding domains in the elephant shark MC2R orthologs would make the cartilaginous fish MC2R chimeric proteins exclusively selective for ACTH, and in the converse experiments, would the teleost/tetrapod chimeric MC2R proteins have more permissive ligand selectivity properties. Given Malik et al. (51) observations on the importance of extracellular domains in human MC2R for interaction with mouse MRAP1, co-expression of these MC2R

A

```
                            N-TERMINAL          [----------TM1----------]     IC1    [---------TM2--------
.  MC2R M---------------------------AVNETDCKEVKIPNEIFFAITMVSLTENLLVVVAVIKNKNLHSPMYCFICSLALFNVLSSVSKAL   93
   MC5R MNSSDKMLMQGPLATSSSNSQSNFTDLPGKTKPTACEQVNIATEVFLTLGIVSLLENILVICAIVKNKNLHSPMYFFVCSLAVADMLVSVSNAW
        ----]       EC1        [----------TM3----------]       IC2          [----------TM4--------] EC2
   MC2R ENTMLVFTDAGRLDSRGKFETKTDDVMDTLLCMSFTGSIFSLSAIAVDRYITIFHALRYHNIMTMKRVAVILGSIWTFCAGSGVVMIIFFRATV 186
   MC5R ETIVIYLLNNRQLIMEDNFIRQVDNVFDSMICISVVASMCSLLAIAVDRYVTIFYALRYHNIMTVRRAGFIIAGIWTFCTGCGIVFIIYSDTTP
            [--------TM5--------]           IC3           [----------TM6----------]       EC3      [---
   MC2R IMTCFIALFLVSLVLILILYVHIFQLARTHVWKIASLPG-NRSRQKNNMKGAITLTILFGVFIICWSPFFFHLLILMVCPLNPYCECYRSLFQV 279
   MC5R VIICLISMFFGMLVLMASLYSHMFLLARSHVKRIAALPGYNSIHQRASMKAAVTLTILLGIFIVCWAPFFLHLILMISCPRNLYCVCFMSHFNM
        ------TM7---------] C-TERMINAL
   MC2R HVILLMCNAVIDPVIYAFRSAELRNTLRKMFFCSGTREPVSIICCDNQSVLSSLSILFHLKQDNPT                          344
   MC5R YLILIMCNSVIDPLIYAFRSQE-----------MRKTFKEIICCYSLRNACGLPSKY
```

B

```
                                N-TERMINAL          [----------TM1----------]    IC1    [----------TM2----
.  MC4R MNTTHHHGLIHNYHSRNFSSGAFTVNNDSNEKDSSSGCYEQLLISTEVFLTLGIVSLLENILVIAAIIKNKNLHSPMYFFICSLAVADMLVSVS   93
   MC5R MNSS---DKMLMQGPLATSSSNSQSNFTDLPGKTKPTACEQVNIATEVFLTLGIVSLLENILVICAIVKNKNLHSPMYFFVCSLAVADMLVSVS
        ------]       EC1        [----------TM3----------]   IC2            [---------TM4---------]
   MC4R NAWETIVMALITSGHLTIQDNLIKNMDNVFDSMICSSLLASICSLLAIAIDRYITIFYALRYHNIMTMRRAMMIITTIWAFCTISGILFIIYSE 186
   MC5R NAWETIVIYLLNNRQLIMEDNFIRQVDNVFDSMICISVVASMCSLLAIAVDRYVTIFYALRYHNIMTVRRAGFIIAGIWTFCTGCGIVFIIYSD
         EC2  [----------TM5------]            IC3            [----------TM6----------]       EC3
   MC4R STTVIICLITMFFTMLALMASLYVHMFMLARLHMKRIAALPGNGTIHQGANMKGAITLTILLGVFVVCWAPFFLHLILMIACPRNPYCVCFMS  278
   MC5R TTPVIICLISMFFGMLVLMASLYSHMFLLARSHVKRIAALPGYNSIHQRASMKAAVTLTILLGIFIVCWAPFFLHLILMISCPRNLYCVCFMS
        [---------TM7--------]        C-TERMINAL
   MC4R HFNMYLILIMCNSVIDPLIYAFRSQEMRKTFKEIFCWYGLPGFCVCELPSKY                                          330
   MC5R HFNMYLILIMCNSVIDPLIYAFRSQEMRKTFKEIICCYSLRNAC--GLPSKY
```

FIGURE 4 | Amino Acid alignment of Gar MC2R, MC4R, and MC5R. The amino acid sequences of gar MC2R (ENSLOCT00000011667), gar MC4R (ENSLOCT00000022303), and gar MC5R (ENSLOCG00000018340) were aligned and positions that were identical are marked in red. **(A)** alignment of gar MC2R and gar MC5R; **(B)** alignment of gar MC4R and gar MC5R.

chimeric proteins with a class-specific MRAP1 ortholog may reveal the domain within the MC2R orthologs that makes contact with MRAP1.

MELANOCORTIN RECEPTOR GENOME AND GENE DUPLICATIONS

The successive genome duplications during the radiation of the chordates theoretically should yield four paralogous genes in the genomes of extant cartilaginous fishes, non-teleost ray finned fishes, and tetrapods. However, in the genomes of the Japanese stingray (39), the spotted gar[5], or the mouse (6), there are five paralogous MCR genes. The conclusion drawn from these observations is that one of the paralogous *mcr* genes underwent a local gene duplication (52). While there is general agreement that the *mc5r* gene was the result of the local gene duplication, the original *mcr* paralog that was duplicated has not been resolved. The issues associated with the origin of the *mc5r* gene can be seen in the spotted gar (sg) genome. Chromosome mapping indicates that the *sgmc1r* gene is located on chromosome 21, the *sgmc2r* gene is located on chromosome 11, the *sgmc3r* gene is located on chromosome 18, the *sgmc4r* gene is located on chromosome 9, and the *sgmc5r* gene is also located on chromosome 11. The presence of paralogous genes on different chromosomes is considered an indication of a genome duplication event(s) (4). The presence of two genes on the same chromosome is generally construed as a result of a local gene duplication. In this regard, synteny studies found that the *mc2r* and the *mc5r* genes were on the same chromosome in the genomes of teleost fishes, the chicken (*Gallus gallus*), and several mammals (43, 52, 53). Based on these observations, it seemed reasonable to conclude that the *mc2r* and *mc5r* genes were the result of a local gene duplication (54, 55). In this scenario, the paralogous *mc2r* and *mc5r* genes would accumulate mutations independently, and based on selection pressures diverge in terms of amino acid sequence, and perhaps in terms of function. The divergence in amino acid sequence can be seen from an alignment of gar MC2R and gar MC5R (**Figure 4A**). The amino acid identity for the two paralogs is 42%. From an evolutionary

[5] http://www.ensembl.org/Lepisosteus_oculatus/Info/Index

```
A
                                    N-TERMINAL                                       [----------TM1-----------]   IC1
hMC2R M-----------------------------------------KHIINSYENINNTARNNSDCPRVVLPEEIFFTISIVGVLENLIVLLAVFKNKNLQA   97
sMC2R MPDMMIPGYGTLLDSNGILPMPPDATISPHSHPTISPWLPYGTEVVIDTINQTNMNATEECSQIEIPTEVYLILGLVSLLENLLVVIAVLKNKKLHF

      [-----------TM2----------]         EC1          [----------TM3-----------]        IC2        [---------
hMC2R PMYFFICSLAISDMLGSLYKILENILIILRNMGYLKPRGSFETTADDIIDSLFVLSLLGSIFSLSVIAADRYITIFHALRYHSIVTMRRTVVVLTVI  194
sMC2R PMYFFICSLAVSDILLCLSKAWEAFTISLVNNHEDLFTQTFLLSLDNVFDTLICISFLASIFNLAAITTDRYISIFHCLRYHNIMTGKRVAFAIAGI
                          *                     *    *  **

      ----TM4-----]   EC2   [-------TM5---------]            IC3             [----------TM6----------]
hMC2R WTFCTGTGITMVIFSHHVPTVITFTSLFPLMLVFILCLYVHMFLLARSH------TRKISTLPRANMKGAITLTILLGVFIFCWAPFVLHVLLMTFC  291
sMC2R WVFCTATGILMINFHNSQGIISFYIIFFLLSVVLIVSLYIYMFLLAQMHARKIRILPGHTAHQGINFKGAFTVTVLLGVFIFCWAPLSLHFILFLLC
                                                                                          *  *  *

        EC3       [-------TM7-----------]        C-terminal
hMC2R PSNPYCACYMSLFQVNGMLIMCNAVIDPFIYAFRSPELRDAFKKMIFCSRYW
sMC2R PSDPYCACFMSLFQIDLIFIMCHSIIDPLIYAFRDPELSNTFKKMMFCHKKQWYFHASPSFLNI                                353

B
          N-TERMINAL      [----------TM1-----------]  IC1  [-----------TM2----------]            EC1
gMC2R M-------AVNETDCKEVKIPNEIFFAITMVSLTENLLVVVAVIKNKNLHSPMYCFICSLALFNVLSSVSKALENTMLVFTDAGRLDSRGKFETKT   97
zMC2R MNPSAESPSSIHTDCAEVQVPGQVFLVIAVASLSENLLVIVAVIKNKNLHSPMYCFICNLAVFNTISSFSKALENILLLFKDAGRLNSRGPFELKI
                                                                                *

      [----------TM3-----------]        IC2       [---------TM4---------]  EC2  [-------TM5---------]
gMC2R DDVMDTLLCMSFTGSIFSLSAIAVDRYITIFHALRYHNIMTMKRVAVILGSIWTFCAGSGVVMIIFFRATVIMTCFIALFLVSLVLILILYVHIFQ  194
zMC2R DDIMDSLLCMCFLGSIFSILAIAVDRYISIFHALRYHMLMTMRRVLIILFTIWVLCGTSGALMVGFFEAATVKIFFIVLFFTALLLILLLYVHMFL
      *   *  **

                 IC3             [----------TM6----------]      EC3     [-------TM7-----------]
gMC2R LARTHVWKIASLPGNRSRQKNNMKGAITLTILFGVFIICWSPFFFHLLILMVCPLNPYCECYRSLFQVHVILLMCNAVIDPVIYAFRSAELRNTLR  291
zMC2R LARHHANRIASMPGAAQHRKSGLRGALTLTILIGVFVACWAPFSLHLLIMMICPENPYCECYRSLFQLHVVLLVSHAVIDPAIYAFRSVELRNTYK
                                            *  *  *

                 C-terminal
gMC2R KMFFCSGTREPVSIICCDNQSVLSSLSILFHLKQDNPT                                                              328
zMC2R KMLLSSASRICKRCA
```

FIGURE 5 | Amino acid sequence identity of MC2R orthologs. (A) The amino acid sequences of human (h) MC2R and stingray (s) MC2R were aligned. **(B)** The amino acid sequences of gar (g) MC2R and zebrafish (z) MC2R (XP_005158229) were aligned. The position of critical amino acids in the proposed HFRW-binding site (47) are marked with a star. Amino acid positions that are identical are marked in red.

perspective, the local gene duplication may have occurred after the 2R genome duplication event in the ancestral gnathostomes prior to the divergence of the ancestral cartilaginous fishes and the ancestral bony fishes.

However, Vastermark and Schioth (1) have pointed out that in phylogenetic analyses, MC5R orthologs form a clade with MC4R orthologs, and do not form a clade with MC2R orthologs. These observations have led to the conclusion that the *mc5r* gene was the result of a duplication of the *mc4r* gene (1). In support of this conclusion, an alignment of gar MC4R and gar MC5R indicates 70% sequence identity (**Figure 4B**). In this scenario, the presence of the *mc2r* and *mc5r* paralogous genes on the same chromosome of extant teleost and tetrapods could have been the result of an exchange of chromosome fragments in the last common ancestor to the ancestral ray-finned fishes (Class Actinopterygii) and the ancestral lobe-finned fishes (Class Sarcopterygii), the lineage which gave rise to the tetrapods, approximately 410 million years ago (56).

While either scenario (i.e., MC2R/MC5R or MC4R/MC5R) can be supported by the current evidence, there are at least two issues that neither scenario adequately addresses. As shown in **Figure 5A**, a comparison of stingray MC2R and human MC2R, vertebrates that last shared a common ancestor over 420 million years ago, the amino acid sequence identity is 37% (positions in red). Given the apparent role of the Hypothalamus/Pituitary/Adrenal (HPA) axis and the Hypothalamus/Pituitary/Interrenal (HPI) axis in maintaining the fitness of vertebrates (57–60), this lack of primary sequence conservation is difficult to comprehend. While divergence is expected, this degree of divergence is difficult to rationalize. It would appear that during the radiation of the gnathostomes, the *mc2r* gene sequence has drifted to the current state, while still maintaining functional capabilities.

For ray-finned fishes, such as the gar or zebrafish (Class Actinopterygii), MC2R primary sequence conservation is higher (55%; **Figure 5B**), and this condition may reflect the close interaction with MRAP1. That interaction most likely

```
A                                N-TERMINAL          [----------TM1----------]   IC1  [------TM2----------
hMC5R MNSSFHLHFLDLNLNATEGNLSGPNVKNKSSPCEDMGIAVEVFLTLGVISLLENILVIGAIVKNKNLHSPMYFFVCSLAVADMLVSMSSAWE  92
sMC5R MN-----LTKLSLMSVTLAEAMVNGTRSSTALCEQVSVAVEVFLILGIISLLENILVIAAIIKNRNLHSPMYFFVCSLAVADMLVSVSNAWE
                                                                                              *

      ---]     EC1      [----------TM3----------]    IC2      [----------TM4--------] EC2
hMC5R TITIYLLNNKHLVIADAFVRHIDNVFDSMICISVVASMCSLLAIAVDRYVTIFYALRYHHIMTARRSGAIIAGIWAFCTGCGIVFILYSEST  184
sMC5R TIVITLLHSRHLVVKDSFVKHVDNVFDSMICTSVVASMCSLLAIAVDRYITIFYALRYHHIMSMKRAAFIIAGIWALCIGCGIIFIIYSESP
                           *   *  **

          [--------TM5--------]         IC3        [----------TM6----------]       EC3
hMC5R YVILCLISMFFAMLFLLVSLYIHMFLLARTHVKRIAALPGASSARQRTSMQGAVTVTMLLGVFTVCWAPFFLHLTLMLSCPQNLYCSRFMSH  276
sMC5R TVIICLVTMFFIMLLIMASLYSHMFLLARSHAKRIAAMSSSNSIHQQASMKGAITLTILLGIFIVCWAPLFLHLILMISCPRNLYCTCFMSH
                                                                        *   * *

      [---------TM7---------] C-TERMINAL
hMC5R FNMYLILIMCNSVMDPLIYAFRSQEMRKTFKEIICCRGFRIACSFPRRD                                            332
sMC5R FNLYLILIMCNSIIDPLIYSFRSQEMRKTLKEIICCHSLRAVCRLTVK
       *  *

B                                     N-TERMINAL        [----------TM1----------]   IC1  [------TM2--
gMC5R MNSS--------DKMLMQGPLATSSSNSQSNFTDLPGKTKPTACEQVNIATEVFLTLGIVSLLENILVICAIVKNKNLHSPMYFFVCSLAVA  92
fMC5R MNTSHRSSDPQEGIMGNSTWNPLSYQPNFTLSPPLLPKTKTAACEQLHIAIEVFLTLGIISLLENILVIMAIVKNKNLHSPMYFFVCSLAVA

      --------------]     EC1      [----------TM3----------]    IC2      [----------TM4---
gMC5R DMVLVSSNAWETIVIYLLNNRQLIMEDNFIRQVDNVFDSMICISVVASMCSLLAIAVDRYVTIFYALRYHNIMTVRRAGFIIAGIWTFCTGC  184
fMC5R DMLVSVSNASETIIIYLLNNKQLIAEDHLIRQLDNVFDSMICISVVASMCSLLAIAVDRYVTIFYALRYHNIMTVRRAGCIIGGIWTFCTGC
               *                   *   *  **

      -----] EC2   [--------TM5--------]         IC3        [----------TM6----------]
gMC5R GIVFIIYSDTTPVIICLISMFFGMLVLMASLYSHMFLLARSHVKRIAALPGYNSIHQRASMKAAVTLTILLGIFIVCWAPFFLHLILMISCP  276
fMC5R GIVFIIYSDTTPVIICLVCMFFAMLLIMASLYSHMFMLARSHVKRIAALPGSNSIHQRASMKGAITLTILLGIFIICWAPFFLHLILMISCP
                                                                                 *   * *

        EC3   [---------TM7---------] C-TERMINAL
gMC5R RNLYCVCFMSHFNMYLILIMCNSVIDPLIYAFRSQEMRKTFKEIICCYSLRNACGLPSKY
fMC5R RNLYCMCFMSHFNMYLILIMCNSVIDPLIYAFRSQEMRKTFKEIIFCYSLRNTCSTICTLPGKY                            339
                *  *
```

FIGURE 6 | Amino Acid Sequence Identity of MC5R Orthologs. **(A)** The amino acid sequences of human (h) MC5R (NP_ 005904.1) and stingray (s) MC5R (AY562212) are aligned. **(B)** The amino acid sequences of gar (g) MC5R and *Takifugu rubripes* (f) MC5R (AA06553.1; fugu) were aligned. The position of critical amino acids in the proposed HFRW-binding site (47) is marked with a star. Amino acid positions that are identical are marked in red.

started in the ancestral bony fishes, and while the interaction may not have "rescued" MC2R functionality, the interaction appears to have stabilized the functional capabilities of teleost and tetrapod MC2R orthologs. Tetrapod MC2R orthologs show a similar level of primary sequence conservation. As a result, selection pressures on teleost and tetrapod MC2R orthologs may involve maintaining the close interaction between MRAP1 and MC2R. For the cartilaginous fishes, the MRAP1/MC2R relationship is unclear or may not exit, and the selection pressures to maintain MC2R primary sequence identity does not appear to be as strong. For example, in a recent study, on stingray MCRs (39), *mc2r* and *mc5r* mRNA levels were detected in the interrenal tissue of this species. However, the EC_{50} value of the stingray MC5R for ACTH (1–24) was in the 10^{-9}M range, whereas the EC_{50} value for stingray MC2R was in the 10^{-7}M range. In this example, MC5R rather MC2R may be the "ACTH" receptor in the HPI axis of the stingray.

The diminished primary sequence conservation for MC2R orthologs is in sharp contrast to the higher degree of primary sequence conservation for stingray and human MC5R orthologs (55%; **Figure 6A**). In addition, for two very distantly related bony fish MC5R orthologs (gar and fugu) the sequence identity was 73% (**Figure 6B**). These observations beg the question of the functional significance of the stability of MC5R orthologs during the radiation of the gnathostomes. For mammals, MC5R plays a role in exocrine gland secretion (61). However, the role of the MC5R receptor in non-mammalian vertebrates is largely unknown. Perhaps a renewed focus on the distribution of MC5 receptors in various tissues of non-mammalian vertebrates will yield some answers.

CONCLUSION

While it has been nearly 25 years since the cloning of the first MCRs (6, 11), and nearly 40 years since the structure/function studies on ACTH (41), there are still many aspects of the pharmacology and physiology of the melanocortin peptides and the MCRs that have not been resolved. One of the interesting facets of this receptor family is the interaction with the MRAPs (8, 9, 16, 17). The presence of a *mrap1* ortholog in the genome of a cartilaginous fish suggests that the *mrap1* and the *mrap2* paralogous genes were the result of the 2R genome duplication event (2). There is still a considerable amount of work to be done to clarify the physiological roles of the MRAP1 and MRAP2 in non-mammalian vertebrates, and the contact sites between MRAPs and the MCRs that can influence ligand selectivity.

When considering the functional activation of the MCRs, the paralogs MC1R, MC3R, MC4R, and MC5R are activated through an HFRW-binding site on these receptors that appears to be highly conserved. However, the MC2R orthologs of teleosts and tetrapods appear to utilize an additional binding site for the R/KKRR motif in gnathostome ACTH. Recent studies on cartilaginous fish MC2R orthologs suggest that a single-binding site may be all that is needed for the activation of these receptors (39, 46). Identifying the functional domains within the various gnathostome MC2R orthologs may clarify the ligand selectivity properties of cartilaginous fish and teleost/tetrapod MC2R orthologs.

Finally, while the role for MC2R orthologs in the HPA/HPI axis seems very clear, the role of the MC5R orthologs in the physiology of non-mammalian vertebrates is not resolved. The possibility that MC2R and MC5R may be functioning in the same cells should be considered.

AUTHOR CONTRIBUTIONS

The author confirms being the sole contributor of this work and approved it for publication.

FUNDING

This research was supported by the Long Research Fund (University of Denver).

REFERENCES

1. Vastermark A, Schiöth HB. The early origin of melanocortin receptors, agouti-related peptide, agouti signaling peptide, and melanocortin receptor-accessory proteins, with emphasis on pufferfishes, elephant shark, lampreys, and amphioxus. *Eur J Pharmacol* (2011) 660:61–9. doi:10.1016/j.ejphar.2010.10.106
2. Ohno S, Wolf U, Atkins NB. Evolution from fish to mammals by gene duplication. *Hereditas* (1968) 59:169–87. doi:10.1111/j.1601-5223.1968.tb02169.x
3. Lundin LG. Evolution of the vertebrate genome as reflected in paralogous chromosomal regions in man and the house mouse. *Genomics* (1993) 16:1–19. doi:10.1006/geno.1993.1133
4. Holland PW, Garcia-Fernandez J, Williams NA, Sidow A. Gene duplications and the origins of vertebrate development. *Dev Suppl* (1994):125–33.
5. Gallo-Payet N, Battista M-C. Steroidogenesis – adreanl cells signal transduction. *Compr Physiol* (2014) 4:889–964. doi:10.1002/cphy.c130050
6. Cone RD. Studies on the physiological functions of the melanocortin system. *Endocr Rev* (2006) 27:736–49. doi:10.1210/er.2006-0034
7. Takahashi A, Amemiya Y, Sarashi M, Sower SA, Kawauchi H. Melanotropin and corticotropin are encoded on two distinct genes in the lamprey, the earliest evolved extant vertebrate. *Biochem Biophys Res Commun* (1995) 213:490–8. doi:10.1006/bbrc.1995.2158
8. Hinkle PM, Sebag JA. Structure and function of the melanocortin 2 receptor accessory protein. *Mol Cell Endocrinol* (2009) 300:25–31. doi:10.1016/j.mce.2008.10.041
9. Webb TR, Clark AJ. Mini-review: the melanocortin 2 receptor accessory proteins. *Mol Endocrinol* (2010) 24:475–84. doi:10.1210/me.2009-0283
10. Gantz I, Fong TM. The melanocortin system. *Am J Physiol Endocrinol Metab* (2003) 284:E468–74. doi:10.1152/ajpendo.00434.2002
11. Mountjoy KG, Robbins LS, Mortrud MT, Cone RD. The cloning of a family of genes that encode the melanocortin receptors. *Science* (1992) 257:1248–51. doi:10.1126/science.1325670
12. Noon LA, Franklin JM, King PJ, Goulding NJ, Hunyady L, Clark AJ. Failed export of the adrenocorticotropin receptor from the endoplasmic reticulum in non-adrenal cells: evidence in support of a requirement for a specific adrenal accessory factor. *J Endocrinol* (2002) 174:17–25. doi:10.1677/joe.0.1740017
13. Rached M, El Mourabit H, Buronfosse A, Blondet A, Naville D, Begeot M, et al. Expression of the human melanocortin-2 receptor in different eukaryotic cells. *Peptides* (2005) 26:1842–7. doi:10.1016/j.peptides.2004.11.037
14. Kilianova Z, Basora N, Kilian P, Payet MD, Gallo-Payet N. Human melanocortin receptor 2 expression and functionality: effects of protein kinase A and protein kinase C on desensitization and internalization. *Endocrinology* (2006) 147:2325–37. doi:10.1210/en.2005-0991

15. Roy S, Rached M, Gallo-Payet N. Differential regulation of the human adrenocorticotropin receptor [melanocortin-2 receptor (MC2R)] by human MC2R accessory protein isoforms α and β in isogenic human embryonic kidney 293 cells. *Mol Endocrinol* (2007) 21:1656–69. doi:10.1210/me.2007-0041
16. Metherell LA, Chapple JP, Cooray S, David A, Becker C, Ruschendorf F, et al. Mutations in MRAP, encoding a new interacting partner of the ACTH receptor, cause familial glucocorticoid deficiency type 2. *Nat Genet* (2005) 37:166–70. doi:10.1038/ng1501
17. Chan LF, Webb TR, Chung T-T, Meimaridou E, Cooray SN, Guasti L, et al. MRAP and MRAP2 are bidirectional regulators of the melanocortin receptor family. *Proc Natl Acad Sci U S A* (2009) 106:6146–51. doi:10.1073/pnas.0809918106
18. Sebag JA, Hinkle PM. Regions of melanocortin (MC2) receptor accessory protein necessary for duel topology and MC2 receptor trafficking and signaling. *J Biol Chem* (2009) 284:610–8. doi:10.1074/jbc.M804413200
19. Barlock TK, Gehr DT, Dores RM. Analysis of the pharmacological properties of chicken melanocortin-2 receptor (cMC2R) and chicken melanocortin-2 accessory protein (cMRAP). *Gen Comp Endocrinol* (2014) 205:260–7. doi:10.1016/j.ygcen.2014.03.045
20. Agulleiro MA, Roy S, Sanchez E, Puchol S, Gallo-Payet N, Cerda-Reverter JM. Role of melanocortin receptor accessory proteins in the function of zebrafish melanocortin receptor type 2. *Mol Cell Endocrinol* (2010) 320:145–52. doi:10.1016/j.mce.2010.01.032
21. Liang L, Sebag JA, Eagelston L, Serasinghe MN, Veo K, Reinick C, et al. Functional expression of frog and rainbow trout melanocortin 2 receptors using heterologous MRAP1s. *Gen Comp Endocrinol* (2011) 174:5–14. doi:10.1016/j.ygcen.2011.07.005
22. Sebag JA, Hinkle PM. Melanocortin-2 receptor accessory protein MRAP forms antiparallel homodimers. *Proc Natl Acad Sci U S A* (2007) 104:20244–9. doi:10.1073/pnas.0708916105
23. Dores RM, Garcia Y. Views on the co-evolution of the melanocortin-2 receptor, MRAPs, and the hypothalamus/pituitary/adrenal-interrenal axis. *Mol Cell Endocrinol* (2015) 408:12–22. doi:10.1016/j.mce.2014.12.022
24. Dores RM, Liang L, Hollmann RE, Sandhu N, Vijayan MM. Identifying the activation motif in the N-terminal of rainbow trout and zebrafish melanocortin-2 receptor accessory protein 1 (MRAP1) orthologs. *Gen Comp Endocrinol* (2016). doi:10.1016/j.ygcen.2015.12.031
25. Boston BA, Cone RD. Characterization of melanocortin receptor subtypes expression in murine adipose tissue and in 3T3-L1 cell line. *Endocrinology* (1996) 137:2043–50. doi:10.1210/en.137.5.2043
26. Nimura M, Udagawa J, Hatta T, Hashimodo R, Otani H. Spacial and temporal patterns of expression of melanocortin type 2 and 5 receptors in the fetal mouse tissues and organs. *Anat Embryol (Berl)* (2006) 211:109–17. doi:10.1007/s00429-005-0066-9
27. Sebag JA, Hinkle PM. Opposite effects of the melanocortin-2(MC2) receptor accessory protein MRAP on MC2 and MC5 receptor dimerization and trafficking. *J Biol Chem* (2009) 284:22641–8. doi:10.1074/jbc.M804413200
28. Takeuchi S, Takahashi S. Melanocortin receptor genes in the chicken – tissue distributions. *Gen Comp Endocrinol* (1998) 112:210–9. doi:10.1006/gcen.1998.7167
29. Haitina T, Klovins J, Andersson J, Fredriksson R, Lagerstrom MC, Larhammar D, et al. Cloning, tissue distribution, pharmacology and three-dimensional modeling of melanocortin receptors 4 and 5 in rainbow trout suggest close evolutionary relationship of these subtypes. *Biochem J* (2004) 380:475–86. doi:10.1042/bj20031934
30. Huszar D, Lynch CA, Fairchild-Huntress V, Dunmore JH, Fang Q, Berkemeier LR, et al. Targeted disruption of the melanocortin-4 receptor results in obesity in mice. *Cell* (1997) 88:131–41. doi:10.1016/S0092-8674(00)81865-6
31. Sebag JA, Zhang C, Hinkle PM, Bradshaw AM, Cone RD. Developmental control of the melanocortin-4 receptor by MRAP2 proteins in zebrafish. *Science* (2013) 341:278–81. doi:10.1126/science.1232995
32. Asai M, Ramachandrappa S, Joachim M, Shen Y, Zhang R, Nuthalapati N, et al. Loss of function of the melanocortin 2 receptor accessory protein 2 is associated with mammalian obesity. *Science* (2013) 34(1):275–8. doi:10.1126/science.1233000
33. Kay EI, Botha R, Montgomery JM, Mountjoy KG. hMRAPα, but not hMRAP2, enhances hMC4R constitutive activity in HEK293 cells and this is not dependent on hMRAPα induced changes in hMC4R complex N-linked glycosylation. *PLoS One* (2015) 10(10):e0140320. doi:10.1371/journal.pone.0140320
34. Aguilleiro MA, Cortes R, Fernandez-Duran B, Navarro S, Guillot R, Meimmaridou E, et al. Melanocortin 4 receptor becomes an ACTH receptor by coexpression of melanocortin receptor accessory protein 2. *Mol Endocrinol* (2013) 27:1934–45. doi:10.1210/me.2013-1099
35. Meyer A, Van de Peer Y. From 2R to 3R: evidence for a fish-specific genome duplication (FSGD). *Bioessays* (2005) 27:937–45. doi:10.1002/bies.20293
36. Zhu M, Xiaobo Y, Choo B, Lu J, Qiao T, Qu Q, et al. A Silurian placoderm with osteichthyan-like marginal jaw bones. *Nature* (2013) 502:188–93. doi:10.1038/nature12617
37. Davis P, Franquemont S, Liang L, Angleson JK, Dores RM. Review: evolution of the melanocortin-2 receptor in tetrapods: studies on *Xenopus tropicalis* MC2R and *Anolis carolinensis* MC2R. *Gen Comp Endocrinol* (2013) 188:75–84. doi:10.1016/j.ygcen.2013.04.007
38. Reinick CL, Liang L, Angleson JK, Dores RM. Identification of an MRAP-independent melanocortin-2 receptor: functional expression of the cartilaginous fish, *Callorhinchus milii*, melanocortin-2 receptor in CHO cells. *Endocrinology* (2012) 153:4757–65. doi:10.1210/en.2012-1482
39. Takahashi A, Davis P, Reinick C, Mizusawa K, Sakamoto T, Dores RM. Characterization of melanocortin receptors from stingray *Dasyatis akajei*, an elasmobranchs. *Gen Comp Endocrinol* (2016). doi:10.1016/j.ygcen.2016.03.030
40. Ling MK, Hotta E, Kilanova Z, Haitina T, Ringholm A, Johansson L, et al. The melanocortin receptor subtypes in chicken have high preference to ACTH-derived peptides. *Br J Pharmacol* (2004) 143:626–37. doi:10.1038/sj.bjp.0705900
41. Schwyzer R. ACTH: a short introductory review. *Ann N Y Acad Sci* (1977) 297:3–26. doi:10.1111/j.1749-6632.1977.tb41843.x
42. Dores RM, Londraville RL, Prokop J, Davis P, Dewey N, Lesinski N. The evolution of melanocortin receptor: the relationship between pharmacology and physiology. *J Mol Endocrinol* (2014) 52:T29–42. doi:10.1530/JME-14-0050
43. Klovins J, Haitina T, Fridmanis D, Kilianova Z, Kapa K, Fredriksson R, et al. The melanocortin system in *Fugu*: determination of POMC/AGRP/MCR gene repertoire and synteny, as well as pharmacology and anatomical distribution of the MCRs. *Mol Biol Evol* (2004) 21:563–79. doi:10.1093/molbev/msh050
44. Ringholm A, Klovins J, Fredriksson R, Poliakova N, Larson ET, Kukkonen JP, et al. Presence of melanocortin (MC4) receptor in spiny dogfish suggests an ancient vertebrate origin of central melanocortin system. *Eur J Biochem* (2003) 270:213–21. doi:10.1046/j.1432-1033.2003.03371.x
45. Klovins J, Haitina T, Ringholm A, Lowgren M, Fridmanis D, Slaidina M, et al. Cloning of two melanocortin (MC) receptors in spiny dogfish. *Eur J Biochem* (2004) 271:4320–31. doi:10.1111/j.1432-1033.2004.04374.x
46. Reinick CL, Liang L, Angleson JK, Dores RM. Functional expression of *Squalus acanthias* melanocortin 5 receptor in CHO cells, ligand selectivity and interaction with MRAP. *Eur J Pharmacol* (2012) 680:1–7. doi:10.1016/j.ejphar.2012.01.021
47. Pogozheva ID, Chai B-X, Lomize AL, Fong TM, Weinberg DH, Nargund RP, et al. Interactions of human melanocortin 4 receptors with nonpeptide and peptide agonists. *Biochemistry* (2005) 44:11329–41. doi:10.1021/bi0501840
48. Fridmanis D, Petrovska R, Kalnina I, Slaidina M, Peculis R, Schiöth HB, et al. Identification of domains responsible for specific membrane transport and ligand specificity of the ACTH receptor (MC2R). *Mol Cell Endocrinol* (2010) 321:175–83. doi:10.1016/j.mce.2010.02.032
49. Hinkle PM, Serasinghe MN, Jakebowski A, Sebag JE, Wilson KA, Haskell-Luevano C. Use of chimeric melanocortin-2 and -4 receptors to identity regions responsible for ligand specificity and dependence on melanocortin 2 accessory protein. *Eur J Pharmacol* (2011) 660:94–102. doi:10.1016/j.ejphar.2010.10.113
50. Dores RM, Liang L, Davis P, Thomas AL, Petko B. Melanocortin receptors: evolution of ligand selectivity for melanocortin peptides. *J Mol Endocrinol* (2016) 56:T1–16. doi:10.1530/JME-15-0292
51. Malik S, Dolan TM, Maben J, Hinkle PM. ACTH responses require actions of the melanocortin-2 receptor accessory protein on the extracellular surface of the plasma membrane. *J Biol Chem* (2015) 290:27972–85. doi:10.1074/jbc.M115.668491
52. Schiöth HB, Haitina T, Ling MK, Ringholm A, Fredricksson R, Cerda-Reverter JM, et al. Evolutionary conservation of the structural, pharmacological, and

genomic characteristics of the melanocortin receptor subtypes. *Peptides* (2005) 26:1886–900. doi:10.1016/j.peptides.2004.11.034

53. Schiöth HB, Raudsepp T, Ringholm A, Fredriksson R, Takeuchi S, Larhammar D, et al. Remarkable synteny conservation of melanocortin receptors in chicken, human, and other vertebrates. *Genomics* (2003) 81:504–9. doi:10.1016/S0888-7543(03)00028-4
54. Baron A, Veo K, Angleson J, Dores RM. Modeling the evolution of the MC2R and MC5R genes: studies on the cartilaginous fish, *Heterondotus francisci*. *Gen Comp Endocrinol* (2009) 161:13–9. doi:10.1016/j.ygcen.2008.11.026
55. Dores RM. Observations on the evolution of the melanocortin receptor gene family: distinctive features of the melanocortin-2 receptor. *Front Endocrinol* (2013) 10(7):28. doi:10.3389/fnins.201300028
56. Rasmussen A-S, Arnason U. Molecular studies suggest that cartilaginous fishes have a terminal position in the piscine tree. *Proc Natl Acad Sci U S A* (1999) 96:2177–82. doi:10.1073/pnas.96.5.2177
57. Munck A, Guyre PM, Holbrook NJ. Physiological functions of glucocorticoids in stress and their relation to pharmacological actions. *Endocr Rev* (1984) 5:25–44. doi:10.1210/edrv-5-1-25
58. Smith SM, Valle WW. The role of the hypothalamus-pituitary-adrenal axis in neuroendocrine responses to stress. *Dialogues Clin Neurosci* (2006) 8:383–95.
59. Flik G, Klaven PHM, Van den Burg EH, Metz JR, Huising MO. CRF and stress in fish. *Gen Comp Endocrinol* (2006) 146:36–44. doi:10.1016/j.ygcen.2005.11.005
60. Crespi EJ, Williams TD, Jessop TS, Delehanty B. Life history and the ecology of stress: how do glucocorticoid hormones influence life-history variation in animals? *Funct Ecol* (2013) 27:93–116. doi:10.1111/1365-2435.12009
61. Zhang L, Li WH, Anthonavage M, Pappas A, Rossetti D, Cavender D, et al. Melanocortin-5 receptor and sebogenesis. *Eur J Pharmacol* (2011) 660:202–6. doi:10.1016/j.ejphar.2010.10.100

9

ACTH Regulation of Adrenal SR-B1

Wen-Jun Shen[1,2], Salman Azhar[1,2] and Fredric B. Kraemer[1,2]*

[1] The Division of Endocrinology, Stanford University, Stanford, CA, USA, [2] Geriatric Research, Education and Clinical Center, Veterans Affairs Palo Alto Health Care System, Palo Alto, CA, USA

***Correspondence:**
Fredric B. Kraemer
fbk@stanford.edu

The adrenal gland is one of the prominent sites for steroid hormone synthesis. Lipoprotein-derived cholesterol esters (CEs) delivered *via* SR-B1 constitute the dominant source of cholesterol for steroidogenesis, particularly in rodents. Adrenocorticotropic hormone (ACTH) stimulates steroidogenesis through downstream actions on multiple components involved in steroidogenesis. Both acute and chronic ACTH treatments can modulate SR-B1 function, including its transcription, posttranscriptional stability, phosphorylation and dimerization status, as well as the interaction with other protein partners, all of which result in changes in the ability of SR-B1 to mediate HDL-CE uptake and the supply of cholesterol for conversion to steroids. Here, we provide a review of the recent findings on the regulation of adrenal SR-B1 function by ACTH.

Keywords: adrenal, cholesterol, ACTH, SR-B1

The adrenal gland, in addition to the gonads, is one of the prominent sites where steroid hormones are synthesized (1–5). Cholesterol is the common precursor for steroidogenesis, which involves the contribution from multiple enzymes and requires the conversion of cholesterol to pregnenolone as the initial step of a multistep process. Pregnenolone is subsequently metabolized to produce various biologically active steroids in a tissue-specific manner. In general, this process is thought to involve five major steps: (1) cholesterol acquisition through *de novo* synthesis and/or uptake from lipoproteins and stored as cholesterol esters (CEs) in lipid droplets (LDs), (2) cholesterol mobilization from CEs that are stored in LDs, (3) trafficking of cholesterol to the cytochrome P450 side-chain cleavage enzyme (P450scc, CYP11A1) at the inner mitochondrial membrane (IMM), following cholesterol trafficking to the outer mitochondrial membrane (OMM), (4) production of pregnenolone by CYP11A1 through cleavage of the cholesterol side-chain, and (5) efflux of pregnenolone from the mitochondria to the endoplasmic reticulum (ER), where enzymes convert it into intermediates that shuttle between mitochondria and ER to produce progestins, estrogens, androgens, glucocorticoids, or mineralocorticoids in a tissue-specific manner (2, 5).

The adrenal gland is a compound endocrine gland composed of two developmentally unrelated tissues, an outer layer of adrenal cortex and an inner layer of adrenal medulla. The adrenal cortex is the site of steroid hormone synthesis and produces three classes of steroid hormones. These are glucocorticoids (cortisol and corticosterone), mineralocorticoids (aldosterone), and androgens [androstenedione and dehydroepiandrosterone (DHEA)]. The cells of the adrenal zona glomerulosa, which is the outermost layer of the adrenal cortex, synthesize aldosterone in response to angiotensin II (1, 2), whereas the cells of the adrenal cortical zona fasciculata–reticularis produce cortisol, corticosterone, or androgens [androstenedione and DHEA/dehydroepiandrostenedione sulfate (DHEAS)] in response to adrenocorticotropic hormone (ACTH) stimulation. Humans synthesize cortisol, but because CYP17 is poorly expressed in the zona fasciculata in rats and mice, consequently, corticosterone is the dominant glucocorticoid produced in rodents. The adrenal steroidogenic pathways are illustrated in **Figure 1**.

All the steroid hormones synthesized within the adrenal cortex utilize cholesterol as the common precursor. For cells that produce polypeptide hormones, large amounts of mature hormones

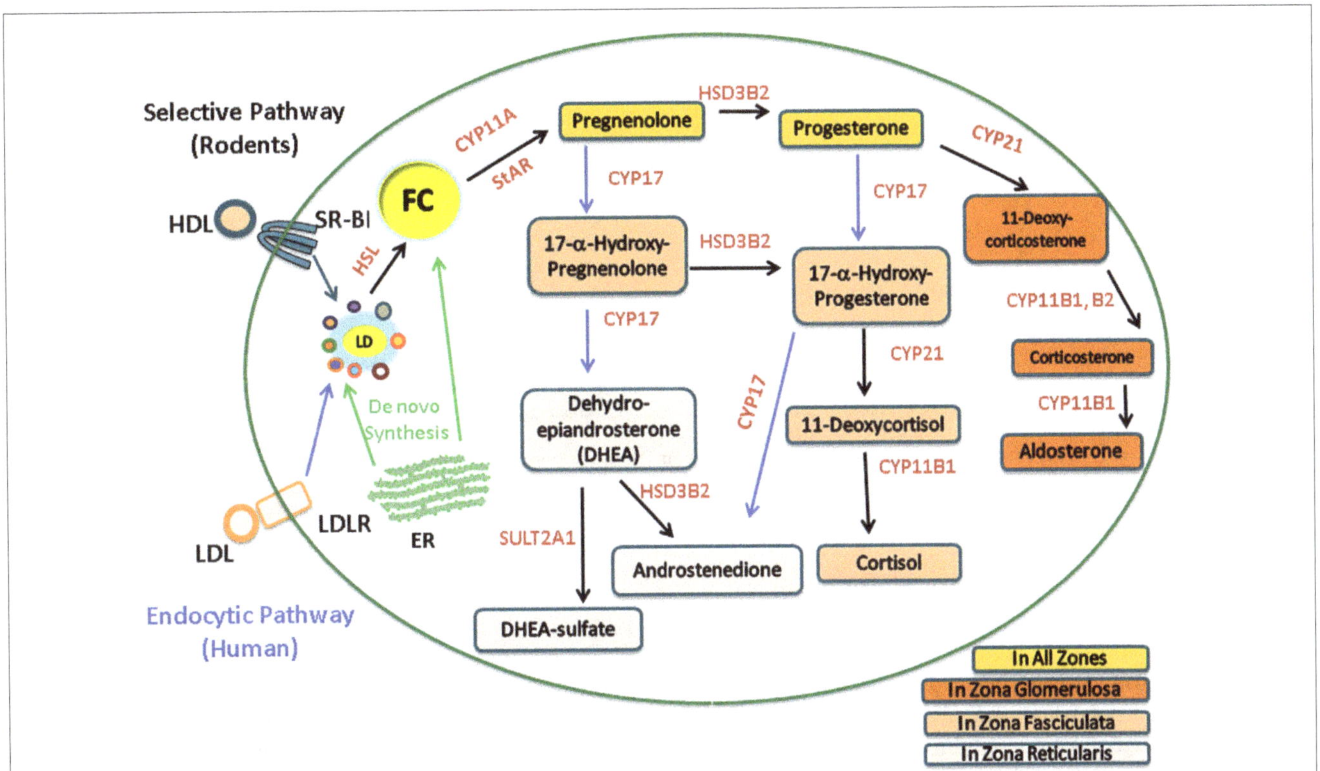

FIGURE 1 | Human and rodent adrenal steroidogenic pathways. In the adrenal, upon stimulation, cholesterol esters (CE) from the LDL endocytic pathway (human) or the SR-B1 selective pathway (rodents) are hydrolyzed by hormone-sensitive lipase (HSL) to release free cholesterol (FC) as the common precursor for steroidogenesis. FC, which can also be synthesized *de novo* within the ER, traffics to the outer mitochondrial membrane and is then transported into the inner mitochondrial membrane by StAR, where it is cleaved by CYP11A to pregnenolone, a common precursor for all other steroid hormones. The adrenal cortex is the site of steroid hormone synthesis and different steroidogenic enzymes are expressed in cells located within different zones of the adrenal cortex, resulting in different classes of steroid hormones being released from different layers. The cells of the zona glomerulosa synthesize aldosterone, the cells of the zona fasciculata synthesize cortisol, and the cells of the zona reticularis produce androgens. In rodents, there is a very low level of CYP17; consequently, corticosterone is the dominant glucocorticoid produced.

can be stored ready for rapid release; however, there is very little steroid hormone storage in steroidogenic cells. Therefore, upon stimulation, there is a rapid response from the steroidogenic cells to synthesize new steroids (3, 4), and with this a requirement for a constant supply of the precursor cholesterol to be converted to steroid hormones. The precursor cholesterol for steroidogenesis can be derived from a combination of sources (5–7): (1) *de novo* cellular cholesterol synthesis, (2) the mobilization of CEs stored in LDs, and (3) lipoprotein-derived CEs delivered through endocytic uptake, which is mediated by the LDL receptor or "selective" cellular uptake *via* the scavenger receptor, class B type 1 (SR-B1).

SR-B1 has been shown to be a HDL receptor and can mediate selective uptake of lipoprotein (HDL)-derived CEs both *in vitro* and *in vivo* (8–11). In the selective CE uptake pathway that is mediated by SR-B1, CE-rich lipoproteins bind on the cell surface and deliver the CEs from the hydrophobic core of the lipoproteins to the inside of the cells. The lipoprotein particles remain intact at the cell surface and can be further recycled to deliver more CEs to the cells (12). In contrast, CEs delivered *via* LDL receptor-mediated lipoprotein uptake are hydrolyzed by lysosomal acid lipase, releasing unesterified free cholesterol (FC) from lysosomes that traffics to the ER and plasma membrane (PM) and is then available to traffic to mitochondria (13, 14). CEs delivered *via* SR-B1 appear to be incorporated directly into LDs (15, 16) and must be hydrolyzed to FC before being used in steroidogenesis. Upon ACTH treatment, adrenal CE stores within LDs are rapidly depleted (17) through the action of hormone-sensitive lipase (HSL), the major neutral cholesteryl ester hydrolase expressed in the adrenal gland (18). This newly released FC from stored LDs is the preferred source of cholesterol. Following LD depletion, lipoprotein-derived CEs delivered *via* SR-B1 become the dominant source of cholesterol for steroidogenesis in rodents (19–21).

Adrenal fasciculata–reticularis cell steroidogenesis is under the regulation of tropic hormone ACTH and is subject to both acute (14, 22–25) and chronic regulation (14, 26–29). ACTH binds to its G protein-coupled receptors, leading to the activation of adenylate cyclase, which generates cAMP and activates cAMP-dependent protein kinase (PKA) (30–33). Stimulation of the cAMP–PKA signaling cascade exerts both acute and chronic effects on the regulation of steroid hormone production (**Figure 2**). On the other hand, angiotensin (AII) stimulates aldosterone biosynthesis in adrenal glomerulosa cells, and its

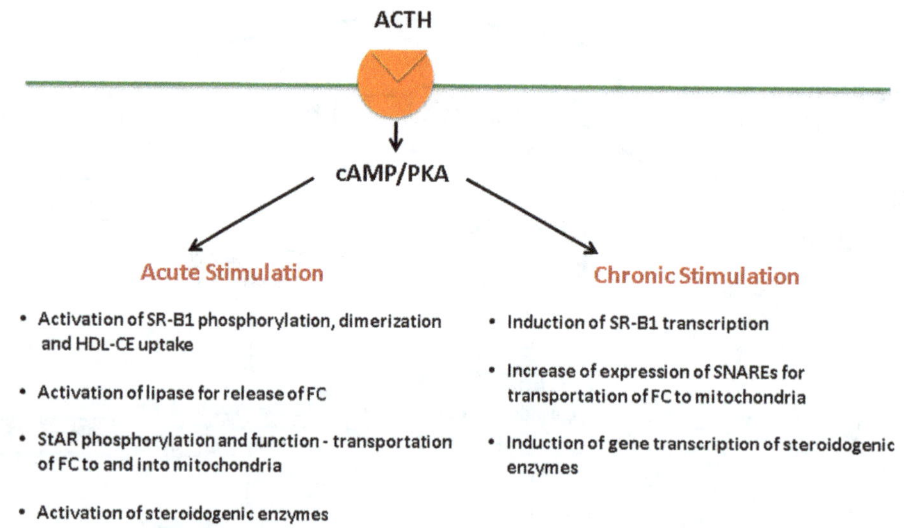

FIGURE 2 | ACTH regulation of steroidogenesis in the adrenal.

actions are primarily mediated by the protein kinase C signaling cascade, whereas potassium can also stimulate aldosterone production through Ca^{2+}-calmodulin-dependent kinase (34). Both acute and chronic ACTH treatments can modulate SR-B1, including its expression levels as well as its phosphorylation status, dimerization, and the interaction with other protein partners, all of which result in changes of SR-B1 function. Here, we aim at providing a review of the most recent findings relevant to these aspects.

ACTH STIMULATION REGULATES THE EXPRESSION OF SR-B1

Initial studies established a functional correlation between SR-B1 expression, HDL-CE uptake, and the ability of steroidogenic cells to produce steroid hormones (8, 35–40). Also, in both lower vertebrates (i.e., turtle) and the fruit fly, there is an increase in SR-B1 expression that correlates with the peak cholesterol flux required during their developmental stages (41). Follow-up studies revealed that the bulk of the cholesterol for steroidogenesis is provided from the selective uptake pathway, which is mediated by SR-B1.

Both rodent and human adrenals express exceptionally high levels of SR-B1; indeed, the highest expression level of SR-B1 per gram of tissue has been reported for rodent adrenals (42, 43). *In vivo* treatment of rats and mice and *in vitro* treatment of cultured rodent adrenocortical cells with ACTH increased SR-B1 expression both at the mRNA level and that of SR-B1 protein (8, 44). In one of our recent studies, the level of SR-B1 protein in rat adrenals shows a trend for increased SR-B1 expression as early as 1 h after treatment with ACTH (45). Similar stimulation of SR-B1 expression and regulation by ACTH was also demonstrated for cultured human adrenal cells (8, 43, 46, 47). Indeed, low levels of SR-B1 mRNA expression seen in normal adrenal tissue adjacent to adenomas causing Cushing's syndrome, where plasma ACTH levels are reduced, is consistent with the notion that the regulation of human SR-B1 is possibly similar to that reported for rodents (43).

Much of the regulation of SR-B1 expression is at the level of transcriptional control. The promoter region of both human and rat SR-B1 contains binding sites for steroidogenic factor-1 (SF-1) (48), which is one of the major transcription factors involved in cAMP regulation of the *SR-B1* gene (49). In addition, the rat promoter has two sterol-responsive elements (SREs) that can bind sterol-responsive element-binding protein (SREBP)-1a and regulate *SR-B1* gene expression in response to altered intracellular sterol levels (50).

Further studies demonstrated that the promoter region of SR-B1 contains sites that can bind both positive and negative regulators. For the expression of SR-B1 in liver and adipose tissue, transcription factors, such as the liver X receptors α and β (LXRα and LXRβ) and the peroxisome proliferator-activated receptor α (PPARα), have been shown to positively regulate the expression of the human *SR-B1* gene in response to oxysterols and fibrates, respectively (51, 52). Other positive regulators include the liver receptor homolog 1 (LRH-1) (53) as well as the estrogen receptors α and β (ERα and ERβ), which bind to three different estrogen-responsive elements on the rat SR-B1 promoter and regulate its activity in response to estrogens (54). The negative regulators of SR-B1 include the nuclear receptor dorsal-sensitive sex adrenal hypoplasia congenital critical region on the X chromosome gene 1 (DAX-1), a protein that plays an important role in adrenal development (49), the Yin Yang 1 (YY1) transcription factor, which represses the activity of the SR-B1 promoter by inhibiting the binding of SREBP-1a (55), and the pregnane X receptor, which represses the human SR-B1 promoter activity in response to the pregnane X receptor agonists rifampicin and lithocholic acid (56). Most of the binding sites for these transcription factors reside within the 2.2 kb proximal 5′-flanking region of the SR-B1 promoter.

In steroidogenic tissues, SR-B1 expression was shown to be upregulated by ACTH (8, 44, 46, 57–59). As mentioned above, SF-1 was shown to mediate the regulation of SR-B1 gene expression through the cAMP–PKA pathway by binding to the promoter region of SR-B1. The SF-1 binding site in the human SR-B1 promoter (5′-CCAAGGCT-3′) resides 77 bp upstream of the transcription start site, and the SF-1 binding site (5′-TCAAGGCC-3′) in the rat SR-B1 promoter is located at −645 bp upstream of the translation start site. These two sites share 75% identity (48, 49). Both the human and rat SR-B1 promoters were shown to be active in mouse adrenocortical tumor Y1 cells, and mutagenesis analysis confirmed the involvement of SF-1 in regulating their promoter activity. The SF-1 binding motif in the rat SR-B1 promoter was shown to be involved in both basal and cAMP-induced regulation of SR-B1 gene expression. Further analysis of the functional domains in SF-1 revealed that both amino acids 448–461 and phosphorylation at Ser430 by PKA are involved in regulating the binding to the consensus sequence in the rat SR-B1 promoter. A recent report showed that when glucocorticoid levels are elevated, SR-B1 expression can also be inhibited by feedback regulation by glucocorticoid (60). In corticosterone-insufficient corticotrophin-releasing hormone knockout Crh (−/−) mice, there is an increase of SR-B1 mRNA levels in adrenal, and oral administration of corticosterone inhibited SR-B1 gene expression. Further studies reveal that the glucocorticoid receptor (GR) can suppress SR-B1 promoter activity. The region between −201 and −62 of the human SR-B1 promoter was shown to contain putative binding sites for transcriptional repressors that are involved in mediating glucocorticoid regulation of SR-B1 expression. However, examination into the mechanism of suppression suggested that GR suppression of SR-B1 in adrenal cells occurs through an indirect mechanism since no direct binding of GR to the SR-B1 promoter was observed. This was the first report showing that by suppressing SR-B1-mediated HDL cholesterol uptake, steroidogenic tissues maintain steroid hormone homeostasis when the endogenous levels of glucocorticoids are elevated.

Recently, in the search for the cellular and molecular mechanisms involved in the regulation of SR-B1 expression and function in steroidogenic cells, we demonstrated that two microRNAs, miRNA-125a and miRNA-455, can bind to specific sites in the 3′ UTR of SR-B1 mRNA and regulate the expression of SR-B1 (61). The expression of miRNA-125a and miRNA-455 is detected in steroidogenic tissue/cells, including adrenal, primary ovarian granulosa cells, and model Leydig cell lines. Both ACTH and cAMP downregulate the expression of miRNA-125a and miRNA-455. When either miRNA-125a or miRNA-455 is overexpressed or inhibited, the amount of SR-B1 protein expressed on the cell surface is decreased or increased, respectively, leading to SR-B1-mediated selective HDL uptake and SR-B1-supported steroid hormone synthesis being inhibited and stimulated, respectively. Therefore, our findings suggest that miRNA-125a and miRNA-455, in response to ACTH stimulation, act as SR-B1 attenuators to negatively regulate SR-B1 expression and SR-B1-mediated selective delivery of lipoprotein cholesterol in steroidogenic cells and, consequently, inhibition of SR-B1-supported steroidogenesis.

MODULATION OF SR-B1 PROTEIN FUNCTION BY ACTH

SR-B1 facilitates HDL-CE selective uptake in two separate independent steps: binding of the lipid-rich lipoprotein to the extracellular domain (ECD) of SR-B1 and the delivery of the CEs from the hydrophobic core of the lipoprotein to the PM (62, 63). A specialized cell surface structure, termed "microvillar channels," was reported to be induced by SR-B1 and shown to facilitate selective lipid transfer to inside the cell (64–67). Studies using electron microscopy demonstrated the presence of microvillar membrane domains in rat ovarian luteal, testicular Leydig, and adrenocortical cells. These domains form channels at the PM and various lipoproteins, including HDL, get trapped within the channels. Immunostaining using specific antibodies for SR-B1 revealed that SR-B1 is preferentially localized on these domains (65, 66). SR-B1 was also shown to be able to facilitate the formation of specific lipid rafts, hence change the properties of the PM and, in turn, affect the flux of free cholesterol (67). These lipid rafts were indicated to be necessary for the formation of the membrane microvillar channels, which are considered a trap for HDL particles for enhancing the efficiency of the selective uptake of HDL-CE. Interestingly, expression of SR-B1 and microvilli are under hormonal regulation; ACTH treatment increases, whereas dexamethasone treatment decreases, SR-B1 expression. Furthermore, the steady-state levels of adrenal microvilli are dictated by SR-B1. In response to SR-B1 deficiency, mouse adrenal microvilli become disorganized, and microvillar channels show a disrupted appearance along with substantially reduced binding of HDL particles to the cell surface (64–67).

In addition, experiments utilizing mutational analysis of SR-B1 or chimeras of CD36/SR-B1 have demonstrated that high affinity binding of lipoproteins to the ECD of SR-B1 is important, but not sufficient to mediate efficient lipid uptake (68). However, at the same time the ECD of SR-B1 does influence the efficient transfer of lipid by SR-B1 (69). This dichotomy is highlighted by the findings that some chemicals can increase lipoprotein binding to SR-B1 while actually blocking lipid transfer (70). Further studies show that the dominant characteristic of lipoprotein binding to SR-B1 involves protein–protein interactions between ligand and receptor. Many of the CE donors (HDL, apoA-I/phospholipid bilayer disks, and lipid-free apoA-I) for SR-B1 all share class A amphipathic helices that could be the structural feature to which SR-B1 is binding (68, 69). In addition, SR-B1 occurs as a multimeric complex with itself or other membrane proteins on the cell surface to facilitate lipid transfer, and the ECD of SR-B1 is essential for efficient CE transfer. ACTH has been shown to induce changes in the oligomeric status as well as protein interaction of SR-B1 and hence modulates SR-B1 protein function.

ACTH Stimulation Modulates the Oligomerization of SR-B1

In response to ACTH stimulation, SR-B1 changes its oligomeric status to facilitate CE uptake (for simplicity, here, we use the term dimerization to include the multiple forms of the SR-B1 protein; i.e., dimers and higher order oligomers). In one of the earliest direct demonstrations of protein–protein interactions involving SR-B1, SR-B1 was shown to exist as homodimers in PMs isolated from rat adrenals stimulated with 17α-ethinyl estradiol (70). Subsequently, dimeric and higher order oligomeric forms of SR-B1 were shown to exist in all cells and tissues that display HDL-CE selective uptake activity (65, 71, 72). In normal rat adrenal tissue, SR-B1 exists primarily in a monomeric form with some dimer formation. Upon ACTH stimulation, there is a significant increase in the dimerization/oligomerization of SR-B1 along with increased selective CE uptake. On the other hand, dexamethasone-mediated suppression of ACTH leads to dramatic loss of SR-B1, SR-B1 dimers/oligomers, and HDL-CE selective uptake activity. When combined with the substantial architectural alterations of the cell surface as related to microvillar formation, these findings indicate that SR-B1 dimer/oligomer formation appears to have significant implications for the expression of the functional properties of SR-B1.

Studies in adrenal cells and other steroidogenic tissues have established a strong correlation between the levels of SR-B1 dimers and enhanced HDL-CE selective uptake activity. Co-immunoprecipitation with differentially epitope-tagged SR-B1s further confirmed that SR-B1 can exist as homodimers (71). In addition, in both native steroidogenic cell lines (endogenous) and in a heterologous insect cell overexpressing SR-B1, dimers/oligomers of SR-B1 were seen when cross-linking agents were added to the cell lysates (65). When cellular extracts from SR-B1 transfected HEK-293 cells or ACTH-treated Y1-BS1 cells were analyzed by size-exclusion chromatography and sucrose density centrifugation, a significant portion of SR-B1 eluted at peaks that correlate with the size of dimeric and oligomeric forms of SR-B1. Immunoelectron microscopy was used as an independent means for confirming the homodimerization of SR-B1. For these experiments, differentially epitope-tagged-SR-B1 proteins were co-expressed in HEK-293 cells, and the epitope-tagged proteins were subsequently immunostained and identified using two differently sized gold particles. The observed mixing and clustering of gold particles suggested that the proteins were localized to the same regions of the cell and that many of the gold particles were in extremely close proximity, i.e., within a distance for protein–protein interactions, as detected by fluorescent resonance energy transfer (FRET) technique. Similar results were obtained when Y1-BS1 mouse adrenocortical cells were transfected with differentially epitope-tagged-SR-B1 constructs. Interestingly, transfection of Y1-BS1 cells with SR-B1 in these experiments resulted in substantial architectural changes with the formation of microvillar structures. Gold-labeled secondary antibodies localized SR-B1 to these sites and revealed substantial dimer formation of this protein – shown by close contact between gold particles (71, 72).

Further investigations concentrated on the contribution of the cysteine residues in the ECD of SR-B1 either independently or in cooperation with the C-terminal domain on SR-B1 dimerization. SR-B1 contains a total of eight cysteine (C) residues (C21, C251, C280, C321, C323, C334, C384, and C470) and six of them are located in the ECD. Mutagenesis studies showed that C280, C321, C323, and C334 residues in the ECD are necessary for preserving normal SR-B1 (HDL) binding activity, selective CE uptake, and/or cell surface expression. Interestingly, mutation of any of these four cysteine residues to serine resulted in a robust induction of SR-B1 dimer formation, but, in contrast to normal SR-B1, these SR-B1 mutants lost their ability to mediate HDL-CE selective uptake. These results indicate that these cysteine residues are most likely essential for optimal HDL binding and selective CE uptake (73).

ACTH Stimulation Regulates SR-B1 Interaction with Accessory Proteins

Adrenocorticotropic hormone treatment activates the cAMP–PKA signaling cascade, and we have recently shown that the expression of salt-inducible kinase 1 (SIK1), a serine/threonine kinase that belongs to the stress- and energy-sensing AMPK family of kinases, is also rapidly induced in Y1 adrenal cells in response to ACTH *via* the cAMP–PKA signaling cascade. Previously, it had been suggested that an increased level of SIK1 expression inhibits adrenal steroidogenesis by repressing the cAMP-dependent transcription of steroidogenic proteins, CYP11A1 and StAR, by attenuating CREB transcriptional activity (74). In contrast, we showed that SIK1 stimulates adrenal steroidogenesis by modulating the selective HDL-CE transport activity of SR-B1. Overexpression of SIK1 increases cAMP-stimulated and SR-B1-mediated selective HDL-BODIPY-CE uptake in cell lines without impacting SR-B1 protein levels, whereas knockdown of SIK1 attenuated cAMP-stimulated selective HDL-BODIPY-CE uptake. SIK1 forms a complex with SR-B1 by interacting with its cytoplasmic C-terminal domain, and *in vitro* kinase activity measurements indicate that SIK1 can phosphorylate the C-terminal domain of SR-B1. Among potential phosphorylation sites, SIK1-catalyzed phosphorylation of Ser496 is critical for SIK1 stimulation of the selective CE transport activity of SR-B1. Mutational studies further demonstrated that both the intact catalytic activity of SIK1 and its PKA-catalyzed phosphorylation are essential for SIK1 stimulation of SR-B1 activity. Finally, overexpression of SIK1 caused time-dependent increases in SR-B1-mediated and HDL-supported steroid production in Y1 cells; however, these effects were lost with knockdown of SR-B1. It should be noted that, as opposed to these stimulatory effects of SIK1 on SR-B1 function, we confirmed that SIK1 does suppress CREB activity, which could contribute to the inhibition of steroidogenesis under some conditions. Taken together, these studies establish a role for SIK1 in the positive regulation of selective HDL-CE transport function of SR-B1 and steroidogenesis and suggest a potential mechanism for SIK1 signaling in modulating SR-B1-mediated selective CE uptake and associated steroidogenesis.

Many studies have also indicated that accessory proteins are crucial for the proper cellular expression of SR-B1 and SR-B1-mediated HDL-CE transport as well as other functions (75–83). For example, it has been shown that PDZK1/NHERF3 regulates hepatic SR-B1 stability and steady-state protein levels. Interestingly, PDZK1/NHERF3 is neither expressed nor essential for SR-B1 abundance or its cellular localization in steroidogenic cells of the adrenal gland, ovary, and testis (77). Recently, we have shown that two other NHERF family members, NHERF1 and NHERF2, negatively regulate the expression and function of SR-B1 in steroidogenic cells of the adrenal and gonads in response to ACTH (84). Specifically, we showed that ACTH treatment decreases NHERF1 and NHERF2 protein levels in rat adrenals and increases SR-B1 function. Co-immunoprecipitation, colocalization, bimolecular fluorescence complementation, and mutational analysis all indicated that NHERF1 and NHERF2 form complexes with SR-B1 protein and, as a result, inhibit SR-B1-mediated selective CE transport and steroidogenesis. Moreover, we demonstrated that the structural components required for NHERF1/2 to interact with SR-B1 included an intact COOH-terminal PDZ recognition motif (EAKL) in SR-B1 as well as the PDZ1 or PDZ2 domain of NHERF1, the PDZ2 domain of NHERF2, or the MERM domains of NHERF1/2. The *de novo* synthesis of SR-B1 was also inhibited by both NHERF1 and NHERF2 (84). In contrast to NHERF1 and NHERF2, NHERF4 had no effect on selective HDL-CE uptake or steroidogenesis. Altogether, these experiments demonstrated that NHERF1 and NHERF2 bind SR-B1 and negatively regulate SR-B1 expression, selective CE transport, and steroidogenesis (84).

ACTH AND REGULATION OF SR-B1 UNDER PATHOPHYSIOLOGICAL CONDITIONS

Since ACTH tightly regulates SR-B1 gene transcription, it should be expected that any pathophysiological conditions that affect ACTH levels would also impact SR-B1 gene expression in an identical manner. However, there is the possibility that altered SR-B1 function may represent an adaptive response to cope with stressful conditions. Indeed, results from studies of mice that underwent chronic psychosocial stress exhibited an exaggerated adrenal corticosterone response along with elevated SR-B1 protein levels (85). On the other hand, since adrenal cholesterol uptake is required for the production of anti-inflammatory glucocorticoids, gene deletion of functional SR-B1 in adrenals results in impaired steroid synthesis (86). Other studies using SR-B1 knockout mice demonstrated that SR-B1 can protect mice against endotoxemia (87). There is an uncontrolled robust inflammatory cytokine response in the SR-B1 deficient animals, and they exhibit higher lethality when challenged with LPS-doses that induce endotoxic shock. Furthermore, these animals also exhibit a dysregulated adrenal glucocorticoid-mediated stress response to fasting. In addition, fasting-induced elevated levels of serum ACTH were the consequence of adrenal glucocorticoid insufficiency in SR-B1 knockout mice (86). Finally, when SR-B1 was only selectively deleted in adrenocortical cells in a tissue-specific manner, the animals had impaired rates of glucocorticoid secretion in response to stress, especially when they were subjected to an endotoxin challenge; these animals with SR-B1 ablated only in adrenocortical cells showed enhanced local and systematic inflammatory response, blunted activation of atrophy genes in skeletal muscle, and have a high incidence of mortality (88). In the setting of acute stress, where the release of corticosterone in

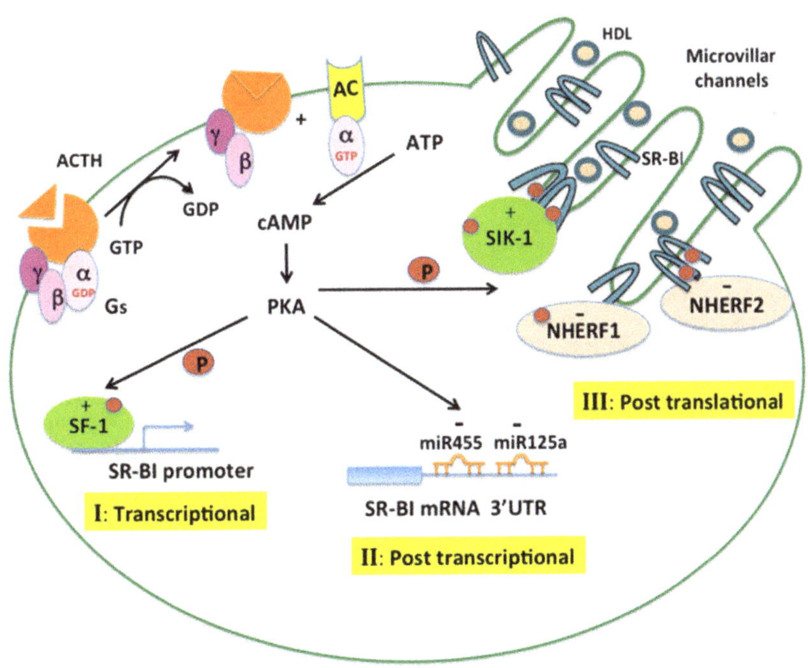

FIGURE 3 | ACTH regulation of SR-B1 in the adrenal. ACTH binds to its G protein-coupled receptor, leading to the activation of adenylate cyclase, which generates cAMP and activates cAMP-dependent protein kinase (PKA). The cAMP–PKA signaling cascade can regulate SR-B1 expression and function at different levels. (I) Transcriptional control: PKA increases the phosphorylation of transcription factors, such as SF1, leading to increased promoter activity of SR-B1. (II) Posttranscriptional control: PKA increases the expression of miRNA-125a and miRNA-455, which can bind to the 3′ UTR of SR-B1 mRNA and negatively regulate SR-B1 expression. (III) Posttranslational control: PKA induces the oligomerization of SR-B1 and stimulates an interaction with SIK1, leading to phosphorylation of SR-B1, both events resulting in increased SR-B1 protein function. PKA can also increase the interaction of SR-B1 with NHERF1 and NHERF2, which negatively regulate SR-B1 function.

rodents or cortisol in humans peaks rapidly and declines quickly, it is likely that posttranslational regulation of SR-B1, such as protein phosphorylation and dimerization, could be more important in the regulation of steroidogenesis than transcriptional control. In contrast, under chronic stress conditions, mechanisms regulating SR-B1 at the transcriptional level and/or through miRNAs would appear to be more relevant.

Some of the adrenal steroid hormones, i.e., glucocorticoids, display robust daily variations in circulation under the circadian control by ACTH, and their rhythmic activity is considered to play important roles in whole body health and disease (89, 90). Ablation of one of the genes involved in circadian control, BMAL1, results in loss of circadian regulation of glucocorticoids. The BMAL1-deficient animals showed impaired response to ACTH regulation of adrenal function and downregulation of genes involved in cholesterol transport, such as StAR and LDLR, in adrenals (89). There is a well-accepted concept of the adrenal clock, with evidence of differential responses between males and females (91). While studies have shown a circadian variation in the expression of several genes involved in regulating the steroid production, no publications have specifically examined whether SR-B1 expression and/or function displays a circadian rhythm, but this is likely in view of the known regulation of SR-B1 by ACTH.

In summary, through binding to its G protein-coupled receptors, leading to the activation of adenylate cyclase, which generates cAMP and activates PKA, ACTH exerts tight regulation of SR-B1 function in the adrenal at three different levels. As illustrated in **Figure 3**, increased cAMP–PKA signaling can increase the phosphorylation of transcription factors, such as SF1, and stimulate promoter activity of SR-B1. ACTH can increase the expression of miRNA-125 and miRNA-455, which can bind to the 3′ UTR of SR-B1 and result in suppressed expression and function of SR-B1 protein. Increased cAMP–PKA signaling can induce oligomerization of SR-B1 as well as stimulate phosphorylation of SIK1, which, in turn, increases the phosphorylation of SR-B1 and results in increased function of SR-B1 protein. Meanwhile, ACTH can also induce the expression of NHERF1 and NHERF2, both of which can bind to SR-B1 and negatively regulate SR-B1 function. Altered SR-B1 function may represent an adaptive response to cope with stressful conditions, as demonstrated by ablation of SR-B1 resulting in disturbed anti-inflammatory glucocorticoid homeostasis and impaired steroid synthesis.

AUTHOR CONTRIBUTIONS

All authors listed, have made substantial, direct and intellectual contribution to the work, and approved it for publication.

FUNDING

This work was supported by the Office of Research and Development, Medical Service, Department of Veterans Affairs and by the National Institutes of Health, NHLBI, grant 2R01HL33881.

REFERENCES

1. McKenna T, Fearon U, Clarke D, Cunningham S. A critical review of the origin and control of adrenal androgens. *Baillieres Clin Obstet Gynecol* (1997) **11**:229–48. doi:10.1016/S0950-3552(97)80035-1
2. Miller W. Androgen biosynthesis from cholesterol to DHEA. *Mol Cell Endocrinol* (2002) **198**:7–14. doi:10.1016/S0303-7207(02)00363-5
3. Davis WW, Garren LD. On the mechanism of action of adrenocorticotropic hormone. The inhibitory site of cycloheximide in the pathway of steroid biosynthesis. *J Biol Chem* (1968) **243**:5153–7.
4. Garren LD, Ney RL, Davis WW. Studies on the role of protein synthesis in the regulation of corticosterone production by adrenocorticotropic hormone in vivo. *Proc Natl Acad Sci U S A* (1965) **53**:1443–50. doi:10.1073/pnas.53.6.1443
5. Andersen JM, Dietschy JM. Relative importance of high and low density lipoproteins in the regulation of cholesterol synthesis in the adrenal gland, ovary, and testis of the rat. *J Biol Chem* (1978) **253**:9024–32.
6. Gwynne JT, Strauss JF III. The role of lipoproteins in steroidogenesis and cholesterol metabolism in steroidogenic glands. *Endocr Rev* (1982) **3**:299–329. doi:10.1210/edrv-3-3-299
7. Kraemer FB. Adrenal cholesterol utilization. *Mol Cell Endocrinol* (2007) **26**(5–266):42–5. doi:10.1016/j.mce.2006.12.001
8. Rigotti A, Edelmann E, Seifert P, Iqbal S, DeMattos R, Temel R, et al. Regulation by adrenocorticotropic hormone of the in vivo expression of scavenger receptor class B type I (SR-BI), a high density lipoprotein receptor, in steroidogenic cells of the murine adrenal gland. *J Biol Chem* (1996) **271**:33545–9. doi:10.1074/jbc.271.52.33545
9. Connelly M, Klein S, Azhar S, Abumrad N. Comparison of class B scavenger receptors, CD36, and scavenger receptor BI (SR-BI), shows that both receptors mediate high-density lipoprotein-cholesteryl ester selective uptake bu SR-BI exhibits a unique enhancement of cholesteryl ester uptake. *J Biol Chem* (1999) **274**:41–7. doi:10.1074/jbc.274.1.41
10. Stangl H, Cao G, Wyne KL, Hobbs HH. Scavenger receptor, class B, type I-dependent stimulation of cholesterol esterification by high density lipoproteins, low density lipoproteins, and nonlipoprotein cholesterol. *J Biol Chem* (1998) **273**:31002–8. doi:10.1074/jbc.273.47.31002
11. Swarnakar S, Temel RE, Connelly MA, Azhar S, Williams DL. Scavenger receptor class B, type I, mediates selective uptake of low density lipoprotein cholesteryl ester. *J Biol Chem* (1999) **274**:29733–9. doi:10.1074/jbc.274.42.29733
12. Simpson E, Lauber M, Demeter M, Means G, Mahendroo M, Kilgore M, et al. Regulation of expression of the genes encoding steroidogenic enzymes in the ovary. *J Steroid Biochem Mol Biol* (1992) **41**:409–13. doi:10.1016/0960-0760(92)90366-Q
13. Faust JR, Goldstein JL, Brown MS. Receptor-mediated uptake of low density lipoprotein and utilization of its cholesterol for steroid synthesis in cultured mouse adrenal cells. *J Biol Chem* (1977) **252**:4861–71.
14. Miller WL, Bose HS. Early steps in steroidogenesis: intracellular cholesterol trafficking thematic review series: genetics of human lipid diseases. *J Lipid Res* (2011) **52**:2111–35. doi:10.1194/jlr.R016675
15. Connelly MA, Kellner-Weibel G, Rothblat GH, Williams DL. SR-BI-directed HDL-cholesteryl ester hydrolysis. *J Lipid Res* (2003) **44**:331–41. doi:10.1194/jlr.M200186-JLR200
16. Kraemer FB, Shen WJ, Harada K, Patel S, Osuga J, Ishibashi S, et al. Hormone-sensitive lipase is required for high-density lipoprotein cholesteryl ester-supported adrenal steroidogenesis. *Mol Endocrinol* (2004) **18**:549–57. doi:10.1210/me.2003-0179
17. Vahouny GV, Chanderbhan R, Hinds R, Hodges VA, Treadwell CR. ACTH-induced hydrolysis of cholesteryl esters in rat adrenal cells. *J Lipid Res* (1978) **19**:570–7.
18. Kraemer FB, Shen WJ, Natu V, Patel S, Osuga J, Ishibashi S, et al. Adrenal neutral cholesteryl hydrolase: identification, subcellular distribution and sex differences. *Endocrinology* (2002) **143**:801–6. doi:10.1210/endo.143.3.8693
19. Kraemer FB, Shen WJ, Patel S, Osuga J, Ishibashi S, Azhar S. The LDL receptor is not necessary for acute adrenal steroidogenesis in mouse adrenocortical cells. *Am J Physiol Endocrinol Metab* (2007) **292**:E408–12. doi:10.1152/ajpendo.00428.2006

20. Verschoor-Klootwyk AH, Verchoor L, Azhar S, Reaven GM. Role of exogenous cholesterol in regulation of adrenal steroidogenesis in the rat. *J Biol Chem* (1982) **257**:7666–71.
21. Xie C, Richardson JA, Turley SD, Dietschy JM. Cholesterol substrate pools and steroid hormone levels are normal in the face of mutational inactivation of NPC1 protein. *J Lipid Res* (2006) **47**:953–63. doi:10.1194/jlr.M500534-JLR200
22. Pon LA, Hartigan JA, Orme-Johnson NR. Acute ACTH regulation of adrenal corticosteroid biosynthesis. Rapid accumulation of a phosphoprotein. *J Biol Chem* (1986) **261**:13309–16.
23. Pon LA, Orme-Johnson NR. Acute stimulation of corpus luteum cells by gonadotrophin or adenosine 3′,5′-monophosphate causes accumulation of a phosphoprotein concurrent with acceleration of steroid synthesis. *Endocrinology* (1988) **123**:1942–8. doi:10.1210/endo-123-4-1942
24. Epstein L, Orme-Johnson N. Regulation of steroid hormone biosynthesis: identification of precursors of a phosphoprotein targeted to the mitochondrion in stimulated rat adrenal cortex cells. *J Biol Chem* (1991) **266**:19739–45.
25. Stocco D, Clark B. Regulation of the acute production of steroids in steroidogenic cells. *Endocr Rev* (1996) **17**:221–44. doi:10.1210/er.17.3.221
26. Miller WL. Molecular biology of steroid hormone synthesis. *Endocr Rev* (1988) **9**:295–318. doi:10.1210/edrv-9-3-295
27. Simpson ER, Waterman MR. Regulation of the synthesis of steroidogenic enzymes in adrenal cortical cells by ACTH. *Annu Rev Physiol* (1988) **50**:427–40. doi:10.1146/annurev.ph.50.030188.002235
28. PayneAH, YoungbloodGL, ShaL, Burgos-TrinidadM, HammondSH. Hormonal regulation of steroidogenic enzyme gene expression in Leydig cells. *J Steroid Biochem Mol Biol* (1992) **43**:895–906. doi:10.1016/0960-0760(92)90317-C
29. LaVoie H, King S. Transcriptional regulation of steroidogenic genes: STARD1, CYP11A1 and HSD3B. *Exp Biol Med (Maywood)* (2009) **234**:880–907. doi:10.3181/0903-MR-97
30. JM M. The role of cyclic AMP in gonadal arteroidogenesis. *Biol Reprod* (1976) **14**:30–53. doi:10.1095/biolreprod14.1.30
31. Simpson E, Waternan M. Regulation by ACTH of steroid hormone biosynthesis in the adrenal cortex. *Can J Biochem Cell Biol* (1983) **61**:692–707. doi:10.1139/o83-088
32. Sanorn B, Heindel J, Robinson G. The role of cyclic nucleotides in the reproductive processes. *Ann Rev Physiol* (1980) **42**:37–57. doi:10.1146/annurev.ph.42.030180.000345
33. Strauss J, Golos T, Silavin S, Soto E, Takagi K. Involvement of cyclic AMP in the functions of granulosa and luteal cells: regulation of steroidogenesis. *Prog Clin Biol Res* (1988) **267**:177–200.
34. Spat A, Hunyady L. Control of aldosterone secretion: a model for convergence in cellular signaling pathways. *Physiol Rev* (2004) **84**:489–539. doi:10.1152/physrev.00030.2003
35. Reaven E, Spicher M, Azhar S. Microvillar channels: a unique plasma membrane compartment for concentrating lipoproteins on the surface of rat adrenal cortical cells. *J Lipid Res* (1989) **30**:1551–60.
36. Plump AS, Erickson SK, Weng W, Partin JS, Breslow JL, Williams DL. Apolipoprotein A-I is required for cholesteryl ester accumulation in steroidogenic cells and for normal adrenal steroid production. *J Clin Invest* (1996) **97**:2660–71. doi:10.1172/JCI118716
37. Landschulz K, Pathak R, Rigotti A, Krieger M, Hobb H. Regulation of scavenger receptor, class B, type I, a high density lipoprotein receptor, in liver and steroidogenic tissues of the rat. *J Clin Invest* (1996) **98**:984–5. doi:10.1172/JCI118883
38. Azhar S, Nomoto A, Leers-Sucheta S, Reaven E. Simultaneous induction of an HDL receptor protein (SR-BI) and the selective uptake of HDL-cholesteryl esters in a physiologically relevant steroiodgenic cell model. *J Lipid Res* (1998) **39**:1616–28.
39. Gwynne JT, Hughes T, Hess B. Characterization of high density lipoprotein binding activity in rat adrenocortical cells. *J Lipid Res* (1984) **25**:1059–71.
40. Gwynne JT, Hess B. The role of high density lipoproteins in rat adrenal cholesterol metabolism and steroidogenesis. *J Biol Chem* (1980) **255**:10875–83.
41. Duggan A, Marie R, Callard I. Expression of SR-BI (scavenger receptor class B type I) in turtle (*Chrysemys picta*) tissues and other nonmammalian vertebrates. *J Exp Zool* (2002) **292**:430–4. doi:10.1002/jez.10067
42. Acton S, Rigotti A, Landschultz K, Xu S, Hobs H, Krieger M. Identification of scavenger receptor SR-BI as a high density lipoprotein receptor. *Science* (1996) **271**:518–20. doi:10.1126/science.271.5248.518
43. Liu J, Voutilainen R, Heikkila P, Kahri AI. Ribonucleic acid expression of the CLA-1 gene, a human homolog to mouse high density lipoprotein receptor SR-BI, in human adrenal tumors and cultured adrenal cells. *J Clin Endocrinol Metab* (1997) **82**:2522–7. doi:10.1210/jcem.82.6.3968
44. Wang N, Weng W, Breslow JL, Tall AR. Scavenger receptor BI (SR-BI) is up-regulated in adrenal gland in apolipoprotein A-I and hepatic lipase knock-out mice as a response to depletion of cholesterol stores. In vivo evidence that SR-BI is a functional high density lipoprotein receptor under feedback control. *J Biol Chem* (1996) **271**:21001–4.
45. Hu Z, Hu J, Shen WJ, Kraemer FB, Azhar S. A novel role of salt-inducible kinase 1 (SIK1) in the post-translational regulation of scavenger receptor class B type 1 activity. *Biochemistry* (2015) **54**:6917–30. doi:10.1021/acs.biochem.5b00147
46. Sun Y, Wang N, Tall AR. Regulation of adrenal scavenger receptor-BI expression by ACTH and cellular cholesterol pools. *J Lipid Res* (1999) **40**:1799–805.
47. Martin G, Pilon A, Albert C, Valle M, Hum DW, Fruchart JC, et al. Comparison of expression and regulation of the high-density lipoprotein receptor SR-BI and the low-density lipoprotein receptor in human adrenocortical carcinoma NCI-H295 cells. *Eur J Biochem* (1999) **261**:481–91. doi:10.1046/j.1432-1327.1999.00296.x
48. Cao G, Garcia CK, Wyne KL, Schultz RA, Parker KL, Hobbs HH. Structure and localization of the human gene encoding SR-BI/CLA-1. Evidence for transcriptional control by steroidogenic factor 1. *J Biol Chem* (1997) **272**:33068–76. doi:10.1074/jbc.272.52.33068
49. Lopez D, Sandhoff TW, McLean MP. Steroidogenic factor-1 mediates cyclic 3′,5′-adenosine monophosphate regulation of the high density lipoprotein receptor. *Endocrinology* (1999) **140**:3034–44. doi:10.1210/en.140.7.3034
50. Lopez D, McLean MP. Sterol regulatory element-binding protein-1a binds to cis elements in the promoter of the rat high density lipoprotein receptor SR-BI gene. *Endocrinology* (1999) **140**:5669–81. doi:10.1210/endo.140.12.7220
51. Malerod L, Juvet LK, Hanssen-Bauer A, Eskild W, Berg T. Oxysterol-activated LXRalpha/RXR induces hSR-BI-promoter activity in hepatoma cells and preadipocytes. *Biochem Biophys Res Commun* (2002) **299**:916–23. doi:10.1016/S0006-291X(02)02760-2
52. Lopez D, McLean MP. Activation of the rat scavenger receptor class B type I gene by PPARalpha. *Mol Cell Endocrinol* (2006) **251**:67–77. doi:10.1016/j.mce.2006.02.011
53. Schoonjans K, Annicotte JS, Huby T, Botrugno OA, Fayard E, Ueda Y, et al. Liver receptor homolog 1 controls the expression of the scavenger receptor class B type I. *EMBO Rep* (2002) **3**:1181–7. doi:10.1093/embo-reports/kvf238
54. Lopez D, Sanchez MD, Shea-Eaton W, McLean MP. Estrogen activates the high-density lipoprotein receptor gene via binding to estrogen response elements and interaction with sterol regulatory element binding protein-1A. *Endocrinology* (2002) **143**:2155–68. doi:10.1210/endo.143.6.8855
55. Shea-Eaton W, Lopez D, McLean MP. Yin yang 1 protein negatively regulates high-density lipoprotein receptor gene transcription by disrupting binding of sterol regulatory element binding protein to the sterol regulatory element. *Endocrinology* (2001) **142**:49–58. doi:10.1210/endo.142.4.8075
56. Sporstol M, Tapia G, Malerod L, Mousavi SA, Berg T. Pregnane X receptor-agonists down-regulate hepatic ATP-binding cassette transporter A1 and scavenger receptor class B type I. *Biochem Biophys Res Commun* (2005) **331**:1533–41. doi:10.1016/j.bbrc.2005.04.071
57. Temel RE, Trigatti B, DeMattos RB, Azhar S, Krieger M, Williams DL. Scavenger receptor class B, type I (SR-BI) is the major route for the delivery of high density lipoprotein cholesterol to the steroidogenic pathway in cultured mouse adrenocortical cells. *Proc Natl Acad Sci U S A* (1997) **94**:13600–5. doi:10.1073/pnas.94.25.13600
58. Cao G, Zhao L, Stangl H, Hasegawa T, Richardson J, Parker K, et al. Developmental and hormonal regulation of murine scavenger receptor, class B, type 1. *Mol Endocrinol* (1999) **13**:1460–73. doi:10.1210/mend.13.9.0346
59. Vieira-van Bruggen D, Kalkman I, van Gent T, van Tol A, Jansen H. Induction of adrenal scavenger receptor BI and increased high density lipoprotein-cholesteryl ether uptake by in vivo inhibition of hepatic lipase. *J Biol Chem* (1998) **273**:32038–41. doi:10.1074/jbc.273.48.32038
60. Mavridou S, Venihaki M, Rassouli O, Tsatsanis C, Kardassis D. Feedback inhibition of human scavenger receptor class B type I gene expression by glucocorticoid in adrenal and ovarian cells. *Endocrinology* (2010) **151**:3214–24. doi:10.1210/en.2009-1302

61. Hu Z, Shen W, Kraemer F, Azhar S. MicroRNAs 125a and 455 repress lipoprotein-supported steroidogenesis by targeting scavenger receptor class B type I in steroidogenic cells. *Mol Cell Biol* (2012) **32**:5035–45. doi:10.1128/MCB.01002-12
62. Rigotti A, Miettinen H, Krieger M. The role of the high-density lipoprotein receptor SR-BI in the lipid metabolism of endocrine and other tissues. *Endocr Rev* (2003) **24**:357–87. doi:10.1210/er.2001-0037
63. Gu X, Trigatti B, Xu S, Acton S, Babitt J, Krieger M. The efficient cellular uptake of high density lipoprotein lipids via scavenger receptor class B type I requires not only receptor-mediated surface binding but also receptor-specific lipid transfer mediated by its extracellular domain. *J Biol Chem* (1998) **273**:26338–48. doi:10.1074/jbc.273.41.26338
64. Reaven E, Zhan L, Nomoto A, Leers-Sucheta S, Azhar S. Expression and microvillar localization of scavenger receptor class B, type I (SR-BI) and selective cholesteryl ester uptake in Leydig cells from rat testis. *J Lipid Res* (2000) **41**:343–56.
65. Reaven E, Leers-Sucheta S, Nomoto A, Azhar S. Expression of scavenger receptor class B type 1 (SR-BI) promotes microvillar channel formation and selective cholesteryl ester transport in a heterologous reconstituted system. *Proc Natl Acad Sci U S A* (2001) **98**:1613. doi:10.1073/pnas.98.4.1613
66. Williams DL, Wong JS, Hamilton RL. SR-BI is required for microvillar channel formation and the localization of HDL particles to the surface of adrenocortical cells in vivo. *J Lipid Res* (2002) **43**:544–9.
67. Peng Y, Akmentin W, Connelly M, Lund-Katz S, Phillips M, Williams D. Scavenger receptor BI (SR-BI) clustered on microvillar extensions suggests that this plasma membrane domain is a way station for cholesterol trafficking between cells and high-density lipoprotein. *Mol Biol Cell* (2004) **15**:384–96. doi:10.1091/mbc.E03-06-0445
68. Bocharov A, Baranova I, Vishnyakova T, Remaley A, Csako G, Thomas F, et al. Targeting of scavenger receptor class B type I by synthetic amphipathic alpha-helical-containing peptides blocks lipopolysaccharide (LPS) uptake and LPS-induced pro-inflammatory cytokine responses in THP-1 monocyte cells. *J Biol Chem* (2004) **279**:36072–82. doi:10.1074/jbc.M314264200
69. Thuahnai S, Lund-Katz S, Anantharamaiah G, Williams D, Phillips M. A quantitative analysis of apolipoprotein binding to SR-BI: multiple binding sites for lipid-free and lipid-associated apolipoproteins. *J Lipid Res* (2003) **44**:1132–42. doi:10.1194/jlr.M200429-JLR200
70. Azhar S, Nomoto A, Reaven E. Hormonal regulation of adrenal microvillar channel formation. *J Lipid Res* (2002) **43**:861–71.
71. Reaven E, Nomoto A, Cortez Y, Azhar S. Consequences of over-expression of rat scavenger receptor, SR-BI, in an adrenal cell model. *Nutr Metab (Lond)* (2006) **3**:43. doi:10.1186/1743-7075-3-43
72. Reaven E, Cortez Y, Leers-Sucheta S, Nomoto A, Azhar S. Dimerization of the scavenger receptor class B type I: formation, function, and localization in diverse cells and tissues. *J Lipid Res* (2004) **45**:513–28. doi:10.1194/jlr.M300370-JLR200
73. Hu J, Zhang Z, Shen W, Nomoto A, Azhar S. Differential roles of cysteine residues in the cellular trafficking, dimerization, and function of the high-density lipoprotein receptor, SR-BI. *Biochemistry* (2011) **50**:10860–75. doi:10.1021/bi201264y
74. Spiga F, Liu Y, Aguilera G, Lightman SL. Temporal effect of adrenocorticotrophic hormone on adrenal glucocorticoid steroidogenesis: involvement of the transducer of regulated cyclic AMP-response element-binding protein activity. *J Neuroendocrinol* (2011) **23**:136–42. doi:10.1111/j.1365-2826.2010.02096.x
75. Ikemoto M, Arai H, Feng D, Tanaka K, Aoki J, Dohmae N, et al. Identification of a PDZ-domain-containing protein that interacts with the scavenger receptor class B type I. *Proc Natl Acad Sci U S A* (2000) **97**:6538–43. doi:10.1073/pnas.100114397
76. Silver D. A carboxyl-terminal PDZ-interacting domain of scavenger receptor B, type I is essential for cell surface expression in liver. *J Biol Chem* (2002) **277**:34042–7. doi:10.1074/jbc.M206584200
77. Kocher O, Yesilaltay A, Cirovic C, Pal R, Rigotti A, Krieger M. Targeted disruption of the PDZK1 gene in mice causes tissue-specific depletion of the high density lipoprotein receptor scavenger receptor class B type I and altered lipoprotein metabolism. *J Biol Chem* (2003) **278**:52820–5. doi:10.1074/jbc.M310482200
78. Komori H, Arai H, Kashima T, Huby T, Kita T, Ueda Y. Coexpression of CLA-1 and human PDZK1 in murine liver modulates HDL cholesterol metabolism. *Arterioscler Thromb Vasc Biol* (2008) **28**:1298–303. doi:10.1161/ATVBAHA.108.165845
79. Robichaud J, Francis G, Vance D. A role for hepatic scavenger receptor class B, type I in decreasing high density lipoprotein levels in mice that lack phosphatidylethanolamine N-methyltransferase. *J Biol Chem* (2008) **283**:35496–506. doi:10.1074/jbc.M807433200
80. Zhu W, Saddar S, Seetharam D, Chambliss K, Longoria C, Silver D, et al. The scavenger receptor class B type I adaptor protein PDZK1 maintains endothelial monolayer integrity. *Circ Res* (2008) **102**(4):480–7. doi:10.1161/CIRCRESAHA.107.159079
81. Fenske S, Yesilaltay A, Pal R, Daniels K, Barker C, Quiñones V, et al. Normal hepatic cell surface localization of the high density lipoprotein receptor, scavenger receptor class B, type I, depends on all four PDZ domains of PDZK1. *J Biol Chem* (2009) **284**:5797–806. doi:10.1074/jbc.M808211200
82. Eyre N, Drummer H, Beard M. The SR-BI partner PDZK1 facilitates hepatitis C virus entry. *PLoS Pathog* (2010) **6**:e1001130. doi:10.1371/journal.ppat.1001130
83. Kocher O, Krieger M. Role of the adaptor protein PDZK1 in controlling the HDL receptor SR-BI. *Curr Opin Lipidol* (2009) **20**:236–41. doi:10.1097/MOL.0b013e32832aee82
84. Hu Z, Hu J, Zhang Z, Shen W, Yun C, Berlot C, et al. Regulation of expression and function of scavenger receptor class B, type I (SR-BI) by Na+/H+ exchanger regulatory factors (NHERFs). *J Biol Chem* (2013) **2013**(288):11416–35. doi:10.1074/jbc.M112.437368
85. Fuchsl AM, Uschold-Schmidt N, Reber SO. Chronic psychosocial stress in male mice causes an up-regulation of scavenger receptor class B type 1 protein in the adrenal glands. *Stress* (2013) **16**:461–8. doi:10.3109/10253890.2013.793303
86. Hoekstra M, Meurs I, Koenders M, Out R, Hildebrand RB, Kruijt JK, et al. Absence of HDL cholesteryl ester uptake in mice via SR-BI impairs an adequate adrenal glucocorticoid-mediated stress response to fasting. *J Lipid Res* (2008) **49**:738–45. doi:10.1194/jlr.M700475-JLR200
87. Cai L, Ji A, de Beer FC, Tannock LR, van der Westhuyzen DR. SR-BI protects against endotoxemia in mice through its roles in glucocorticoid production and hepatic clearance. *J Clin Invest* (2008) **118**:364–75. doi:10.1172/JCI31539
88. Gilibert S, Galle-Treger L, Moreau M, Saint-Charles F, Costa S, Ballaire R, et al. Adrenocortical scavenger receptor class B type I deficiency exacerbates endotoxic shock and precipitates sepsis-induced mortality in mice. *J Immunol* (2014) **193**:817–26. doi:10.4049/jimmunol.1303164
89. Leliavski A, Shostak A, Husse J, Oster H. Impaired glucocorticoid production and response to stress in Arntl-deficient male mice. *Endocrinology* (2014) **155**:133–42. doi:10.1210/en.2013-1531
90. Kil IS, Lee SK, Ryu KW, Woo HA, Hu MC, Bae SH, et al. Feedback control of adrenal steroidogenesis via H2O2-dependent, reversible inactivation of peroxiredoxin III in mitochondria. *Mol Cell* (2012) **46**:584–94. doi:10.1016/j.molcel.2012.05.030
91. Kloehn I, Pillai SB, Officer L, Klement C, Gasser PJ, Evans JA. Sexual differentiation of circadian clock function in the adrenal gland. *Endocrinology* (2016):en20151968. doi:10.1210/en.2015-1968

10

Adrenal Mitochondria and Steroidogenesis: From Individual Proteins to Functional Protein Assemblies

Andrew Midzak[1†] and Vassilios Papadopoulos[1,2,3*]*

[1]Research Institute of the McGill University, Montreal, QC, Canada, [2]Department of Biochemistry, McGill University, Montreal, QC, Canada, [3]Department of Pharmacology and Therapeutics, McGill University, Montreal, QC, Canada

***Correspondence:**
Andrew Midzak
midzak1982@gmail.com;
Vassilios Papadopoulos
vassilios.papadopoulos@mcgill.ca

†Present address:
Andrew Midzak,
USAMRMC, Ft. Detrick,
Frederick, MD, USA

The adrenal cortex is critical for physiological function as the central site of glucocorticoid and mineralocorticoid synthesis. It possesses a great degree of specialized compartmentalization at multiple hierarchical levels, ranging from the tissue down to the molecular levels. In this paper, we discuss this functionalization, beginning with the tissue zonation of the adrenal cortex and how this impacts steroidogenic output. We then discuss the cellular biology of steroidogenesis, placing special emphasis on the mitochondria. Mitochondria are classically known as the "powerhouses of the cell" for their central role in respiratory adenosine triphosphate synthesis, and attention is given to mitochondrial electron transport, in both the context of mitochondrial respiration and mitochondrial steroid metabolism. Building on work demonstrating functional assembly of large protein complexes in respiration, we further review research demonstrating a role for multimeric protein complexes in mitochondrial cholesterol transport, steroidogenesis, and mitochondria–endoplasmic reticulum contact. We aim to highlight with this review the shift in steroidogenic cell biology from a focus on the actions of individual proteins in isolation to the actions of protein assemblies working together to execute cellular functions.

Keywords: cholesterol transport, translocator protein, steroidogenic acute regulatory protein, voltage-dependent anion channels, cytochrome P450 enzyme system, mitochondria, endoplasmic reticulum

INTRODUCTION

The cortex of the adrenal is the principal site of synthesis of vertebrate glucocorticoid and mineralocorticoid steroid hormones (1). These hormones are two of the five classes of steroid hormones which are indispensable for mammalian development and physiology, the remaining including the estrogens, progestins, and androgens (2). The steroidogenic capacity of the adrenal gland is highly compartmentalized, performed by specialized cells, organelles, and proteins. The biosynthesis of steroids has been authoritatively reviewed (3), and this manuscript looks to focus attention on the compartmentalization of steroidogenesis of the adrenal mitochondria. To this end, several topics will be covered, including adrenal tissue zonation, mitochondrial organellar organization, and macromolecular protein complexes, all contributing to the regulation and optimization of adrenal endocrine signaling. Special attention will be devoted to our increasing understanding of multiprotein assemblies in mitochondrial function.

ADRENAL GLAND ZONATION

The adrenal gland is composed of two anatomically and functionally distinct compartments: the cortex and the medulla. The adrenal medulla is innervated with chromaffin cells and plays a key role in catecholamine synthesis and the sympathetic stress response (4), while the cortex contains the steroidogenic cells responsible for the adrenal's contribution to the endocrine system (5). The adrenal cortex is further compartmentalized, in humans functionally and morphologically divided into three concentric layers: the zona glomerulosa, the zona fasciculata, and the zona reticularis (**Figure 1**).

The zona glomerulosa, lying under the adrenal capsule (**Figure 1**), functions as part of the renin–angiotensin–aldosterone endocrine axis and contributes to organismal electrolyte balance (6). In response to the peptide angiotensin-II, or elevated plasma potassium, the cells of the zona glomerulosa secrete aldosterone. Aldosterone, such as all steroids, is synthesized from cholesterol *via* a multienzyme pathway particular to each steroidogenic tissue, resulting in successive modifications to the sterol backbone (**Figure 2**). Aldosterone, a mineralocorticoid, in turn promotes sodium and water retention, as well as potassium excretion by the kidney (7). Ultrastructurally, glomerulosa cells are characteristically contain numerous mitochondria with lamelli form cristae and some lipid droplets in the cytoplasm (8). The zona fasciculata, the next layer of the adrenal cortex (**Figure 1**), is responsible for organismal glucocorticoid production – cortisol in humans, corticosterone in rodents (**Figure 2**) (3). The cells of the zona fasciculata participate in the hypothalamic–pituitary–adrenal endocrine signaling axis and respond to pituitary adrenocorticotropic hormone (ACTH) signaling through the ACTH receptor (M2CR) and its accessory protein, the melanocortin 2 receptor accessory protein (MRAP). The fasciculata cells are organized in cord-like bundles – the fascicles – surrounded by fenestrated capillaries (8). Ultrastructurally, these cells also contain numerous mitochondria, although their cristae take a more tubulovesicular form. Fasciculata cells, consistent with their prolific capacity to synthesize glucocorticoids, contain prominent smooth endoplasmic reticulum (ER) and large numbers of lipid droplets (9). The layer of the cortex abutting the medulla in humans, the zona reticularis, is not part of currently well-defined endocrine axis, but does secrete significant amounts of the androgen dehydroepiandrosterone (DHEA; **Figure 2**) (10). The cells of the zona reticularis resemble those of the fasciculata ultrastructurally, although contain relatively fewer lipid droplets with comparatively greater numbers of lysosomes (9).

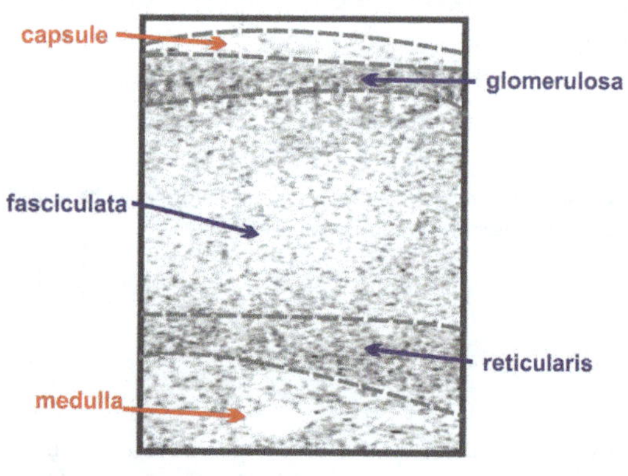

FIGURE 1 | Schematic of adrenal zonation. The different functional zones of the human adrenal gland are depicted with the outermost capsule layer overlying the mineralocorticoid-synthesizing glomerulosa layer. The fasciculata layer lies under the granulosa layer and is responsible for the synthesis of the glucocorticoid cortisol. The final layer of the cortex, the reticularis, synthesizes the androgen dehydroepiandrosterone (DHEA), while the innermost layer of the schematic, the medulla, is composed of chromaffin cells, responsible for the production of the catecholamine epinephrine.

Developmentally, the adrenal cortex arises from the adrenocortical primordium, itself derived from the urogenital ridge, a specialized region of the embryonic coelomic epithelium that also serves as the developmental precursor of the kidneys and hematopoietic progenitors (11). Cells in the adrenocortical primordium express the transcription factor genes Wilms tumor suppressor-1 (WT1), GATA-binding protein 4 (GATA4), and steroidogenicfactor-1 (SF1/NR5A1) (8, 12, 13). As development proceeds, adrenal progenitor cells in the migrate dorsomedially from the adrenocortical primordium into subjacent mesenchyme, concurrently upregulating expression of SF1, and downregulating expression of WT1 and GATA4 (13, 14). The developing adrenal gland is subsequently innervated by sympathoblasts from the neural crest, the precursors of the chromaffin cells of the medulla (15), and finally enveloped by capsule cells derived from the surrounding mesenchyme.

CELLULAR COMPARTMENTALIZATION AND MITOCHONDRIAL RESPIRATION

Eukaryotic cells are characteristically compartmentalized, containing numerous membrane-bounded organelles, each with specialized functions. These organelles achieve their specialization through non-uniform segregation of molecules, whether they are nucleic acids, proteins, lipids, or carbohydrates. The mitochondria are famously known as the "powerhouse of the cell" for their respiratory capacity and synthesis of adenosine triphosphate (ATP). Although mitochondrial energetics have traditionally served an ancillary role in steroidogenic research (16), the recent finding that mitochondrial function directly impacts neuroendocrine, metabolic, inflammatory, and transcriptional responses to acute psychological stress (17) prompts a brief review. We will introduce individual proteins involved and use the mitochondrial respiratory chain serves an example of higher order functional protein assemblies.

The mitochondria generate ATP by oxidizing hydrogens derived from carbohydrates (through the tricyclic acid cycle) and fats (through fatty acid β-oxidation). Electrons from nicotinamide adenine dinucleotide (NADH) are donated to the iron–sulfur (Fe–S) clusters of mitochondrial complex I (NADH

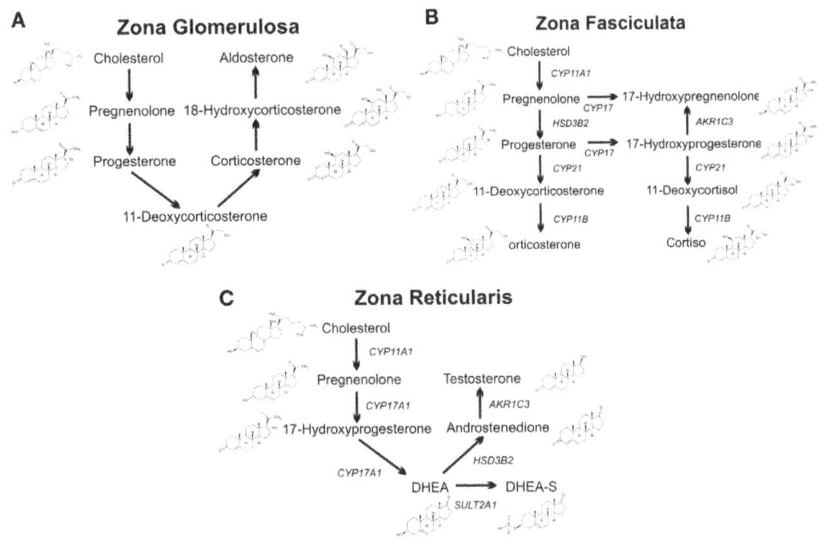

FIGURE 2 | Schematics of adrenal steroidogenic pathways. The metabolism of cholesterol to pregnenolone by the mitochondrial CYP11A1 is common to all three zones of the human adrenal. **(A)** The mitochondrial/microsomal enzyme HSD3B converts pregnenolone to progesterone, which is metabolized to 11-deoxycorticosterone by the microsomal CYP21. The final reactions of aldosterone synthesis are catalyzed by the mitochondrial CYP11B2, which converts 11-deoxycorticosterone to corticosterone, which is hydroxylated at C18 to form 18-hydroxycorticosterone which is then finally converted to aldosterone. **(B)** In the zona fasciculata, the microsomal CYP17 and the mitochondrial/microsomal HSD3B can generate 17-hydroxyprogesterone, progesterone, and 17-hydroxyprogesterone. The microsomal CYP21 preferentially metabolizes 17-hydroxyprogesterone to 11-deoxycortisol, which is finally metabolized to the glucocorticoid cortisol by the microsomal CYP11B2. CYP21 can also metabolize progesterone to 11-deoxycorticosterone, which CYP11B2 converts to the glucocorticoid corticosterone, although this pathway is secondary in humans (although the principal pathway in rodents). **(C)** In the zona reticularis, CYP17 hydroxylates pregnenolone to 17-hydroxypregnenolone, and then DHEA. DHEA is the major steroid product of the reticularis, with sulfated DHEA (DHEA-S), androstenedione, and testosterone serving as only minor steroidogenic products.

dehydrogenase), a multimeric inner mitochondrial membrane (IMM) protein complex. From Complex I, the electrons are sequentially shuttled to ubiquinone (coenzyme Q/CoQ), giving rise to ubiquinol ($CoQH_2$). Ubiquinol transfers its electrons to a cytochrome-containing IMM protein complex, Complex III (ubiquinol/cytochrome *c* oxidoreductase), which further shuttles the electrons to cytochrome *c*. From cytochrome *c*, the electrons flow to the cytochrome-containing Complex IV (cytochrome *c* oxidase, COX), the terminal IMM protein complex of the mitochondrial respiratory chain, which uses the electrons to reduce O_2 to yield H_2O. The free energy of electron movement through the ETC is used to pump protons (H^+) out of the mitochondrial matrix into the mitochondrial intermembrane space (IMS), creating a capacitance across the IMM. This potential energy is utilized to drive ATP synthesis by the IMM Complex V (ATP synthase), which condenses ADP + P_i to form ATP while pumping protons back into the matrix. Matrix ATP is then exchanged with cytosolic ADP by the adenine nucleotide translocator (ANT/SLC25), which works in conjunction with the outer mitochondrial membrane (OMM) voltage-dependent anion channel (VDAC) to form an energy-transducing mitochondrial contact site (18).

An interesting development in mitochondrial respiratory electron transport and one that, as discussed below, offers insight into mitochondrial steroidogenesis, began at the beginning of the twenty-first century with the proposal that the mitochondrial respiratory chain was organized in supramolecular assemblies termed "respirasomes" (19). This paradigm shift changed the view of mitochondrial electron transport from one of randomly organized respiratory chain complexes – in which components associated *via* random diffusion (20) – to one of respiratory chain supercomplexes locally transferring electrons between restricted components (21). Numerous studies utilizing blue native gel electrophoresis, preserving the fidelity of weakly associated members of protein complexes (22), have repeatedly shown that the oxidative phosphorylation complexes associate in supercomplexes of the three proton-translocating units: Complex I, Complex III, and Complex IV (19, 23, 24). Moreover, these supercomplexes have been demonstrated to be functional *in vitro*, further supporting a role for complex molecular assemblies in cellular function (25).

The conceptual justification of such supercomplexes derives from theoretical work indicating that spatial proximity of chemical reactions fosters efficiency, providing fitness advantages for evolutionary selection. This concept was originally proposed by Welch in the 1970s (26) as the concept of the "metabolon," and subsequently popularized by Srere (27), among others. This is not a novel concept for steroidogenic research, as Lieberman and Prasad utilized the metabolon construct in their work on steroidogenic metabolism (28). The crux of the metabolon is that groups of enzymes and/or proteins within metabolic pathways physically associate. This association, as noted above, would facilitate metabolite channeling, increasing the regulation, control, and speed of metabolic pathways. The metabolon appeals to common sense and biological evolutionary arguments, as increased efficiency is a requirement of biological survival in hostile environments. However, the metabolon has been difficult to demonstrate experimentally. Biochemical pull-down experiments have been reticent to demonstrate large biological metabolic complexes (29), and it has been argued that metabolic protein complex association is weak to easily facilitate regulation. The development of non-denaturing molecular assays, such as the blue native PAGE described above, as well as high-resolution fluorescent microscopy, has supported research into transient, but functionally critical, aspects of protein–protein interactions. Indeed, increasing evidence of such interactions in cellular metabolism is receiving attention, ranging from descriptions of cytoplasmic purinosomes – regulating purine biosynthesis (30, 31) – to mitochondrial fatty acid translocation machinery – contributing to mitochondrial fatty acid beta-oxidation and energetics (32, 33). The following sections describe the molecular components of mitochondrial steroidogenic machinery, first introducing individual proteins before transitioning description of a model of steroidogenesis functionally incorporating these proteins into larger protein assemblies, much akin to what has been observed for mitochondrial respiration.

STEROIDOGENIC CELLS, PROTEINS, AND MITOCHONDRIA

Cholesterol serves as the metabolic precursor of all adrenal steroids, and as such, the adrenal cortex can be viewed as a highly specialized lipid processing organ. Cholesterol possesses fascinating structural characteristics, making it one of the most studied and versatile molecules in biological systems. Steroid hormones, in turn, are oxygenated forms of cholesterol, a characteristic they share with bile acids and oxysterols (2), and one which changes their chemical properties from highly hydrophobic to modestly hydrophilic. This change in chemical properties underlies the shift in their biological role from structural (as cholesterol plays in lipid membranes) to informational (as steroids play in biological signaling).

Any discussion of the steroidogenic mitochondria of the adrenal gland must revolve around the mitochondrial steroidogenic enzymes. These steroidogenic enzymes fall into two broad families: the cytochrome P450 (CYP) and hydroxysteroid dehydrogenase/ketosteroid reductase (HSD/KSR) enzymes. The CYP enzymes represent the majority of the steroidogenic enzymes and will receive the greatest attention here as they are the most abundant steroidogenic enzymes of mitochondria. A highly diverse superfamily of enzymes, the CYPs are characterized by a single heme prosthetic group and the ability to absorb light at 450 nm when reduced with carbon monoxide. Enzymatically, P450 enzymes exhibit an extraordinary ability to insert oxygen into non-activated carbon–hydrogen bonds at the same time exhibiting high structural selectively. They accomplish this feat through their ability to activate molecular oxygen, although the iron atom of their heme tetrapyrrole prosthetic group with the aid of an ancillary redox partner (34).

Thousands of CYPs have been identified, in all domains of life, suggesting that this class of protein has ancient roots. There are 57 CYP genes encoding CYP enzymes in humans, subdivided into 18 clades. The majority of the CYP enzymes are localized to the ER, but one clade is localized to the mitochondria. While ER-localized CYPs obtain their electrons from a single P450 oxidoreductase, the mitochondrial CYPs utilize an electron transport chain containing the ferredoxin reductase (FDXR) and ferredoxin proteins (34). There are seven mitochondrial CYPs in humans, namely CYP11A1, CYP11B1, CYP11B2, CYP24A1, CYP27A1, CYP27B1, and CYP27C1. Of these, CYP11A1, CYP11B1, and CYP11B2 are involved in steroidogenesis, metabolizing cholesterol and steroids. Interestingly, CYP24A1 and the three CYP27 isozymes are all involved in cholesterol metabolism, playing roles in bile acid, oxysterol, and vitamin D biosynthesis (35, 36), suggestive that the ancestor of the mitochondrial clade of enzymes was involved in sterol metabolism. Interestingly, however, phylogenomic analysis of the CYP enzymes has repeatedly shown that the CYP11 family appears with, or shortly before, the emergence of vertebrates (37, 38) (**Figure 3**). Indeed, it has been postulated that the advent of steroidogenesis and steroid hormone receptor signaling and the increased developmental complexity of vertebrates are intimately linked (39). Moreover, evolution of the mitochondrial CYP11 family is itself of interest within the vertebrate lineage, for while homologs of the CYP11 family, responsible for the first step of synthesis for all steroids, are observed throughout vertebrata from fish to mammals (37, 38) (**Figure 3**), the CYP11B family, responsible for glucocorticoid and mineralocorticoid synthesis, is underrepresented throughout this subphylum (**Figure 3**). Thus, while the molecular details of adrenal mitochondrial steroid biosynthesis are well understood, as described below, the evolution of this system remains an important and poorly understood area of research (7, 40).

CHOLESTEROL SIDE CHAIN CLEAVAGE: CYP11A1

CYPA11A1 is absolutely essential for the synthesis of all vertebrate steroids, which are all characterized by the CYP11A1 reaction, namely cleavage of the cholesterol aliphatic side chain. The proposed reaction mechanism of CYP11A1 involves three sequential modifications of cholesterol. In the first step, CYP11A1 hydroxylates cholesterol at carbon 22 of the aliphatic tail; in the second step, cholesterol is hydroxylated at the carbon 20 of the aliphatic tail; finally, in the third step, oxidative scission of the C20–22 bond of the subsequent 20,22-dihydroxycholesterol yields the steroid pregnenolone and the reactive aldehyde, isocaproaldehyde (44). This reaction mechanism, originally proposed in the 1970s based on purified enzyme catalysis of hydroxycholesterol (45), has found support in the publishing of x-ray crystal structures of bovine and human CYP11A1 (46, 47), which indicate that the heme prosthetic group lies proximally to the 20′ and 22′ carbons of cholesterol. Recent high-resolution temporal enzymatic work further indicates that transient cholesterol hydroperoxyl serves as reaction intermediates (48, 49), further supporting the sequential oxidative cleavage model of this enzyme.

The cellular expression CYP11A1 is hormonally regulated in the steroidogenic tissues of the adrenal and gonads, with circulating pituitary hormones stimulating intracellular cAMP production, which in turn promotes CYP11A1 expression (50). A number of paracrine and endocrine factors affect the expression

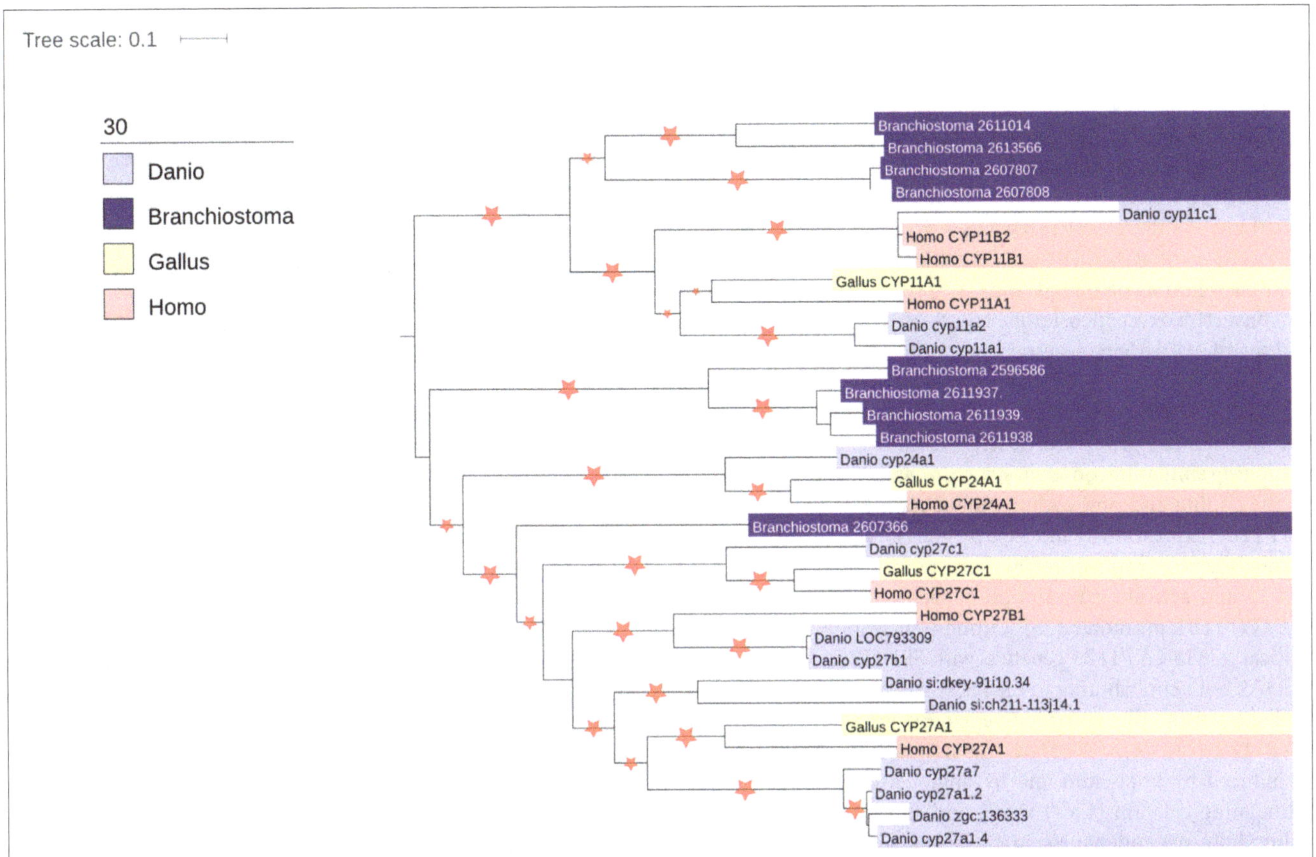

FIGURE 3 | Phylogenetic analysis of vertebrate mitochondrial CYP evolution. Homologs of the seven human mitochondrial CYPs (CYP11A1, CYP11B2, CYP11B3, CYP24A1, CYP27A1, CYP27B1, and CYP27C1) were identified using the nucleotide BLAST tool (41). Organisms chosen for search included the fully sequenced chicken (*Gallus gallus*), zebrafish (*Danio rerio*), and lancelet (*Branchiostoma floridae*), as they represented divergent vertebrate sequences (chicken vs. human vs. zebrafish) that could be compared with a non-vertebrate chordate (lancelet). The genomes of the Western clawed frog (*Xenopus tropicalis*) and anole lizard (*Anolis carolinesis*) were also searched, but sequences from these organisms were not included in the analysis as surprisingly no homologs of CYP11B1 or CYP11B2 were found (*data not shown*). Nucleotide sequences were aligned using MUSCLE (42), and phylogenetic trees constructed using PHyML (43).

of CYP11A1. Pituitary hormones, such as ACTH or angiotensin-II, stimulate CYP11A1 expression through a cAMP-dependent mechanism (51, 52), and the human CYP11A1 promoter contains two cAMP-responsive regions (53). Additional factors that stimulate cAMP in adrenocortical cells, such as activin (54), are also able to stimulate CYP11A1 expression. In contrast to cAMP, intracellular signaling pathways activated by Ca^{2+} and protein kinase C (PKC) can suppress CYP11A1 transactivation (55). In addition to the cAMP-responsive sites (CRSs) in the CYP11A1 promoter, the transcription factor SF-1 also contains an activating site (56, 57), which modulates the basal and cAMP-stimulated levels of CYP11A1 expression through association with the transcription factors p300 and CREB-binding protein (CBP) (58).

GLUCOCORTICOID AND MINERALOCORTICOID SYNTHESIS: CYP11B1 AND CYP11B2

The final steps in the synthesis of glucocorticoids and mineralocorticoids are catalyzed by two closely related mitochondrial enzymes: CYP11B1 and CYP11B2 (59). Similar to CYP11A1 and the other mitochondrial CYPs, CYP11B1 and CYP11B2 are associated with the IMM and are expressed with leader peptides targeting them to the mitochondrial matrix (60). CYP11B1 is the more abundantly expressed of the two proteins and is expressed predominantly in the zona fasciculata, and to a lesser extent in the zona reticularis, but not in the zona glomerulosa (61). CYP11B1 catalyzes the 11β-hydroxylation of 11-deoxycorticosterone and 11-deoxycortisol yielding corticosterone and cortisol, respectively (**Figure 2**) (44). CYP11B1 also has the capacity to hydroxylate C18 of 11-deoxycorticosterone or corticosterone to form 18-hydroxycorticosterone (62); however, it cannot catalyze the oxidation of the 18-hydroxy group to form aldosterone. This last reaction is catalyzed by CYP11B2, which is able to catalyze the sequential 11β-hydroxylation of 11-deoxycorticosterone, the hydroxylation of C18 and the subsequent oxidation of C18 to yield the C18 aldehyde group of aldosterone (**Figure 2**) (63–65). CYP11B2 inefficiently catalyzes oxidation of corticosterone; this finding has lent support to the zonation theory of mineralocorticoid and glucocorticoid synthesis, as the products of CYP11B1 would not be sequentially catalyzed to aldosterone (65).

Although it is unclear whether the CYP11B clade of mitochondrial CYPs emerged with the advent of vertebrates or mammals, within the mammalian lineage, the CYP11B clade exhibits significant diversity. While humans possess the two enzymes discussed above, cattle and pigs possess a single enzyme, CYP11B (66, 67), which is able to catalyze all of the reactions of CYP11B1 and CYP11B2. Conversely, within the rodent lineage, rats (but not mice) possess three CYP11B genes - CYP11B1, CYP11B2, and CYP11B3 - with CYP11B1 and B2 exhibiting homologous activity to their human orthologs, and CYP11B3 possessing the ability to convert deoxycorticosterone to 18-deoxycorticosterone, but lacking the 18 activity necessary to synthesize aldosterone (68).

CYP11B1 and CYP11B2 are located on human chromosome 8q21–22 (59, 69). Consistent with a tandem duplication event, the two human genes are closely linked, separated by 40 kb, exhibiting similar intron/exon structure, and 90 and 95% identity in the coding and non-coding sequences, respectively (59, 70). CYP11B1 expression is induced by ACTH *via* cAMP (71, 72), through a mechanism relying on cAMP response element (CRE) and activating transcription factor (ATF) sequences in the CYP11B1 promoter (73). Orphan nuclear receptors play a critical role in CYP11B1 genetics, with SF1/NR5A1 and LRH-1/NR5A2 both contributing to the relative expression of CYP11B1 and regulating the comparative expression of CYP11B1 vs. CYP11B2 (73, 74). CYP11B2 transcription in granulosa cells is induced by potassium and by angiotensin-II, in both cases stimulating calcium (Ca^{2+}) influx and stimulation of PKC and calmodulin-dependent protein kinase kinase (CAMKK) intracellular signaling (75, 76). CYP11B2 expression requires the action of the transcription factors NURR1 and NGF1B, but interestingly contrasts with CYP11B1 in its relationship with the transcription factor SF-1 (77, 78). Transcriptional regulation of CYP11B2 is also influenced by the activity of chicken ovalbumin upstream promoter transcription factor I (COUP-TF1), which itself is coactivated by the small ubiquitin-related modifier-1 (SUMO-1) conjugase and ligase Ubc9 and PIAS1 (79).

ELECTRON TRANSFER TO CYP11A1: FERREDOXIN REDUCTASE AND FERREDOXIN

The mitochondrial clade of CYP enzymes uses two sequential electron-transfer donors - ferredoxin (FDX) and FDXR - as intermediates in electron donation from NADPH (**Figure 4**). These are ancient proteins, with orthologs expressed in all domains of life and involved in numerous processes outside of steroidogenesis (80). FDXR is a 54.5-kDa flavoprotein affixed to the IMM that reduces NADPH and contains of two domains (81): (1) a NADPH-binding domain and (2) a flavin adenine dinucleotide-binding domain, with electron transfer occurring between the two. This cleft possesses a number of basic residues, residues essential for interaction with acidic residues on its electron donor partner, FDX (82). FDXR is broadly expressed in numerous tissues, but is comparatively abundant in steroidogenic tissues (83), where its abundance contributes to the catalytic activity of the mitochondrial CYPs (84). High SF-1 expression

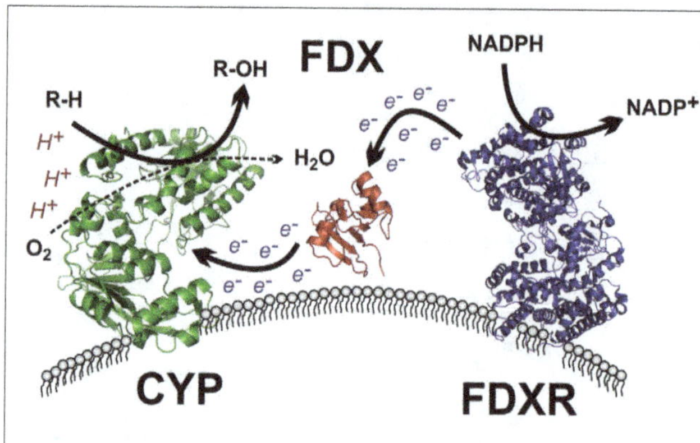

FIGURE 4 | Mitochondrial cytochrome P450 electron transport chain. The membrane-bound flavin-containing ferredoxin reductase (FDXR) accepts two electrons from NADPH, yielding $NADP^+$. These electrons are passed to the iron–sulfur cluster of ferredoxin (FDX), which donates the electrons to the heme prosthetic group of the mitochondrial cytochrome P450 (CYP), which uses protons and molecular oxygen to hydroxylate its target substrate (R–H) yielding the final hydroxylated product (R–OH) and water.

in steroidogenic tissue likely contributes this preponderance of FDXR, as SF-1-binding sites are present in the FDXR promoter and SF-1 overexpression in adrenal cell models drives FDXR expression (85).

The electron donor partner of FDXR, FDX, is a 14-kDa mitochondrial matrix-localized protein containing a Fe–S cluster tethered by four cysteine residues (86). Two ferredoxins exist in humans, with FDX1 supporting steroidogenesis and FDX2 participating in heme and Fe/S cluster protein synthesis (87). After obtaining electrons from FDXR, FDX1 subsequently transfers its electrons to mitochondrial P450 enzymes, including CYP11A1, CYP11B1, and CYP11B2, among others (**Figure 4**). FDX has been described as a mobile, indiscriminate, diffusible electron shuttle (3), much as cytochrome *c* and ubiquinol have been described previously (20).

IDENTIFICATION OF STEROIDOGENIC PROTEIN COMPLEXES

Research on CYP enzymes has contributed to the emerging picture of CYPs operating in functional complexes with other CYPs (88) as well as with their cognate electron donor partners (89). As noted in the previous section, the mitochondrial CYPs and the FDX and FDXR redox partners have been considered to interact randomly in the mitochondrial inner membrane (3). However, examination of native protein complexes in steroidogenic mitochondria from tumor Leydig cells using BN-PAGE and mass spectroscopy suggested that CYP11A1 and FDXR physically associate (90). In addition, these natively isolated CYP11A1 complexes were functionally active, cleaving the aliphatic tail of a fluorescent cholesterol reporter. Taken together, these findings support a model for CYP11A1–FDXR electron transport occurring in a physically associated metabolon, much akin to the electron transport of the respirasomes discussed above (24). This CYP11A1 metabolon model integrates with work on the steroidogenic transduceosome, a multiprotein complex traversing the OMM and IMM of the steroidogenic mitochondria integrating the movement of cholesterol with intracellular signaling to CYP111A1 (90, 91) (**Figure 5**). The steroidogenic transduceosome and metabolon complexes contain a number of cytoplasmic and mitochondrial components (**Figure 5**): cytoplasmic proteins include the steroidogenic acute regulatory (StAR) protein, the protein kinase cAMP-dependent type I regulatory subunit alpha (PRKAR1A), the diazepam-binding inhibitor (DBI), and the acyl-CoA-binding domain containing 3 (ACBD3); mitochondrial proteins include the VDAC, the translocator protein (TSPO), ATPase family, AAA domain containing 3A (ATAD3A), CYP family 11 subfamily A member 1 (CYP11A1), and FDXR. In addition, functional partners of the transduceosome have been identified, including mitochondria-associated members of the 14-3-3 adaptor protein family (92, 93) as well as kinase signalers such as extracellular signal-regulated kinase (ERK) 1/2 (94); the physical association and temporal interaction of these proteins with the transduceosome remain an active area of research. Because the focus of this review is upon mitochondrial contributions to steroidogenesis, the mitochondrial components of the transduceosome and metabolon are focused upon below.

VOLTAGE-DEPENDENT ANION CHANNEL

Voltage-dependent anion channel is the most abundant protein of the mitochondrial outer membrane and is widely accepted as the principal route and control of metabolic flux between the cytosol and mitochondria (95). VDAC is a 32-kDa beta barrel protein and has been implicated in numerous cellular processes, ranging from cellular energetics to apoptosis (96). Three VDAC isoforms are expressed in the human genome, with VDAC1 located on chromosome 5q31, VDAC2 located on chromosome 10q22, and VDAC3 located on chromosome 8p11 (97). The relative abundance of the different VDAC isoforms vary by tissue, by VDAC1 is the predominant form, followed by VDAC2, with VDAC3 expression low in comparison. Although functional redundancy is believed to exist between the isoforms, significant differences in roles of the VDAC proteins has been slowly teased out through biochemical and genetic investigations (98). Interestingly, mice null for *Vdac1* and *Vdac3* are viable and display little overt phenotypical changes; however, on this particular murine genetic background, *Vdac2*$^{-/-}$ mice were embryonically lethal (99, 100). Moreover, although the VDAC proteins have been recurrently implicated in apoptosis, mitochondria from *Vdac1*$^{-/-}$ and *Vdac3*$^{-/-}$ null mice, as well as cell lines null for all three isozymes fail to show changes in mitochondrial permeability transition and Bcl-2 family member-driven cell death compared with wild-type mitochondria.

Voltage-dependent anion channel is found at contact sites between the OMM and the IMM (101) where it may complex with energetics-related proteins, such as hexokinase, ANT, and creatine kinase, or with apoptotic proteins of the Bcl-2 family (18), and as noted above, and discussed below in greater detail, appears

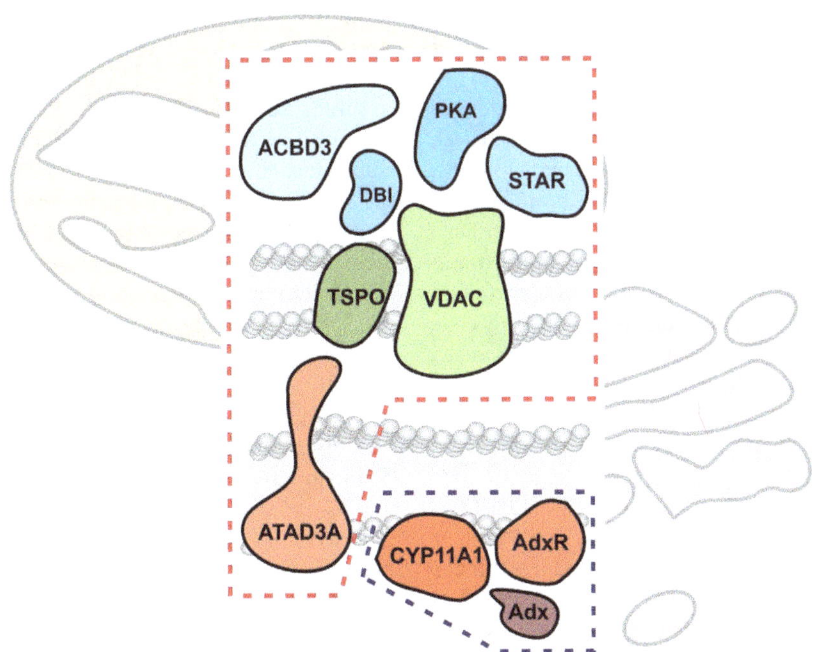

FIGURE 5 | Mitochondrial cholesterol transport and metabolism machinery. The mitochondrial cholesterol import and metabolism machinery are shown, demarcated by red (transduceosome) and blue (metabolon) dashed lines, respectively. The transduceosome contains cytoplasmic (StAR, ACBD3, DBI, and PRKARI; colored blue), OMM (VDAC and TSPO; colored green), and IMM (ATAD3A; colored red) components which assemble in response to hormonal stimulation and transduce the resultant cAMP signal to the mitochondria for cholesterol import. It is important to note, however, that molecular details of cholesterol import are still lacking. Once cholesterol is imported into the mitochondria, the IMM metabolon (CYP11A1, FDX, and FDXR; colored red) metabolizes cholesterol to pregnenolone, the precursor to all other steroids, including adrenal glucocorticoids and mineralocorticoids.

to play a central role in facilitating mitochondrial steroidogenic cholesterol transport through interactions with several key proteins. Moreover, VDAC also appears to play a significant, albeit poorly understood, role in cellular cholesterol homeostasis (102). Structural characterization of VDAC indicates that it is a cholesterol-binding protein; whether this cholesterol binding is a non-specific artifact of VDAC hydrophobicity, or whether this cholesterol binding plays a physiological role in steroidogenesis or other processes remains to be determined. It is unlikely that VDAC itself participates as a cholesterol channel, as the center of its ring-like structure is hydrophilic, suitable for anion transport but unsuitable for hydrophobic molecule transport (103, 104). After nearly half a century of work on this ubiquitous protein, much remains to be understood, especially in the context of mitochondrial cholesterol metabolism.

TRANSLOCATOR PROTEIN, 18 kDa

In the 1970s and 1980s, studies of benzodiazepine drug binding to sites outside of the central nervous system led to the identification of a peripheral benzodiazepine-binding site, generally expressed throughout the body, but concentrated in the steroidogenic cells of the adrenal and gonad (105–107). Isolation of this benzodiazepine-binding site led to the identification of an 18-kDa integral OMM protein, originally named the peripheral benzodiazepine receptor (PBR) (106). Subsequent research demonstrated that benzodiazepine and other chemical distinct PBR ligands were able to stimulate steroid biosynthesis by mobilizing mitochondrial cholesterol transport in isolated mitochondria, cell cultures, as well as in humans (108–111), and based on work implying the involvement of this protein in mitochondrial cholesterol and heme tetrapyrrole import, the PBR was renamed the TSPO (112).

Biochemical evidence and recent structural determinations of the TSPO protein indicate that TSPO is predominantly α-helical, containing five helices clustered into a barrel-like shape (113–115). Although antioxidant properties of TSPO have been demonstrated (115), no classical redox enzymatic or prosthetic groups, such as transition metals or active thiols, have been observed, and functional analysis of the protein has been difficult owing to its hydrophobicity (116). TSPO does contain an evolutionarily conserved C-terminal cholesterol recognition amino acid concensus (CRAC) motif (117, 118), which has been shown to facilitate cholesterol binding through a conserved tyrosine residue (119). This cholesterol-binding activity for TSPO has been implicated in steroidogenesis, as small molecules targeting the CRAC motif inhibit steroid production in cell and animal models (120, 121), and a naturally occurring human polymorphism in the protein proximal to the C-terminal CRAC motif (A147T) reduces cellular steroid production (122).

Hormonal stimulation of steroidogenesis in a steroidogenic cell model resulted in increased TSPO polymerization in correlation with increased ligand-binding affinity and steroid production (123, 124). Much like VDAC discussed above, TSPO has been identified as concentrated at OMM–IMM contact sites (125), and in addition to homooligomerization, TSPO has been consistently shown to physically associate with VDAC (126–128). Moreover, VDAC–TSPO interaction affects binding of TSPO ligands (127), suggestive of a functional relationship between the two proteins. The TSPO–VDAC platform appears to serve as an OMM base for the steroidogenic transduceosome cholesterol-transfer machinery (90, 91), a complex which appears to predominantly contain the polymerized form of TSPO (90). However, the mechanistic details of TSPO involvement in this complex are unclear at this time. Recent genetic mouse models in which TSPO had been deleted tissue specifically and globally have yielded conflicting results regarding steroidogenesis, ranging from no effect on steroidogenesis to severe compromise of ACTH-stimulated production of corticosterone (129–131). The complex effects of genetic background and selection for compensatory changes likely play a role in the experimental variability, however, especially in light of skewed embryonic Mendelian ratios in TSPO null mice (131).

STEROIDOGENIC ACUTE REGULATORY PROTEIN

Pharmacological inhibition of protein synthesis by compounds, such as cycloheximide, was long known as an inhibitor of steroidogenesis (132), suggesting that rapid protein synthesis was a necessary driver of steroid biosynthesis. The StAR protein was originally identified as a labile protein factor rapidly induced in response to hormonal stimulation of steroidogenic cells in correlation with increased steroid production (133, 134). Moreover, a number of studies have demonstrated that StAR is a direct target of hormonally stimulated cellular kinase signaling pathways, including the protein kinase A (PKA) and ERK kinase pathways (94, 135, 136). The necessity of StAR for steroidogenesis derived from work in humans showing that a broad spectrum of mutations in StAR contribute to congenital adrenal lipoid hyperplasia, a condition characterized by the inability to synthesize steroids, resulting in impaired sexual development and adrenal dysfunction leading to infant death unless treated with glucocorticoid supplementation (137).

Steroidogenic acute regulatory protein is located on chromosome 8p11 and is expressed as a 37-kDa mitochondrial pre-protein containing a mitochondrial targeting leader sequence, and subsequently imported into mitochondria, where the presequence is cleaved by Lon proteases in the matrix to a 30-kDa mature protein (although it is interesting to note that theoretical calculation of StAR protein molecular mass indicate 30 and 25 kDa masses for the pre- and mature proteins, although the reason for this discrepancy is unclear at this time). Surprisingly, StAR was found to stimulate steroid production in cell model systems without its leader sequence and import into the mitochondria (138). This led to elegant work on StAR action involving its molecular tether to the OMM, IMS, and IMM which indicated that StAR acts on the OMM and that mitochondrial import to the matrix inactivates StAR activity (139). Interestingly, however, *in vivo* work has demonstrated that the StAR mitochondrial presequence has biological necessity, as mouse models in which full-length StAR has been replaced by StAR that lacks the mitochondrial targeting sequence stochastically exhibit the CAH phenotype of steroidogenic failure (140). Moreover, CAH-causing mutations have been found in the leader sequence of human StAR-mutation patients (141), collectively arguing that the StAR relationship with its leader peptide is more complex than previously thought. The finding that StAR physically interacts with VDAC1 (142) and can be found in the OMM transduceosome complex when proteins are crosslinked after steroidogenic stimulation (91) supports a model in which StAR serves as a "key" acting to "start" the mitochondrial cholesterol import machinery. However, the precise molecular details of this model remain to be determined.

ATPase FAMILY, AAA DOMAIN CONTAINING 3A

The ATAD3A protein belongs to the AAA$^+$ family of ATPases, a broadly conserved family of ATPases implicated in various cellular processes (1, 3–5). ATAD3A is characterized by two N-terminal coiled-coil domains: a central transmembrane helix and a conserved C-terminal AAA$^+$-type ATPase domain (143). Several studies have localized ATAD3A to the mitochondria (143, 144), where is appears to be involved in mitochondrial membrane dynamics. Trypsin digestion assays have been used to study the membrane topology of ATAD3A, suggesting that the C-terminal ATPase domain is localized in the mitochondrial matrix, the transmembrane segment traverses the IMM, and the N-terminal coiled-coils anchor the protein the OMM. ATAD3A appears capable of homooligomerization, and as noted above, appears to be a partner protein in the mitochondrial transduceosome of steroidogenic cells, critical for cholesterol import into mitochondria and steroidogenesis (90, 145).

MITOCHONDRIA-ASSOCIATED MEMBRANES: SITES OF ER–MITOCHONDRIAL MEMBRANE INTERACTION

The ER is a complex cellular organelle, formed by an interconnected network of cisternae (146), is distributed across the cell and is involved in numerous processes, including lipid and protein synthesis. The ER is well known in steroidogenic research as the site of action of numerous steroidogenic CYP and HSD/KSR enzymes (3), but recently, the ER has attracted recent interest in mitochondrial cholesterol metabolism as a possible source of cholesterol (147). The ER and mitochondria are considered cholesterol poor organelles, especially in contrast to the high levels present in plasma membranes and endosomes. However, the ER appears to be a staging platform for cellular cholesterol homeostasis, as endogenous cellular cholesterol is synthesized in the ER, and cholesterol taken up by cells from circulating lipoproteins makes its way to the ER before incorporation into lipid droplets. In addition, the ER houses the sterol regulatory element-binding protein (SREBP) sensory machinery, which senses ER sterol levels and subsequently regulates transcription of genes involved in cholesterol and fatty acid synthesis and uptake (148). Although lipid droplets have been considered the classic source of steroidogenic cholesterol, the intimate relationship between lipid droplets, the ER and mitochondria, suggest a complex relationship in mitochondrial cholesterol delivery for steroidogenesis (149).

Almost 30 years ago, Vance demonstrated phospholipid synthesis in cellular fractions enriched in mitochondrial and ER markers (150). Electron microscopic investigations of mitochondria–ER association have consistently revealed the existence of specific regions of close apposition between the ER membranes and the OMM, with these regions representing between 5 and 20% of the mitochondrial surface (151–153). These mitochondria-associated membrane (MAM) sites have become recognized as possessing their own particular makeup, characterized by a number of resident proteins (154). Interestingly, several of these proteins have been demonstrated to participate in mitochondrial cholesterol transport and steroid biosynthesis. VDAC itself has been demonstrated to be present in MAMs (155), and, interestingly, StAR appears to interact with VDAC2 in steroidogenic cell model MAMs, an interaction necessary for its steroidogenic activity and mitochondrial import (156). In addition to VDAC, which is predominantly localized to mitochondria, several highly enriched resident MAM proteins have been demonstrated to play a key role in mitochondrial cholesterol transport. The first of these proteins, the sigma-1 receptor (SIGMAR1), was found to coimmunoprecipitate with VDAC2 in a steroidogenic cell model as well as disrupt mitochondrial cholesterol metabolism when its expression was reduced by short interfering RNA (siRNA) (157). Interestingly, SIGMAR1 appears to promote the compartmentalization of cholesterol in ER membranes (158), although depletion of cholesterol promoted mitochondrial–ER association in *in vitro* membrane association assays and cell models (159). A second resident MAM protein, acyl-CoA synthetase 4 (ACSL4), an enzyme involved in cellular arachidonic acid metabolism, participates in mitochondrial arachidonic acid movement (160). Of note, silencing the expression of ACSL4 inhibits steroidogenesis in a cell model, overexpression of ACSL4 promotes steroidogenesis (161), and cAMP signaling promotes increased mitochondrial colocalization of ACSL4 (162), collectively suggestive of a MAM relationship to mitochondrial arachidonic acid and cholesterol import. Finally, ATAD3A, in addition to forming a physical link between the IMM and OMM, may be involved in linking the mitochondria to the ER at MAMs. A long isoform of ATAD3A was found to be present in the MAMs of steroidogenic cells (145), and this work, in conjunction with the VDAC–StAR–MAM work cited above (156), suggesting that the transduceosome complex may serve to link not only the membranes of the mitochondria to the CYP metabolon but also the metabolon to cholesterol reserves in the ER and beyond.

CONCLUSION

Steroidogenesis begins with the mobilization and movement of cholesterol from intracellular stores into mitochondria. Control of steroidogenic output is organized at two levels: substrate availability and targeting, and enzyme expression and localization. Past and recent studies in hormone-inducible steroidogenic cells showed that cholesterol trafficking and targeting into mitochondria is rate limiting and driven by intracellular protein networks, referred to as the transduceosome, which amplifies the cAMP signal at the OMM, and the steroidogenic metabolon. This mitochondrial metabolon prevents unwanted crosstalk of the substrate cholesterol with other pathways, optimizing substrate concentration and targeting to CYP11A1. Deciphering the organization and regulation of intracellular protein assemblies that interact with the steroidogenic machinery will provide insight into the intracellular events involved in normal and disease states, facilitating diagnosis and treatment. These studies suggest a shift in focus in steroidogenic cell biology from the actions of individual proteins in isolation to the actions of protein assemblies working together to execute specialized cellular functions, in this case adrenal steroid formation.

AUTHOR CONTRIBUTIONS

All authors listed have made substantial, direct, and intellectual contribution to the work and approved it for publication.

FUNDING

This work was supported by grants from the Canadian Institutes of Health Research (MOP102647 and MOP125983) and a Canada Research Chair in Biochemical Pharmacology to VP.

REFERENCES

1. Vinson G. The adrenal cortex and life. *Mol Cell Endocrinol* (2009) 300(1–2):2–6. doi:10.1016/j.mce.2008.09.008
2. Midzak A, Papadopoulos V. Binding domain-driven intracellular trafficking of sterols for synthesis of steroid hormones, bile acids and oxysterols. *Traffic* (2014) 15(9):895–914. doi:10.1111/tra.12177
3. Miller W, Auchus R. The molecular biology, biochemistry, and physiology of human steroidogenesis and its disorders. *Endocr Rev* (2011) 32(1):81–151. doi:10.1210/er.2010-0013
4. Kvetnansky R, Sabban E, Palkovits M. Catecholaminergic systems in stress: structural and molecular genetic approaches. *Physiol Rev* (2009) 89(2):535–606. doi:10.1152/physrev.00042.2006
5. Miller W. A brief history of adrenal research: steroidogenesis – the soul of the adrenal. *Mol Cell Endocrinol* (2013) 371(1–2):5–14. doi:10.1016/j.mce.2012.10.023
6. Spät A, Hunyady L. Control of aldosterone secretion: a model for convergence in cellular signaling pathways. *Physiol Rev* (2004) 84(2):489–539. doi:10.1152/physrev.00030.2003
7. Rossier B, Baker M, Studer R. Epithelial sodium transport and its control by aldosterone: the story of our internal environment revisited. *Physiol Rev* (2015) 95(1):297–340. doi:10.1152/physrev.00011.2014
8. Pihlajoki M, Dörner J, Cochran RS, Heikinheimo M, Wilson DB. Adrenocortical zonation, renewal, and remodeling. *Front Endocrinol* (2015) 5(6):27. doi:10.3389/fendo.2015.00027
9. Nussdorfer G. Cytophysiology of the adrenal cortex. *Int Rev Cytol* (1986) 98:1–405.
10. Warner M, Gustafsson J. DHEA – a precursor of ERβ ligands. *J Steroid Biochem Mol Biol* (2015) 145:245–7. doi:10.1016/j.jsbmb.2014.08.003
11. Ariza L, Carmona R, Cañete A, Cano E, Muñoz-Chápuli R. Coelomic epithelium-derived cells in visceral morphogenesis. *Dev Dyn* (2016) 245(3):307–22. doi:10.1002/dvdy.24373
12. Yates R, Katugampola H, Cavlan D, Cogger K, Meimaridou E, Hughes C, et al. Adrenocortical development, maintenance, and disease. *Curr Top Dev Biol* (2013) 106:239–312. doi:10.1016/B978-0-12-416021-7.00007-9
13. Bandiera R, Vidal VP, Motamedi FJ, Clarkson M, Sahut-Barnola I, von Gise A, et al. WT1 maintains adrenal-gonadal primordium identity and marks a population of AGP-like progenitors within the adrenal gland. *Dev Cell* (2013) 27(1):5–18. doi:10.1016/j.devcel.2013.09.003
14. Val P, Martinez-Barbera J, Swain A. Adrenal development is initiated by Cited2 and Wt1 through modulation of Sf-1 dosage. *Development* (2007) 134(12):2349–58. doi:10.1242/dev.004390
15. Lumb R, Schwarz Q. Sympathoadrenal neural crest cells: the known, unknown and forgotten? *Dev Growth Differ* (2015) 57(2):146–57. doi:10.1111/dgd.12189
16. Midzak AS, Chen H, Aon MA, Papadopoulos V, Zirkin BR. ATP synthesis, mitochondrial function, and steroid biosynthesis in rodent primary and tumor Leydig cells. *Biol Reprod* (2011) 84(5):976–85. doi:10.1095/biolreprod.110.087460
17. Picard M, McManus MJ, Gray JD, Nasca C, Moffat C, Kopinski PK, et al. Mitochondrial functions modulate neuroendocrine, metabolic, inflammatory, and transcriptional responses to acute psychological stress. *Proc Natl Acad Sci U S A* (2015) 112(48):E6614–23. doi:10.1073/pnas.1515733112
18. Brdiczka D, Zorov D, Sheu S. Mitochondrial contact sites: their role in energy metabolism and apoptosis. *Biochim Biophys Acta* (2006) 1762(2):148–63. doi:10.1016/j.bbadis.2005.09.007
19. Schägger H, Pfeiffer K. Supercomplexes in the respiratory chains of yeast and mammalian mitochondria. *EMBO J* (2000) 19(8):1777–83. doi:10.1093/emboj/19.8.1777
20. Hackenbrock C, Chazotte B, Gupte S. The random collision model and a critical assessment of diffusion and collision in mitochondrial electron transport. *J Bioenerg Biomembr* (1986) 18(5):331–68. doi:10.1007/BF00743010
21. Wittig I, Carrozzo R, Santorelli FM, Schägger H. Supercomplexes and subcomplexes of mitochondrial oxidative phosphorylation. *Biochim Biophys Acta* (2006) 1757(9–10):1066–72. doi:10.1016/j.bbabio.2006.05.006
22. Wittig I, Schägger H. Features and applications of blue-native and clear-native electrophoresis. *Proteomics* (2008) 8(19):3974–90. doi:10.1002/pmic.200800017
23. Lenaz G, Genova M. Kinetics of integrated electron transfer in the mitochondrial respiratory chain: random collisions vs. solid state electron channeling. *Am J Physiol Cell Physiol* (2007) 292(4):C1221–39. doi:10.1152/ajpcell.00263.2006
24. Genova M, Lenaz G. Functional role of mitochondrial respiratory supercomplexes. *Biochim Biophys Acta* (2014) 1837(4):427–43. doi:10.1016/j.bbabio.2013.11.002
25. Acín-Pérez R, Fernández-Silva P, Peleato ML, Pérez-Martos A, Enriquez JA. Respiratory active mitochondrial supercomplexes. *Mol Cell* (2008) 32(4):529–39. doi:10.1016/j.molcel.2008.10.021
26. Welch G. On the role of organized multienzyme systems in cellular metabolism: a general synthesis. *Prog Biophys Mol Biol* (1977) 32(2):103–91. doi:10.1016/0079-6107(78)90019-6
27. Srere P. Complexes of sequential metabolic enzymes. *Annu Rev Biochem* (1987) 56:89–124. doi:10.1146/annurev.bi.56.070187.000513
28. Lieberman S, Prasad V. Heterodox notions on pathways of steroidogenesis. *Endocr Rev* (1990) 11(4):469–93. doi:10.1210/edrv-11-4-469
29. Williamson M, Sutcliffe M. Protein-protein interactions. *Biochem Soc Trans* (2010) 38(4):875–8. doi:10.1042/BST0380875
30. An S, Kumar R, Sheets ED, Benkovic SJ. Reversible compartmentalization of de novo purine biosynthetic complexes in living cells. *Science* (2008) 320(5872):103–6. doi:10.1126/science.1152241
31. Deng Y, Gam J, French JB, Zhao H, An S, Benkovic SJ. Mapping protein-protein proximity in the purinosome. *J Biol Chem* (2012) 287(43):36201–7. doi:10.1074/jbc.M112.407056
32. Lee K, Kerner J, Hoppel C. Mitochondrial carnitine palmitoyltransferase 1a (CPT1a) is part of an outer membrane fatty acid transfer complex. *J Biol Chem* (2011) 286(29):25655–62. doi:10.1074/jbc.M111.228692
33. Rone MB, Midzak AS, Martinez-Arguelles DB, Fan J, Ye X, Blonder J, et al. Steroidogenesis in MA-10 mouse Leydig cells is altered via fatty acid import into the mitochondria. *Biol Reprod* (2014) 91(4):96. doi:10.1095/biolreprod.114.121434
34. Nebert D, Wikvall K, Miller W. Human cytochromes P450 in health and disease. *Philos Trans R Soc Lond B Biol Sci* (2013) 368(1612):20120431. doi:10.1098/rstb.2012.0431
35. Miller W. Genetic disorders of Vitamin D biosynthesis and degradation. *J Steroid Biochem Mol Biol* (2016). doi:10.1016/j.jsbmb.2016.04.001

36. Heverin M, Ali Z, Olin M, Tillander V, Joibari MM, Makoveichuk E, et al. On the regulatory importance of 27-hydroxycholesterol in mouse liver. *J Steroid Biochem Mol Biol* (2016). doi:10.1016/j.jsbmb.2016.02.001
37. Nelson D, Goldstone J, Stegeman J. The cytochrome P450 genesis locus: the origin and evolution of animal cytochrome P450s. *Philos Trans R Soc Lond B Biol Sci* (2013) 368(1612):20120474. doi:10.1098/rstb.2012.0474
38. Markov GV, Tavares R, Dauphin-Villemant C, Demeneix BA, Baker ME, Laudet V. Independent elaboration of steroid hormone signaling pathways in metazoans. *Proc Natl Acad Sci U S A* (2009) 106(29):11913–8. doi:10.1073/pnas.0812138106
39. Baker M. Origin and diversification of steroids: co-evolution of enzymes and nuclear receptors. *Mol Cell Endocrinol* (2011) 334(1–2):14–20. doi:10.1016/j.mce.2010.07.013
40. Baker M, Nelson D, Studer R. Origin of the response to adrenal and sex steroids: roles of promiscuity and co-evolution of enzymes and steroid receptors. *J Steroid Biochem Mol Biol* (2015) 151:12–24. doi:10.1016/j.jsbmb.2014.10.020
41. Johnson M, Zaretskaya I, Raytselis Y, Merezhuk Y, McGinnis S, Madden TL. NCBI BLAST: a better web interface. *Nucleic Acids Res* (2008) 36(Web Server issue):W5–9. doi:10.1093/nar/gkn201
42. Edgar R. MUSCLE: multiple sequence alignment with high accuracy and high throughput. *Nucleic Acids Res* (2004) 32(5):1792–7. doi:10.1093/nar/gkh340
43. Guindon S, Gascuel O. A simple, fast, and accurate algorithm to estimate large phylogenies by maximum likelihood. *Syst Biol* (2003) 52(5):696–704. doi:10.1080/10635150390235520
44. Payne A, Hales D. Overview of steroidogenic enzymes in the pathway from cholesterol to active steroid hormones. *Endocr Rev* (2004) 25(6):947–70. doi:10.1210/er.2003-0030
45. Shikita M, Hall P. The stoichiometry of the conversion of cholesterol and hydroxycholesterols to pregnenolone (3beta-hydroxypregn-5-en-20-one) catalysed by adrenal cytochrome P-450. *Proc Natl Acad Sci U S A* (1974) 71(4):1441–5. doi:10.1073/pnas.71.4.1441
46. Mast N, Annalora AJ, Lodowski DT, Palczewski K, Stout CD, Pikuleva IA. Structural basis for three-step sequential catalysis by the cholesterol side chain cleavage enzyme CYP11A1. *J Biol Chem* (2011) 286(7):5607–13. doi:10.1074/jbc.M110.188433
47. Strushkevich N, MacKenzie F, Cherkesova T, Grabovec I, Usanov S, Park HW. Structural basis for pregnenolone biosynthesis by the mitochondrial monooxygenase system. *Proc Natl Acad Sci U S A* (2011) 108(25):10139–43. doi:10.1073/pnas.1019441108
48. Davydov R, Gilep AA, Strushkevich NV, Usanov SA, Hoffman BM. Compound I is the reactive intermediate in the first monooxygenation step during conversion of cholesterol to pregnenolone by cytochrome P450scc: EPR/ENDOR/cryoreduction/annealing studies. *J Am Chem Soc* (2012) 134(41):17149–56. doi:10.1021/ja3067226
49. Davydov R, Strushkevich N, Smil D, Yantsevich A, Gilep A, Usanov S, et al. Evidence that compound I is the active species in both the hydroxylase and lyase steps by which P450scc converts cholesterol to pregnenolone: EPR/ENDOR/cryoreduction/annealing studies. *Biochemistry* (2015) 54(48):7089–97. doi:10.1021/acs.biochem.5b00903
50. Lavoie H, King S. Transcriptional regulation of steroidogenic genes: StARD1, CYP11A1 and HSD3B. *Exp Biol Med (Maywood)* (2009) 234(8):880–907. doi:10.3181/0903-MR-97
51. John ME, John MC, Ashley P, MacDonald RJ, Simpson ER, Waterman MR. Identification and characterization of cDNA clones specific for cholesterol side-chain cleavage cytochrome P-450. *Proc Natl Acad Sci U S A* (1984) 81(18):5628–32. doi:10.1073/pnas.81.18.5628
52. Lebrethon MC, Jaillard C, Defayes G, Begeot M, Saez JM. Human cultured adrenal fasciculata-reticularis cells are targets for angiotensin-II: effects on cytochrome P450 cholesterol side-chain cleavage, cytochrome P450 17 alpha-hydroxylase, and 3 beta-hydroxysteroid-dehydrogenase messenger ribonucleic acid and proteins and on steroidogenic responsiveness to corticotropin and angiotensin-II. *J Clin Endocrinol Metab* (1994) 78(5):1212–9.
53. Guo IC, Huang CY, Wang CK, Chung BC. Activating protein-1 cooperates with steroidogenic factor-1 to regulate 3',5'-cyclic adenosine 5'-monophosphate-dependent human CYP11A1 transcription in vitro and in vivo. *Endocrinology* (2007) 148(4):1804–12. doi:10.1210/en.2006-0938
54. Suzuki J, Otsuka F, Inagaki K, Takeda M, Ogura T, Makino H. Novel action of activin and bone morphogenetic protein in regulating aldosterone production by human adrenocortical cells. *Endocrinology* (2004) 145(2):639–49. doi:10.1210/en.2003-0968
55. Moore C, Brentano S, Miller W. Human P450scc gene transcription is induced by cyclic AMP and repressed by 12-O-tetradecanoylphorbol-13- acetate and A23187 through independent cis elements. *Mol Cell Biol* (1990) 10(11):6013–23. doi:10.1128/MCB.10.11.6013
56. Lala D, Rice D, Parker K. Steroidogenic factor I, a key regulator of steroidogenic enzyme expression, is the mouse homolog of fushi tarazu-factor I. *Mol Endocrinol* (1992) 6(8):1249–58. doi:10.1210/me.6.8.1249
57. Liu Z, Simpson E. Molecular mechanism for cooperation between Sp1 and steroidogenic factor-1 (SF-1) to regulate bovine CYP11A gene expression. *Mol Cell Endocrinol* (1999) 153(1–2):183–96. doi:10.1016/S0303-7207(99)00036-2
58. Monté D, DeWitte F, Hum D. Regulation of the human P450scc gene by steroidogenic factor 1 is mediated by CBP/p300. *J Biol Chem* (1998) 273(8):4585–91. doi:10.1074/jbc.273.8.4585
59. Mornet E, Dupont J, Vitek A, White PC. Characterization of two genes encoding human steroid 11 beta-hydroxylase (P-450(11) beta). *J Biol Chem* (1989) 264(35):20961–7.
60. Midzak A, Rone M, Aghazadeh Y, Culty M, Papadopoulos V. Mitochondrial protein import and the genesis of steroidogenic mitochondria. *Mol Cell Endocrinol* (2011) 336(1–2):70–9. doi:10.1016/j.mce.2010.12.007
61. Nishimoto K, Nakagawa K, Li D, Kosaka T, Oya M, Mikami S, et al. Adrenocortical zonation in humans under normal and pathological conditions. *J Clin Endocrinol Metab* (2010) 95(5):2296–305. doi:10.1210/jc.2009-2010
62. Mulatero P, Curnow KM, Aupetit-Faisant B, Foekling M, Gomez-Sanchez C, Veglio F, et al. Recombinant CYP11B genes encode enzymes that can catalyze conversion of 11-deoxycortisol to cortisol, 18-hydroxycortisol, and 18-oxocortisol. *J Clin Endocrinol Metab* (1998) 83(11):3996–4001. doi:10.1210/jcem.83.11.5237
63. Ogishima T, Shibata H, Shimada H, Mitani F, Suzuki H, Saruta T, et al. Aldosterone synthase cytochrome P-450 expressed in the adrenals of patients with primary aldosteronism. *J Biol Chem* (1991) 266(17):10731–4.
64. Curnow KM, Tusie-Luna MT, Pascoe L, Natarajan R, Gu JL, Nadler JL, et al. The product of the CYP11B2 gene is required for aldosterone biosynthesis in the human adrenal cortex. *Mol Endocrinol* (1991) 5(10):1513–22. doi:10.1210/mend-5-10-1513
65. Kawamoto T, Mitsuuchi Y, Toda K, Yokoyama Y, Miyahara K, Miura S, et al. Role of steroid 11 beta-hydroxylase and steroid 18-hydroxylase in the biosynthesis of glucocorticoids and mineralocorticoids in humans. *Proc Natl Acad Sci U S A* (1992) 89(4):1458–62. doi:10.1073/pnas.89.4.1458
66. Yanagibashi K, Haniu M, Shively JE, Shen WH, Hall P. The synthesis of aldosterone by the adrenal cortex. Two zones (fasciculata and glomerulosa) possess one enzyme for 11 beta-, 18-hydroxylation, and aldehyde synthesis. *J Biol Chem* (1986) 261(8):3556–62.
67. Morohashi K, Yoshioka H, Gotoh O, Okada Y, Yamamoto K, Miyata T, et al. Molecular cloning and nucleotide sequence of DNA of mitochondrial cytochrome P-450(11 beta) of bovine adrenal cortex. *J Biochem* (1987) 102(3):559–68.
68. Mellon S, Bair S, Monis H. P450c11B3 mRNA, transcribed from a third P450c11 gene, is expressed in a tissue-specific, developmentally, and hormonally regulated fashion in the rodent adrenal and encodes a protein with both 11-hydroxylase and 18-hydroxylase activities. *J Biol Chem* (1995) 270(4):1643–9. doi:10.1074/jbc.270.4.1643
69. Chua SC, Szabo P, Vitek A, Grzeschik KH, John M, White PC. Cloning of cDNA encoding steroid 11 beta-hydroxylase (P450c11). *Proc Natl Acad Sci U S A* (1987) 84(20):7193–7. doi:10.1073/pnas.84.20.7193
70. Lifton RP, Dluhy RG, Powers M, Rich GM, Cook S, Ulick S, et al. A chimaeric 11 beta-hydroxylase/aldosterone synthase gene causes glucocorticoid-remediable aldosteronism and human hypertension. *Nature* (1992) 355(6357):262–5. doi:10.1038/355262a0
71. Kramer RE, Rainey WE, Funkenstein B, Dee A, Simpson ER, Waterman MR. Induction of synthesis of mitochondrial steroidogenic enzymes of bovine adrenocortical cells by analogs of cyclic AMP. *J Biol Chem* (1984) 259(2):707–13.

72. Denner K, Rainey WE, Pezzi V, Bird IM, Bernhardt R, Mathis JM. Differential regulation of 11 beta-hydroxylase and aldosterone synthase in human adrenocortical H295R cells. *Mol Cell Endocrinol* (1996) 121(1):87–91. doi:10.1016/0303-7207(96)03853-1
73. Wang XL, Bassett M, Zhang Y, Yin S, Clyne C, White PC, et al. Transcriptional regulation of human 11beta-hydroxylase (hCYP11B1). *Endocrinology* (2000) 141(10):3587–94. doi:10.1210/en.141.10.3587
74. Wang Z, Bassett M, Rainey W. Liver receptor homologue-1 is expressed in the adrenal and can regulate transcription of 11 beta-hydroxylase. *J Mol Endocrinol* (2001) 27(2):255–8. doi:10.1677/jme.0.0270255
75. Clyne CD, Zhang Y, Slutsker L, Mathis JM, White PC, Rainey WE. Angiotensin II and potassium regulate human CYP11B2 transcription through common cis-elements. *Mol Endocrinol* (1997) 11(5):638–49. doi:10.1210/mend.11.5.9920
76. Nanba K, Chen A, Nishimoto K, Rainey WE. Role of Ca(2+)/calmodulin-dependent protein kinase kinase in adrenal aldosterone production. *Endocrinology* (2015) 156(5):1750–6. doi:10.1210/en.2014-1782
77. Bassett MH, Zhang Y, Clyne C, White PC, Rainey WE. Differential regulation of aldosterone synthase and 11beta-hydroxylase transcription by steroidogenic factor-1. *J Mol Endocrinol* (2002) 28(2):125–35. doi:10.1677/jme.0.0280125
78. Ye P, Nakamura Y, Lalli E, Rainey WE. Differential effects of high and low steroidogenic factor-1 expression on CYP11B2 expression and aldosterone production in adrenocortical cells. *Endocrinology* (2009) 150(3):1303–9. doi:10.1210/en.2008-0667
79. Kurihara I, Shibata H, Kobayashi S, Suda N, Ikeda Y, Yokota K, et al. Ubc9 and protein inhibitor of activated STAT 1 activate chicken ovalbumin upstream promoter-transcription factor I-mediated human CYP11B2 gene transcription. *J Biol Chem* (2005) 280(8):6721–30. doi:10.1074/jbc.M411820200
80. Ewen KM, Hannemann F, Iametti S, Morleo A, Bernhardt R. Functional characterization of Fdx1: evidence for an evolutionary relationship between P450-type and ISC-type ferredoxins. *J Mol Biol* (2011) 413(5):940–51. doi:10.1016/j.jmb.2011.09.010
81. Ziegler GA, Vonrhein C, Hanukoglu I, Schulz GE. The structure of adrenodoxin reductase of mitochondrial P450 systems: electron transfer for steroid biosynthesis. *J Mol Biol* (1999) 289(4):981–90. doi:10.1006/jmbi.1999.2807
82. Heinz A, Hannemann F, Müller JJ, Heinemann U, Bernhardt R. The interaction domain of the redox protein adrenodoxin is mandatory for binding of the electron acceptor CYP11A1, but is not required for binding of the electron donor adrenodoxin reductase. *Biochem Biophys Res Commun* (2005) 338(1):491–8. doi:10.1016/j.bbrc.2005.08.077
83. Brentano ST, Black SM, Lin D, Miller WL. cAMP post-transcriptionally diminishes the abundance of adrenodoxin reductase mRNA. *Proc Natl Acad Sci U S A* (1992) 89(9):4099–103. doi:10.1073/pnas.89.9.4099
84. Harikrishna JA, Black SM, Szklarz GD, Miller WL. Construction and function of fusion enzymes of the human cytochrome P450scc system. *DNA Cell Biol* (1993) 12(5):371–9. doi:10.1089/dna.1993.12.371
85. Imamichi Y, Mizutani T, Ju Y, Matsumura T, Kawabe S, Kanno M, et al. Transcriptional regulation of human ferredoxin reductase through an intronic enhancer in steroidogenic cells. *Biochim Biophys Acta* (2014) 1839(1):33–42. doi:10.1016/j.bbagrm.2013.11.005
86. Müller A, Müller JJ, Muller YA, Uhlmann H, Bernhardt R, Heinemann U. New aspects of electron transfer revealed by the crystal structure of a truncated bovine adrenodoxin, Adx(4-108). *Structure* (1998) 6(3):269–80. doi:10.1016/S0969-2126(98)00031-8
87. Sheftel AD, Stehling O, Pierik AJ, Elsässer HP, Mühlenhoff U, Webert H, et al. Humans possess two mitochondrial ferredoxins, Fdx1 and Fdx2, with distinct roles in steroidogenesis, heme, and Fe/S cluster biosynthesis. *Proc Natl Acad Sci U S A* (2010) 107(26):11775–80. doi:10.1073/pnas.1004250107
88. Davydov DR, Davydova NY, Sineva EV, Halpert JR. Interactions among cytochromes P450 in microsomal membranes: oligomerization of cytochromes P450 3A4, 3A5, and 2E1 and its functional consequences. *J Biol Chem* (2015) 290(6):3850–64. doi:10.1074/jbc.M114.615443
89. Szczesna-Skorupa E, Mallah B, Kemper B. Fluorescence resonance energy transfer analysis of cytochromes P450 2C2 and 2E1 molecular interactions in living cells. *J Biol Chem* (2003) 278(33):31269–76. doi:10.1074/jbc.M301489200
90. Rone MB, Midzak AS, Issop L, Rammouz G, Jagannathan S, Fan J, et al. Identification of a dynamic mitochondrial protein complex driving cholesterol import, trafficking, and metabolism to steroid hormones. *Mol Endocrinol* (2012) 26(11):1868–82. doi:10.1210/me.2012-1159
91. Liu J, Rone M, Papadopoulos V. Protein-protein interactions mediate mitochondrial cholesterol transport and steroid biosynthesis. *J Biol Chem* (2006) 281(50):38879–93. doi:10.1074/jbc.M608820200
92. Aghazadeh Y, Rone MB, Blonder J, Ye X, Veenstra TD, Hales DB, et al. Hormone-induced 14-3-3γ adaptor protein regulates steroidogenic acute regulatory protein activity and steroid biosynthesis in MA-10 Leydig cells. *J Biol Chem* (2012) 287(19):15380–94. doi:10.1074/jbc.M112.339580
93. Aghazadeh Y, Martinez-Arguelles DB, Fan J, Culty M, Papadopoulos V. Induction of androgen formation in the male by a TAT-VDAC1 fusion peptide blocking 14-3-3ε protein adaptor and mitochondrial VDAC1 interactions. *Mol Ther* (2014) 22(10):1779–91. doi:10.1038/mt.2014.116
94. Poderoso C, Converso DP, Maloberti P, Duarte A, Neuman I, Galli S, et al. A mitochondrial kinase complex is essential to mediate an ERK1/2-dependent phosphorylation of a key regulatory protein in steroid biosynthesis. *PLoS One* (2008) 3(1):e1443. doi:10.1371/journal.pone.0001443
95. Colombini M, Mannella C. VDAC, the early days. *Biochim Biophys Acta* (2012) 1818(6):1438–43. doi:10.1016/j.bbamem.2011.11.014
96. Mertins B, Psakis G, Essen L. Voltage-dependent anion channels: the wizard of the mitochondrial outer membrane. *Biol Chem* (2014) 395(12):1435–42. doi:10.1515/hsz-2014-0203
97. Blachly-Dyson E, Baldini A, Litt M, McCabe ER, Forte M. Human genes encoding the voltage-dependent anion channel (VDAC) of the outer mitochondrial membrane: mapping and identification of two new isoforms. *Genomics* (1994) 20(1):62–7. doi:10.1006/geno.1994.1127
98. Messina A, Reina S, Guarino F, De Pinto V. VDAC isoforms in mammals. *Biochim Biophys Acta* (2012) 1818(6):1466–76. doi:10.1016/j.bbamem.2011.10.005
99. Raghavan A, Sheiko T, Graham BH, Craigen WJ. Voltage-dependant anion channels: novel insights into isoform function through genetic models. *Biochim Biophys Acta* (2012) 1818(6):1477–85. doi:10.1016/j.bbamem.2011.10.019
100. Baines CP, Kaiser RA, Sheiko T, Craigen WJ, Molkentin JD. Voltage-dependent anion channels are dispensable for mitochondrial-dependent cell death. *Nat Cell Biol* (2007) 9(5):550–5. doi:10.1038/ncb1575
101. Mannella C, Forte M, Colombini M. Toward the molecular structure of the mitochondrial channel, VDAC. *J Bioenerg Biomembr* (1992) 24(1):7–19. doi:10.1007/BF00769525
102. Campbell A, Chan S. The voltage dependent anion channel affects mitochondrial cholesterol distribution and function. *Arch Biochem Biophys* (2007) 466(2):203–10. doi:10.1016/j.abb.2007.06.012
103. Hiller S, Garces RG, Malia TJ, Orekhov VY, Colombini M, Wagner G. Solution structure of the integral human membrane protein VDAC-1 in detergent micelles. *Science* (2008) 321(5893):1206–10. doi:10.1126/science.1161302
104. Bayrhuber M, Meins T, Habeck M, Becker S, Giller K, Villinger S, et al. Structure of the human voltage-dependent anion channel. *Proc Natl Acad Sci U S A* (2008) 105(40):15370–5. doi:10.1073/pnas.0808115105
105. Anholt RR, De Souza EB, Oster-Granite ML, Snyder SH. Peripheral-type benzodiazepine receptors: autoradiographic localization in whole-body sections of neonatal rats. *J Pharmacol Exp Ther* (1985) 233(2):517–26.
106. Braestrup C, Squires R. Specific benzodiazepine receptors in rat brain characterized by high-affinity (3H)diazepam binding. *Proc Natl Acad Sci U S A* (1977) 74(9):3805–9. doi:10.1073/pnas.74.9.3805
107. Gavish M, Bachman I, Shoukrun R, Katz Y, Veenman L, Weisinger G, et al. Enigma of the peripheral benzodiazepine receptor. *Pharmacol Rev* (1999) 51(4):629–50.
108. Krueger K, Papadopoulos V. Peripheral-type benzodiazepine receptors mediate translocation of cholesterol from outer to inner mitochondrial membranes in adrenocortical cells. *J Biol Chem* (1990) 265(25):15015–22.
109. Papadopoulos V, Mukhin AG, Costa E, Krueger KE. The peripheral-type benzodiazepine receptor is functionally linked to Leydig cell steroidogenesis. *J Biol Chem* (1990) 265(7):3772–9.
110. Lacapere J, Papadopoulos V. Peripheral-type benzodiazepine receptor: structure and function of a cholesterol-binding protein in steroid and bile acid biosynthesis. *Steroids* (2003) 68(7–8):569–85. doi:10.1016/S0039-128X(03)00101-6
111. Rupprecht R, Rammes G, Eser D, Baghai TC, Schüle C, Nothdurfter C, et al. Translocator protein (18 kD) as target for anxiolytics without

benzodiazepine-like side effects. *Science* (2009) 325(5939):490–3. doi:10.1126/science.1175055

112. Papadopoulos V, Baraldi M, Guilarte TR, Knudsen TB, Lacapère JJ, Lindemann P, et al. Translocator protein (18kDa): new nomenclature for the peripheral-type benzodiazepine receptor based on its structure and molecular function. *Trends Pharmacol Sci* (2006) 27(8):402–9. doi:10.1016/j.tips.2006.06.005
113. Joseph-Liauzun E, Delmas P, Shire D, Ferrara P. Topological analysis of the peripheral benzodiazepine receptor in yeast mitochondrial membranes supports a five-transmembrane structure. *J Biol Chem* (1998) 273(4):2146–52. doi:10.1074/jbc.273.4.2146
114. Li F, Liu J, Zheng Y, Garavito RM, Ferguson-Miller S. Protein structure. Crystal structures of translocator protein (TSPO) and mutant mimic of a human polymorphism. *Science* (2015) 347(6221):555–8. doi:10.1126/science.1260590
115. Guo Y, Kalathur RC, Liu Q, Kloss B, Bruni R, Ginter C, et al. Protein structure. Structure and activity of tryptophan-rich TSPO proteins. *Science* (2015) 347(6221):551–5. doi:10.1126/science.aaa1534
116. Lacapère JJ, Delavoie F, Li H, Péranzi G, Maccario J, Papadopoulos V, et al. Structural and functional study of reconstituted peripheral benzodiazepine receptor. *Biochem Biophys Res Commun* (2001) 284(2):536–41. doi:10.1006/bbrc.2001.4975
117. Li H, Papadopoulos V. Peripheral-type benzodiazepine receptor function in cholesterol transport. Identification of a putative cholesterol recognition/interaction amino acid sequence and consensus pattern. *Endocrinology* (1998) 139(12):4991–7. doi:10.1210/en.139.12.4991
118. Fan J, Papadopoulos V. Evolutionary origin of the mitochondrial cholesterol transport machinery reveals a universal mechanism of steroid hormone biosynthesis in animals. *PLoS One* (2013) 8(10):e76701. doi:10.1371/journal.pone.0076701
119. Li H, Yao Z, Degenhardt B, Teper G, Papadopoulos V. Cholesterol binding at the cholesterol recognition/interaction amino acid consensus (CRAC) of the peripheral-type benzodiazepine receptor and inhibition of steroidogenesis by an HIV TAT-CRAC peptide. *Proc Natl Acad Sci U S A* (2001) 98(3):1267–72. doi:10.1073/pnas.98.3.1267
120. Midzak A, Akula N, Lecanu L, Papadopoulos V. Novel androstenetriol interacts with the mitochondrial translocator protein and controls steroidogenesis. *J Biol Chem* (2011) 286(11):9875–87. doi:10.1074/jbc.M110.203216
121. Midzak AS, Akula N, Rone MB, Papadopoulos V. Computational modeling and biological validation of novel non-steroidal ligands for the cholesterol recognition/interaction amino acid consensus (CRAC) motif of the mitochondrial translocator protein (TSPO). *Pharmacol Res* (2015) 99:393–403. doi:10.1016/j.phrs.2015.03.023
122. Costa B, Pini S, Gabelloni P, Da Pozzo E, Abelli M, Lari L, et al. The spontaneous Ala147Thr amino acid substitution within the translocator protein influences pregnenolone production in lymphomonocytes of healthy individuals. *Endocrinology* (2009) 150(12):5438–45. doi:10.1210/en.2009-0752
123. Boujrad N, Vidic B, Papadopoulos V. Acute action of choriogonadotropin on Leydig tumor cells: changes in the topography of the mitochondrial peripheral-type benzodiazepine receptor. *Endocrinology* (1996) 137(12):5727–30. doi:10.1210/en.137.12.5727
124. Delavoie F, Li H, Hardwick M, Robert JC, Giatzakis C, Péranzi G, et al. In vivo and in vitro peripheral-type benzodiazepine receptor polymerization: functional significance in drug ligand and cholesterol binding. *Biochemistry* (2003) 42(15):4506–19. doi:10.1021/bi0267487
125. Culty M, Li H, Boujrad N, Amri H, Vidic B, Bernassau JM, et al. In vitro studies on the role of the peripheral-type benzodiazepine receptor in steroidogenesis. *J Steroid Biochem Mol Biol* (1999) 69(1–6):123–30. doi:10.1016/S0960-0760(99)00056-4
126. McEnery MW, Snowman AM, Trifiletti RR, Snyder SH. Isolation of the mitochondrial benzodiazepine receptor: association with the voltage-dependent anion channel and the adenine nucleotide carrier. *Proc Natl Acad Sci U S A* (1992) 89(8):3170–4. doi:10.1073/pnas.89.8.3170
127. Garnier M, Dimchev AB, Boujrad N, Price JM, Musto NA, Papadopoulos V. In vitro reconstitution of a functional peripheral-type benzodiazepine receptor from mouse Leydig tumor cells. *Mol Pharmacol* (1994) 45(2):201–11.
128. Gatliff J, East D, Crosby J, Abeti R, Harvey R, Craigen W, et al. TSPO interacts with VDAC1 and triggers a ROS-mediated inhibition of mitochondrial quality control. *Autophagy* (2014) 10(12):2279–96. doi:10.4161/15548627.2014.991665
129. Tu LN, Morohaku K, Manna PR, Pelton SH, Butler WR, Stocco DM, et al. Peripheral benzodiazepine receptor/translocator protein global knock-out mice are viable with no effects on steroid hormone biosynthesis. *J Biol Chem* (2014) 289(40):27444–54. doi:10.1074/jbc.M114.578286
130. Banati RB, Middleton RJ, Chan R, Hatty CR, Kam WW, Quin C, et al. Positron emission tomography and functional characterization of a complete PBR/TSPO knockout. *Nat Commun* (2014) 5:5452. doi:10.1038/ncomms6452
131. Fan J, Campioli E, Midzak A, Culty M, Papadopoulos V. Conditional steroidogenic cell-targeted deletion of TSPO unveils a crucial role in viability and hormone-dependent steroid formation. *Proc Natl Acad Sci U S A* (2015) 112(23):7261–6. doi:10.1073/pnas.1502670112
132. Crivello J, Jefcoate C. Intracellular movement of cholesterol in rat adrenal cells. Kinetics and effects of inhibitors. *J Biol Chem* (1980) 255(17):8144–51.
133. Pon L, Hartigan J, Orme-Johnson N. Acute ACTH regulation of adrenal corticosteroid biosynthesis. Rapid accumulation of a phosphoprotein. *J Biol Chem* (1986) 261(28):13309–16.
134. Pon L, Orme-Johnson N. Acute stimulation of steroidogenesis in corpus luteum and adrenal cortex by peptide hormones. Rapid induction of a similar protein in both tissues. *J Biol Chem* (1986) 261(14):6594–9.
135. Arakane F, King SR, Du Y, Kallen CB, Walsh LP, Watari H, et al. Phosphorylation of steroidogenic acute regulatory protein (StAR) modulates its steroidogenic activity. *J Biol Chem* (1997) 272(51):32656–62. doi:10.1074/jbc.272.51.32656
136. Duarte A, Castillo AF, Podestá EJ, Poderoso C. Mitochondrial fusion and ERK activity regulate steroidogenic acute regulatory protein localization in mitochondria. *PLoS One* (2014) 9(6):e100387. doi:10.1371/journal.pone.0100387
137. Bose HS, Sugawara T, Strauss JF III, Miller WL; International Congenital Lipoid Adrenal Hyperplasia Consortium. The pathophysiology and genetics of congenital lipoid adrenal hyperplasia. *N Engl J Med* (1996) 335(25):1870–8. doi:10.1056/NEJM199612193352503
138. Arakane F, Sugawara T, Nishino H, Liu Z, Holt JA, Pain D, et al. Steroidogenic acute regulatory protein (StAR) retains activity in the absence of its mitochondrial import sequence: implications for the mechanism of StAR action. *Proc Natl Acad Sci U S A* (1996) 93(24):13731–6. doi:10.1073/pnas.93.24.13731
139. Bose H, Lingappa V, Miller W. Rapid regulation of steroidogenesis by mitochondrial protein import. *Nature* (2002) 417(6884):87–91. doi:10.1038/417087a
140. Sasaki G, Ishii T, Jeyasuria P, Jo Y, Bahat A, Orly J, et al. Complex role of the mitochondrial targeting signal in the function of steroidogenic acute regulatory protein revealed by bacterial artificial chromosome transgenesis in vivo. *Mol Endocrinol* (2008) 22(4):951–64. doi:10.1210/me.2007-0493
141. Baquedano MS, Guercio G, Marino R, Berensztein E, Costanzo M, Bailez M, et al. Unique dominant negative mutation in the N-terminal mitochondrial targeting sequence of StAR, causing a variant form of congenital lipoid adrenal hyperplasia. *J Clin Endocrinol Metab* (2013) 98(1):E153–61. doi:10.1210/jc.2012-2865
142. Bose M, Whittal RM, Miller WL, Bose HS. Steroidogenic activity of StAR requires contact with mitochondrial VDAC1 and phosphate carrier protein. *J Biol Chem* (2008) 283(14):8837–45. doi:10.1074/jbc.M709221200
143. Gilquin B, Taillebourg E, Cherradi N, Hubstenberger A, Gay O, Merle N, et al. The AAA+ ATPase ATAD3A controls mitochondrial dynamics at the interface of the inner and outer membranes. *Mol Cell Biol* (2010) 30(8):1984–96. doi:10.1128/MCB.00007-10
144. Da Cruz S, Xenarios I, Langridge J, Vilbois F, Parone PA, Martinou JC. Proteomic analysis of the mouse liver mitochondrial inner membrane. *J Biol Chem* (2003) 278(42):41566–71. doi:10.1074/jbc.M304940200
145. Issop L, Fan J, Lee S, Rone MB, Basu K, Mui J, et al. Mitochondria-associated membrane formation in hormone-stimulated Leydig cell steroidogenesis: role of ATAD3. *Endocrinology* (2015) 156(1):334–45. doi:10.1210/en.2014-1503
146. Hu J, Prinz W, Rapoport T. Weaving the web of ER tubules. *Cell* (2011) 147(6):1226–31. doi:10.1016/j.cell.2011.11.022
147. Martin L, Kennedy B, Karten B. Mitochondrial cholesterol: mechanisms of import and effects on mitochondrial function. *J Bioenerg Biomembr* (2016) 48(2):137–51. doi:10.1007/s10863-014-9592-6

148. Brown M, Goldstein J. Cholesterol feedback: from Schoenheimer's bottle to Scap's MELADL. *J Lipid Res* (2009) 50(Suppl):S15–27. doi:10.1194/jlr.R800054-JLR200
149. Issop L, Rone M, Papadopoulos V. Organelle plasticity and interactions in cholesterol transport and steroid biosynthesis. *Mol Cell Endocrinol* (2013) 371(1–2):34–46. doi:10.1016/j.mce.2012.12.003
150. Vance J. Phospholipid synthesis in a membrane fraction associated with mitochondria. *J Biol Chem* (1990) 265(13):7248–56.
151. Mannella CA, Buttle K, Rath BK, Marko M. Electron microscopic tomography of rat-liver mitochondria and their interaction with the endoplasmic reticulum. *Biofactors* (1998) 8(3–4):225–8. doi:10.1002/biof.5520080309
152. Rizzuto R, Pinton P, Carrington W, Fay FS, Fogarty KE, Lifshitz LM, et al. Close contacts with the endoplasmic reticulum as determinants of mitochondrial Ca2+ responses. *Science* (1998) 280(5370):1763–6. doi:10.1126/science.280.5370.1763
153. Csordás G, Várnai P, Golenár T, Roy S, Purkins G, Schneider TG, et al. Imaging interorganelle contacts and local calcium dynamics at the ER-mitochondrial interface. *Mol Cell* (2010) 39(1):121–32. doi:10.1016/j.molcel.2010.06.029
154. Raturi A, Simmen T. Where the endoplasmic reticulum and the mitochondrion tie the knot: the mitochondria-associated membrane (MAM). *Biochim Biophys Acta* (2013) 1833(1):213–24. doi:10.1016/j.bbamcr.2012.04.013
155. Szabadkai G, Bianchi K, Várnai P, De Stefani D, Wieckowski MR, Cavagna D, et al. Chaperone-mediated coupling of endoplasmic reticulum and mitochondrial Ca2+ channels. *J Cell Biol* (2006) 175(6):901–11. doi:10.1083/jcb.200608073
156. Prasad M, Kaur J, Pawlak KJ, Bose M, Whittal RM, Bose HS. Mitochondria-associated endoplasmic reticulum membrane (MAM) regulates steroidogenic activity via steroidogenic acute regulatory protein (StAR)-voltage-dependent anion channel 2 (VDAC2) interaction. *J Biol Chem* (2015) 290(5):2604–16. doi:10.1074/jbc.M114.605808
157. Marriott KS, Prasad M, Thapliyal V, Bose HS. σ-1 receptor at the mitochondrial-associated endoplasmic reticulum membrane is responsible for mitochondrial metabolic regulation. *J Pharmacol Exp Ther* (2012) 343(3):578–86. doi:10.1124/jpet.112.198168
158. Hayashi T, Su T. Sigma-1 receptors (sigma(1) binding sites) form raft-like microdomains and target lipid droplets on the endoplasmic reticulum: roles in endoplasmic reticulum lipid compartmentalization and export. *J Pharmacol Exp Ther* (2003) 306(2):718–25. doi:10.1124/jpet.103.051284
159. Fujimoto M, Hayashi T, Su T. The role of cholesterol in the association of endoplasmic reticulum membranes with mitochondria. *Biochem Biophys Res Commun* (2012) 417(1):635–9. doi:10.1016/j.bbrc.2011.12.022
160. Lewin TM, Kim JH, Granger DA, Vance JE, Coleman RA. Acyl-CoA synthetase isoforms 1, 4, and 5 are present in different subcellular membranes in rat liver and can be inhibited independently. *J Biol Chem* (2001) 276(27):24674–9. doi:10.1074/jbc.M102036200
161. Maloberti P, Castilla R, Castillo F, Cornejo Maciel F, Mendez CF, Paz C, et al. Silencing the expression of mitochondrial acyl-CoA thioesterase I and acyl-CoA synthetase 4 inhibits hormone-induced steroidogenesis. *FEBS J* (2005) 272(7):1804–14. doi:10.1111/j.1742-4658.2005.04616.x
162. Duarte A, Poderoso C, Cooke M, Soria G, Cornejo Maciel F, Gottifredi V, et al. Mitochondrial fusion is essential for steroid biosynthesis. *PLoS One* (2012) 7(9):e45829. doi:10.1371/journal.pone.0045829

11

Impact of ACTH Signaling on Transcriptional Regulation of Steroidogenic Genes

Carmen Ruggiero[1,2,3] and Enzo Lalli[1,2,3]**

[1] *Institut de Pharmacologie Moléculaire et Cellulaire CNRS UMR 7275, Valbonne, France,* [2] *Laboratoire International Associé (LIA) CNRS NEOGENEX, Valbonne, France,* [3] *Université de Nice, Valbonne, France*

***Correspondence:**
Carmen Ruggiero
cruggiero@ipmc.cnrs.fr;
Enzo Lalli
ninino@ipmc.cnrs.fr*

The trophic peptide hormone adrenocorticotropic (ACTH) stimulates steroid hormone biosynthesis evoking both a rapid, acute response and a long-term, chronic response, via the activation of cAMP/protein kinase A (PKA) signaling. The acute response is initiated by the mobilization of cholesterol from lipid stores and its delivery to the inner mitochondrial membrane, a process that is mediated by the steroidogenic acute regulatory protein. The chronic response results in the increased coordinated transcription of genes encoding steroidogenic enzymes. ACTH binding to its cognate receptor, melanocortin 2 receptor (MC2R), stimulates adenylyl cyclase, thus inducing cAMP production, PKA activation, and phosphorylation of specific nuclear factors, which bind to target promoters and facilitate coactivator protein recruitment to direct steroidogenic gene transcription. This review provides a general view of the transcriptional control exerted by the ACTH/cAMP system on the expression of genes encoding for steroidogenic enzymes in the adrenal cortex. Special emphasis will be given to the transcription factors required to mediate ACTH-dependent transcription of steroidogenic genes.

Keywords: adrenal cortex, steroidogenesis, cAMP, transcription factors, gene regulation

INTRODUCTION

The adrenal gland is a key component of the hypothalamus–pituitary–adrenal (HPA) axis, thus playing a crucial role in the adaptation of organism to stressors. The adrenocorticotropic hormone (ACTH) belongs to this regulatory circuitry, being one of the most potent physiological modulators of adrenal cortex steroidogenesis and trophicity (1, 2). It exerts its role through the binding to the G protein-coupled receptor (GPCR) melanocortin 2 receptor (MC2R), which activates adenylyl cyclase cascade leading to cAMP production and subsequent activation of cAMP-dependent protein kinase A (PKA). PKA is the main kinase responsible for the phosphorylation of specific transcription factors, which in turn regulate free cholesterol availability and activate steroidogenic enzyme expression (3, 4). Among those transcription factors, steroidogenic factor 1 (SF-1), cAMP response element-binding protein (CREB), CRE modulator (CREM), CCAAT/enhancer-binding proteins (C/EBPs), and activator protein 1 (AP-1) have been extensively described for their implication in regulating the expression of the genes encoding for steroidogenic acute regulatory (StAR) protein and steroidogenic enzymes (5–8). Any perturbation of this ACTH/cAMP/PKA-dependent cascade may cause alteration in adrenocortical cell proliferation and dysregulation of steroidogenesis as occur in various human diseases. The aim of the present review is to provide an overview of the ACTH/cAMP-dependent transcriptional regulation of the steroidogenic process in the adrenal cortex.

ADRENAL STEROIDOGENESIS

Steroid hormones are implicated in the regulation of a plethora of developmental and physiological processes from fetal life to adulthood. Cholesterol is the precursor of all those hormones that hence share a closely related structure based on the cyclopentanophenanthrene 4-ring hydrocarbon nucleus. Cholesterol can be synthesized *de novo* from acetate in the adrenal (9). However, the main adrenal source of cholesterol is plasma low-density lipoproteins (LDLs) provided by dietary cholesterol (10). The sterol response element-binding proteins (SREBPs) are a family of transcription factors implicated in the regulation of genes participating in the biosynthesis of cholesterol and fatty acids (11). They are the main regulators of intracellular cholesterol metabolism. ACTH promotes the activation of 3-hydroxy-3-methylglutaryl coenzyme A reductase, the rate-limiting enzyme in cholesterol synthesis. It also stimulates the uptake of LDL cholesterol esters, which, once taken up by receptor-mediated endocytosis can be converted to free cholesterol for steroid hormone biosynthesis (12) or directly stored. Moreover, ACTH stimulates hormone-sensitive lipase (HSL) and inhibits acyl-coenzyme A (CoA):cholesterol acyltransferase (ACAT), thereby increasing the free cholesterol pool available for steroid hormone biosynthesis.

The initial step of steroidogenesis occurs in the mitochondria. Whereas the movement of cholesterol from the outer mitochondrial membrane (OMM) to the inner mitochondrial membrane (IMM) is known to be promoted by StAR (see below), the molecular mechanism underlying cholesterol transport and loading into the OMM is still under investigation (13). The enzymes that participate in steroid biosynthesis are either cytochrome P450s (CYPs) or hydroxysteroid dehydrogenases (HSDs).

Cytochrome P450s are a group of oxidative enzymes. In the human genome, genes for 57 CYPs enzymes have been described. Seven of them are called "type 1" enzymes. They are targeted to mitochondria and receive electrons from NADPH via a flavoprotein (ferrodoxin reductase) and a small iron-sulfur protein (ferredoxin). "Type 2" enzymes are localized in the endoplasmic reticulum and received electrons form NADPH via a single 2-flavin protein called P450 oxidoreductase (14). Six P450 enzymes participate in steroidogenesis. The mitochondrial P450 side chain cleavage (SCC, encoded by the *CYP11A1* gene) catalyzes breakage of the bond between positions 20 and 22 in the cholesterol side chain (20, 22 desmolase). P450c11β (11β-hydroxylase, encoded by the *CYP11B1* gene) and P450c11AS (aldosterone synthase, encoded by the *CYP11B2* gene) catalyze 11β-hydroxylase, 18-hydroxylase, and 18-methyl oxidase activities. At the level of the endoplasmic reticulum, we distinguish: P450c17 (encoded by the *CYP17A1* gene) that catalyzes both 17α-hydroxylase and 17,20-lyase activities; P450c21 (encoded by the *CYP21A1* gene) that catalyzes 21-hydroxylation in the synthesis of both glucocorticoids and mineralocorticoids; and P450-Aro (encoded by the *CYP19A1* gene) that catalyzes the aromatization of androgens to estrogens.

The HSDs use nicotinamide adenine dinucleotides or their phosphate forms ($NADH/NAD^+$ or $NADPH/NADP^+$) as cofactors to either reduce or oxidize a steroid through a hydride transfer mechanism (15). Differently from steroidogenic reactions catalyzed by P450 enzymes, which are mediated by a single form of P450, each reaction catalyzed by HSDs involves at least two, often different isozymes. On the basis of their structures, those enzymes are divided into: short-chain dehydrogenase/reductase (SDR) family, which include 11β-HSDs 1, 2, and 17β-HSDs 1, 2, and 3 and aldo-keto reductase (AKR) family, which include 17β-HSD5 (15, 16). Under a physiological point of view, it is preferable to classify the HSDs as dehydrogenases or reductases. The former use NAD^+ as cofactors to oxidize hydroxysteroids to ketosteroids, whereas the latter mainly use NADPH to reduce ketosteroids to hydroxysteroids. Those enzymes act *in vitro* typically bidirectionally on the basis of the pH and cofactor concentration, while in intact cells they work mainly in one direction, with the direction established by the cofactors available (15, 16).

The pattern of steroid hormones secreted by each adrenal zone is determined by the enzymes expressed in each zone (17). Specifically, adrenal *zona glomerulosa* expresses angiotensin II receptors and P450c11AS, whereas it does not express P450c17. Indeed, *zona glomerulosa* produces aldosterone under the regulation of the renin–angiotensin system. In contrast, at the levels of *zona fasciculata*, angiotensin II receptors, and P450c11AS are not detected, whereas the ACTH receptor MC2R and P450c11β are expressed (18). The *zona fasciculata* also expresses P450c17, which catalyzes 17α-hydroxylation, exhibiting only little 17,20-lyase activity. Indeed, *zona fasciculata* secretes the two glucocorticoids, cortisol and corticosterone, under the influence of ACTH, but very little dehydroepiandrosterone (DHEA). Interestingly, patients displaying mutations in P450c17 are not able to produce cortisol, but show increased corticosterone production (19), like in rodents, which normally do not express P450c17 in their adrenals. Regarding the *zona reticularis*, it also expresses MC2R and large amounts of P450c17 and cytochrome b_5, thus displaying 17,20-lyase activity with subsequent DHEA production, the most part of which is sulfated to DHEAS by SULT2A1. In general, small amounts of DHEA are converted to androstenedione, and very little amounts of androstenedione are converted to testosterone, likely through AKR1C3/17βHSD5. In contrast, *zona reticularis* expresses very little P450c21 and P450c11β (thus producing only a minimal amount of cortisol) and relatively little 3βHSD2.

ACUTE RESPONSE TO ACTH: THE STEROIDOGENIC ACUTE REGULATORY PROTEIN

Steroidogenic cells are able to store very little amounts of steroids, which imply a rapid synthesis of new steroids in response to a sudden demand. ACTH exerts its role in promoting steroidogenic cell growth and stimulating steroidogenesis at three distinct levels. We first distinguish a long-term exposure to ACTH. It takes weeks or months to stimulate adrenal growth and it is mediated by ACTH-dependent production of cAMP, which in turn triggers IGF-II (20), fibroblast growth factor (FGF) (21), and epidermal growth factor (EGF) (22) synthesis. The concerted action of those growth factors is to promote adrenal cellular hypertrophy and hyperplasia. Second, ACTH can act over days through cAMP to stimulate the transcription of genes, which encode for different steroidogenic enzymes (see below). Third, ACTH can mediate an acute response, which occurs within minutes and is inhibited by protein synthesis inhibitors (like puromycin or cycloheximide). This ACTH-mediated acute response is accompanied by a rapid stimulation of the StAR gene transcription in steroidogenic cells of the adrenal cortex, testis, and ovary (5, 23) and by the phosphorylation of Ser195 in the existent pool of StAR (24). Those events promote cholesterol flow from the OMM to the IMM, where cholesterol is converted to pregnenolone in the first and rate limiting step of steroid hormone biosynthesis. The first to show that ACTH acute steroidogenic response involved the rapid synthesis of a 37-kDa phosphoprotein were Orme-Johnson and coworkers (25, 26). Just a few years later, Stocco and colleagues cloned this protein and they gave it the name of "StAR" (27). StAR is an acutely regulated, cycloheximide-sensitive protein exhibiting a mitochondrial leader sequence by which it is directed to the mitochondria. Once inside the mitochondria, StAR is cleaved to a 30-kDa protein. It has been shown that the overexpression of a mouse StAR in the mouse Leydig MA-10 cells increased their basal steroidogenesis (27). Moreover, when expression vectors for both StAR and P450scc enzyme are cotransfected in non-steroidogenic COS-1 cells, the synthesis of pregnenolone is augmented respect to that obtained with P450scc alone (28). The pivotal role of StAR in the regulation of steroidogenesis was strengthened after the identification of mutations causing premature stop codons in the StAR gene of patients affected by the most common form of congenital lipoid adrenal hyperplasia (CAH) (28, 29), a rare disorder of steroid biosynthesis. In this disorder, glucocorticoid, mineralocorticoid, and sex steroids biosynthesis is impaired, which may lead to adrenal failure, severe salt wasting crisis and hyperpigmentation in phenotypical female infants irrespective of genetic sex (29). Moreover, it has been shown that in mice the targeted disruption of the *Star* gene causes defects in steroidogenesis, with consequent male pseudohermaphroditism and lethality within 1 week after birth (30, 31).

Several studies have been carried out to understand the mechanism of action of StAR (32), which still remains to be fully elucidated. It was hypothesized that the "mature" 30-kDa intramitochondrial form of StAR was the biologically active portion of the protein, due to its longer half-life respect to the short one of the 37 kDa precursor. However, when the two StAR forms are expressed in the cytoplasm or added to mitochondria *in vitro*, they are equally active (33). Moreover, while constitutively active when it is localized on the OMM, StAR results to be inactive at the level of the mitochondrial intramembranous space or the matrix (34). That evidence suggested that StAR exerts its action on the OMM, its steroidogenesis-promoting function tightly depending on the residency time on the OMM itself (33, 34). This implies that StAR activity is linked to its localization rather than to its cleavage to the "mature" form. When StAR interacts with the OMM, it undergoes to conformational changes (35, 36) that allow StAR to accept and discharge cholesterol molecules. Interestingly, steroidogenesis-promoting and cholesterol-transfer activities of StAR are distinct. Indeed, StAR-mediated transfer of cholesterol between synthetic membranes *in vitro* (37) is maintained also by the inactive R182L mutant, which impairs steroidogenesis, causing lipoid CAH (38). Finally, StAR activity on the OMM requires the translocator protein TSPO, also called peripheral benzodiazepine receptor (PBR) (39, 40), which has been identified as a key player in the flow of cholesterol into mitochondria to permit the initiation of steroid hormone synthesis. Moreover, it has been demonstrated that phosphorylated StAR interacts with voltage-dependent anion channel 1 (VDAC1) on the OMM, which in turn promotes processing of the 37-kDa phospho-StAR to the 32-kDa intermediate (41). In the absence of VDAC1, phospho-StAR undergoes degradation by cysteine proteases prior to mitochondrial import and subsequent cleavage to the 30-kDa protein. StAR phosphorylation by PKA requires phosphate carrier protein on the OMM, which seems to interact with StAR before it interacts with VDAC1 (41). Importantly, although StAR is necessary for the ACTH-mediated acute steroidogenic response, steroidogenesis still occurs in the absence of StAR (around 14% of StAR-induced rate) (29, 42). This may account for the steroidogenic capacity of tissues lacking StAR, like placenta and brain.

CHRONIC RESPONSE TO ACTH

The transcription of steroidogenic genes depends on the slower, chronic response to ACTH in the adrenal cortex. Indeed, ACTH interaction with specific membrane receptors leads to the activation of coupled G proteins, with subsequent stimulation of membrane-associated adenylyl cyclase catalyzing cAMP formation. cAMP-activated PKA hence phosphorylates multiple transcription factors, whose concerted action and interaction with different *cis*-regulatory elements direct StAR and steroidogenic gene expression. Furthermore, after transcription factor binding to gene promoters, posttranslational modifications, like phosphorylation/dephosphorylation and coactivator proteins binding, are required to activate gene expression. In the following section, the main transcription factors that direct the transcription of steroidogenic genes in response to ACTH will be described (**Table 1**; **Figure 1**).

Steroidogenic Factor 1

Steroidogenic factor-1 (SF-1; NR5A1) is an orphan member of the nuclear receptor superfamily, which acts as a key regulator of adrenogonadal development and tissue-specific gene expression in steroidogenic cells. Parker and Morohashi groups identified SF-1 by its capacity to bind to and activate transcription from multiple P450 steroidogenic enzyme promoters, which display one or more SF-1-binding sequences in close proximity to the TATA box (72, 73). Furthermore, it has been shown that SF-1 interacts with multiple coactivator and corepressor proteins that function as bridges between transcription factors and the basal transcription system (74–76).

In the human adrenocortical cancer cell line H295R *StAR* gene transcription is induced by both angiotensin II and cAMP via increased SF-1-binding to a cAMP-responsive region within the first 350 bp upstream of the transcription initiation site (45, 77–79). On the other hand, the mutation of the SF-1 response elements in the mouse promoter of the StAR gene does not impair cAMP-dependent StAR induction in MA-10 Leydig cells or Y1 adrenocortical cells (78).

TABLE 1 | Promoter elements implicated in basal and ACTH/cAMP-regulated expression of steroidogenic genes.

	Basal regulation	ACTH/cAMP-dependent regulation
StAR	Three SF-1-binding sites [−135; −95; −45; **mouse** promoter, Ref. (7)] Three SF-1-binding sites [−926/−918; −105/−96; −43/−36; **human** promoter, Ref. (43, 44)] Two Sp1-binding sites [−1159/−1153; −157/−151; **human** promoter, Ref. (44, 45)]	CRE2/AP-1 [−81/−75, **mouse** promoter; Ref. (6)] Two C/EBPs putative-binding sites [−119/−100; −50/−41; **human** promoter, Ref. (43)] Two SF-1-binding sites [−105/−65; −43/−36; **human** promoter, Ref. (43)] Highly conserved overlapping motif [−81/−72, **mouse** promoter, which recognizes the CRE/AP1 and C/EBPs family of proteins, Ref. (7, 46–48)]
CYP11A1	Proximal SF-1-binding site [P site, −46/−38; **human** promoter, reviewed in Ref. (49)] Imperfect Sp1-binding site [−111/−101; **human** promoter, reviewed in Ref. (49)] TReP-132 [−155/−131; **human** promoter, reviewed in Ref. (49)] Adrenal enhancer (AdE, −1850) composed of two binding regions (a) AdE1 (−1845) containing an imperfect Sp1 and an NF-1-binding site [**human** promoter, reviewed in Ref. (49)] (b) AdE2 (−1898) containing an imperfect Sp1-binding site [**human** promoter, reviewed in Ref. (49)] AP-1 motif [−319/−313; **mouse** promoter, Ref. (50)] TGAGTCA motif [termed SF-3-binding site, −120/−114; **mouse** promoter, Ref. (50, 51)] AGGTCA motif [termed SF-2-binding site, −73/−68; **mouse** promoter, Ref. (50, 51)] AGCCTTG motif [termed SF-1-binding site, −45/−39; **mouse** promoter, Ref. (50, 51)]	Proximal SF-1-binding site [P site, −46/−38; **human** promoter, reviewed in Ref. (49)] Upstream cAMP responsive sequence (U-CRS, −1600 bp), which includes (a) SF-1-binding site (−1617/−1609) (b) CREB/ATF-binding site (CRE; −1685/−1606) (c) Two AP-1-binding sites (−1559/−1553; −1633/−1626) (a)/(b)/(c) **human** promoter, reviewed in Ref. (49) AP-1 motif [−319/−313; **mouse** promoter, Ref. (50), although available data indicate that this motif is not a major contributor to the induction of CYP11A1 expression by ACTH/cAMP] TGAGTCA motif [termed SF-3-binding site, −120/−114; **mouse** promoter, Ref. (50, 51)] AGGTCA motif [termed SF-2-binding site, −73/−68; **mouse** promoter, Ref. (50, 51)] AGCCTTG motif [termed SF-1-binding site, −45/−39; **mouse** promoter, Ref. (50, 51)] (mutation of those elements reduced the expression levels of *Cyp11A1* gene following treatment with 8-Br-cAMP, although all mutated plasmids retained appreciable responsiveness to cAMP)
CYP11B1	CRE-binding site [termed Ad1/CRE and resembling a consensus CRE, −71/−64; **human** promoter, Ref. (52, 53) reviewed in Ref. (54)] Ad5 [−119/−111; **human** promoter, ERRalpha has been shown to be the nuclear protein interacting with this element under basal conditions, reviewed in Ref. (54)] SF-1-binding site [termed Ad4, −242/−234; **human** promoter, it seems to be less important for both CYP11B1 and CYP11B2 basal expression, reviewed in Ref. (54)] CRE-binding site [−74/−67; **mouse** promoter, reviewed in Ref. (54)] Two Ad5-binding sites [one at −122/−114 and the other one at −208/−200; **mouse** promoter, reviewed in Ref. (54)] SF-1-binding site [−247/−240; **mouse** promoter, reviewed in Ref. (54)]	CRE-binding site [termed Ad1/CRE and resembling a consensus CRE, −71/−64; **human** promoter, Ref. (52, 53), reviewed in Ref. (54)] Functional CRE consensus sequence [−56/−49, **mouse** promoter, Ref. (55)]
CYP11B2	CRE-binding site [termed Ad1/CRE and resembling a consensus CRE, −71/−64; **human** promoter; Ref. (53), reviewed in Ref. (54)] Ad5 [−119/−111; **human** promoter, ERRalpha has been shown to be the nuclear protein interacting with this element under the basal conditions, reviewed in Ref. (54)] Two SF-1-binding sites [one at −129/−114, **human** promoter, Ref. (56)]; The other one termed Ad4, −344/−337, **human** promoter. It seems to be less important for both CYP11B1 and CYP11B2 basal expression; reviewed in Ref. (54) Chicken ovalbumin upstream promoter transcription factor [COUP-TF, −129/−114; **human** promoter, Ref. (56)] CRE-binding site [−67/−60; **mouse** promoter, reviewed in Ref. (54)] Ad5 [−108/−100; **mouse** promoter, reviewed in Ref. (54)] SF-1 [−330/−323; **mouse** promoter, reviewed in Ref. (54)]	CRE-binding site [termed Ad1/CRE and resembling a consensus CRE, −71/−64; **human** promoter; Ref. (53, 56) reviewed in Ref. (54)] SF-1-binding site [−129/−114; **human** promoter, Ref. (56)] Chicken ovalbumin upstream promoter transcription factor [COUP-TF, −129/−114; **human** promoter, Ref. (56)] CRE-binding site [−67/−60; **mouse** promoter, Ref. (56), reviewed in Ref. (54)]
CYP17A1	ASP/Sp1-binding site [−8/−19; **human** promoter, Ref. (57)] SF-1-binding site [−58/−50; **human** promoter, Ref. (57)] Two nuclear factor 1 (NF-1)-binding sites [−107/−85; −178/−152, **human** promoter, Ref. (59)] −184/−206 region [The site within this sequence that confers basal activity is not known, although it does contain a sequence resembling an SF-1 site at −195/−200; **human** promoter, Ref. (57)] Sp1/Sp3-binding site [−227/−184, **human** promoter; Ref. (59)] SF-1 (−62/−40), Sp1 (−186/−177), and Pbx/Meis (−243/−225) binding sites [**bovine** promoter; Ref. (59–63)]	cAMP-regulatory sequence [CRS, −57/−38: SF-1, p54nrb/NonO, and poly-pyrimidine tract-binding protein-associated splicing factor (PSF) are the transcription factors shown to be associated to this region; **human** promoter, Ref. (58)] SF-1 (−62/−40)- and Pbx/Meis (−243/−225)-binding sites [**bovine** promoter; Ref. (60–63)]

(Continued)

TABLE 1 | Continued

	Basal regulation	ACTH/cAMP-dependent regulation
CYP21	Two Sp1-binding sites [−118/−112 and −106/−100 within the recognition site −129/−96; **human** promoter, Ref. (64)] Two SF-1-binding sites [a putative one within the −300 bp proximal promoter and a second one within a distal region, lying approximately 4.8 kb upstream of the transcription start site; **human** promoter, Ref. (65)] Enhancer element [−330/−150; **mouse** promoter, Ref. (51)] Essential regulatory element [−210/−170; **mouse** promoter, highly conserved in the genes from human and bovine; Ref. (51, 66, 67)] A and B elements located 5.3 and 6 kb upstream of the transcriptional start site [**mouse** promoter, Ref. (69)]	Adrenal-specific protein (ASP)-binding site [−129/−113, within the recognition site −129/−96; **human** promoter, Ref. (64)] Enhancer element [−330/−150; **mouse** promoter, Ref. (51)] Essential regulatory element [−210/−170; **mouse** promoter, highly conserved in the genes from human and bovine; Ref. (51, 66, 67)] cAMP consensus sequence [−68/−62; **mouse** promoter, it matches part of the consensus sequence proposed for cAMP-regulated expression of other genes, Ref. (68)] Nuclear-binding response element (NBRE)/Nurr77 binding site [−65, **mouse** promoter, Ref. (66)] Regulatory elements containing variation of an AGGTCA motif at −170, −210, −140, −65 [**mouse** promoter; they show similarity to the CRE consensus, although they do not function as classical CREs, Ref. (68); variations of these same AGGTCA-bearing elements are also involved in the expression of *Cyp11a* and *Cyp11b* in Y1 adrenocortical cells, see above and Ref. (70)]
HSD3B2	Two SF-1/LRH-1-binding sites [−64/−56; −315/−307; **human** promoter, reviewed in Ref. (71)] Nuclear-binding response element (NBRE)/Nurr77 binding site [−131; **human** promoter, reviewed in Ref. (71)] GATA-binding site [−196/−190; **human** promoter, reviewed in Ref. (71)]	Nuclear-binding response element (NBRE)/Nurr77 binding site [−131, **human** promoter, reviewed in Ref. (71)]

Blue, red and green colours distinguish the different species (human, mouse and bovine, respectively).

Adrenocorticotropic hormone/cAMP-dependent transcription of the human *CYP11A1* gene, encoding for the mitochondrial enzyme P450scc responsible for cholesterol conversion to pregnenolone, requires the binding of SF-1 at two sites (−40 and −1600 bp) on the gene promoter (80). Remarkably, Omura and Chung laboratories have shown that the upstream promoter elements confer a large portion of CYP11A1 responsiveness to cAMP in Y1 or I-10 Leydig tumor cells and primary adrenal cells of transgenic mice (80, 81). SF-1-dependent activation of the *CYP11A1* promoter can be potentiated by cotransfection with c-Jun in steroidogenic JEG3 cells, but not in COS-1 cells (82). Thus, c-Jun and SF-1 act synergistically to activate the transcription of *CYP11A1*. It has also been shown that in the human adrenal cortex *CYP11A1* can be strongly activated by GATA-6 in a SF-1-dependent and DAX1-sensitive fashion (83).

Moreover, it has been shown that SF-1 interacts with the homeodomain-containing transcription factor pituitary homeobox 1 (Ptx/Pitx1) to synergistically promote *CYP11B1* gene transcription (84). Interestingly, in the bovine adrenal only one *CYP11B1* gene is expressed. Its promoter is characterized by the presence of both a SF-1- and a CRE (cAMP-response element)-like binding site, which are essential for cAMP-driven transcription (85, 86).

Adrenocorticotropic hormone/cAMP signaling also regulates the expression of the human *CYP11B2* gene in the *zona glomerulosa*, where it is responsible for mineralocorticoid production via an SF-1-binding site and a CRE (56).

Furthermore, SF-1 is implicated in the transcriptional regulation of *CYP17A1*, the gene encoding the P450c17 enzyme, which catalyzes both the 17α-hydroxylation of pregnenolone and progesterone (required for cortisol biosynthesis) and the 17,20-lyase reaction of 17α-hydroxylated steroids (leading to androgen production). Studies carried out on H295R cells revealed that CREs are located within the first 63 bp upstream of the transcriptional initiation site and that a second basal transcription element lies between −184 and −206 bp (87). SF-1 forms a complex with $p54^{nrb}$/NonO and polypyrimidine tract-binding protein-associated splicing factor (PSF), which binds within those first 60-bp upstream of the transcriptional start site, stimulating CYP17 expression in response to ACTH/cAMP signaling (58). As for *CYP11A1*, GATA-6 promotes the SF-1-dependent transcription of *CYP17* in H295R cells (83).

Many studies have revealed that the ACTH-regulated expression of the *CYP21A1* gene, coding for the P450c21 enzyme, which has a key role in the production of cortisol and aldosterone, requires the binding of the nuclear receptors SF-1 and Nur77 to its promoter (88–90). Interestingly, SF-1 binds to a distal region that lies approximately 4.8 kb upstream of the *CYP21A1* transcription start site driving adrenal-specific expression of the human gene (65).

cAMP Response Element/Binding Protein/CRE Modulator/Activating Transcription Factor

A family of cAMP-responsive nuclear factors mediates transcriptional regulation by ACTH/cAMP signaling pathway. This family is composed by a large number of proteins, which are encoded by the CREB, CREM, and ATF genes. Those proteins recognize and bind the 8-bp 5′-TGACGTCA-3′ palindromic sequence or a minor variation, called the CRE, which lie within 100 nucleotides of the TATA box in the promoters of eukaryotic cAMP responsive genes (91–93). The members of the CREB family are characterized by their DNA-binding leucine zipper (bZIP) domains and generally they interact with each other to mediate cAMP-dependent transcriptional response (91). Interestingly, the sequences of the mouse (27), human (94), and rat *StAR* promoters, which exhibit an extensive homology, lack a consensus CRE, similarly

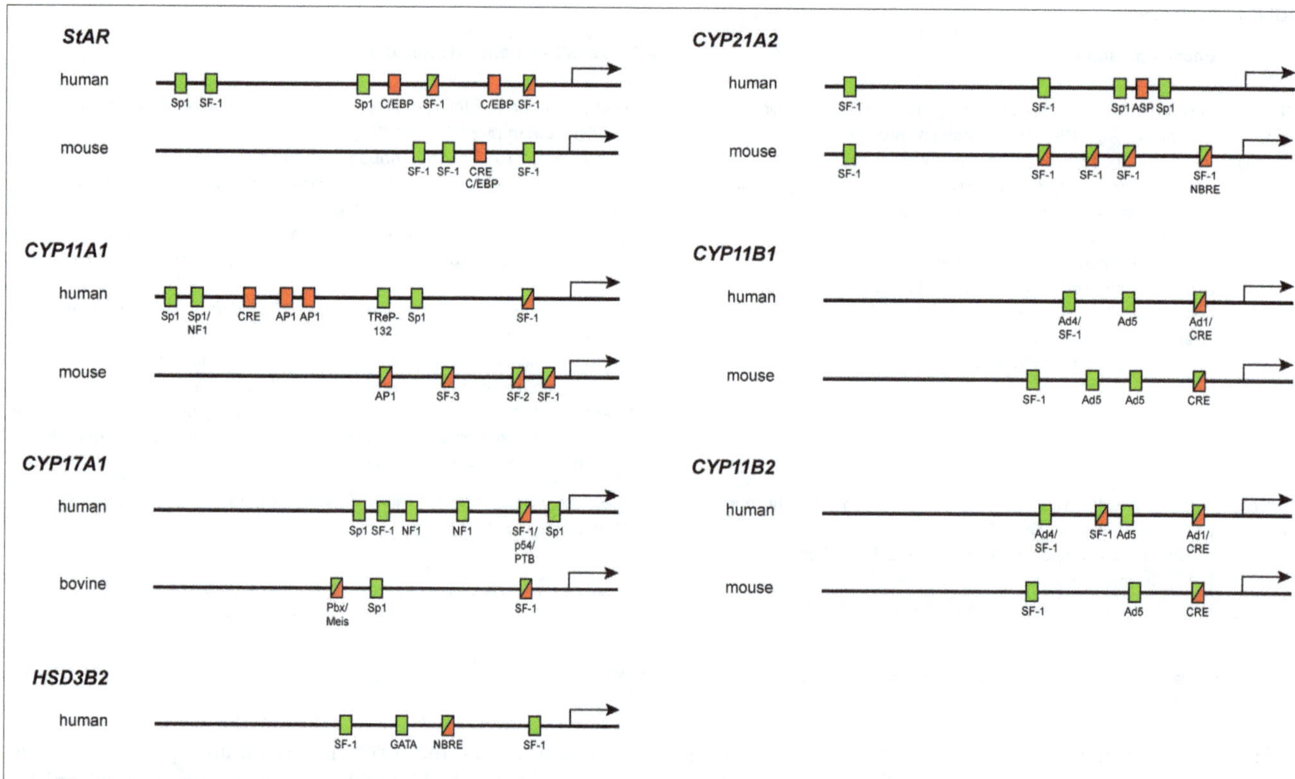

FIGURE 1 | Diagram showing the localization of elements required for basal activity (green rectangles), cAMP-regulated activity (red rectangles) or both basal and cAMP-regulated activities (green–red rectangles) in steroidogenic gene promoters.

to the promoters of different steroid hydroxylase genes whose transcription is regulated by ACTH/cAMP signaling (57). It has been shown that the cAMP-responsive region of the StAR gene promoter exhibits a highly conserved motif (50-TGACTGATGA-30 corresponding to 281/272 bp in the mouse promoter) to which different bZIP families of transcription factors, like not only CREB, CREM, and ATF1, but also AP-1 and C/EBPs (see below) bind to drive StAR transcription (7, 46, 47, 95, 96).

cAMP response element-binding protein has been demonstrated to be the principal player in mediating stimulus-transcription coupling in the ACTH/cAMP pathway. However, knockout mouse CREB studies showed that this action can be compensated by other CRE-binding proteins like CREM and ATF-1 (97). This mechanism also seems to work in the regulation of steroiodogenesis, as CREB family members directly induce *StAR* gene transcription (6, 7, 47). Interestingly, whereas CREB gene products usually function as positive transactivators, CREM can either activate or repress CRE-mediated transcription (98, 99). Alternative splicing of the CREM gene originates multiple isoforms that can act as either activators (τ, τ1, and τ2) or repressors (α, β, and γ) of transcription (100). Identical functional regions have been identified in CREB and CREMτ proteins (99). When overexpressed, either CREB or CREMτ display qualitatively comparable effects toward cAMP-dependent StAR gene transcription in murine adrenal and gonadal cells (6, 7, 101), whereas CREMα and CREMβ have been shown to repress StAR transcription (7). Further, CREM proteins can bind to CREs as homodimers or as heterodimers with CREB/ATF displaying similar functional outcomes to those of CREB (91). Remarkably, it has been shown that CREB and CREM associate with the proximal rather than the distal StAR promoter upon cAMP analog treatment (47, 48). Sugawara and coworkers compared the implication of CREB and CREM in cAMP-mediated StAR gene expression and identified CREM as the main mediator in H295R cells (101). In contrast, another group showed that CREB and ATF-1, but not CREM, mainly bound to the StAR promoter upon ACTH/cAMP stimulation (47). Besides CREB and CREM, also the CRE-binding protein, ATF-1 is a key regulator of StAR gene expression. ATF-1 differs from CREB and CREM as it lacks the glutamine-rich Q1 domain, although this does not affect its ability to work as a transcriptional activator (91, 102). Interestingly, two paralogs of ATF-1, called CRE-binding protein 1(CRE-BP1 or ATF-2) and ATF-a, display alternative exon splicing and bind to CREs, but they are not able to mediate cAMP-responsive transactivations (91).

cAMP response element-binding protein/CREM/ATF are activated by PKA, PKC, and other kinases that phosphorylate them at specific residues within their N-terminus. Indeed, phosphorylation of CREB at Ser133/119 or CREM at Ser117 leads to CREB–CREM interaction with coactivators like CREB-binding protein/p300 (CBP/p300) (see below) with subsequent stimulation of their transcriptional activity (47, 103–105). It has been reported that cAMP analogs increase CREB phosphorylation in a time-dependent manner in steroidogenic cells. This phosphorylation event correlates with the association of both phosphorylated CREB and CBP to the proximal promoter of the StAR gene (47, 48, 106). The phosphorylation of Ser133 is required for CREB activation; however, it is not sufficient for full activation of the protein. Indeed, it has been shown that a short region C-terminal to the PKA phosphorylation site within CREB protein is required for CREB transcriptional activation (91, 107, 108). The crucial role of CREB phosphorylation by PKA has been also observed *in vivo* where transgenic mice, which express a non-phosphorylatable mutant of CREB (called CREB-M1, Ser133Ala), exhibit somatotroph hypoplasia and dwarfism (109). Moreover, expression of CREB-M1 in adrenal and gonadal cells strongly decreases cAMP-induced StAR gene expression (6, 7, 101).

cAMP response element-binding protein participates together with GATA-6 and AP-1 to the SF-1- and AP-2-dependent *CYP11A1* gene transcription in rodent placenta and ovary (110). Interestingly, the ACTH-stimulated transcription of the human *CYP11B1* gene depends on the CREB family member ATF-2 (52). Moreover, as reported above, ACTH/cAMP signaling regulates *CYP11B2* gene transcription via a CRE and a SF-1-binding site (56). Similarly, CREB binds to a CRE at the level of the mouse *Cyp11b1* gene promoter to drive ACTH-dependent transcription (55).

CCAT/Enhancer-Binding Proteins

CCAT/enhancer-binding proteins are a family of transcription factors containing a highly conserved bZIP at the C-terminus that is involved in dimerization and DNA binding. C/EBPs bind with different affinities to a consensus site consisting of a dyad symmetrical repeat (A/GTTGCGC/TAAC/T) (111). At least six members of the family have been cloned and characterized, named from C/EBPα to C/EBPζ. C/EBPα and C/EBPβ are expressed in steroidogenic cells, the expression levels of C/EBPβ being increased in the nucleus by the action of LH and analogs of cAMP (112, 113). The cAMP-inducible domains of C/EBPs, with the exception for C/EBPβ, lack a PKA phosphorylation site, which implies that C/EBPs are able to mediate cAMP-dependent responses by indirect mechanisms. In contrast, C/EBPβ phosphorylation by PKA within its bZIP domain affects its DNA-binding activity (114).

C/EBPβ targets a binding region in the promoter of the mouse *Star* gene (281/272 bp), which is also bound by CREB/ATF (see above) and Fos/Jun (see below). Further, two putative C/EBP-binding sites have been identified within the human StAR promoter (43). Consequently, an implication for both C/EBPα and C/EBPβ in StAR gene transcription has been reported (43, 115, 116). C/EBPβ phosphorylation on Thr325 increases its association to the proximal StAR promoter, thus inducing StAR transcription (117, 118). Interestingly, it has been shown that GATA-4 and C/EBPβ directly interact *in vitro* and *in vivo* and synergistically activate the StAR promoter only in the presence of PKA (95, 117). This suggests that GATA-C/EBP transcriptional cooperation might promote ACTH/cAMP-dependent StAR transcription in all steroidogenic tissues, as this kind of PKA-dependent synergy has been shown for other members of GATA and C/EBP families. Finally, the disruption of either C/EBPα or C/EBPβ impairs normal reproductive development in female mice, with consequent reduced or altered ovulation and corpus luteum formation inability (112, 119).

AP-1 Family of Transcription Factors

The AP-1 family of transcription factors participates in the regulation of cellular responses to multiple stimuli regulating proliferation, transformation, and cell death (120). It recognizes and binds to a DNA sequence known as the AP-1/phorbol 12-*O*-tetradecanoate 13-acetate responsive element [AP-1/TRE; TGA(C/G)TCA]. AP-1 is composed by a mixture of homo- and hetero-dimers formed between Jun (c-Jun, JunB, and JunD) and Fos (c-Fos, FosB, Fra1, and Fra2) family members (121–123). Fos members heterodimerize with Jun proteins and with specific members of the CREB/ATF family, but they are not able to form homodimers, whereas Jun members function as homodimers or heterodimers among themselves or with members of the Fos and CREB/ATF families (124). Both Jun and Fos family proteins belong to the bZIP group of DNA-binding transcription factors and their dimerization is necessary for specific and high affinity binding to the palindromic DNA sequence TGAC/GTCA (see above) (125). Studies carried out on the mouse *Star* promoter identified a highly conserved element (TGACTGA, −81/−75 bp), which shows homology with the AP-1/TRE sequence and overlaps also with the CRE2 sequence (6). Interestingly, it has been shown that Fos and Jun bind to this element, called CRE2/AP-1, thus regulating *Star* gene transcription (46, 96, 126). Moreover, two additional putative AP-1-binding sites have been identified within the rat *Star* promoter. c-Fos reduces basal, cAMP-, and c-Jun-mediated rat *Star* gene transcription in Y-1 adrenocortical cells (127). Indeed, a functional comparison between Fos and Jun revealed that c-Jun is the most powerful AP-1 family member for *Star* gene transactivation. Accordingly to this, it has been shown that only c-Jun, but not other AP-1 members, plays a pivotal role in the regulation of PKC-mediated *Star* transcription and steroidogenesis in Leydig and adrenal cells (96, 128).

Not only Protein kinase A but also PKC phosphorylate several Ser and Thr residues on c-Jun and c-Fos. In particular, the treatment with a cAMP analog or a growth factor increases the phosphorylation of c-Jun Ser63 and c-Fos Thr325. Those phosphorylation events are associated to StAR gene transcription and steroidogenesis in mouse Leydig cells (47, 96, 126, 129). Interestingly, ACTH/cAMP-dependent c-Jun and c-Fos phosphorylation increases the association between p-c-Jun/p-c-Fos and the CBP/p300 cofactors (see below), with consequent recruitment of CBP/p300 to the StAR promoter (47, 96, 126). The phosphorylation of c-Fos and c-Jun can alter their capacity to interact with other transcription factors, affecting their dimerization and DNA-binding specificity (124). This explains why the crosstalk between CREB and c-Fos/c-Jun can be associated with both gain and loss of function on the same *cis*-element in the context of a fine regulation of the transregulatory elements which participate in StAR gene transcription (126).

Sp Family of Transcription Factors

The Sp family of transcription factors is characterized by the presence of three conserved Cys2His2-type zinc fingers at their

C-terminus that form the sequence-specific DNA-binding domain (130). They can bind and exert their action through GC/GT-rich promoter elements to regulate the expression of multiple target genes (130, 131). Sp1 is the most well characterized member of the family and it exhibits similar structure and a high homology with Sp3 at the level of its DNA-binding domains, both being able to enhance ore repress promoter activity. However, although Sp1 and Sp3 recognize the same consensus-binding sites, it has been reported that both their DNA-binding properties and regulatory functions differ and depend on the promoter context and cellular background (130, 132, 133).

Regulatory elements for Sp1 and Sp3 have been identified within the human TSPO proximal promoter (134). They have been demonstrated to be strong positive elements for the promoter activity, although differences have been detected in the mechanism by which TSPO is regulated in non-steroidogenic versus steroidogenic cells (134). Sp1 is also involved in the cAMP-dependent transcription of the *CYP11A1* gene in human (135), bovine (136, 137), and porcine (138) adrenals. Furthermore, a cooperation between SF-1, Sp1, and CBP has been reported to drive cAMP-dependent *CYP11A1* transcription in bovine adrenal (136). Sp1 and Sp3, together with the nuclear fator-1C (NF-1C), bind to the second basal element of the *CYP17* gene promoter. This event is crucial for optimal basal transcription (59). Sp1 can also form a complex with GATA-4 or GATA-6 to regulate the expression of *CYP17* in the adrenal gland (139). Finally, Sp1 and adrenal-specific protein (ASP) bind to the *CYP21* gene promoter to regulate its cAMP-dependent transcription (140). This synergistic action seems to be required for maximal *CYP21* induction (140).

DAX-1

DAX-1/NR0B1 encodes an unusual member of the nuclear hormone receptor family of transcription factors. Its mutations cause adrenal hypoplasia congenita (AHC) associated with hypogonadotropic hypogonadism (HHG) (141, 142). *DAX-1* expression pattern, mostly restricted to steroidogenic tissues, suggested that it may have a role in the regulation of steroidogenesis. Indeed, in adrenocortical cells, DAX-1 works as a global negative regulator of basal and cAMP-regulated transcription of steroidogenic genes, both through direct binding to gene promoters and interaction with SF-1 and other transcription factors [(143–145); reviewed in Ref. (146)]. In addition, consistently with DAX-1 negative action on steroidogenesis, activation of the PKA pathway by ACTH in adrenocortical cells (147) and FSH in Sertoli cells (148) down-regulates Dax-1 expression.

ROLE OF COREGULATORS

Transcriptional coregulators are crucially implicated in nuclear receptor-mediated transcriptional activation (149–151) and transactivation by other factors, exerting their roles in multiples processes, like histone modification (152–154), chromatin remodeling (155), post-translational modification of transactivation complex members (156, 157), and ordered recruitment of basal transcriptional machinery (158, 159).

The role of coactivators and corepressors in the transcriptional regulation of steroid hydroxylase genes and *StAR* has been shown by several studies (74, 76). CBP and its functional homolog p300 are transcriptional coactivators that contain multiple functional domains and display intrinsic histone acetyltransferase activity (151, 160), by which they increase transcription factor accessibility to nucleosomal DNA. Classically, ACTH/cAMP signaling triggers the phosphorylation of specific transcription factors, which in turn can bind and recruit CBP/p300 (105, 160–162). As already reported (see above), when phosphorylated at Ser133 CREB is able to interact with CBP (104, 105). Interestingly, CBP/p300 contain PKA consensus sites, the phosphorylation of which is involved in regulating their functions. CBP/p300 play a key role in the transcriptional regulation of the *StAR* gene. Different studies have shown that cAMP-dependent phosphorylation of CREB at Ser133, c-Jun at Ser63, and c-Fos at Thr325 promotes the association and recruitment of CBP/p300 to the proximal *StAR* promoter (47, 48, 95, 126). cAMP-stimulated phosphorylation of C/EBPβ at Thr325 also increases C/EBPβ association to the proximal *StAR* promoter (117). Other factors like SF-1 and GATA-4 (see above), that are bound to the proximal *StAR* promoter, once phosphorylated in response to ACTH might enhance CBP/p300 recruitment to the promoter. This correlates with the CBP/p300-dependent increased effects of C/EBPβ and GATA-4 on *StAR* expression (95). Further, when overexpressed, CBP/p300 potentiated CREB, Fos/Jun, C/EBPβ, and GATA-4 transcriptional activity on the *StAR* gene (95, 126). This event is attenuated by the adenovirus E1A oncoprotein, which acts impairing CBP/p300 histone acetyltransferase activity and/or their interaction with other transcription factors or with the basal transcription machinery.

As already reported, coactivators and corepressors also play a key role in the transcriptional regulation of steroid hydroxylase genes. We report here some examples. Coexpression of CBP/p300 with the zinc finger protein TReP-132 has an additive effect on human *CYP11A1* gene promoter activity (163). Similarly, it has been shown that the coactivators CBP/p300, steroid receptor coactivator (SRC)-1, and transcriptional intermediary factor-2 (TIF-2) enhance SF-1-mediated bovine *CYP17* transcription, whereas the corepressors nuclear receptor corepressor (N-CoR) and the silencing mediator of retinoic acid and thyroid hormone receptor (SMRT) increase the repressive activity of chicken ovalbumin upstream-transcription factor 1(COUP-TF-1) (164).

Finally, Sewer and coworkers have shown that a corepressor protein called mSin3A inhibits human *CYP17* gene transcription by the recruitment of a histone deacetylase to the SF-1/NonO/PSF complex that binds to the *CYP17* promoter (58). They have also described that coregulator exchange and sphingosine-sensitive cooperativity of SF-1, general control non-derepressed 5 (GCN5), p54, and p160 coactivators regulate cAMP-dependent *CYP17* transcription rate in H295R cells (165). The same group has shown that ACTH/cAMP signaling pathway promotes acid ceramidase (*ASAH1*) gene transcription via the binding of CREB to multiple region of the *ASAH1* promoter. This event triggers the recruitment of CBP/p300 with a related increase in the trimethylation of Lys4 on histone H3 (H3K4) on the *ASAH1* promoter in H295R cells (166).

ROLE OF PHOSPHATASE ACTIVITY ON ACTH/cAMP-DEPENDENT STEROIDOGENIC GENE TRANSCRIPTION

As already discussed, the ACTH-dependent increase in intracellular cAMP levels leads to the activation of PKA, which, in turn, phosphorylates specific nuclear factors to drive steroidogenic gene transcription. Remarkably, in the adrenal cortex ACTH regulation of steroidogenesis depends not only on PKA-mediated Ser/Thr phosphorylation, but also on the activity of protein tyrosine phosphatases (PTPs), which have been implicated in *StAR* expression and steroidogenesis (167–172). Indeed, the phospho-dephosphorylation of intermediate proteins is considered as a key event in the regulation of steroid biosynthesis. In 1999, Paz and coworkers showed that *in vivo* treatment with ACTH leads to an increase in total PTPs activity in adrenal *zona fasciculata*. The stimulation was characterized by a rapid onset (5 min), reached a peak after 15 min of ACTH administration (around twofold) and returned to basal levels after 30 min (168). They showed that the increase in PTPs correlated with a decrease in phosphotyrosine proteins (168). Moreover, the PTPs inhibitors pervanadate (PV) and phenylarsine oxide (PAO) inhibited ACTH- and 8Br-cAMP (a permeant analog of adenosine 3′,5′-phosphate)-dependent steroidogenesis in a dose-dependent fashion, whereas they did not affect steroid production supported by a cell-permeant analog of cholesterol (168). Those studies clearly indicated that PTPs activity has a key role in ACTH/cAMP signaling pathway, acting downstream of PKA activation and upstream of cholesterol transport across the mitochondrial membrane. The same group evaluated steroid production and StAR protein levels in Y1 cells upon PTP inhibition. They reported that PAO reduced ACTH-dependent stimulated steroidogenesis in those cells in a concentration-dependent manner and abrogated StAR protein induction (169). Those effects have been reproduced by a second PTPs inhibitor, benzyl phosphonic acid, which has a different mechanism of action (169). Altogether, those results show that PKA-mediated PTP activation in the steroidogenic system exerts the functional role of mediating StAR protein induction (169). The ACTH/cAMP/PKA signaling pathway stimulates also the release of arachidonic acid (AA) in adrenal and Leydig cells by the concerted action of two enzymes: an acylCoA-thioesterase (Acot2) and an acyl-CoA-synthetase (ACS4) (170, 173). Several reports have shown that AA and its metabolites play a key role in the hormonal control of steroidogenesis by regulating both the expression and function of StAR protein (174, 175). The ACTH/PKA system has been shown to control this pathway upregulating the ACS4 protein levels in adrenal and Leydig cells (175). Two PTP inhibitors both abrogate the ACTH/PKA-dependent ACS4 induction and reduced the effects of cAMP on steroidogenesis and StAR protein levels (175). Interestingly, exogenous AA is able to overcome this PTP-dependent inhibitory effect on StAR protein expression and steroidogenesis (176, 177). Furthermore, Sewer and Waterman have shown that PTP activity is essential for cAMP-dependent transcription of the human *CYP17* gene in H295R cells (178). They also investigated whether the inhibition of PTP activity can impair cAMP-dependent mRNA expression of other steroidogenic genes in the adrenal cortex. They have reported that *CYP11A1*, *CYP11B1/2*, and *CYP21A1* also require PTPs for cAMP-dependent mRNA expression, as the inhibition of both serine/threonine and tyrosine phosphatase activities negatively affected this event (178). Those evidences led those authors to propose a model whereby PKA phosphorylates and activates a dual-specificity phosphatase (DSP), which is able to mediate ACTH/cAMP/PKA-dependent transcription of steroidogenic genes (178, 179). The specific DSP has been identified as mitogen-activated protein phosphatase 1 (MKP-1), whose levels are increased by ACTH and cAMP in H295R cells (180). Moreover, the evidence showing that MKP1 overexpression promotes the transcriptional activity of a human *CYP17* promoter-reporter construct and its silencing decreases cAMP-stimulated *CYP17* gene expression, suggest a role for MKP-1 in cAMP-dependent *CYP17* transcriptional activation (180).

SUMMARY AND CONCLUSION

The studies outlined here have given an important contribution to the understanding of the impact of ACTH on the regulation of steroidogenic gene expression in the adrenal cortex. Given the pivotal role played by ACTH/cAMP signaling in the acute and chronic regulation of steroid secretion and the implication of those hormones in diverse arrays of fundamental physiological processes, an in-depth investigation is needed to completely elucidate the ACTH-dependent transcriptional regulatory mechanisms that control steroid secretion. Indeed, some aspects addressed in this review still represent a challenge for future studies, which might provide the scientific community with a broader picture of the complex signaling pathways and the intricate transcriptional circuitries that coordinately ensure optimal hormonal output.

AUTHOR CONTRIBUTIONS

All authors listed, have made substantial, direct, and intellectual contribution to the work, and approved it for publication.

REFERENCES

1. Simpson ER, Waterman MR. Regulation of the synthesis of steroidogenic enzymes in adrenal cortical cells by ACTH. *Annu Rev Physiol* (1988) **50**:427–40. doi:10.1146/annurev.ph.50.030188.002235
2. Markowska A, Rebuffat P, Rocco S, Gottardo G, Mazzocchi G, Nussdorfer GG. Evidence that an extrahypothalamic pituitary corticotropin releasing hormone (CRH)/adrenocorticotropin (ACTH) system controls adrenal growth and secretion in rats. *Cell Tissue Res* (1993) **272**:439–45. doi:10.1007/BF00318550
3. Miller WL, Bose HS. Early steps in steroidogenesis: intracellular cholesterol trafficking. *J Lipid Res* (2011) **52**:2111–35. doi:10.1194/jlr.R016675
4. Sewer MB, Waterman MR. ACTH modulation of transcription factors responsible for steroid hydroxylase gene expression in the adrenal cortex. *Microsc Res Tech* (2003) **61**:300–7. doi:10.1002/jemt.10339
5. Stocco DM. Tracking the role of a StAR in the sky of the new millennium. *Mol Endocrinol* (2001) **15**:1245–54. doi:10.1210/mend.15.8.0697
6. Manna PR, Dyson MT, Eubank DW, Clark BJ, Lalli E, Sassone-Corsi P, et al. Regulation of steroidogenesis and the steroidogenic acute regulatory protein

by a member of the cAMP response-element binding protein family. *Mol Endocrinol* (2002) **16**:184–99. doi:10.1210/mend.16.1.0759

7. Manna PR, Eubank DW, Lalli E, Sassone-Corsi P, Stocco DM. Transcriptional regulation of the mouse steroidogenic acute regulatory protein gene by the cAMP response-element binding protein and steroidogenic factor 1. *J Mol Endocrinol* (2003) **30**:381–97. doi:10.1677/jme.0.0300381
8. Manna PR, Dyson MT, Stocco DM. Regulation of the steroidogenic acute regulatory protein gene expression: present and future perspectives. *Mol Hum Reprod* (2009) **15**:321–33. doi:10.1093/molehr/gap025
9. Mason JI, Rainey WE. Steroidogenesis in the human fetal adrenal: a role for cholesterol synthesized de novo. *J Clin Endocrinol Metab* (1987) **64**:140–7. doi:10.1210/jcem-64-1-140
10. Gwynne JT, Strauss JF 3rd. The role of lipoproteins in steroidogenesis and cholesterol metabolism in steroidogenic glands. *Endocr Rev* (1982) **3**:299–329. doi:10.1210/edrv-3-3-299
11. Horton JD, Goldstein JL, Brown MS. SREBPs: activators of the complete program of cholesterol and fatty acid synthesis in the liver. *J Clin Invest* (2002) **109**:1125–31. doi:10.1172/JCI15593
12. Brown MS, Kovanen PT, Goldstein JL. Receptor-mediated uptake of lipoprotein-cholesterol and its utilization for steroid synthesis in the adrenal cortex. *Recent Prog Horm Res* (1979) **35**:215–57. doi:10.1126/science.6261329
13. Chang TY, Chang CC, Ohgami N, Yamauchi Y. Cholesterol sensing, trafficking and esterification. *Annu Rev Cell Dev Biol* (2006) **22**:129–57. doi:10.1146/annurev.cellbio.22.010305.104656
14. Miller WL. Regulation of steroidogenesis by electron transfer. *Endocrinology* (2005) **146**:2544–50. doi:10.1210/en.2005-0096
15. Agarwal AK, Auchus RJ. Cellular redox state regulates hydroxysteroid dehydrogenase activity and intracellular hormone potency. *Endocrinology* (2005) **146**:2531–8. doi:10.1210/en.2005-0061
16. Penning TM. Molecular endocrinology of hydroxysteroid dehydrogenases. *Endocr Rev* (1997) **18**:281–305. doi:10.1210/edrv.18.3.0302
17. Auchus RJ, Rainey WE. Adrenarche – physiology, biochemistry and human disease. *Clin Endocrinol (Oxf)* (2004) **60**:288–96. doi:10.1046/j.1365-2265.2003.01858
18. Mulatero P, Curnow KM, Aupetit-Faisant B, Foekling M, Gomez-Sanchez C, Veglio F, et al. Recombinant CYP11B genes encode enzymes that can catalyze conversion of 11-deoxycortisol to cortisol, 18-hydroxycortisol, and 18-oxocortisol. *J Clin Endocrinol Metab* (1998) **83**:3996–4001. doi:10.1210/jcem.83.11.5237
19. Kater CE, Biglieri EG. Disorders of steroid 17α-hydroxylase deficiency. *Endocrinol Metab Clin North Am* (1994) **23**:341–57.
20. Voutilainen R, Miller WL. Coordinate tropic hormone regulation of mRNAs for insulin-like growth factor II and the cholesterol side-chain cleavage enzyme, P450scc, in human steroidogenic tissues. *Proc Natl Acad Sci U S A* (1987) **84**:1590–4. doi:10.1073/pnas.84.6.1590
21. Mesiano S, Mellon SH, Gospodarowicz D, Di Blasio AM, Jaffe RB. Basic fibroblast growth factor expression is regulated by corticotropin in the human fetal adrenal: a model for adrenal growth regulation. *Proc Natl Acad Sci U S A* (1991) **88**:5428–32. doi:10.1073/pnas.88.12.5428
22. Coulter CL, Read LC, Carr BR, Tarantal AF, Barry S, Styne DM. A role for epidermal growth factor in the morphological and functional maturation of the adrenal gland in the fetal rhesus monkey *in vivo*. *J Clin Endocrinol Metab* (1996) **81**:1254–60. doi:10.1210/jcem.81.3.8772608
23. Clark BJ, Soo SC, Caron KM, Ikeda Y, Parker KL, Stocco DM. Hormonal and developmental regulation of the steroidogenic acute regulatory (StAR) protein. *Mol Endocrinol* (1995) **9**:1346–55. doi:10.1210/mend.9.10.8544843
24. Arakane F, King SR, Du Y, Kallen CB, Walsh LP, Watari H, et al. Phosphorylation of steroidogenic acute regulatory protein (StAR) modulates its steroidogenic activity. *J Biol Chem* (1997) **272**:32656–62. doi:10.1074/jbc.272.51.32656
25. Pon LA, Hartigan JA, Orme-Johnson NR. Acute ACTH regulation of adrenal corticosteroid biosynthesis: rapid accumulation of a phosphoprotein. *J Biol Chem* (1986) **261**:13309–16.
26. Epstein LF, Orme-Johnson NR. Regulation of steroid hormone biosynthesis: identification of precursors of a phosphoprotein targeted to the mitochondrion in stimulated rat adrenal cortex cells. *J Biol Chem* (1991) **266**:19739–45.
27. Clark BJ, Wells J, King SR, Stocco DM. The purification, cloning and expression of a novel luteinizing hormone-induced mitochondrial protein in MA-10 mouse Leydig tumor cells. Characterization of the steroidogenic acute regulatory protein (StAR). *J Biol Chem* (1994) **269**:28314–22.
28. Lin D, Sugawara T, Strauss JF III, Clark BJ, Stocco DM, Saenger P, et al. Role of steroidogenic acute regulatory protein in adrenal and gonadal steroidogenesis. *Science* (1995) **267**:1828–31. doi:10.1126/science.7892608
29. Bose HS, Sugawara T, Strauss JF III, Miller WL; International Congenital Lipoid Adrenal Hyperplasia Consortium. The pathophysiology and genetics of congenital lipoid adrenal hyperplasia. *N Engl J Med* (1996) **335**:1870–8. doi:10.1056/NEJM199612193352503
30. Caron KM, Soo SC, Wetsel WC, Stocco DM, Clark BJ, Parker KL. Targeted disruption of the mouse gene encoding steroidogenic acute regulatory protein provides insights into congenital lipoid adrenal hyperplasia. *Proc Natl Acad Sci U S A* (1997) **94**:11540–5. doi:10.1073/pnas.94.21.11540
31. Hasegawa T, Zhao L, Caron KM, Majdic G, Suzuki T, Shizawa S, et al. Developmental roles of the steroidogenic acute regulatory protein (StAR) as revealed by StAR knockout mice. *Mol Endocrinol* (2000) **14**:1462–71. doi:10.1210/mend.14.9.0515
32. Miller WL. Steroidogenic acute regulatory protein (StAR), a novel mitochondrial cholesterol transporter. *Biochim Biophys Acta* (2007) **1771**:663–76. doi:10.1016/j.bbalip.2007.02.012
33. Arakane F, Sugawara T, Nishino H, Liu Z, Holt JA, Pain D, et al. Steroidogenic acute regulatory protein (StAR) retains activity in the absence of its mitochondrial targeting sequence: implications for the mechanism of StAR action. *Proc Natl Acad Sci U S A* (1996) **93**:13731–6. doi:10.1073/pnas.93.24.13731
34. Bose HS, Lingappa VR, Miller WL. Rapid regulation of steroidogenesis by mitochondrial protein import. *Nature* (2002) **417**:87–91. doi:10.1038/417087a
35. Bose HS, Whittal RM, Baldwin MA, Miller WL. The active form of the steroidogenic acute regulatory protein, StAR, appears to be a molten globule. *Proc Natl Acad Sci U S A* (1999) **96**:7250–5. doi:10.1073/pnas.96.13.7250
36. Baker BY, Yaworsky DC, Miller WL. A pH-dependent molten globule transition is required for activity of the steroidogenic acute regulatory protein, StAR. *J Biol Chem* (2005) **280**:41753–60. doi:10.1074/jbc.M510241200
37. Tuckey RC, Headlam MJ, Bose HS, Miller WL. Transfer of cholesterol between phospholipid vesicles mediated by the steroidogenic acute regulatory protein (StAR). *J Biol Chem* (2002) **277**:47123–8. doi:10.1074/jbc.M206965200
38. Baker BY, Epand RF, Epand RM, Miller WL. Cholesterol binding does not predict activity of the steroidogenic acute regulatory protein, StAR. *J Biol Chem* (2007) **282**:10223–32. doi:10.1074/jbc.M611221200
39. Papadopoulos V. Peripheral-type benzodiazepine/diazepam binding inhibitor receptor: biological role in steroidogenic cell function. *Endocr Rev* (1993) **14**:222–40. doi:10.1210/edrv-14-2-222
40. Hauet T, Yao ZX, Bose HS, Wall CT, Han Z, Li W, et al. Peripheral-type benzodiazepine receptor-mediated action of steroidogenic acute regulatory protein on cholesterol entry into Leydig cell mitochondria. *Mol Endocrinol* (2005) **19**:540–54. doi:10.1210/me.2004-0307
41. Bose M, Whittal RM, Miller WL, Bose HS. Steroidogenic activity of StAR requires contact with mitochondrial VDAC1 and PCP. *J Biol Chem* (2008) **283**:8837–45. doi:10.1074/jbc.M709221200
42. Miller WL, Strauss JF 3rd. Molecular pathology and mechanism of action of the steroidogenic acute regulatory protein, StAR. *J Steroid Biochem Mol Biol* (1999) **69**:131–41. doi:10.1016/S0960-0760(98)00153-8
43. Christenson LK, Johnson PF, McAllister JM, Strauss JF III. CCAAT/enhancer-binding proteins regulate expression of the human steroidogenic acute regulatory protein (StAR) gene. *J Biol Chem* (1999) **274**:26591–8. doi:10.1074/jbc.274.37.26591
44. Sugawara T, Saito M, Fujimoto S. Sp1 and SF-1 interact and cooperate in the regulation of human steroidogenic acute regulatory protein gene expression. *Endocrinology* (2000) **141**:2895–903. doi:10.1210/endo.141.8.7602
45. Sugawara T, Holt JA, Kiriakidou M, Strauss JR III. Steroidogenic factor 1-dependent promoter activity of the human steroidogenic acute regulatory protein (StAR) gene. *Biochemistry* (1996) **35**:9052–9. doi:10.1021/bi960057r
46. Manna PR, Eubank DW, Stocco DM. Assessment of the role of activator protein-1 on transcription of the mouse steroidogenic acute regulatory protein gene. *Mol Endocrinol* (2004) **18**:558–73. doi:10.1210/me.2003-0223
47. Clem BF, Hudson EA, Clark BJ. Cyclic adenosine 3′,5′-monophosphate (cAMP) enhances cAMP-responsive element binding (CREB) protein phosphorylation and phospho-CREB interaction with the mouse steroidogenic acute regulatory protein gene promoter. *Endocrinology* (2005) **146**:1348–56. doi:10.1210/en.2004-0761

48. Hiroi H, Christenson LK, Chang L, Sammel MD, Berger SL, Strauss JF III. Temporal and spatial changes in transcription factor binding and histone modifications at the steroidogenic acute regulatory protein (StAR) locus associated with StAR transcription. *Mol Endocrinol* (2004) **18**:791–806. doi:10.1210/me.2003-0305
49. Shih MC, Chiu YN, Hu MC, Guo IC, Chung BC. Regulation of steroid production: analysis of *Cyp11a1* promoter. *Mol Cell Endocrinol* (2011) **10**:80–4. doi:10.1016/j.mce.2010.12.017
50. Rice DA, Kirkman MS, Aitken LD, Mouw AR, Schimmer BP, Parker KL. Analysis of the promoter region of the gene encoding mouse cholesterol side-chain cleavage enzyme. *J Biol Chem* (1990) **15**:11713–20.
51. Handler JD, Schimmer BP, Flynn TR, Szyf M, Seidman JG, Parker KL. An enhancer element and a functional cyclic AMP-dependent protein kinase are required for expression of adrenocortical 21-hydroxylase. *J Biol Chem* (1988) **263**:13068–73.
52. Wang XL, Bassett M, Zhang Y, Yin S, Clyne C, White PC, et al. Transcriptional regulation of human 11beta-hydroxylase (hCYP11B1). *Endocrinology* (2000) **141**:3587–94. doi:10.1210/endo.141.10.7689
53. Bassett MH, Zhang Y, White PC, Rainey WE. Regulation of human *CYP11B2* and *CYP11B1*: comparing the role of the common CRE/Ad1 element. *Endocr Res* (2000) **26**:941–51. doi:10.3109/07435800009048620
54. Cheng LC, Pai TW, Li LA. Regulation of human *CYP11B1* and *CYP11B2* promoters by transposable elements and conserved cis elements. *Steroids* (2012) **77**:100–9. doi:10.1016/j.steroids.2011.10.010
55. Rice DA, Aitken LD, Vandenbark GR, Mouw AR, Franklin A, Schimmer BP, et al. A cAMP-responsive element regulates expression of the mouse steroid 11 betahydroxylase gene. *J Biol Chem* (1989) **264**:14011–5.
56. Clyne CD, Zhang Y, Slutsker L, Mathis JM, White PC, Rainey WE. Angiotensin II and potassium regulate human CYP11B2 transcription through common cis-elements. *Mol Endocrinol* (1997) **11**:638–49. doi:10.1210/mend.11.5.9920
57. Waterman MR. Biochemical diversity of cAMP-dependent transcription of steroid hydroxylase genes in the adrenal cortex. *J Biol Chem* (1994) **269**:27783–6.
58. Sewer MB, Nguyen V, Huang C, Tucker PW, Kagawa N, Waterman MR. Transcriptional activation of human CYP17 in H295R adrenocortical cells depends on complex formation between p54nrb/NonO, PSF and SF-1, a complex which also participates in repression of transcription. *Endocrinology* (2002) **143**:1280–90. doi:10.1210/endo.143.4.8748
59. Lin CJ, Martens JWM, Miller WL. NF-1C, Sp1, and Sp3 are essential for transcription of the human gene for P450c17 (steroid 17a-hydroxylase/17,20 lyase) in human adrenal NCI-H295A cells. *Mol Endocrinol* (2001) **15**:1277–93. doi:10.1210/mend.15.8.0679
60. Lund J, Ahlgren R, Wu D, Kagimoto M, Simpson ER, Waterman MR. Transcriptional regulation of the bovine *CYP17* (P-$450_{17\alpha}$) gene. *J Biol Chem* (1990) **265**:3304–12.
61. Bakke M, Lund J. Mutually exclusive interactions of two nuclear orphan receptors determine activity of a cyclic adenosine 3′,5′-monophosphate-responsive sequence in the bovine *CYP17* gene. *Mol Endocrinol* (1995) **9**:327–9. doi:10.1210/mend.9.3.7776979
62. Kagawa N, Ogo A, Takahashi Y, Iwamatsu A, Waterman M. A cAMP-regulatory sequence (CRS1) of CYP17 is a cellular target for the homeodomain protein Pbx1. *J Biol Chem* (1994) **269**:18716–9.
63. Bischof L, Kagawa N, Moskow JJ, Takahashi Y, Iwamatsu A, Buchberg AM, et al. Members of the Meis and Pbx homeodomain proteins families cooperatively bind a cAMP-responsive sequence (CRS1) from bovine *CYP17*. *J Biol Chem* (1998) **273**:7941–8. doi:10.1074/jbc.273.14.7941
64. Kagawa N, Waterman MR. Purification and characterization of a transcription factor which appears to regulate cAMP responsiveness of the human *CYP21B* gene. *J Biol Chem* (1992) **15**:25213–9.
65. Wijesuriya SD, Zhang G, Dardis A, Miller WL. Transcriptional regulatory elements of the human gene for cytochrome P450c21 (steroid 21-hydroxylase) lie within intron 35 of the linked C4B gene. *J Biol Chem* (1999) **274**:38097–106. doi:10.1074/jbc.274.53.38097
66. Wilson TE, Mouw AR, Weaver CA, Milbrandt J, Parker KL. The orphan nuclear receptor NGFI-B regulates expression of the gene encoding steroid 21-hydroxylase. *Mol Cell Biol* (1993) **13**:861–8. doi:10.1128/MCB.13.2.861
67. Parker KL, Schimmer BP, Chaplin DD, Seidman JG. Characterization of a regulatory region of the steroid 21-hydroxylase gene. *J Biol Chem* (1986) **261**:15353–5.
68. Schimmer BP, Parker KL. Promoter elements of the mouse 21-hydroxylase (Cyp-21) gene involved in cell-selective and cAMP-dependent gene expression. *J Steroid Biochem Mol Biol* (1992) **43**:937–50. doi:10.1016/0960-0760(92)90322-A
69. Milstone DS, Shaw SK, Parker KL, Szyf M, Seidman JG. An element regulating adrenal-specific steroid 21-hydroxylase expression is located within the slp gene. *J Biol Chem* (1992) **267**:21924–7.
70. Rice DA, Mouw AR, Bogerd AM, Parker KL. A shared promoter element regulates the expression of three steroidogenic enzymes. *Mol Endocrinol* (1991) **5**:1552–61. doi:10.1210/mend-5-10-1552
71. Udhane S, Kempna P, Hofer G, Mullis PE, Flück CE. Differential regulation of human 3β-hydroxysteroid dehydrogenase type 2 for steroid hormone biosynthesis by starvation and cyclic AMP stimulation: studies in the human adrenal NCI-H295R cell model. *PLoS One* (2013) **9**:e68691. doi:10.1371/journal.pone.0068691
72. Lala DS, Rice DA, Parker KL. Steroidogenic factor I, a key regulator of steroidogenic enzyme expression, is the mouse homolog of fushi tarazu-factor I. *Mol Endocrinol* (1992) **6**:1249–58. doi:10.1210/mend.6.8.1406703
73. Morohashi K, Honda S, Inomata Y, Handa H, Omura T. A common trans-acting factor, Ad4-binding protein, to the promoters of steroidogenic P-450s. *J Biol Chem* (1992) **25**:17913–9.
74. Hammer GD, Krylova I, Zhang Y, Darimont BD, Simpson K, Weigel NL, et al. Phosphorylation of the nuclear receptor SF-1 modulates cofactor recruitment: integration of hormone signalling in reproduction and stress. *Mol Cell* (1999) **3**:521–6. doi:10.1016/S1097-2765(00)80480-3
75. Ito M, Yu RN, Jameson JL. Steroidogenic factor-I contains a carboxy-terminal transcriptional activation domain that interacts with steroid receptor coactivator-1. *Mol Endocrinol* (1998) **12**:290–301. doi:10.1210/mend.12.2.0059
76. Monte D, DeWitte F, Hum DW. Regulation of the human P450scc gene by steroidogenic factor 1 is mediated by CBP/p300. *J Biol Chem* (1998) **273**:4585–91. doi:10.1074/jbc.273.8.4585
77. Clark BJ, Combs R. Angiotensin II and cyclic adenosine 3′,5′-monophosphate induce human steroidogenic acute regulatory protein transcription through a common steroidogenic factor-1 element. *Endocrinology* (1999) **140**:4390–8. doi:10.1210/endo.140.10.7085
78. Caron KM, Ikeda Y, Soo SC, Stocco DM, Parker KL, Clark BJ. Characterization of the promoter region of the mouse gene encoding the steroidogenic acute regulatory protein. *Mol Endocrinol* (1997) **11**:137–47. doi:10.1210/mend.11.2.9880
79. Sandhoff TW, Hales DB, Hales KH, McLean MP. Transcriptional regulation of steroidogenic acute regulatory protein gene by steroidogenic factor 1. *Endocrinology* (1998) **139**:4820–31. doi:10.1210/endo.139.12.6345
80. Hu MC, Hsu NC, Pai CI, Wang CK, Chung B. Functions of the upstream and proximal steroidogenic factor 1 (SF-1)-binding sites in the CYP11A1 promoter in basal transcription and hormonal response. *Mol Endocrinol* (2001) **15**:812–28. doi:10.1210/me.2002-0055
81. Takayama K, Morohashi K, Honda S, Hara N, Omura T. Contribution of Ad4BP, a steroidogenic cell-specific transcription factor, to regulation of the human CYP11A and bovine CYP11B genes through their distal promoters. *J Biochem* (1994) **116**:193–203.
82. Huang Y, Hu M, Hsu N, Wang CL, Chung B. Action of hormone responsive sequence in 2.3 kb promoter of CYP11A1. *Mol Cell Endocrinol* (2001) **175**:205–10. doi:10.1016/S0303-7207(01)00388-4
83. Jimenez P, Saner K, Mayhew B, Rainey WE. GATA-6 is expressed in the human adrenal and regulates transcription of genes required for adrenal androgen biosynthesis. *Endocrinology* (2003) **144**:4285–8. doi:10.1210/en.2003-0472
84. Hiroi N, Kino T, Bassett M, Rainey WE, Phung M, Abu-Asab M, et al. Pituitary homeobox factor 1, a novel transcription factor in the adrenal regulating steroid 11beta-hydroxylase. *Horm Metab Res* (2003) **35**:273–8. doi:10.1055/s-2003-41301
85. Hashimoto T, Morohashi K, Takayama K, Honda S, Wada T, Handa H, et al. Cooperative transcription activation between Ad1, CRE-like element, and other elements in the CYP11B gene promoter. *J Biochem* (1992) **12**:573–5.
86. Morohashi K, Zanger UM, Honda S, Hara M, Waterman MR, Omura T. Activation of CYP11A and CYP11B gene promoters by the steroidogenic cell-specific transcription factor, Ad4BP. *Mol Endocrinol* (1993) **7**:1196–204. doi:10.1210/mend.7.9.8247022

87. Rodriguez H, Hum DW, Staels B, Miller WL. Transcription of the human genes for cytochrome P450scc and P450c17 is regulated differently in human adrenal NCI-H295 cells than in mouse adrenal Y1 cells. *J Clin Endocrinol Metab* (1997) **82**:365–71. doi:10.1210/jcem.82.2.3721
88. Rice DA, Kronenberg MS, Mouw AR, Aitken LD, Franklin A, Schimmer BP, et al. Multiple regulatory elements determine adrenocortical expression of steroid 21-hydroxylase. *J Biol Chem* (1990) **265**:8052–8.
89. Parissenti AM, Parker KL, Schimmer BP. Identification of promoter elements in the mouse 21-hydroxylase (Cyp21) gene that require a functional cyclic adenosine 3′,5′-monophosphate-dependent protein kinase. *Mol Endocrinol* (1993) **7**:283–90. doi:10.1210/mend.7.2.8385740
90. Parker KL, Schimmer BP. Transcriptional regulation of the genes encoding the cytochrome P-450 steroid hydroxylases. *Vitam Horm* (1995) **51**:339–70. doi:10.1016/S0083-6729(08)61044-4
91. Meyer TE, Habener JF. Cyclic adenosine 3′,5′-monophosphate response element binding protein (CREB) and related transcription-activating deoxyribonucleic acid-binding proteins. *Endocr Rev* (1993) **14**:269–90. doi:10.1210/edrv-14-3-269
92. Montminy M. Transcriptional regulation by cyclic AMP. *Annu Rev Biochem* (1997) **66**:807–22. doi:10.1146/annurev.biochem.66.1.807
93. Lalli E, Sassone-Corsi P. Signal transduction and gene regulation: the nuclear response to cAMP. *J Biol Chem* (1994) **269**:17359–62.
94. Sugawara T, Holt JA, Driscoll D, Strauss JF III, Lin D, Miller WL, et al. Human steroidogenic acute regulatory protein: functional activity in COS-1 cells, tissue-specific expression, and mapping of the structural gene to 8p11.2 and a pseudogene to chromosome 13. *Proc Natl Acad Sci U S A* (1995) **92**:4778–82. doi:10.1073/pnas.92.11.4778
95. Silverman E, Yivgi-Ohana N, Sher N, Bell M, Eimerl S, Orly J. Transcriptional activation of the steroidogenic acute regulatory protein (StAR) gene: GATA-4 and CCAAT/enhancer-binding protein beta confer synergistic responsiveness in hormone-treated rat granulosa and HEK293 cell models. *Mol Cell Endocrinol* (2006) **252**:92–101. doi:10.1016/j.mce.2006.03.008
96. Manna PR, Stocco DM. The role of JUN in the regulation of PRKCC-mediated STAR expression and steroidogenesis in mouse Leydig cells. *J Mol Endocrinol* (2008) **41**:329–41. doi:10.1677/JME-08-0077
97. Hummler E, Cole TJ, Blendy JA, Ganss R, Aguzzi A, Schmid W, et al. Targeted mutation of the CREB gene: compensation within the CREB/ATF family of transcription factors. *Proc Natl Acad Sci U S A* (1994) **91**:5647–51. doi:10.1073/pnas.91.12.5647
98. Foulkes NS, Sassone-Corsi P. More is better: activators and repressors from the same gene. *Cell* (1992) **68**:411–4. doi:10.1016/0092-8674(92)90178-F
99. Meyer TE, Habener JF. Cyclic AMP response element binding protein CREB and modulator protein CREM are products of distinct genes. *Nucleic Acids Res* (1992) **20**:6106. doi:10.1093/nar/20.22.6106
100. Walker WH, Habener JF. Role of transcription factors CREB and CREM in cAMP-regulated transcription during spermatogenesis. *Trends Endocrinol Metab* (1996) **7**:133–8. doi:10.1016/1043-2760(96)00035-5
101. Sugawara T, Sakuragi N, Minakami H. CREM confers cAMP responsiveness in human steroidogenic acute regulatory protein expression in NCI-H295R cells rather than SF-1/Ad4BP. *J Endocrinol* (2006) **191**:327–327. doi:10.1677/joe.1.06601
102. Della Fazia MA, Servillo G, Sassone-Corsi P. Cyclic AMP signalling and cellular proliferation: regulation of CREB and CREM. *FEBS Lett* (1997) **410**:22–4. doi:10.1016/S0014-5793(97)00445-6
103. Gonzalez GA, Montminy MR. Cyclic AMP stimulates somatostatin gene transcription by phosphorylation of CREB at serine 133. *Cell* (1989) **59**:675–80. doi:10.1016/0092-8674(89)90013-5
104. Chrivia JC, Kwok RP, Lamb N, Hagiwara M, Montminy MR, Goodman RH. Phosphorylated CREB binds specifically to the nuclear protein CBP. *Nature* (1993) **365**:855–9. doi:10.1038/365855a0
105. Parker D, Ferreri K, Nakajima T, LaMorte VJ, Evans R, Koerber SC, et al. Phosphorylation of CREB at Ser-133 induces complex formation with CREB-binding protein via a direct mechanism. *Mol Cell Biol* (1996) **16**:694–703. doi:10.1128/MCB.16.2.694
106. Hiroi H, Christenson LK, Strauss JF III. Regulation of transcription of the steroidogenic acute regulatory protein (StAR) gene: temporal and spatial changes in transcription factor binding and histone modification. *Mol Cell Endocrinol* (2004) **215**:119–26. doi:10.1016/j.mce.2003.11.014
107. Bonni A, Ginty DD, Dudek H, Greenberg ME. Serine 133-phosphorylated CREB induces transcription via a cooperative mechanism that may confer specificity to neurotrophin signals. *Mol Cell Neurosci* (1995) **6**:168–83. doi:10.1006/mcne.1995.1015
108. Johannessen M, Delghandi MP, Moens U. What turns CREB on? *Cell Signal* (2004) **16**:1211–27. doi:10.1016/j.cellsig.2004.05.001
109. Struthers RS, Vale WW, Arias C, Sawchenko PE, Montminy MR. Somatotroph hypoplasia and dwarfism in transgenic mice expressing a nonphosphorylatable CREB mutant. *Nature* (1991) **350**:622–4. doi:10.1038/350622a0
110. Sher N, Yivgi-Ohana N, Orly J. Transcriptional regulation of the cholesterol side chain cleavage cytochrome P450 gene (*CYP11A1*) revisited: binding of GATA, cyclic adenosine 3′,5′-monophosphate response element-binding protein and activating protein (AP)-1 proteins to a distal novel cluster of cis-regulatory elements potentiates AP-2 and steroidogenic Factor-1-dependent gene expression in the rodent placenta and ovary. *Mol Endocrinol* (2007) **21**:948–62. doi:10.1210/en.2008-054
111. Osada S, Yamamoto H, Nishihara T, Imagawa M. DNA binding specificity of the CCAAT/enhancer-binding protein transcription factor family. *J Biol Chem* (1996) **271**:3891–6. doi:10.1074/jbc.271.7.3891
112. Piontkewitz Y, Enerback S, Hedin L. Expression of CCAAT enhancer binding protein-alpha (C/EBP alpha) in the rat ovary: implications for follicular development and ovulation. *Dev Biol* (1996) **179**:288–96. doi:10.1006/dbio.1996.0258
113. Nalbant D, Williams SC, Stocco DM, Khan SA. Luteinizing hormone dependent gene regulation in Leydig cells may be mediated by CCAAT/enhancer-binding protein-beta. *Endocrinology* (1998) **139**:272–9. doi:10.1210/endo.139.1.5663
114. Wilson HL, Roesler WJ. CCAAT/enhancer binding proteins: do they possess intrinsic cAMP-inducible activity? *Mol Cell Endocrinol* (2002) **188**:15–20. doi:10.1016/S0303-7207(01)00754-7
115. Reinhart AJ, Williams SC, Clark BJ, Stocco DM. SF-1 (steroidogenic factor-1) and C/EBP beta (CCAAT/enhancer binding protein-b) cooperate to regulate the murine StAR (steroidogenic acute regulatory) promoter. *Mol Endocrinol* (1999) **13**:729–41. doi:10.1210/mend.13.5.0279
116. Silverman E, Eimerl S, Orly J. CCAAT enhancer-binding protein beta and GATA-4 binding regions within the promoter of the steroidogenic acute regulatory protein (StAR) gene are required for transcription in rat ovarian cells. *J Biol Chem* (1999) **274**:17987–96. doi:10.1074/jbc.274.25.17987
117. Tremblay JJ, Hamel F, Viger RS. Protein kinase A-dependent cooperation between GATA and CCAAT/enhancer-binding protein transcription factors regulates steroidogenic acute regulatory protein promoter activity. *Endocrinology* (2002) **143**:3935–45. doi:10.1210/en.2002-220413
118. Hsu CC, Lu CW, Huang BM, Wu MH, Tsai SJ. Cyclic adenosine 3′,5′-monophosphate response element-binding protein and CCAAT/enhancer-binding protein mediate prostaglandin E2-induced steroidogenic acute regulatory protein expression in endometriotic stromal cells. *Am J Pathol* (2008) **173**:433–41. doi:10.2353/ajpath.2008.080199
119. Sterneck E, Tessarollo L, Johnson PF. An essential role for C/EBPbeta in female reproduction. *Genes Dev* (1997) **11**:2153–62. doi:10.1101/gad.11.17.2153
120. Shaulian E, Karin M. AP-1 as a regulator of cell life and death. *Nat Cell Biol* (2002) **4**:131–6. doi:10.1038/ncb0502-e131
121. Sassone-Corsi P, Lamph WW, Kamps M, Verma IM. Fos-associated cellular p39 is related to nuclear transcription factor AP-1. *Cell* (1988) **54**:553–60. doi:10.1016/0092-8674(88)90077-3
122. Curran T, Franza BR Jr. Fos and Jun: the AP-1 connection. *Cell* (1998) **55**:395–7. doi:10.1016/0092-8674(88)90024-4
123. Halazonetis TD, Georgopoulos K, Greenberg ME, Leder P. c-Jun dimerizes with itself and with c-Fos, forming complexes of different DNA binding affinities. *Cell* (1988) **55**:917–24. doi:10.1016/0092-8674(88)90147-X
124. Hai T, Curran T. Cross-family dimerization of transcription factors Fos/Jun and ATF/CREB alters DNA binding specificity. *Proc Natl Acad Sci U S A* (1991) **1**:3720–4. doi:10.1016/0092-8674(88)90147-X
125. Gentz R, Rauscher FJ III, Abate C, Curran T. Parallel association of Fos and Jun leucine zippers juxtaposes DNA binding domains. *Science* (1989) **243**:1695–9. doi:10.1126/science.2494702
126. Manna PR, Stocco DM. Crosstalk of CREB and Fos/Jun on a single cis-element: transcriptional repression of the steroidogenic acute regulatory protein gene. *J Mol Endocrinol* (2007) **39**:261–77. doi:10.1677/JME-07-0065

127. Shea-Eaton W, Sandhoff TW, Lopez D, Hales DB, McLean MP. Transcriptional repression of the rat steroidogenic acute regulatory (StAR) protein gene by the AP-1 family member c-Fos. *Mol Cell Endocrinol* (2002) **188**:161–70. doi:10.1016/S0303-7207(01)00715-88
128. Lehoux JG, Fleury A, Ducharme L. The acute and chronic effects of adrenocorticotropin on the levels of messenger ribonucleic acid and protein of steroidogenic enzymes in rat adrenal in vivo. *Endocrinology* (1998) **139**:3913–22. doi:10.1210/endo.139.9.6196
129. Manna PR, Chandrala SP, Jo Y, Stocco DM. cAMP-independent signaling regulates steroidogenesis in mouse Leydig cells in the absence of StAR phosphorylation. *J Mol Endocrinol* (2006) **37**:81–95. doi:10.1677/jme.1.02065
130. Suske G. The Sp-family of transcription factors. *Gene* (1999) **238**:291–300. doi:10.1016/S0378-1119(99)00357-1
131. Kadonaga JT, Jones KA, Tjian R. Promoter-specific activation of RNA polymerase II transcription by Sp1. *Trends Biochem Sci* (1986) **11**:20–3. doi:10.1016/0968-0004(86)90226-4
132. Majello B, De Luca P, Suske G, Lania L. Differential transcriptional regulation of c-myc promoter through the same DNA binding sites targeted by Sp1-like proteins. *Oncogene* (1995) **10**:1841–8.
133. Yu B, Datta PK, Bagchi S. Stability of the Sp3-DNA complex is promoter-specific: Sp3 efficiently competes with Sp1 for binding to promoters containing multiple Sp-sites. *Nucleic Acids Res* (2003) **102**:5368–76. doi:10.1093/nar/gkg706
134. Giatzakis C, Papadopoulos V. Differential utilization of the promoter of peripheral-type benzodiazepine receptor by steroidogenic versus nonsteroidogenic cell lines and the role of Sp1 and Sp3 in the regulation of basal activity. *Endocrinology* (2004) **145**:1113–23. doi:10.1210/en.2003-1330
135. Chou SJ, Lai KN, Chung BC. Characterization of the upstream sequence of the human CYP11A1 gene for cell type-specific expression. *J Biol Chem* (1996) **271**:22125–9. doi:10.1074/jbc.271.36.22125
136. Ahlgren R, Suske G, Waterman MR, Lund J. Role of Sp1 in cAMP-dependent transcriptional regulation of the bovine CYP11A gene. *J Biol Chem* (1999) **274**:19422–8. doi:10.1074/jbc.274.27.19422
137. Liu Z, Simpson ER. Molecular mechanism for cooperation between Sp1 and steroidogenic factor-1 (SF-1) to regulate bovine CYP11A gene expression. *Mol Cell Endocrinol* (1999) **153**:183–96. doi:10.1016/S0303-7207(99)00036-2
138. Urban RJ, Bodenburg Y, Kurosky A, Wood TG, Gasic S. Polypyrimidine tract-binding protein-associated splicing factor is a negative regulator of transcriptional activity of the porcine P450scc insulin-like growth factor response element. *Mol Endocrinol* (2000) **14**:774–82. doi:10.1210/mend.14.6.0485
139. Fluck CE, Miller WL. GATA-4 and GATA-6 modulate tissue-specific transcription of the human gene for P450c17 by direct interaction with Sp1. *Mol Endocrinol* (2004) **18**:1144–57. doi:10.1210/me.2003-0342
140. Zanger UM, Kagawa N, Lund J, Waterman MR. Distinct biochemical mechanisms for cAMP-dependent transcription of CYP17 and CYP21. *FASEB J* (1992) **6**:719–23.
141. Zanaria E, Muscatelli F, Bardoni B, Strom TM, Guioli S, Guo W, et al. An unusual member of the nuclear hormone receptor superfamily responsible for X-linked adrenal hypoplasia congenita. *Nature* (1994) **372**:635–41. doi:10.1038/372635a0
142. Muscatelli F, Strom TM, Walker AP, Zanaria E, Récan D, Meindl A, et al. Mutations in the DAX-1 gene give rise to both X-linked adrenal hypoplasia congenita and hypogonadotropic hypogonadism. *Nature* (1994) **372**:672–6. doi:10.1038/372672a0
143. Zazopoulos E, Lalli E, Stocco DM, Sassone-Corsi P. DNA binding and transcriptional repression by DAX-1 blocks steroidogenesis. *Nature* (1997) **390**:311–5. doi:10.1038/36899
144. Ito M, Yu R, Jameson JL. DAX-1 inhibits SF-1-mediated transactivation via a carboxy-terminal domain that is deleted in adrenal hypoplasia congenita. *Mol Cell Biol* (1997) **17**:1476–83. doi:10.1128/MCB.17.3.1476
145. Lalli E, Melner MH, Stocco DM, Sassone-Corsi P. DAX-1 blocks steroid production at multiple levels. *Endocrinology* (1998) **139**:4237–43. doi:10.1210/en.139.10.4237
146. Lalli E. Role of orphan nuclear receptor DAX-1 in development, physiology and disease. *Adv Biol* (2014). doi:10.1155/2014/582749
147. Ragazzon B, Lefrançois-Martinez AM, Val P, Sahut-Barnola I, Tournaire C, Chambon C, et al. Adrenocorticotropin-dependent changes in SF-1/DAX-1 ratio influence steroidogenic genes expression in a novel model of glucocorticoid-producing adrenocortical cell lines derived from targeted tumorigenesis. *Endocrinology* (2006) **147**:1805–18. doi:10.1210/en.2005-1279
148. Tamai KT, Monaco L, Alastalo TP, Lalli E, Parvinen M, Sassone-Corsi P. Hormonal and developmental regulation of DAX-1 expression in Sertoli cells. *Mol Endocrinol* (1996) **10**:1561–9. doi:10.1210/me.10.12.1561
149. McKenna NJ, O'Malley BW. Nuclear receptor coregulators. *Pure Appl Chem* (2003) **75**:1665–9. doi:10.1351/pac200375111665
150. McKenna NJ, Xu J, Nawaz Z, Tsai SY, Tsai M-J, O'Malley BW. Nuclear receptor coactivators: multiple enzymes, multiple complexes, multiple functions. *J Steroid Biochem Mol Biol* (1999) **69**:3–12. doi:10.1016/S0960-0760(98)00144-7
151. Lonard DM, O'Malley BW. Expanding functional diversity of the coactivators. *Trends Biochem Sci* (2005) **30**:126–32. doi:10.1016/j.tibs.2005.01.001
152. Spencer TE, Jenster G, Burcin MM, Allis CD, Zhou J, Mizzen CA, et al. Steroid receptor coactivator-1 is a histone acetyltransferase. *Nature* (1997) **389**:194–8. doi:10.1038/38304
153. Chen H, Lin RJ, Schiltz RL, Chakravarti D, Nash A, Nagy L, et al. Nuclear receptor coactivator ACTR is a novel histone acetyltransferase and forms a multimeric activation complex with P/CAF and CBP/p300. *Cell* (1997) **90**:569–80. doi:10.1016/S0092-8674(00)80516-4
154. Vo N, Goodman RH. CREB-binding protein and p300 in transcriptional regulation. *J Biol Chem* (2001) **276**:13505–8. doi:10.1074/jbc.R000025200
155. Chen J, Kinyamu K, Archer TK. Changes in attitude, changes in latitude: nuclear receptors remodeling chromatin to regulate transcription. *Mol Endocrinol* (2006) **20**:1–13. doi:10.1210/me.2005-0192
156. Chen H, Lin R, Xie W, Wilpitz D, Evans R. Regulation of hormone-induced histone hyperacetylation and gene activation via acetylation of an acetylase. *Cell* (1999) **98**:675–86. doi:10.1016/S0092-8674(00)80054-9
157. Chen WY, Juan LJ, Chung BC. SF-1 (nuclear receptor 5A1) activity is activated by cyclic AMP via p300-mediated recruitment to active foci, acetylation, and increased DNA binding. *Mol Cell Biol* (2005) **25**:10442–53. doi:10.1128/MCB.25.23.10442-10453.2005
158. An W, Kim J, Roeder RG. Ordered cooperative functions of PRMT1, p300, and CARM1 in transcriptional activation by p53. *Cell* (2004) **117**:735–48. doi:10.1016/j.cell.2004.05.009
159. Perissi V, Rosenfeld MG. Controlling nuclear receptors: the circular logic of cofactor cycles. *Nat Rev Mol Cell Biol* (2005) **6**:542–54. doi:10.1038/nrm1682
160. Bannister AJ, Kouzarides T. The CBP co-activator is a histone acetyltransferase. *Nature* (1996) **384**:641–3. doi:10.1038/384641a0
161. Fronsdal K, Engedal N, Slagsvold T, Saatcioglu F. CREB binding protein is a coactivator for the androgen receptor and mediates cross-talk with AP-1. *J Biol Chem* (1998) **273**:31853–9. doi:10.1074/jbc.273.48.31853
162. Kovacs KA, Steinmann M, Magistretti PJ, Halfon O, Cardinaux JR. CCAAT/enhancer-binding protein family members recruit the coactivator CREBbinding protein and trigger its phosphorylation. *J Biol Chem* (2003) **278**:36959–65. doi:10.1074/jbc.M303147200
163. Gizard F, Lavallee B, DeWitte F, Hum DW. A novel zinc finger protein TReP-132 interacts with CBP/p300 to regulate human CYP11A1 gene expression. *J Biol Chem* (2001) **276**:33881–92. doi:10.1074/jbc.M100113200
164. Shibata H, Ando T, Kurihara I, Suzuki T, Lund J, Morohashi K, et al. Functional role of COUP-TF1, SF-1, and nuclear receptor coregulators in the steroidogenesis of adrenocortical adenomas. In: Nawata H, editor. *Molecular Steroidogenesis. Okamoto MIY*. Tokyo: J Universal Academy Press (2000). p. 345–8.
165. Dammer EB, Leon A, Sewer MB. Coregulator exchange and sphingosine-sensitive cooperativity of steroidogenic factor-1, general control non-derepressed 5, p54, and p160 coactivators regulate cyclic adenosine 3′,5′-monophosphate-dependent cytochrome P450c17 transcription rate. *Mol Endocrinol* (2007) **21**:415–38. doi:10.1210/me.2006-0361
166. Lucki N, Sewer M. The cAMP-responsive element binding protein (CREB) regulates the expression of acid ceramidase (ASAH1) in H295R human adrenocortical cells. *Biochim Biophys Acta* (2009) **1791**:706–13. doi:10.1016/j.bbalip.2009.03.005
167. Sayed SB, Jones PM, Persaud SJ, Whitehouse BJ. Effects of phosphoprotein phosphatase inhibitors on steroidogenesis and StAR protein expression in Y1 cells. *Endocr Res* (1998) **24**:413–4. doi:10.3109/07435809809032624
168. Paz C, Cornejo Maclel F, Mendez C, Podesta EJ. Corticotropin increases protein tyrosine phosphatase activity by a cAMP-dependent

mechanism in rat adrenal gland. *Eur J Biochem* (1999) **265**:911–8. doi:10.1046/j.1432-1327.1999.00759.x

169. Poderoso C, Cornejo Maciel F, Gorostizaga A, Bey P, Paz C, Podestá EJ. The obligatory action of protein tyrosine phosphatases in ACTH-stimulated steroidogenesis is exerted at the level of StAR protein. *Endocr Res* (2002) **28**:413–7. doi:10.1081/ERC-120016816
170. Castillo F, Cano F, Maloberti P, Castilla R, Neuman I, Poderoso C, et al. Tyrosine phosphates act on steroidogenesis through the activation of arachidonic acid release. *Endocr Res* (2004) **30**:623–7. doi:10.1081/ERC-200043795
171. Gorostizaga A, Cornejo Maciel F, Brion L, Maloberti P, Podestá EJ, Paz C. Tyrosine phosphatases in steroidogenic cells: regulation and function. *Mol Cell Endocrinol* (2007) **26**(5–266):131–7. doi:10.1016/j.mce.2006.12.009
172. Cooke M, Mele P, Maloberti P, Duarte A, Poderoso C, Orlando U, et al. Tyrosine phosphatases as key regulators of StAR induction and cholesterol transport: SHP2 as a potential tyrosine phosphatase involved in steroid synthesis. *Mol Cell Endocrinol* (2011) **336**:63–9. doi:10.1016/j.mce.2010.11.030
173. Maloberti P, Castilla R, Castillo F, Cornejo Maciel F, Mendez CF, Paz C, et al. Silencing the expression of mitochondrial acyl-CoA thioesterase I and acyl-CoA synthetase 4 inhibits hormone-induced steroidogenesis. *FEBS J* (2005) **272**:1804–14. doi:10.1111/j.1742-4658.2005.04616.x
174. Mele PG, Dada LA, Paz C, Cymeryng CB, Cornejo Maciel MF, Neuman MI, et al. Site of action of proteinases in the activation of steroidogenesis in rat adrenal gland. *Biochim Biophys Acta* (1996) **29**:260–8. doi:10.1016/0167-4889(95)00177-8
175. Wang XJ, Dyson MT, Jo Y, Eubank DW, Stocco DM. Involvement of 5-lipoxygenase metabolites of arachidonic acid in cyclic AMP-stimulated steroidogenesis and steroidogenic acute regulatory protein gene expression. *J Steroid Biochem Mol Biol* (2003) **85**:159–66. doi:10.1016/S0960-0760(03)00189-4
176. Cornejo Maciel F, Maloberti P, Neuman I, Cano F, Castilla R, Castillo F, et al. An arachidonic acid-preferring acyl-CoA synthetase is a hormone-dependent and obligatory protein in the signal transduction pathway of steroidogenic hormones. *J Mol Endocrinol* (2005) **3**:655–66. doi:10.1677/jme.1.01691
177. Cano F, Poderoso C, Cornejo Maciel F, Castilla R, Maloberti P, Castillo F, et al. Protein tyrosine phosphatases regulate arachidonic acid release, StAR induction and steroidogenesis acting on a hormone-dependent arachidonic acid-preferring acyl-CoA synthetase. *J Steroid Biochem Mol Biol* (2006) **99**:197–202. doi:10.1016/j.jsbmb.2006.01.003
178. Sewer MB, Waterman MR. Adrenocorticotropin/cyclic adenosine 3′,5′-monophosphate-mediated transcription of the human CYP17 gene in the adrenal cortex is dependent on phosphatase activity. *Endocrinology* (2002) **143**:1769–77. doi:10.1210/endo.143.5.8820
179. Sewer MB, Waterman MR. cAMP-dependent transcription of steroidogenic genes in the human adrenal cortex requires a dual-specificity phosphatase in addition to protein kinase A. *J Mol Endocrinol* (2002) **29**:163–74. doi:10.1677/jme.0.0290163
180. Sewer MB, Waterman MR. cAMP-dependent protein kinase enhances CYP17 transcription via MKP-1 activation in H295R human adrenocortical cells. *J Biol Chem* (2003) **7**:8106–11. doi:10.1074/jbc.M210264200

12

Role of Protein Phosphorylation and Tyrosine Phosphatases in the Adrenal Regulation of Steroid Synthesis and Mitochondrial Function

*Cristina Paz, Fabiana Cornejo Maciel, Alejandra Gorostizaga, Ana F. Castillo, M. Mercedes Mori Sequeiros García, Paula M. Maloberti, Ulises D. Orlando, Pablo G. Mele, Cecilia Poderoso and Ernesto J. Podesta**

Departamento de Bioquímica Humana, Facultad de Medicina, Instituto de Investigaciones Biomédicas (INBIOMED), Universidad de Buenos Aires (UBA-CONICET), Ciudad Autónoma de Buenos Aires, Argentina

Correspondence:
Ernesto J. Podesta
ernestopodesta@yahoo.com.ar,
biohrdc@fmed.uba.ar

In adrenocortical cells, adrenocorticotropin (ACTH) promotes the activation of several protein kinases. The action of these kinases is linked to steroid production, mainly through steroidogenic acute regulatory protein (StAR), whose expression and activity are dependent on protein phosphorylation events at genomic and non-genomic levels. Hormone-dependent mitochondrial dynamics and cell proliferation are functions also associated with protein kinases. On the other hand, protein tyrosine dephosphorylation is an additional component of the ACTH signaling pathway, which involves the "classical" protein tyrosine phosphatases (PTPs), such as Src homology domain (SH) 2-containing PTP (SHP2c), and members of the MAP kinase phosphatase (MKP) family, such as MKP-1. PTPs are rapidly activated by posttranslational mechanisms and participate in hormone-stimulated steroid production. In this process, the SHP2 tyrosine phosphatase plays a crucial role in a mechanism that includes an acyl-CoA synthetase-4 (Acsl4), arachidonic acid (AA) release and StAR induction. In contrast, MKPs in steroidogenic cells have a role in the turn-off of the hormonal signal in ERK-dependent processes such as steroid synthesis and, perhaps, cell proliferation. This review analyzes the participation of these tyrosine phosphates in the ACTH signaling pathway and the action of kinases and phosphatases in the regulation of mitochondrial dynamics and steroid production. In addition, the participation of kinases and phosphatases in the signal cascade triggered by different stimuli in other steroidogenic tissues is also compared to adrenocortical cell/ACTH and discussed.

Keywords: PKA, PTPs, ERK1/2, SHP2, mitochondrial dynamics, MKP-1, Acsl4

Abbreviations: AA, arachidonic acid; ACBD3, acyl CoA-binding domain 3; Acot 2, acyl-CoA thioesterase; Acsl4, acyl-CoA synthetase 4; ACTH, adrenocorticotropin; Ang II, angiotensin II; ERK1/2, extracellular signal-regulated kinases 1 and 2; LH, luteinizing hormone; MAM, mitochondria-associated ER membrane; MAPKs, mitogen-activated protein kinases; MEK1/2, mitogen-activated protein kinase kinase 1 and 2; Mfn, mitofusin; MAKP, mitogen-activated protein kinase phosphatase; PAO, phenylarsine oxide; PKA, cAMP-dependent protein kinase; PKC, protein kinase C; PTPs, protein tyrosine phosphatases; PV, pervanadate; SHP2, Src homology domain 2-containing PTP; StAR, steroidogenic acute regulatory protein; ZF, zona fasciculata.

INTRODUCTION

Steroid hormones are synthesized in steroidogenic cells of the adrenal gland, ovary, testis, placenta, and brain and are required for normal reproductive function and body homeostasis. Unlike cells producing polypeptide hormones, which store large amounts of hormone in secretory vesicles ready for rapid release, steroidogenic cells store low amounts of steroids. Thus, a rapid steroidogenic response requires a rapid synthesis of new steroid molecules.

The transport of cholesterol from the outer to the inner mitochondrial membrane (IMM) is the rate-limiting step of steroidogenesis (1, 2), and it is controlled by a complex mechanism that includes phosphorylation–dephosphorylation processes and the interaction of several proteins. Among these, the steroidogenic acute regulatory protein (StAR along this review, also known as STAR or more precisely STARD1) is the most widely studied (3, 4). Indeed, specialized reviews have focused and deeply covered the role of StAR protein in steroidogenesis (3, 4).

Steroid biosynthesis is finely regulated by the phosphorylation–dephosphorylation of intermediate proteins (5–9). In this regard, it is well accepted that steroidogenic hormones act through the activation of serine/threonine (Ser/Thr) protein kinases. In all steroidogenic tissues, phosphorylation-dependent events are required for the acute stimulation of steroid biosynthesis through the activation of protein kinases, including cAMP-dependent protein kinase (PKA), protein kinase C (PKC), calcium/calmodulin-dependent protein kinase, and mitogen-activated protein kinases (MAPKs). Adrenocorticotropic hormone (ACTH) and luteinizing hormone (LH) [or its surrogate chorionic gonadotropin (CG)] signal transduction pathways include PKA-dependent phosphorylation events in adrenal and Leydig cells, respectively (10–12) In the adrenal zona glomerulosa, aldosterone secretion is stimulated by angiotensin II (Ang II) and K^+, in addition to ACTH. These stimuli promote phosphorylation events, which are not dependent on cAMP/PKA. Indeed, K^+ activates voltage-operated Ca^{2+} channels, while Ang II, bound to Ang II type 1 receptors, acts through the inositol 1,4,5-trisphosphate IP_3–Ca^{2+}/calmodulin system (13). In other words, steroid biosynthesis is modulated by hormones, ions, or growth factors through the posttranslational phosphorylation of proteins, while the question that arises is how these phosphorylation events can lead a specific signal to its mitochondrial site of action.

Signal transduction pathways in eukaryotic cells include protein phosphorylation as an integral component regulated by the delicate balance between protein kinases and phosphatases activity. Thereby, many cellular responses require a coordinated cross talk between Ser/Thr and Tyr kinases and phosphatases activity.

In this context, this article will discuss the role of protein phosphorylation–dephosphorylation in cellular biology and endocrine function of steroidogenic cells.

PROTEIN PHOSPHORYLATION

Kinases Involved in StAR Phosphorylation

Since the middle 80s, Orme-Johnson and her group were pioneers describing the relevance of the rapid induction of a 30-kDa protein in adrenal cortex after ACTH stimulation (14) and Leydig cells stimulated by cAMP (15). After these first discoveries, this group demonstrated that this protein is accumulated in mitochondria after hormone stimulation and processed to render two isoforms of 32 and 30 kDa (16, 17). Later, Stocco and Clark provided important data on the crucial role of this protein on the acute regulation of steroidogenesis and also on its molecular aspects. Since this protein is essential for cholesterol transport to the IMM and consequently for steroid synthesis, it was named StAR (3). Even when StAR has been widely identified as a phosphoprotein, the exact role of phosphorylation in StAR protein activity and hence cholesterol transport to the IMM still remains to be fully elucidated.

It is well established that non-genomic effects of PKA mainly involve posttranslational modifications of StAR protein. In fact, PKA phosphorylates murine and human StAR at specific residues such as Ser56/57 and Ser194/195 (18, 19). Moreover, genomic effects of PKA are known to include not only *STAR* gene (also known as *STARD1* gene) transcription but also the transcriptional regulation of several steroidogenic-related genes (20). Even if cAMP-dependent signaling is the major pathway in steroid biosynthesis stimulated by ACTH and LH/CG, and PKA phosphorylation sites in StAR protein are well described, it is noteworthy that StAR sequence also contains putative phosphorylation sites for PKC, cGMP-dependent protein kinase or protein kinase G (PKG), casein kinase I and II, and cyclin-dependent kinase 5 (Cdk5), as it was described elsewhere for eukaryotic phosphoproteins using database Expasy Prosite[1] (21). Although the presence of these consensus sites might indicate StAR as a possible substrate for the respective kinases, the occurrence of this phosphorylation *in vivo* and its impact on steroid production remain uncertain.

Recent studies by Sasaki et al. – using a transgenic model with a bacterial artificial chromosome expressing either wild-type (WT) StAR or mutant StAR S194A to rescue StAR knockout mice – have demonstrated that Ser194, a conserved site among species, is an essential residue for normal StAR function in mice adrenal cortex and testis (22). These data indicate that phosphorylation of the Ser194/195 residues of StAR may account, at least in part, for the immediate increase in cholesterol side chain cleavage as a result of enhanced StAR protein activity. Consistent with these results, it has been demonstrated that the mutation in Ser195 in human mature StAR protein, which lacks the leader peptide, reduces pregnenolone production, as determined by an *in vitro* assay using mitochondria isolated from MA-10 Leydig cells (23). Strikingly, when cholesterol binding to StAR is measured with fluorescent or radioactive cholesterol, purified mutant S195A and WT StAR display equal binding activity. As determined by StAR structural analyses, Ser195 lies in a short loop opposite to the C-α helix, which is essential for cholesterol binding. Therefore, the addition of phosphate-negative charge in this Ser might influence StAR activity by modifying its interaction with hypothetical mitochondrial partners such as ACBD3 (previously known as peripheral benzodiazepine receptor-associated protein, PAP7)

[1] http://expasy.org

(24). This could, in turn, anchor PKA to Ser194/195, rather than alter cholesterol binding to the sterol-binding pocket (23).

In the same line, work by Stocco's group has explored the regulation mechanism of StAR expression and steroidogenesis in conjunction with PKA and PKC pathways in MA-10 Leydig cells (25). This study shows that PKC-dependent induction of steroid synthesis is low when compared to that observed with PKA signaling, but it is capable of enhance LH/CG- and/or cAMP-stimulated steroidogenic response. On the one hand, the activation of PKC markedly increases StAR expression, but not phospho-StAR, with only a modest increase in progesterone production. On the other hand, PKA activation triggers a substantial increase in the band of StAR phosphorylated in Ser194 (25).

Role of ERKs in the Regulation of StAR Protein and Steroid Biosynthesis

In addition to PKA activation importance for trophic hormone-stimulated steroid biosynthesis, it is also known that extracellular signal-regulated kinases 1 and 2 (ERK1/2) and upstream activator mitogen-activated protein kinase kinase 1 and 2 (MEK1/2) participate in the regulation of steroidogenesis. Indeed, several reports describe the role of members of the MAPK family in the regulation of steroid synthesis acting at both genomic and non-genomic levels.

One of the first published works in the field indicates that cAMP-induced steroid synthesis depends on ERKs phosphorylation and activation (26). These authors show that adenylyl cyclase activation with forskolin promotes a time-dependent increase in ERK activity and translocation of this enzyme to the nucleus in mouse adrenocortical Y1 cells. Similarly, Roy et al. have demonstrated that ACTH receptor activation leads to rapid ERK1/2 phosphorylation in primary cultures of human fasciculata cells (27), an effect also observed in a human adrenocortical H295R cell line (28). Moreover, Ang II also promotes MAPK activation in adrenal glomerulosa cells (29, 30). Thus, ERK activation seems to be a common event in the stimulation of different steroidogenic systems.

Although already demonstrated, PKA involvement in ERK activation continues to generate controversy; Le and Shimmer have shown that ACTH increases MEK and ERK phosphorylation in Y1 adrenocortical murine cells. This effect has also been detected in Kin-8 cells, a PKA-deficient mutant Y1-derived cell line (31), which suggests that ERK activation is independent of PKA activity. H295R adrenocortical cells exhibit only a very modest cAMP response to ACTH, yet ERK1/2 response is immediate and consistent. ERK activation is minimally reduced by PKA inhibitor H89, but unaffected by PKC and calcium inhibitors. Thus, ACTH-induced ERK1/2 activation in H295R cells does not appear to depend on the mechanism by which most G protein-coupled receptors activate ERK1/2, but does seem to depend on receptor internalization (28). On the other hand, Roy et al. have demonstrated the participation of PKA in ERK activation in human fasciculata cells (27).

A role for ERK activity has also been demonstrated in adrenal and gonadal steroidogenesis. Gyles et al. have shown that ERK activation results in enhanced phosphorylation of steroidogenic factor 1 (SF-1) and increased steroid production through increased transcription of the *STAR* gene in Y1 cells (26). The activation of the ERK/MEK pathway correlates with an increase in StAR mRNA levels, StAR protein accumulation, and steroidogenesis. Similarly, ERK inhibition leads to a reduction in the levels of forskolin-stimulated StAR mRNA, StAR protein, and steroid secretion (26).

Luteinizing hormone receptor cascade activation in Leydig cells also promotes ERK1/2 phosphorylation, which is mediated by PKA through Ras activation (32). More recently, and using mice with a Leydig-specific deletion of MEK1/2 as an experimental model, Yamashita et al. have concluded that the MEK/ERK pathway is critical for maintaining a functional population of adult Leydig cells and fertility (33).

In agreement with findings in adrenocortical cells (26), Martinelle et al. have demonstrated the functional role of the ERK cascade in human CG (hCG)-induced steroidogenesis in primary cultures of immature rat Leydig cells (34). In this system, inhibition of MEK1/2 by U0126 suppresses several cellular responses to hCG.

In turn, 3-day treatment with Ang II in cultured rat adrenal glomerulosa cells increases aldosterone secretion through a mechanism involving both ERK1/2 and p38 MAPK pathways (30). In addition, the effect of Ang II on aldosterone synthesis also requires ERK1/2 activity in primary cultures of glomerulosa bovine cells (29).

Even though several reports support a role for ERK1/2 in StAR mRNA induction and steroid biosynthesis, other studies show controversial results. Indeed, it has been demonstrated that MEK1/2 inhibitors, such as U0126 and PD98059, enhance the expression of StAR protein in MTLC-1 and primary Leydig cells (35). Also, in MA-10 Leydig cells stimulated with dibutyryl cAMP, inhibition of ERK1/2 activity increases *STAR* gene expression (25). Similarly, Seger et al. have demonstrated that ERK signaling cascade inhibits CG-stimulated steroidogenesis in granulosa-derived cell lines (36). Taken together, the discrepancies on the role of ERK1/2 in StAR transcription might be due to different experimental conditions and cellular types, which generate different factor availability, such as transcription factors required for StAR expression. Nevertheless, the results of Yamashita et al. strongly support the requirement of ERK for StAR expression and steroidogenesis (33). Indeed, they analyzed the role of ERK1/2 on steroidogenesis and fertility using as experimental models knockout mice carrying a deletion for MEK1/2 in Leydig cells and primary culture of Leydig cells isolated from these knockout mice. This study demonstrates that the deletion of MEK1/2 and concomitant reduction of phospho-ERK1/2 levels decreased testicular expression of several Leydig cells markers, including StAR protein. Then, a similar experimental model based on transgenic mouse should be a powerful tool to univocally demonstrate the role of ERK1/2 on ACTH action on steroidogenesis and cell growth.

Extracellular signal-regulated kinase activity seems to regulate key steroidogenic transcription factors by non-genomic and genomic actions. *STAR* gene transcriptional regulation requires transcription factors already present in the cell, which are activated by posttranslational modifications, such as SF1, and others which must be *de novo* synthesized, e.g., NUR77, encoded by *Nr4a1* gene (37). Finally, it has been pharmacologically and molecularly demonstrated that ERK1/2 participates in cAMP-induced *Nr4a1* expression in both MA-10 Leydig and Y1 adrenocortical cells (38), in addition to SF-1 activation (26).

In addition to their role in steroid biosynthesis, ERK1/2 is also involved in adrenal cell proliferation and growth (39–41). ACTH stimulates adrenal growth *in vivo*, whereas *in vitro* ACTH has an inhibitory effect on adrenal cell proliferation. In serum-starved Y1 cells, a short pulse of ACTH produces a mitogenic effect, which is preceded by the rapid activation of ERK1/2 (39). This result is in accordance with the requirement of ERK activation for cell proliferation. However, it is well documented that ACTH-mediated ERK activation is a transient process in Y1 cells. Thus, the early ERK activation could trigger StAR induction, steroidogenesis, and also cell proliferation, while the following decrease in pERK levels could contribute to the inhibition of cell proliferation mediated by prolonged exposure to ACTH.

ERK-Mediated Phosphorylation of StAR Protein

The activation of the MEK1/2–ERK1/2 cascade appears to enhance steroid synthesis; nevertheless, the requirement of MEK1/2 and ERK1/2 cascade for the induction of *STAR* gene expression is less evident. Although it is well known the regulatory role of PKA on StAR protein activity, also this MEK1/2 and ERK1/2 cascade has been unveiled as a new mechanism of StAR activity modulation.

Our group has reported the role of MEK1/2–ERK1/2 cascade in the hCG/LH stimulation of StAR protein activity and steroidogenesis (42). In line with reports by Manna et al. and Martinelle et al. (25, 34), our work has shown that PKA acts upstream the stimulation of MEK and ERK activities. The inhibition of MEK1/2 on stimulated progesterone synthesis is not mediated by inhibition of PKA, as this enzyme activity is not altered in the presence of both inhibitors, U0126 and PD98095 (42).

Using a different strategy to study the role of active ERK1/2 in steroidogenesis, the overexpression of a WT form of ERK2 in MA-10 Leydig cells was performed. We observed an increase in steroid production stimulated by submaximal concentration of cAMP (42). Furthermore, an inactive form of ERK2, the H230R variant, which fails to interact with MEK1, but retains the ability to interact with MEK2 in a weakened fashion, does not produce the effect of WT ERK2 (42).

In short, both kinases, PKC and PKA, are capable of phosphorylating ERK1/2 through MEK1/2 activation (25, 32). ERK1/2 activity is involved in *STAR* gene expression induced by PKC or PKA activation, while a relevant role in StAR protein phosphorylation is attributed to PKA signaling pathway (25).

In summary, it is recognized that the ERK1/2 signaling cascade involved in regulating StAR expression and steroid synthesis is mediated by multiple factors and pathways, and is stimulus-specific.

MEK1/2 and ERK1/2 at the Mitochondria

The site of action of MEK inhibitors appears to be downstream of PKA activation and before of cholesterol transport, which implies that one of the targets may be located at the mitochondria. Gyles et al. have observed that activation of adenylyl cyclase causes a time-dependent increase in ERK activity and its localization from cytoplasm to nucleus (26), and our group has further proven a temporal ERK1/2 activation localized in the mitochondria, which is obligatory for PKA-mediated steroid synthesis in Leydig cells (42). Worth pointing out, the phosphorylation of mitochondrial ERK occurs before the increase in steroid production, and the hormone dose that is required for ERK activation at the mitochondria is the equivalent for eliciting steroid synthesis. Phosphorylated ERK1/2 (pERK1/2) is located in the cytosol, mitochondria, and, in lower proportion, in the nuclear fractions after cAMP stimulation. In the mitochondria and the cytosol, an early peak in ERK1/2 phosphorylation is followed by a slow progressive signal reduction during the first hour of cAMP incubation, a profile similar to that observed in hCG stimulation, leading to pERK1/2 activation. In contrast, pERK1/2 is mainly localized in the cytosol and nucleus, after epidermal growth factor (EGF) stimulation. Two different pools of MEK1/2 and pMEK1/2 have been found to be constitutively present in the cytosol and mitochondria. Remarkably, MEK1/2 differential distribution triggers different responses upon cellular stimulation (42).

Poderoso and coworkers have also shown that cAMP clearly induces sustained MEK1/2 phosphorylation in mitochondria, with a minor effect on the cytosolic kinases. Conversely, EGF induces a prolonged and strong cytosolic MEK1/2 activation, but only a discrete phosphorylation, in mitochondria. Although both EGF and cAMP increase total cytosolic MEK1/2, only EGF promotes its phosphorylation in this subcellular fraction (42).

The inhibition of PKA activity with the compound H89 and by PKA knockdown experiments diminishes the increase in mitochondrial pMEK1/2 and pERK1/2 after cAMP action (42). In agreement, the increase in mitochondrial PKA activity occurs after 5 min of cAMP action in parallel with the appearance of the phosphorylated forms of MEK1/2 and ERK1/2 in this organelle.

In regard to PKA activity and subcellular organization, a family of proteins named A-kinase anchor proteins (AKAPs) enhances cAMP-dependent pathways (43, 44). AKAPs raise cAMP signal by anchoring PKA near its cellular substrate, while mouse-derived AKAP121 binds PKA to the mitochondrial outer surface (45, 46). In addition, purified AKAP121 KH domain binds the 3′-untranslated regions of transcripts encoding the Fo-f subunit of mitochondrial ATP synthase and manganese superoxide dismutase (47). A special member of the AKAP family, AKAP121, can be anchored to mitochondria and may compartmentalize PKA and other proteins on the outer mitochondria membrane (OMM) (48). In Leydig cells, cAMP-induced StAR expression and steroidogenesis were found to correlate with the extent of AKAP 121 expression (49). Expression and role of AKAP121 in H295R cells deserve elucidation. Another relevant AKAP in steroidogenic tissues is the ACBD3 protein, an acyl CoA-binding protein, known previously as PAP7 (24). Human ACBD3 is highly expressed in steroidogenic tissues, where it follows the pattern of PRKAR1A expression, suggesting that it participates in PRKAR1A-mediated tumorigenesis and hypercortisolism (50). Therefore, StAR protein is likely to be phosphorylated at the mitochondria by the activation of a cascade of kinases, including ERK.

StAR Protein as a Substrate of ERK1/2

Steroidogenic acute regulatory protein structural analyses have revealed a consensus sequence that would allow the docking of StAR protein to ERK1/2 and a consensus site for ERK1/2 phosphorylation. A typical docking site known as the D domain (**KTK**LTWL**LSI**) lies between amino acids 235 and 244 and is conserved among MEK1/2, MAPK phosphatase, and ERK substrates (51). Regarding the ERK1/2 phosphorylation site in StAR protein, it was possible to detect only two Ser-Pro motifs, at Ser232 and Ser277, targets for ERK1/2 phosphorylation in the mature form of the murine StAR protein. In accordance with the database Expasy Prosite,[2] Ser232 (PLAGS[232]PS) has a 90% probability of phopshorylation and is adjacent to the docking D domain, while the probability of Ser277 is only 5%. Besides, Ser277 is relatively less conserved among species. In agreement of a predicted StAR–ERK binding, the treatment of subcellular fractions with pERK–GST has shown that StAR protein interacts with pERK1 just in the mitochondrial fraction, but not in the cytosol. Together, MEK phosphorylation PKA-dependent, mitochondrial StAR and pERK1/2 activity increase cholesterol transport and mitochondrial synthesis of progesterone in cell-free assays (42).

In vitro phosphorylation assays using recombinant 30-kDa form of StAR protein and WT and the inactive mutant K71A forms of ERK1 demonstrated that the StAR protein is indeed phosphorylated by ERK1 and not by the K71A mutant. Remarkably, phosphorylation of StAR by ERK1 is dependent on the presence of cholesterol, while phosphorylation by PKA is not. Besides, StAR phosphorylation by PKA does not require previous ERK phosphorylation. By means of directed mutagenesis of Ser 232 (S232A), we demonstrated that this residue is indeed the target of ERK (42).

Expression of S232A mutated form of StAR partially blocks progesterone production enhanced by cAMP treatment in MA-10 cells. In contrast, the StAR mutant in which Ser 232 is replaced by a glutamic acid (S232E) does not produce such effect, which suggests that the negatively charged amino acid partially mimics the negative charge of the phosphate group present in the phospho-Ser (42).

Taking together, PKA phosphorylates StAR protein and also activates mitochondrial MEK1/2. Then, phosphorylated MEK1/2 activates a non-phosphorylated mitochondrial pool of ERK1/2 when the three kinases interact at the OMM, a crucial site for cholesterol transport forming a mitochondrial multi-complex with StAR.

PROTEIN DEPHOSPHORYLATION

Regulation of Protein Tyrosine Phosphatases by Steroidogenic Hormones

The degree of tyrosine phosphorylation of a given protein is the result of the action of protein tyrosine kinases and protein tyrosine phosphatases (PTPs). Protein kinases have been the focus of the research for a long time. Proportionately much less research has focused on protein phosphatases.

Whereas PTPs were initially regarded as household enzymes with constitutive activity and capable of all-substrate dephosphorylation, evidence in favor of tight regulation of PTP activity by various mechanisms is now accumulating. Like protein phosphorylation, dephosphorylation by PTPs is required in a cell compartment-specific manner. Protein–protein interaction domains and compartment-specific targeting domains in PTPs serve to localize PTPs all over the cell compartments (52).

Based on the amino acid sequence of their catalytic domain, PTPs are classified into four groups, Class I, II, III (all Cys-based PTPs), and IV (Asp-based PTPs), each with a specific range of substrates. The largest family is the Class I (Cys-based PTPs), comprising the 38 "classical" PTPs, and the 61 "dual-specificity" PTPs (DSPs), which is the most diverse group in terms of substrate specificity. The group of the classical PTPs, with strict tyrosine specificity, consists of the receptor-like (transmembrane) and non-receptor (intracellular) classes. In the human genome, these PTPs comprise 21 and 17 genes, respectively (52, 53).

The cross talk between pathways that involve Ser/Thr phosphorylation and Tyr dephosphorylation has been described in the regulation of steroid synthesis. Our group has reported that ACTH treatment causes an increase in the activity of PTPs located in the cytosol of adrenal zona fasciculata (ZF). The stimulation is detected very soon after ACTH stimulation (5 min), reaches a maximum (twofold) after 15 min, and returns to basal levels after 30 min (54). Incubation of adrenal ZF with 8Br-cAMP (permeant analog of cAMP) also produces PTPs activation, suggesting that it can be mediated by PKA-dependent phosphorylation. Moreover, detection of PTP activity by in-gel assays has shown at least two ACTH-stimulated soluble PTPs with molecular masses of 115 and 80 kDa (54).

Protein tyrosine phosphatases are regulated by Ser/Thr or Tyr-kinases. Indeed, several PTPs are known to be phosphoproteins *in vivo* (55, 56), which reflects the potential of cross-regulation between kinases and phosphatases, either PTPs or Ser/Thr phosphatases, for the fine control of cellular activity. Among those phospho-PTPs, there is a membrane-bound form, which can be activated by treatment of intact cells with isoproterenol, forskolin, or cAMP analogs (55), and a soluble form of PTP, known as PTP-PEST, which is inhibited after *in vitro* phosphorylation by PKA and in HeLa cells after forskolin or methylisobutylxanthine treatment (56). Our current studies demonstrate the expression of PTP-PEST in Y1 cells and in rat adrenal ZF and suggest that the ACTH-activated PTP of 115 kDa could be PTP-PEST. Furthermore, when paxillin is precipitated from the cytosol of ACTH-treated rats, a PTP of 115 kDa is coprecipitated according to the analyses of precipitate by in-gel PTP assay (57).

The Src homology domain (SH) 2-containing PTP (SHP2) is classified among the non-receptor, classical PTPs. It is widely expressed and plays an essential role in many organisms from lower eukaryotes to mammals (58). In contrast to other PTPs that inactivate intracellular signaling pathways, SHP2 activates them (59). The ACTH-activated PTP of 80 kDa from adrenal ZF has been recognized by a commercially available antibody against SHP2 in Western blot analyses (unpublished results), which

[2] http://expasy.org/prosite/

suggests that SHP2 is a PTP activated by ACTH in rat adrenal ZF. In line with our results, Rocchi et al. have demonstrated SHP2 expression in bovine adrenocortical cells and its activation by ACTH through PKA-dependent phosphorylation (60). Finally, our group has also shown that SHP2 is expressed in MA-10 Leydig cells (61).

PTP Activity and Steroidogenesis

The rapid increase in PTP activity induced by ACTH may prove that this activity is necessary in the stimulation of steroidogenesis. Studies on PTPs role in the acute steroidogenic response to hormones have been performed using incubation of rat adrenal ZF cells with two powerful cell permeant PTP inhibitors, phenylarsine oxide (PAO) and pervanadate (PV), and evaluation of the steroid production upon stimulation by ACTH and 8Br-cAMP. It has been proven that those PTP inhibitors block ACTH- and cAMP-stimulated corticosterone production, but exert no effects on basal steroidogenesis (54). Similar conclusions were obtained using Y1 cells (62, 63).

Phenylarsine oxide and PV also reduce LH/hCG- and cAMP-stimulated steroid production in testicular interstitial cells (64) and in MA-10 cells (65). PTP inhibitors affect StAR induction at the protein and mRNA levels in MA-10 Leydig cells (65), as well as in Y1 cells (63). PTP inhibitors affect neither cell viability nor mitochondrial enzymatic activity evaluated as steroidogenesis triggered by 22-OH-cholesterol treatment. Thus, hormone-dependent steroid synthesis requires PTP activity in a site localized beyond PKA actions and before cholesterol transport across the IMM.

Phenylarsine oxide oxidizes the thiol group of a cysteine present in the active site of all PTPs. Benzyl phosphonic acid (BPA) has a structure very similar to the PTP substrate, exerting its inhibitory action on PTPs by competitive inhibition of the enzyme. However, both inhibitors, PAO and BPA, inhibit Ang II- or K^+-induced steroid synthesis in a dose-dependent fashion in H295R cells, a cell line derived from human ZG tumor (66), and in Y1 cells (63).

Collectively, our group's work demonstrates that steroidogenic stimulus (ACTH, LH, Ang II, and K^+), acting by different signal transduction pathways, conveys on PTPs as common intermediaries (63–66).

In regard of substrates downstream PTP activity, *in vivo* ACTH treatment decreases phosphotyrosine contents in several proteins, one of them identified as paxillin, a focal adhesion protein (54). In Y1 cells, ACTH and cAMP elicit a rapid morphological transition from a flat epithelioid morphology to rounded cells (11). cAMP causes a rapid and selective Tyr dephosphorylation of paxillin in these cells (67). Moreover, the inhibition of PTP activity blocks changes in cell shape promoted by ACTH (67). Taken together, these results indicate that PTP activity is involved in cAMP-dependent paxillin dephosphorylation and this might mediate hormone-stimulated cell shape changes in adrenocortical cells.

In summary, results presented here support the view that the morphological and functional responses to ACTH in adrenocortical cells are intimately linked to and mediated by PTP activity.

Links between PTP Activity and Arachidonic Acid Release

cAMP- and PKA-dependent pathways triggered by trophic hormones in steroidogenic cells stimulate arachidonic acid (AA) release (68, 69). AA and its metabolites take part in the acute stimulation of steroid production. The effect is exerted on both the expression and function of StAR (70, 71). Previously, we proposed that free AA levels in steroidogenic cells are determined by a novel hormone-regulated mechanism (69, 72, 73). This mechanism involves the concerted action of an acyl-CoA synthetase (Acsl4) and an acyl-CoA thioesterase (Acot2). Acsl4 is a long chain fatty acid acyl-CoA synthetase, with high affinity for AA, and it is preferentially expressed in steroidogenic tissues (72, 74). Acot2, a thioesterase that acts on long chain fatty acyl-CoA, associates with the matrix face of mitochondrial cristae (75–77). Acot2 mRNA and protein are present in adrenal cortex, ovary, testis, placenta, and brain, among other tissues. The activity of both enzymes is acutely modified after hormone stimulation of steroidogenic cells. Acot2 is activated by phosphorylation and substrate availability (78), and Acsl4 is rapidly induced after hormone treatment (79).

The activity of Acsl4 and Acot2 are needed for AA release, StAR induction, and steroidogenesis. This statement is supported by the fact that the reduction of the expression of both, Acsl4 and Acot2, causes an inhibition of steroid production in two steroidogenic systems (79, 80). Moreover, this effect is overcome by addition of exogenous AA (80). On the basis of these results, we propose that upon hormone treatment, Acsl4 would convert free AA in AA–CoA. The action of mitochondrial Acot2 on AA–CoA would release AA, specifically in the mitochondria, to increase StAR and steroidogenesis (69).

Our group has also linked the sequential action of PTPs, Acsl4, and StAR to the hormone-stimulated steroid production (66, 81). In Y1 cells, inhibition of PTP activity prevents Acsl4 and StAR induction exerted by 8Br-cAMP (81). Moreover, the effect of PTP inhibition is overcome by addition of exogenous AA (81). These results indicate that there is a consecutive action of PTP and Acsl4 to release AA before StAR induction. Moreover, the effect of PTPs on Acsl4 is also described in Leydig (81) and adrenocortical ZG cells (66) (**Figure 1**), indicating that the action of PTPs on Acsl4 may be a regulatory event that controls the steroidogenesis.

These results brought about a challenge to determine the identity of the PTP involved in the stimulation of steroid synthesis through AA release.

SHP2 Involvement in Steroid Synthesis

By means of overexpression and suppression approaches, SHP2 has been proven to be at least one of the PTPs playing an obligatory role in steroidogenesis. NSC87877, a specific inhibitor of the tyrosine phosphatase SHP2, has been shown to reduce Acsl4 protein levels in Acsl4-rich breast cancer cells and steroidogenic cells. In addition, overexpression of an active form of SHP2 has increased Acsl4 protein levels in MA-10 Leydig cells. SHP2 has to be activated through a cAMP-dependent pathway to exert its effect on Acsl4, which could be specifically attributed to SHP2, as phosphatase knockdown reduces Acsl4

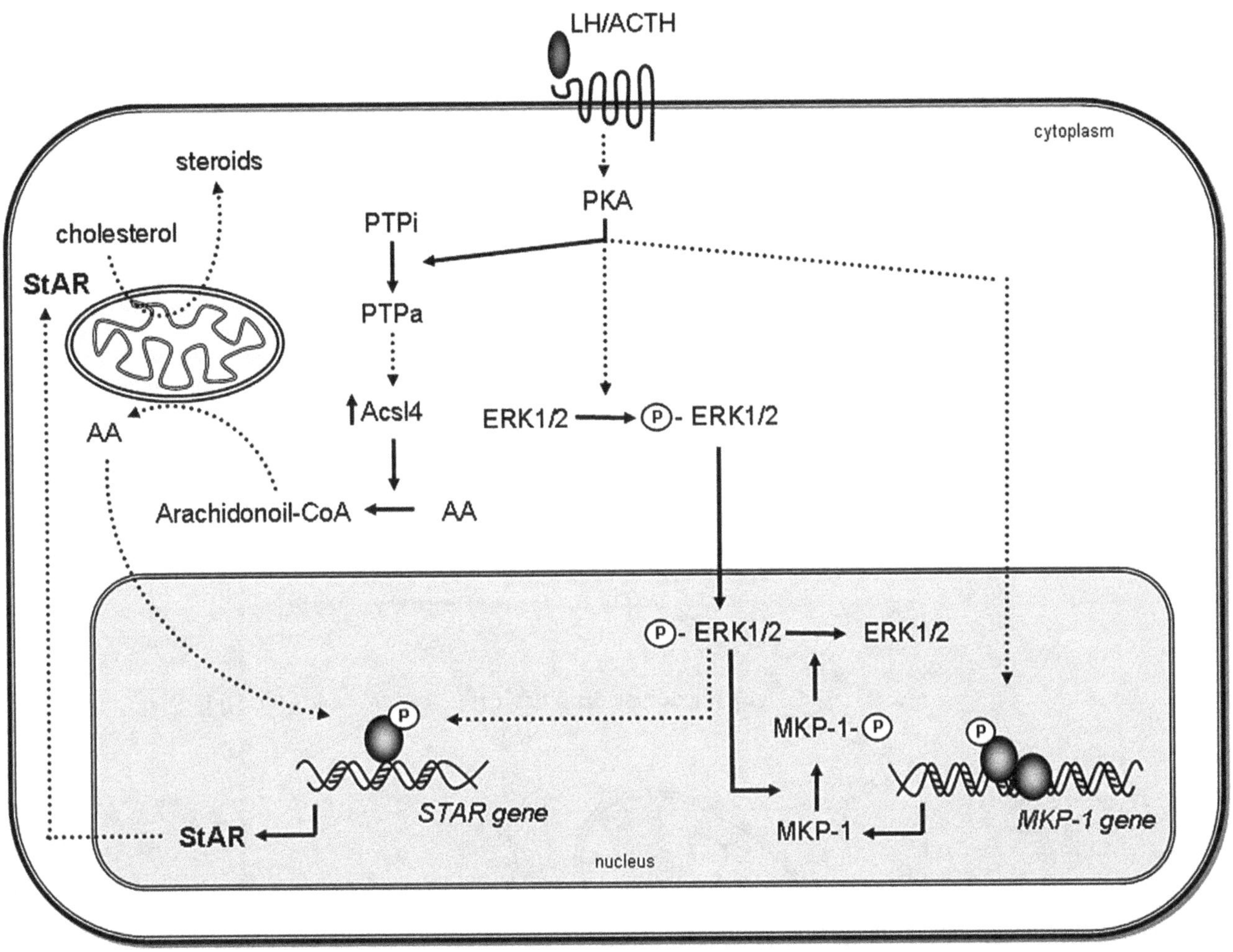

FIGURE 1 | Proposed model for the role of MAPK and phosphatases in steroidogenesis. Steroidogenic hormones trigger the activation of PKA, which leads to the rapid phosphorylation of ERK1/2. Activated ERK (P-ERK) translocates to the nucleus, where it phosphorylates and activates transcription factors, leading to STAR gene induction. Then, StAR protein acts in the mitochondria facilitating steroid synthesis. Simultaneously, activated PKA also induces MKP-1 gene transcription. MKP-1 is stabilized by ERK-mediated phosphorylation; therefore, the stabilization promotes its accumulation in the cell. In turn, MKP-1 dephosphorylates ERK1/2, generating a negative feedback mechanism on its activity, thus terminating MAPK-regulated events involved in steroidogenesis. Inactive PTPs (PTPi) are activated by PKA (PTPa) and participate in Acsl4 regulation, which in turn, through arachidonic acid (AA) metabolism, leads to the increase of StAR gene expression. Direct effects are indicated by solid lines, whereas indirect effects are indicated as dotted lines.

mRNA and protein levels. Through the action on Acsl4 protein levels, SHP2 affects AA–CoA production and metabolism and, finally, the steroidogenic capacity of MA-10 cells: overexpression (or knockdown) of SHP2 leads to increased (or decreased) steroid production (82).

The downregulation of SHP2 also modifies StAR expression. StAR expression increases in MA-10 Leydig cells treated with cAMP, an effect impaired by a short hairpin RNA (shRNA) against SHP2. Also, cAMP treatment causes a significant increase in StAR levels in mock-transfected cells, whereas SHP2 shRNA treatment prevents this effect. The involvement of AA in this process receives strong support from the fact that AA addition to SHP2 shRNA-treated cells bypasses the inhibitory effect produced by SHP2 knockdown (61). In this context, the hypothesis that arises is that a putative transcription factor, inhibited by tyrosine phosphorylation, is involved in ACTH-mediated Acsl4 induction. SHP2 could promote the tyrosine dephosphorylation of this factor, thus increasing steroid synthesis.

The Src homology domain (SH) 2-containing PTP is phosphorylated upon ACTH treatment (60). Moreover, *in vitro* phosphorylation of SHP2 by PKA dramatically increases its phosphatase activity (60). Although the phosphorylation of SHP2 by cAMP-independent kinases has not been demonstrated in steroidogenic cells, SHP2 may be phosphorylated by several different kinases to become Ser/Thr- or Tyr-phosphorylated. Indeed, SHP2 itself is Tyr-phosphorylated and activated through the action of different growth factors (83–86).

The Src homology domain (SH) 2-containing PTP has been identified in mitochondria, being the first evidence of the presence of a tyrosine phosphatase in such organelle (87). Several tyrosine kinases are present in the mitochondria (88). Particularly, c-Src is involved in the modulation of the efficiency of the mitochondrial electron transport chain (88). These data become important as stimulation of steroidogenesis needs energized mitochondria, and AA export and StAR induction need the activity of complexes III and V (73). In case, SHP2 is also located in the mitochondria of steroidogenic cells, this phosphatase would be involved in the regulation of mitochondrial respiration.

The translocation of ERK to mitochondria is abolished by SHP2 knockdown in MA-10 cells. Moreover, the pronounced rearrangement of mitochondria that occurs after hCG stimulation is reduced by the downregulation of SHP2 expression (89). Then, the complete description of the steroid synthesis and secretion after hormone stimulation needs the study of SHP2 activation and mitochondrial reorganization (**Figure 2**).

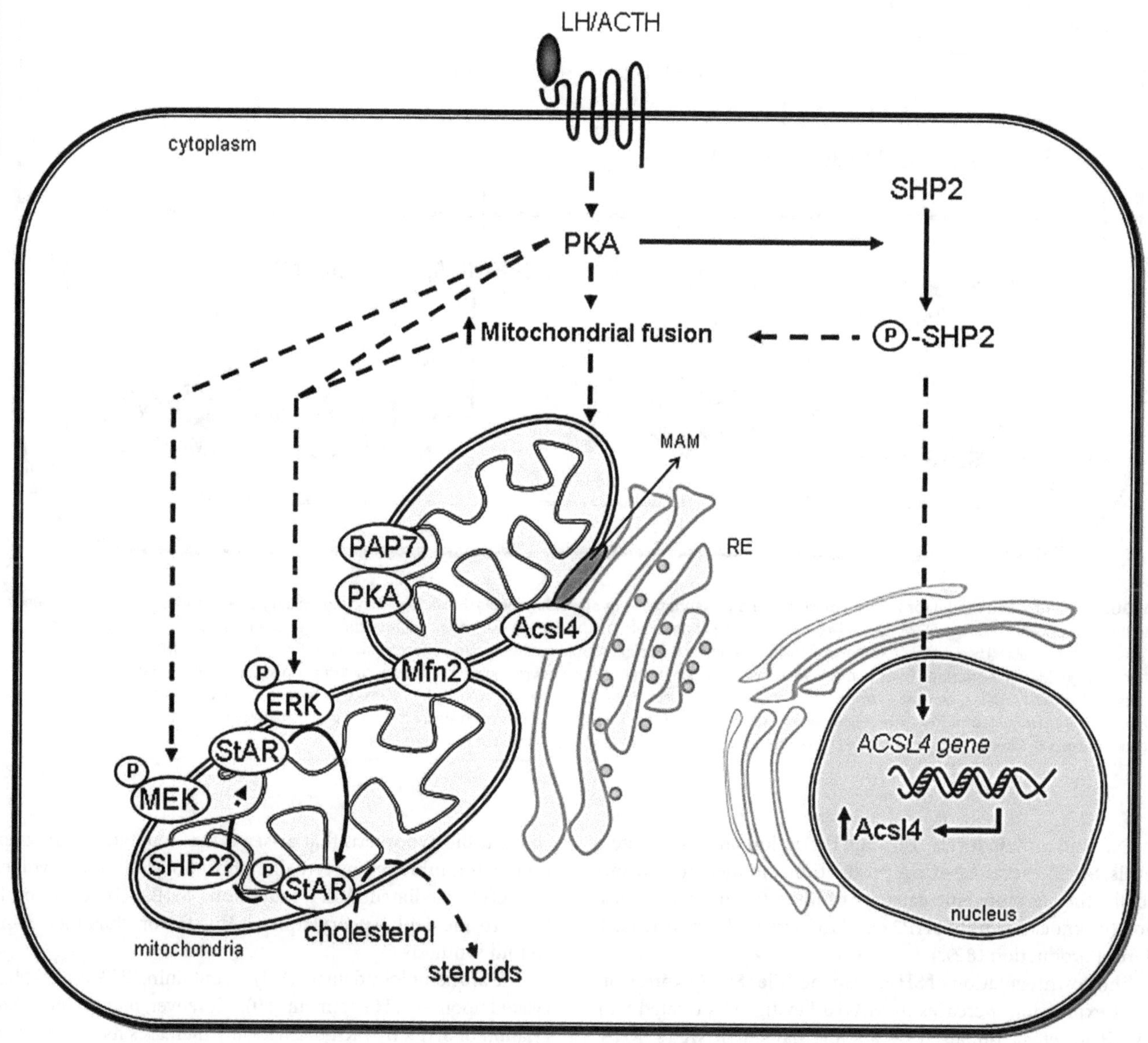

FIGURE 2 | Scheme showing the association between ER and mitochondria in steroidogenic cells. The proposed interaction between organelles and the involved proteins in the regulation of cholesterol delivery is shown. After steroidogenic hormone action, PKA is activated and Mitofusin 2 (Mfn2) is localized in mitochondria. SHP2 is phosphorylated (P-SHP2) by active PKA, then it participates in both ACSL4 gene induction and the increase of mitochondrial fusion. Next, Acsl4 is localized in MAM subdomains in an Mfn2-dependent manner to exert its enzymatic activity. Mitochondrial ERK is activated by phosphorylation (P-ERK) in a PKA- and MEK-dependent mechanism and phosphorylates mitochondrial StAR (P-StAR) to achieve maximal steroid production. A putative mechanism involves StAR dephosphorylation by SHP2 in mitochondria to release a cholesterol molecule to be substrate of P450scc. Direct effects are indicated by solid lines, whereas indirect effects are indicated as dotted lines.

MAPK Phosphatases in Steroidogenic Cells

Given that MAPK activation depends on Thr/Tyr protein phosphorylation, the magnitude and duration of their activity are related to protein phosphatases. MAPK phosphatases (MKPs) are a family of dual activity (Thr/Tyr) protein phosphatases, which dephosphorylate specifically members of MAPKs (90, 91). Several distinct mammalian MKP family members have been identified and characterized and can be divided into two broad classes. One group, typified as MKP-1, comprises nuclear enzymes rapidly induced by growth factors or stress signals. This group also includes MKP-2, a nuclear enzyme induced by the same stimuli that induce MKP-1, but with a slower kinetics. The second group, typified as MKP-3, includes predominantly cytosolic enzymes, and their transcripts are induced with delayed kinetics by specific stimuli, but not by environmental stress.

On the basis of evidence showing that ACTH can regulate the activity of MAPKs (31, 92), the regulation of MKPs by this hormone is expected. Analyses on MKP-1 induction in serum-starved Y1 cells demonstrated that ACTH stimulation results in a transient increase in MKP-1 mRNA followed by an increase in protein levels (93). Sewer and Wateman have also described the regulation of MKP-1 expression by cAMP in H295R cells. In this regard, they demonstrated that MKP-1 mRNA and protein levels are induced by cAMP, and overexpression of this phosphatase stimulates hCYP17 reporter gene activity. Besides, this study also demonstrates that PKA phosphorylates MKP-1 (94).

The hormone-dependent expression of MKP-1 has also been analyzed in MA-10 Leydig cells, where hCG/cAMP rapidly increases MKP-1 gene induction in a transient manner (95). Besides, MKP-1 protein levels increased in both nuclear and mitochondrial compartments. Moreover, MKP-1 increase (95) and ERK1/2 dephosphorylation in the mitochondria (42) are temporally coordinated events. In addition, our group has demonstrated that, in cells expressing flag-MKP-1 protein, hCG/cAMP trigger the phosphorylation and the accumulation of the recombinant protein in a time-dependent manner. Altogether, these results indicate that hCG modulates MKP-1 expression by transcriptional and posttranslational actions.

The functional role of MKP-1 in the regulation of steroidogenesis has also been analyzed in MA-10 Leydig cells. Work by our group demonstrates that MKP-1 overexpression downregulates the effects of cAMP on phospho-ERK1/2 levels, StAR expression, and steroidogenesis, while MKP-1 downregulation produces opposite effects. In summary, these data demonstrate that in Leydig cells, MKP-1 expression is regulated at multiple levels as a negative feedback regulatory mechanism to modulate the hormonal action on ERK1/2 activity and steroidogenesis (95).

Casal et al. have demonstrated the expression and regulation of MPK-1 also in primary cultures of bovine adrenal glomerulosa cells (29). These authors show that Ang II markedly increases MKP-1 protein levels in a time- and concentration-dependent manner. Ang II-induced phosphorylation of ERK1/2 leads to MKP-1 phosphorylation and, in turn, MKP-1 promotes ERK1/2 dephosphorylation. MKP-1 overexpression in bovine adrenal glomerulosa cells results in decreased phosphorylation of ERK1/2 and aldosterone production in response to Ang II stimulation. These results strongly suggest that MKP-1 is induced by Ang II and that it is involved in the negative feedback mechanism, ensuring adequate ERK1/2-mediated aldosterone production in response to the hormone.

In MA-10 Leydig cells, LH receptor stimulation also induces MKP-2 (96) and MKP-3 (97) through multiple mechanisms. While MKP-2 completes the ERK1/2 dephosphorylation in the nucleus initiated by MKP-1, MKP-3 dephosphorylates ERK1/2 in the cytoplasm.

In conclusion, stimuli promoting MAPK activity also regulate MKPs expression at multiple stages as a negative feedback regulatory mechanism to modulate hormonal actions on ERK1/2 activity and steroidogenesis (**Figure 1**).

KINASES AND PHOSPHATASES IN THE REGULATION OF MITOCHONDRIAL DYNAMICS: ROLE IN StAR ACTIVITY AND STEROIDOGENESIS

StAR Structural Changes

Several protein kinases, such as PKA, MEK, and ERK – which are essential to complete steroidogenesis – form a mitochondria-associated complex and are completely required for mitochondrial cholesterol transport along with StAR and other proteins such as Acsl4, voltage-dependent anion channel (VDAC1), and adenine nucleotidetranslocase (ANT) (42, 98).

The precise mechanism of StAR action has been widely explored, but still remains elusive. StAR is synthesized as a 37-kDa protein with a typical mitochondrial leader sequence that directs the protein to the mitochondria for the import and cleavage to an intramitochondrial form of 30-kDa (99–102). After reaching the matrix, the 30-kDa StAR is controlled by the ATP-dependent Lon protease (103) and proteolysed, its half-life being 4–5 h (101, 104). A tight regulation of mitochondrial StAR levels is imperative since excessive accumulation of StAR protein in the matrix provokes mitochondrial damage and a "mitochondria to nucleus" signaling which, in turn, activates transcription of genes that encode mitochondrial proteases crucial for complete clearance of StAR (105). In this regard, we have observed that the presence of mitochondrial ERK is strictly necessary for protecting StAR from unknown proteases to avoid further degradation, which constitutes one of the mechanisms playing a role in mitochondrial StAR levels regulation (106).

This mechanistic model of StAR action suggests that the active form of StAR is partially unfolded, with the N-terminal domain entering the mitochondria and the partially unfolded C-terminus interacting with the OMM. Direct evidence has been presented showing that StAR exists as a molten globule. While certain native structure is retained at the N-terminal domain, the C-terminal domain folding appears to be less tight at the low pH that StAR may undergo on the mitochondrial membrane. Then, the tightly folded N-terminal domain could make StAR halt as it enters the mitochondria, extending the time window for the C-terminus to act.

Steroidogenic acute regulatory protein exhibits constitutive activity on the OMM, but no activity when localized to the intermembrane space (IMS) or to the matrix (107). Mitochondrial StAR protein import experiments using a modified leader peptide confirmed StAR exclusive activity on the OMM, as reflected by a negative correlation between the time of StAR mitochondrial entry and its activity. Once again, StAR role in promoting steroidogenesis is proportional to the time it spends on the OMM (107, 108).

Even when N-62 StAR form (which lacks mitochondrial peptide leader) does not access to the mitochondria, a few molecules of this protein are associated with the OMM as it is shown by immuno-electron microscopy (108, 109). This truncated StAR form would transport several cholesterol molecules, while complete StAR protein is able to bind just one. This suggests that StAR could transport several cholesterol molecules before entering mitochondria and be processed.

Mitochondrial Dynamics and Its Regulation by Protein Kinases in Steroidogenic Cells

"Mitochondrial dynamics," which includes fusion/fission events, is relevant for maintaining mitochondrial integrity. Indeed, mitochondrial plasticity is important for several cellular functions and for protection against aging-related changes. Among these functions, mitochondrial dynamics play a role in mitochondrial replication and repair, propagation of intramitochondrial calcium waves, and in the elimination, *via* mitophagy, of depolarized mitochondria (110). Two GTPases located on the OMM have a crucial role in mitochondrial fusion, mitofusin (Mfn) 1 and 2. These proteins, structurally related to dynamin, are expressed in several tissues, as brain (mainly Mfn2), liver, adrenal glands, and testis. Mfn1 and Mfn2 modulate the interactions mitochondria–mitochondria and endoplasmic reticulum (ER)–mitochondria and also mediate mitochondrial fusion acting in a concerted fashion with another GTPase located in the IMM, optic atrophy 1 (OPA1).

Mitochondria have been shown to be in constant movement within the cells, and this movement can be induced after steroidogenic hormone action. This event would allow the contact between mitochondria and other membranes. It is well known that the contact between mitochondria and ER plays an important role in cell metabolism and signaling transduction pathways. Indeed, it is considered as a unique subdomain termed the mitochondria-associated ER membrane (MAM), with a vast importance in regulation of Ca^{2+} signaling, mitochondrial bioenergetics, apoptosis, and lipid metabolism (111–113).

Mfn2 in the ER bridges mitochondria and ER by forming homotypic and heterotypic complexes, with Mfn2 or Mfn1 on the mitochondrial surface. Therefore, Mfn2 is critical for MAM formation by tethering ER to the mitochondria. A mitochondrial ubiquitin ligase, MITOL, has been described as the regulator of the ER–mitochondria interaction by controlling Mfn2 activity (114). Interestingly, Acsl4, the key enzyme involved in the regulation of steroidogenesis through AA release and induced by steroidogenic hormones (66, 79, 80), is localized and active in the MAM subdomain (115).

Dynamin-related protein 1 (Drp1) is required for mitochondrial fission. It is a cytosolic protein, which is recruited to the OMM by a poorly characterized multiprotein complex. In neurons, Drp1 phosphorylation by PKA in the mitochondria results in its inactivation and concomitant mitochondrial elongation (116). On the other hand, Drp1 phosphorylation by PKCδ at Ser579 increases mitochondrial fragmentation (117). In summary, several works support a key regulatory role for phosphorylation in mitochondrial morphology maintenance.

Although it is well recognized the relevance of mitochondrial dynamics in several cellular processes, its role in steroid synthesis is poorly described. Nevertheless, a work published 30 years ago described hormone-induced changes in intracellular location of the mitochondria and in the morphology of this organelle (118). Later, it was described that mitochondria move across the cell in a PKA-dependent manner after ACTH stimulation in H295R adrenocortical cells (119). This work demonstrates that ACTH/cAMP-stimulated mitochondrial movements depend on microtubules and have a role in the regulation of cortisol production, facilitating the shuttle of steroidoigenic substrates between the ER and mitochondria (119). In this cell line, the reduction of OPA1 facilitates the transfer of cytosolic Ca^{2+} signal into the mitochondrial matrix (120), which results in turn in enhanced aldosterone production (121). The authors stated that this is probably due to the altered diffusion conditions under OPA1 knockout. The study of an extramitochondrial form of OPA1 closely related to the lipid droplets ruled out any role of this fraction of OPA1 in cAMP-mediated steroid hormone production, the specific biological function of adrenocortical cells (66, 120). Moreover, the reduction of OPA1 in Leydig cells did not affect steroid production (98), suggesting that OPA1 is not critical for hormone-induced steroidogenesis. Then, the contribution of OPA1 and cristae remodelation to steroid synthesis needs further investigation.

Mitochondrial Dynamics and Steroidogenesis

Steroid synthesis requires mitochondrial fusion induced by in a hormone-dependent fashion (89). The fact that Mfn2 is rapidly induced after the steroidogenic stimuli, and that blocking mitochondrial fusion by Mfn 2 knockdown expression reduce steroid synthesis, further supports a role of mitochondrial dynamics on steroidogenesis (89). The hormone-induced mitochondrial fusion might also be crucial for the generation of the mitochondrial multiprotein complex that facilitates the access of cholesterol to the P450scc system, since the mitochondrial rearrangement after cell stimulation is necessary for the relocalization of ERK1/2 to mitochondria. Moreover, the abrogation of mitochondrial fusion prevents the association of Acsl4 with the mitochondria, showing clearly that MAM formation depends on mitochondrial fusion (89). As previously mentioned in this review, SHP2 modulates mitochondrial fusion, suggesting that protein tyrosine dephosphorylation could be involved in the mechanism of mitochondrial dynamics (89). According to a published work (119), mitochondrial fusion might represent a limiting step in the onset of processes that require transport of intermediate products, e.g., liposoluble steroid hormones between organelles, probably mediated by MAM. In agreement with the previous results from our group, recent work demonstrate that hormone-induced MAM formation participates in the optimum transfer of cholesterol from the ER into the IMM increasing steroidogenesis rates (122). Then, steroid hormones might reach the plasma membrane without moving across the hydrophilic cytoplasm. Our group has shown that mitochondrial fusion is an essential process in regulating StAR mRNA levels and driving StAR to the mitochondrial context, probably participating in StAR mRNA stabilization and/or tethering the protein to the OMM (106) (**Figure 2**).

Role of StAR Phosphorylation and Mitochondrial Fusion in StAR Localization

In silico molecular modeling has demonstrated that cholesterol binding to StAR could elicit a conformational change in StAR C-terminal domain, which in turn might favor the exposure of StAR Ser 232 and the docking domain for ERK. Therefore, StAR could be a substrate for ERK binding and phosphorylation, only when this protein is bound to cholesterol (42). This model is sustained by the fact that cholesterol binding to StAR promotes a decrease in its helical structure (123). The OMM is the most probable environment for the interaction between StAR and ERK since this submitochondrial domain anchors both StAR and ERK, as demonstrated in the previous work (42, 53). In turn, the overexpression of the mutated form of StAR, S232A, in steroidogenic cells prevents StAR phosphorylation by active ERK, thus proving that the kinase indeed phosphorylates this residue.

Cholesterol acts as an allosteric modulator of its own binding to StAR (123) and is strong stabilizing of the partially unfolded state in the StAR molecule (124). However, when cholesterol has to reach the P450scc, its release from StAR hydrophobic pocket is obligatory. Since ERK phosphorylation of StAR requires cholesterol, it is conceivable to think that StAR phosphorylation at Ser232 occurs after cholesterol binding. Thus, a conformational change in StAR induced by a negative charge at the Ser232 might reduce StAR affinity for cholesterol, favoring its release. This might in turn facilitate cholesterol transport into mitochondria to achieve high rates of pregnenolone synthesis.

Steroidogenic acute regulatory protein molecular structure has been partially studied (123–126), and the Ser232 residue is predicted to be localized in one of the last β barrels of the StAR-related lipid-transfer (START) domain (126, 127). It is well known that protein stability and interaction with several components are modulated by phosphorylation. Phosphorylation of proteins promotes acidic loops formation in their structure, as it has been described (128). The pH-dependent transition to the molten globule structure in the mitochondrial context (OMM) could provoke a weakened association between StAR C-terminal α-helix and lipid molecules, thus releasing cholesterol from StAR hydrophobic pocket. Under acidic pH conditions, the cholesterol affinity for START domain is significantly decreased (127). Thus, the addition of a phosphate group to StAR by ERK could establish a local decrease in pH, directing a conformational change in StAR, to a form with a lower affinity for cholesterol.

Our group has shown that StAR S232A expression significantly diminishes the localization of StAR in the mitochondria induced by hCG or cAMP. ERK phosphorylation affects mitochondrial StAR levels posttranscriptionally, as the expression of transfected StAR S232A is independent of cellular endogenous regulation (106). The mitochondrial module includes MEK, ERK, and cholesterol with a direct physical association between StAR and ERK (42). Their interaction facilitates StAR phosphorylation by ERK. Therefore, it could lead to phospho-StAR retention in the mitochondria, particularly on the OMM where ERK resides (53) (**Figure 2**).

Steroidogenic acute regulatory protein activity is determined by its localization on the OMM, and not its cleavage from the 37- to 30-kDa form (107). Hence, the longest StAR retention time on the OMM might render the maximal StAR activity in cholesterol transport, in agreement with the previous data (102). As described above, ERK is transiently activated after hormone stimulation in MA-10 cells (42). Its dephosphorylation could be mediated by MKP-1, since the temporal profile of mitochondrial MKP-1 and ERK dephosphorylation are compatible (95). Mitochondrial phospho-StAR and ERK interaction could avoid ERK dephosphorylation and inactivation. The temporal frame of ERK activity in this organelle correlates with highest StAR activity and cholesterol transport after hormone stimulation. These results agree with the fact that MKP-1 downregulation leads an increase in progesterone levels (95). The hormone-dependent induction of Mfn2 and mitochondrial fusion play an essential role in localization of ERK and StAR on the OMM and on the steroidogenesis (89, 129).

Taken together, these results offer new insights into StAR regulation by kinases and phosphatases and their impact on StAR site of action. The phosphorylation–dephosphorylation of StAR would contribute to modulate its affinity for cholesterol and to increase pregnenolone synthesis with a few molecules of StAR. In this work, we have reviewed StAR mechanism of action on cholesterol transport to the P450scc to achieve maximal steroid production. We have also described the role of phosphorylation–dephosphorylation events and mitochondrial fusion as novel regulators of the localization of StAR protein in order to carry out its action in steroidogenic cells.

CONCLUDING REMARKS

Serine/threonine phosphatases have an important role in the regulation of adrenocortical cell functions, mainly steroid synthesis. In this context, the participation of PKA and PKC appears relevant, as phosphorylation events mediated by these kinases are involved in the expression and activation of StAR. Although StAR activation mechanism has not been fully described, it is known to require hormonal action on mitochondrial dynamic. Studies from other and our laboratory show that MAPKs, particularly ERK1/2, play an important role in StAR induction as well as in its posttranslational regulation in the mitochondria. In addition, ACTH-activated ERK1/2 regulates adrenal cell proliferation.

A field scarcely described is the role of PTPs in steroidogenic cells. We presented data on PTP activation triggered by ACTH through a PKA-dependent mechanism. In this context, PTP SHP2 has a role in the stimulation of steroidogenesis involving Acsl4 protein induction. In turn, Acsl4 promotes AA release, StAR induction, and steroidogenesis. Moreover, SHP2 along with ERK could also have a role in steroidogenesis promoting mitochondrial fusion. MKPs, a group of dual activity phosphatases that inactivate MAPK, are also regulated by steroidogenic hormones at multiple levels. While MAPK activation is linked to steroid production activation and cell proliferation, MKP induction is associated with the turn-off of hormonal signal through MAPK inactivation and, consequently, the downregulation of ERK-dependent events.

AUTHOR CONTRIBUTIONS

Ernesto J. Podesta, Cristina Paz, Cecilia Poderoso and Ana F. Castillo wrote the paper. All authors provided critical revisions of the paper.

ACKNOWLEDGMENTS

We thank María T. Rancez for providing language help and writing assistance.

FUNDING

The authors were supported by Consejo Nacional de Investigaciones Científicas y Técnicas (CONICET), Universidad de Buenos Aires (UBA), and Agencia Nacional de Promoción Científica y Tecnológica (ANPCyT).

REFERENCES

1. Crivello JF, Jefcoate CR. Intracellular movement of cholesterol in rat adrenal cells. Kinetics and effects of inhibitors. *J Biol Chem* (1980) 255:8144–51.
2. Privalle CT, Crivello JF, Jefcoate CR. Regulation of intramitochondrial cholesterol transfer to side-chain cleavage cytochrome P-450 in rat adrenal gland. *Proc Natl Acad Sci U S A* (1983) 80:702–6. doi:10.1073/pnas.80.3.702
3. Clark BJ, Wells J, King SR, Stocco DM. The purification, cloning, and expression of a novel luteinizing hormone-induced mitochondrial protein in MA-10 mouse Leydig tumor cells. Characterization of the steroidogenic acute regulatory protein (StAR). *J Biol Chem* (1994) 269:28314–22.
4. Stocco DM, Clark BJ. Regulation of the acute production of steroids in steroidogenic cells. *Endocr Rev* (1996) 17:221–44. doi:10.1210/edrv-17-3-221
5. Podesta EJ, Milani A, Steffen H, Neher R. Adrenocorticotropin (ACTH) induces phosphorylation of a cytoplasmic protein in intact isolated adrenocortical cells. *Proc Natl Acad Sci U S A* (1979) 76:5187–91. doi:10.1073/pnas.76.10.5187
6. Podesta EJ, Milani A, Steffen H, Neher R. Steroidogenesis in isolated adrenocortical cells. Correlation with receptor-bound adenosine e 3':5'-cyclic monophosphate. *Biochem J* (1979) 180:355–63. doi:10.1042/bj1800355
7. Rae PA, Gutmann NS, Tsao J, Schimmer BP. Mutations in cyclic AMP-dependent protein kinase and corticotropin (ACTH)-sensitive adenylate cyclase affect adrenal steroidogenesis. *Proc Natl Acad Sci U S A* (1979) 76:1896–900. doi:10.1073/pnas.76.4.1896
8. Sala GB, Hayashi K, Catt KJ, Dufau ML. Adrenocorticotropin action in isolated adrenal cells. The intermediate role of cyclic AMP in stimulation of corticosterone synthesis. *J Biol Chem* (1979) 254:3861–5.
9. Olson MF, Krolczyk AJ, Gorman KB, Steinberg RA, Schimmer BP. Molecular basis for the 3',5'-cyclic adenosine monophosphate resistance of Kin mutant Y1 adrenocortical tumor cells. *Mol Endocrinol* (1993) 7:477–87. doi:10.1210/me.7.4.477
10. Dufau ML, Tsuruhara T, Horner KA, Podesta E, Catt KJ. Intermediate role of adenosine 3':5'-cyclic monophosphate and protein kinase during gonadotropin-induced steroidogenesis in testicular interstitial cells. *Proc Natl Acad Sci U S A* (1977) 74:3419–23. doi:10.1073/pnas.74.8.3419
11. Schimmer BP, Tsao J, Knapp M. Isolation of mutant adrenocortical tumor cells resistant to cyclic nucleotides. *Mol Cell Endocrinol* (1977) 8:135–45. doi:10.1016/0303-7207(77)90025-9
12. Podesta EJ, Dufau ML, Solano AR, Catt KJ. Hormonal activation of protein kinase in isolated Leydig cells. Electrophoretic analysis of cyclic AMP receptors. *J Biol Chem* (1978) 253:8994–9001.
13. Spat A, Hunyady L. Control of aldosterone secretion: a model for convergence in cellular signaling pathways. *Physiol Rev* (2004) 84:489–539. doi:10.1152/physrev.00030.2003
14. Krueger RJ, Orme-Johnson NR. Acute adrenocorticotropic hormone stimulation of adrenal corticosteroidogenesis. Discovery of a rapidly induced protein. *J Biol Chem* (1983) 258:10159–67.
15. Pon LA, Hartigan JA, Orme-Johnson NR. Acute ACTH regulation of adrenal corticosteroid biosynthesis. Rapid accumulation of a phosphoprotein. *J Biol Chem* (1986) 261:13309–16.
16. Epstein LF, Orme-Johnson NR. Regulation of steroid hormone biosynthesis. Identification of precursors of a phosphoprotein targeted to the mitochondrion in stimulated rat adrenal cortex cells. *J Biol Chem* (1991) 266:19739–45.
17. Epstein LF, Orme-Johnson NR. Acute action of luteinizing hormone on mouse Leydig cells: accumulation of mitochondrial phosphoproteins and stimulation of testosterone synthesis. *Mol Cell Endocrinol* (1991) 81:113–26. doi:10.1016/0303-7207(91)90210-J
18. Arakane F, King SR, Du Y, Kallen CB, Walsh LP, Watari H, et al. Phosphorylation of steroidogenic acute regulatory protein (StAR) modulates its steroidogenic activity. *J Biol Chem* (1997) 272:32656–62. doi:10.1074/jbc.272.51.32656
19. Fleury A, Mathieu AP, Ducharme L, Hales DB, LeHoux JG. Phosphorylation and function of the hamster adrenal steroidogenic acute regulatory protein (StAR). *J Steroid Biochem Mol Biol* (2004) 91:259–71. doi:10.1016/j.jsbmb.2004.04.010
20. Tremblay JJ, Hamel F, Viger RS. Protein kinase A-dependent cooperation between GATA and CCAAT/enhancer-binding protein transcription factors regulates steroidogenic acute regulatory protein promoter activity. *Endocrinology* (2002) 143:3935–45. doi:10.1210/en.2002-220413
21. Blom N, Gammeltoft S, Brunak S. Sequence and structure-based prediction of eukaryotic protein phosphorylation sites. *J Mol Biol* (1999) 294:1351–62. doi:10.1006/jmbi.1999.3310
22. Sasaki G, Zubair M, Ishii T, Mitsui T, Hasegawa T, Auchus RJ. The contribution of serine 194 phosphorylation to steroidogenic acute regulatory protein function. *Mol Endocrinol* (2014) 28:1088–96. doi:10.1210/me.2014-1028
23. Baker BY, Epand RF, Epand RM, Miller WL. Cholesterol binding does not predict activity of the steroidogenic acute regulatory protein, StAR. *J Biol Chem* (2007) 282:10223–32. doi:10.1074/jbc.M611221200
24. Fan J, Liu J, Culty M, Papadopoulos V. Acyl-coenzyme A binding domain containing 3 (ACBD3; PAP7; GCP60): an emerging signaling molecule. *Prog Lipid Res* (2010) 49:218–34. doi:10.1016/j.plipres.2009.12.003
25. Manna PR, Jo Y, Stocco DM. Regulation of Leydig cell steroidogenesis by extracellular signal-regulated kinase 1/2: role of protein kinase A and protein kinase C signaling. *J Endocrinol* (2007) 193:53–63. doi:10.1677/JOE-06-0201
26. Gyles SL, Burns CJ, Whitehouse BJ, Sugden D, Marsh PJ, Persaud SJ, et al. ERKs regulate cyclic AMP-induced steroid synthesis through transcription of the steroidogenic acute regulatory (StAR) gene. *J Biol Chem* (2001) 276:34888–95. doi:10.1074/jbc.M102063200

27. Roy S, Pinard S, Chouinard L, Gallo-Payet N. Adrenocorticotropin hormone (ACTH) effects on MAPK phosphorylation in human fasciculata cells and in embryonic kidney 293 cells expressing human melanocortin 2 receptor (MC2R) and MC2R accessory protein (MRAP)beta. *Mol Cell Endocrinol* (2011) 336:31–40. doi:10.1016/j.mce.2010.12.030
28. Janes ME, Chu KM, Clark AJ, King PJ. Mechanisms of adrenocorticotropin-induced activation of extracellularly regulated kinase 1/2 mitogen-activated protein kinase in the human H295R adrenal cell line. *Endocrinology* (2008) 149:1898–905. doi:10.1210/en.2007-0949
29. Casal AJ, Ryser S, Capponi AM, Wang-Buholzer CF. Angiotensin II-induced mitogen-activated protein kinase phosphatase-1 expression in bovine adrenal glomerulosa cells: implications in mineralocorticoid biosynthesis. *Endocrinology* (2007) 148:5573–81. doi:10.1210/en.2007-0241
30. Otis M, Gallo-Payet N. Role of MAPKs in angiotensin II-induced steroidogenesis in rat glomerulosa cells. *Mol Cell Endocrinol* (2007) 26(5–266):126–30. doi:10.1016/j.mce.2006.12.008
31. Le T, Schimmer BP. The regulation of MAPKs in Y1 mouse adrenocortical tumor cells. *Endocrinology* (2001) 142:4282–7. doi:10.1210/endo.142.10.8441
32. Hirakawa T, Ascoli M. The lutropin/choriogonadotropin receptor-induced phosphorylation of the extracellular signal-regulated kinases in Leydig cells is mediated by a protein kinase a-dependent activation of ras. *Mol Endocrinol* (2003) 17:2189–200. doi:10.1210/me.2003-0205
33. Yamashita S, Tai P, Charron J, Ko C, Ascoli M. The Leydig cell MEK/ERK pathway is critical for maintaining a functional population of adult Leydig cells and for fertility. *Mol Endocrinol* (2011) 25:1211–22. doi:10.1210/me.2011-0059
34. Martinelle N, Holst M, Soder O, Svechnikov K. Extracellular signal-regulated kinases are involved in the acute activation of steroidogenesis in immature rat Leydig cells by human chorionic gonadotropin. *Endocrinology* (2004) 145:4629–34. doi:10.1210/en.2004-0496
35. Martinat N, Crepieux P, Reiter E, Guillou F. Extracellular signal-regulated kinases (ERK) 1, 2 are required for luteinizing hormone (LH)-induced steroidogenesis in primary Leydig cells and control steroidogenic acute regulatory (StAR) expression. *Reprod Nutr Dev* (2005) 45:101–8. doi:10.1051/rnd:2005007
36. Seger R, Hanoch T, Rosenberg R, Dantes A, Merz WE, Strauss JF III, et al. The ERK signaling cascade inhibits gonadotropin-stimulated steroidogenesis. *J Biol Chem* (2001) 276:13957–64. doi:10.1074/jbc.M006852200
37. Martin LJ, Boucher N, Brousseau C, Tremblay JJ. The orphan nuclear receptor NUR77 regulates hormone-induced StAR transcription in Leydig cells through cooperation with Ca^{2+}/calmodulin-dependent protein kinase I. *Mol Endocrinol* (2008) 22:2021–37. doi:10.1210/me.2007-0370
38. Mori Sequeiros Garcia M, Gorostizaga A, Brion L, Gonzalez-Calvar SI, Paz C. cAMP-activated Nr4a1 expression requires ERK activity and is modulated by MAPK phosphatase-1 in MA-10 Leydig cells. *Mol Cell Endocrinol* (2015) 408:45–52. doi:10.1016/j.mce.2015.01.041
39. Lotfi CF, Todorovic Z, Armelin HA, Schimmer BP. Unmasking a growth-promoting effect of the adrenocorticotropic hormone in Y1 mouse adrenocortical tumor cells. *J Biol Chem* (1997) 272:29886–91. doi:10.1074/jbc.272.47.29886
40. Otis M, Campbell S, Payet MD, Gallo-Payet N. Angiotensin II stimulates protein synthesis and inhibits proliferation in primary cultures of rat adrenal glomerulosa cells. *Endocrinology* (2005) 146:633–42. doi:10.1210/en.2004-0935
41. Ferreira JG, Cruz CD, Neves D, Pignatelli D. Increased extracellular signal regulated kinases phosphorylation in the adrenal gland in response to chronic ACTH treatment. *J Endocrinol* (2007) 192:647–58. doi:10.1677/joe.1.06961
42. Poderoso C, Converso DP, Maloberti P, Duarte A, Neuman I, Galli S, et al. A mitochondrial kinase complex is essential to mediate an ERK1/2-dependent phosphorylation of a key regulatory protein in steroid biosynthesis. *PLoS One* (2008) 3:e1443. doi:10.1371/journal.pone.0001443
43. Rubin CS. A kinase anchor proteins and the intracellular targeting of signals carried by cyclic AMP. *Biochim Biophys Acta* (1994) 1224:467–79.
44. Feliciello A, Gottesman ME, Avvedimento EV. cAMP-PKA signaling to the mitochondria: protein scaffolds, mRNA and phosphatases. *Cell Signal* (2005) 17:279–87. doi:10.1016/j.cellsig.2004.09.009
45. Angelo RG, Rubin CS. Characterization of structural features that mediate the tethering of *Caenorhabditis elegans* protein kinase A to a novel A kinase anchor protein. Insights into the anchoring of PKAI isoforms. *J Biol Chem* (2000) 275:4351–62. doi:10.1074/jbc.275.6.4351
46. Diviani D, Scott JD. AKAP signaling complexes at the cytoskeleton. *J Cell Sci* (2001) 114:1431–7.
47. Ginsberg MD, Feliciello A, Jones JK, Avvedimento EV, Gottesman ME. PKA-dependent binding of mRNA to the mitochondrial AKAP121 protein. *J Mol Biol* (2003) 327:885–97. doi:10.1016/S0022-2836(03)00173-6
48. Wong W, Scott JD. AKAP signalling complexes: focal points in space and time. *Nat Rev Mol Cell Biol* (2004) 5:959–70. doi:10.1038/nrm1527
49. Dyson MT, Jones JK, Kowalewski MP, Manna PR, Alonso M, Gottesman ME, et al. Mitochondrial A-kinase anchoring protein 121 binds type II protein kinase A and enhances steroidogenic acute regulatory protein-mediated steroidogenesis in MA-10 mouse leydig tumor cells. *Biol Reprod* (2008) 78:267–77. doi:10.1095/biolreprod.107.064238
50. Liu J, Matyakhina L, Han Z, Sandrini F, Bei T, Stratakis CA, et al. Molecular cloning, chromosomal localization of human peripheral-type benzodiazepine receptor and PKA regulatory subunit type 1A (PRKAR1A)-associated protein PAP7, and studies in PRKAR1A mutant cells and tissues. *FASEB J* (2003) 17:1189–91. doi:10.1096/fj.02-1066fje
51. Zhou T, Sun L, Humphreys J, Goldsmith EJ. Docking interactions induce exposure of activation loop in the MAP kinase ERK2. *Structure* (2006) 14:1011–9. doi:10.1016/j.str.2006.04.006
52. den Hertog J, Ostman A, Bohmer FD. Protein tyrosine phosphatases: regulatory mechanisms. *FEBS J* (2008) 275:831–47. doi:10.1111/j.1742-4658.2008.06247.x
53. Alonso M, Melani M, Converso D, Jaitovich A, Paz C, Carreras MC, et al. Mitochondrial extracellular signal-regulated kinases 1/2 (ERK1/2) are modulated during brain development. *J Neurochem* (2004) 89:248–56. doi:10.1111/j.1471-4159.2004.02323.x
54. Paz C, Cornejo MacIel F, Mendez C, Podesta EJ. Corticotropin increases protein tyrosine phosphatase activity by a cAMP-dependent mechanism in rat adrenal gland. *Eur J Biochem* (1999) 265:911–8. doi:10.1046/j.1432-1327.1999.00759.x
55. Brautigan DL, Pinault FM. Activation of membrane protein-tyrosine phosphatase involving cAMP- and Ca^{2+}/phospholipid-dependent protein kinases. *Proc Natl Acad Sci U S A* (1991) 88:6696–700. doi:10.1073/pnas.88.15.6696
56. Garton AJ, Tonks NK. PTP-PEST: a protein tyrosine phosphatase regulated by serine phosphorylation. *EMBO J* (1994) 13:3763–71.
57. Gorostizaga AB, Mori Sequeiros Garcia MM, Acquier AB, Lopez-Costa JJ, Mendez CF, Maloberti PM, et al. ACTH modulates PTP-PEST activity and promotes its interaction with paxillin. *J Cell Biochem* (2016). doi:10.1002/jcb.25566
58. Adachi M, Iwaki H, Shindoh M, Akao Y, Hachiya T, Ikeda M, et al. Predominant expression of the src homology 2-containing tyrosine phosphatase protein SHP2 in vascular smooth muscle cells. *Virchows Arch* (1997) 430:321–5. doi:10.1007/BF01092755
59. Matozaki T, Murata Y, Saito Y, Okazawa H, Ohnishi H. Protein tyrosine phosphatase SHP-2: a proto-oncogene product that promotes Ras activation. *Cancer Sci* (2009) 100:1786–93. doi:10.1111/j.1349-7006.2009.01257.x
60. Rocchi S, Gaillard I, van Obberghen E, Chambaz EM, Vilgrain I. Adrenocorticotrophic hormone stimulates phosphotyrosine phosphatase SHP2 in bovine adrenocortical cells: phosphorylation and activation by cAMP-dependent protein kinase. *Biochem J* (2000) 352(Pt 2):483–90. doi:10.1042/bj3520483
61. Cooke M, Orlando U, Maloberti P, Podesta EJ, Cornejo Maciel F. Tyrosine phosphatase SHP2 regulates the expression of acyl-CoA synthetase ACSL4. *J Lipid Res* (2011) 52:1936–48. doi:10.1194/jlr.M015552
62. Whitehouse BJ, Gyles SL, Burns CJ, Cock MH, Jones PM. Inhibition of protein tyrosine phosphatase activity blocks shape change & steroidogenesis in Y1 cells. *Endocr Res* (2000) 26:617–21. doi:10.3109/07435800009048581
63. Poderoso C, Cornejo Maciel F, Gorostizaga A, Bey P, Paz C, Podesta EJ. The obligatory action of protein tyrosine phosphatases in ACTH-stimulated steroidogenesis is exerted at the level of StAR protein. *Endocr Res* (2002) 28:413–7. doi:10.1081/ERC-120016816
64. Cornejo Maciel F, Poderoso C, Gorostizaga A, Paz C, Podesta EJ. LH/chorionic gonadotropin signaling pathway involves protein tyrosine phosphatase activity downstream of protein kinase A activation: evidence of an obligatory step in steroid production by Leydig cells. *J Endocrinol* (2001) 170:403–11. doi:10.1677/joe.0.1700403

65. Paz C, Cornejo Maciel F, Maloberti P, Walsh LP, Stocco DM, Podesta EJ. Protein tyrosine phosphatases are involved in LH/chorionic gonadotropin and 8Br-cAMP regulation of steroidogenesis and StAR protein levels in MA-10 Leydig cells. *J Endocrinol* (2002) 175:793–801. doi:10.1677/joe.0.1750793
66. Mele PG, Duarte A, Paz C, Capponi A, Podesta EJ. Role of intramitochondrial arachidonic acid and acyl-CoA synthetase 4 in angiotensin II-regulated aldosterone synthesis in NCI-H295R adrenocortical cell line. *Endocrinology* (2012) 153:3284–94. doi:10.1210/en.2011-2108
67. Han JD, Rubin CS. Regulation of cytoskeleton organization and paxillin dephosphorylation by cAMP. Studies on murine Y1 adrenal cells. *J Biol Chem* (1996) 271:29211–5. doi:10.1074/jbc.271.46.29211
68. Solano AR, Dada L, Podesta EJ. Lipoxygenase products as common intermediates in cyclic AMP-dependent and -independent adrenal steroidogenesis in rats. *J Mol Endocrinol* (1988) 1:147–54. doi:10.1677/jme.0.0010147
69. Castillo AF, Cornejo Maciel F, Castilla R, Duarte A, Maloberti P, Paz C, et al. cAMP increases mitochondrial cholesterol transport through the induction of arachidonic acid release inside this organelle in Leydig cells. *FEBS J* (2006) 273:5011–21. doi:10.1111/j.1742-4658.2006.05496.x
70. Mele PG, Dada LA, Paz C, Cymeryng CB, Cornejo Maciel MF, Neuman MI, et al. Site of action of proteinases in the activation of steroidogenesis in rat adrenal gland. *Biochim Biophys Acta* (1996) 1310:260–8. doi:10.1016/0167-4889(95)00177-8
71. Wang XJ, Dyson MT, Jo Y, Eubank DW, Stocco DM. Involvement of 5-lipoxygenase metabolites of arachidonic acid in cyclic AMP-stimulated steroidogenesis and steroidogenic acute regulatory protein gene expression. *J Steroid Biochem Mol Biol* (2003) 85:159–66. doi:10.1016/S0960-0760(03)00189-4
72. Maloberti P, Lozano RC, Mele PG, Cano F, Colonna C, Mendez CF, et al. Concerted regulation of free arachidonic acid and hormone-induced steroid synthesis by acyl-CoA thioesterases and acyl-CoA synthetases in adrenal cells. *Eur J Biochem* (2002) 269:5599–607. doi:10.1046/j.1432-1033.2002.03267.x
73. Duarte A, Castillo AF, Castilla R, Maloberti P, Paz C, Podesta EJ, et al. An arachidonic acid generation/export system involved in the regulation of cholesterol transport in mitochondria of steroidogenic cells. *FEBS Lett* (2007) 581:4023–8. doi:10.1016/j.febslet.2007.07.040
74. Kang MJ, Fujino T, Sasano H, Minekura H, Yabuki N, Nagura H, et al. A novel arachidonate-preferring acyl-CoA synthetase is present in steroidogenic cells of the rat adrenal, ovary, and testis. *Proc Natl Acad Sci U S A* (1997) 94:2880–4. doi:10.1073/pnas.94.7.2880
75. Paz C, Dada LA, Cornejo Maciel MF, Mele PG, Cymeryng CB, Neuman I, et al. Purification of a novel 43-kDa protein (p43) intermediary in the activation of steroidogenesis from rat adrenal gland. *Eur J Biochem* (1994) 224:709–16. doi:10.1111/j.1432-1033.1994.00709.x
76. Finkielstein CV, Maloberti P, Mendez CF, Podesta EJ. A novel arachidonic acid-related thioesterase involved in acute steroidogenesis. *Endocr Res* (1998) 24:363–71. doi:10.3109/07435809809032616
77. Lindquist PJ, Svensson LT, Alexson SE. Molecular cloning of the peroxisome proliferator-induced 46-kDa cytosolic acyl-CoA thioesterase from mouse and rat liver - recombinant expression in *Escherichia coli*, tissue expression, and nutritional regulation. *Eur J Biochem* (1998) 251:631–40. doi:10.1046/j.1432-1327.1998.2510631.x
78. Maloberti P, Mele PG, Neuman I, Cornejo Maciel F, Cano F, Bey P, et al. Regulation of arachidonic acid release in steroidogenesis: role of a new acyl-CoA thioestrase (ARTISt). *Endocr Res* (2000) 26:653–62. doi:10.3109/07435800009048585
79. Cornejo Maciel F, Maloberti P, Neuman I, Cano F, Castilla R, Castillo F, et al. An arachidonic acid-preferring acyl-CoA synthetase is a hormone-dependent and obligatory protein in the signal transduction pathway of steroidogenic hormones. *J Mol Endocrinol* (2005) 34:655–66. doi:10.1677/jme.1.01691
80. Maloberti P, Castilla R, Castillo F, Cornejo Maciel F, Mendez CF, Paz C, et al. Silencing the expression of mitochondrial acyl-CoA thioesterase I and acyl-CoA synthetase 4 inhibits hormone-induced steroidogenesis. *FEBS J* (2005) 272:1804–14. doi:10.1111/j.1742-4658.2005.04616.x
81. Cano F, Poderoso C, Cornejo Maciel F, Castilla R, Maloberti P, Castillo F, et al. Protein tyrosine phosphatases regulate arachidonic acid release, StAR induction and steroidogenesis acting on a hormone-dependent arachidonic acid-preferring acyl-CoA synthetase. *J Steroid Biochem Mol Biol* (2006) 99:197–202. doi:10.1016/j.jsbmb.2006.01.003
82. Cooke M, Mele P, Maloberti P, Duarte A, Poderoso C, Orlando U, et al. Tyrosine phosphatases as key regulators of StAR induction and cholesterol transport: SHP2 as a potential tyrosine phosphatase involved in steroid synthesis. *Mol Cell Endocrinol* (2011) 336:63–9. doi:10.1016/j.mce.2010.11.030
83. Feng GS, Hui CC, Pawson T. SH2-containing phosphotyrosine phosphatase as a target of protein-tyrosine kinases. *Science* (1993) 259:1607–11. doi:10.1126/science.8096088
84. Vogel W, Lammers R, Huang J, Ullrich A. Activation of a phosphotyrosine phosphatase by tyrosine phosphorylation. *Science* (1993) 259:1611–4. doi:10.1126/science.7681217
85. Bennett AM, Tang TL, Sugimoto S, Walsh CT, Neel BG. Protein-tyrosine-phosphatase SHPTP2 couples platelet-derived growth factor receptor beta to Ras. *Proc Natl Acad Sci U S A* (1994) 91:7335–9. doi:10.1073/pnas.91.15.7335
86. Zhang EE, Chapeau E, Hagihara K, Feng GS. Neuronal Shp2 tyrosine phosphatase controls energy balance and metabolism. *Proc Natl Acad Sci U S A* (2004) 101:16064–9. doi:10.1073/pnas.0405041101
87. Salvi M, Stringaro A, Brunati AM, Agostinelli E, Arancia G, Clari G, et al. Tyrosine phosphatase activity in mitochondria: presence of Shp-2 phosphatase in mitochondria. *Cell Mol Life Sci* (2004) 61:2393–404. doi:10.1007/s00018-004-4211-z
88. Miyazaki T, Neff L, Tanaka S, Horne WC, Baron R. Regulation of cytochrome c oxidase activity by c-Src in osteoclasts. *J Cell Biol* (2003) 160:709–18. doi:10.1083/jcb.200209098
89. Duarte A, Poderoso C, Cooke M, Soria G, Cornejo Maciel F, Gottifredi V, et al. Mitochondrial fusion is essential for steroid biosynthesis. *PLoS One* (2012) 7:e45829. doi:10.1371/journal.pone.0045829
90. Boutros T, Chevet E, Metrakos P. Mitogen-activated protein (MAP) kinase/MAP kinase phosphatase regulation: roles in cell growth, death, and cancer. *Pharmacol Rev* (2008) 60:261–310. doi:10.1124/pr.107.00106
91. Caunt CJ, Keyse SM. Dual-specificity MAP kinase phosphatases (MKPs): shaping the outcome of MAP kinase signalling. *FEBS J* (2013) 280:489–504. doi:10.1111/j.1742-4658.2012.08716.x
92. Watanabe G, Pena P, Albanese C, Wilsbacher LD, Young JB, Pestell RG. Adrenocorticotropin induction of stress-activated protein kinase in the adrenal cortex in vivo. *J Biol Chem* (1997) 272:20063–9. doi:10.1074/jbc.272.32.20063
93. Bey P, Gorostizaga AB, Maloberti PM, Lozano RC, Poderoso C, Cornejo Maciel F, et al. Adrenocorticotropin induces mitogen-activated protein kinase phosphatase 1 in Y1 mouse adrenocortical tumor cells. *Endocrinology* (2003) 144:1399–406. doi:10.1210/en.2002-220987
94. Sewer MB, Waterman MR. cAMP-dependent transcription of steroidogenic genes in the human adrenal cortex requires a dual-specificity phosphatase in addition to protein kinase A. *J Mol Endocrinol* (2002) 29:163–74. doi:10.1677/jme.0.0290163
95. Brion L, Maloberti PM, Gomez NV, Poderoso C, Gorostizaga AB, Mori Sequeiros Garcia MM, et al. MAPK phosphatase-1 (MKP-1) expression is up-regulated by hCG/cAMP and modulates steroidogenesis in MA-10 Leydig cells. *Endocrinology* (2011) 152:2665–77. doi:10.1210/en.2011-0021
96. Gomez NV, Gorostizaga AB, Mori Sequeiros Garcia MM, Brion L, Acquier A, Gonzalez-Calvar SI, et al. MAPK phosphatase-2 (MKP-2) is induced by hCG and plays a role in the regulation of CYP11A1 expression in MA-10 Leydig cells. *Endocrinology* (2013) 154:1488–500. doi:10.1210/en.2012-2032
97. Mori Sequeiros Garcia M, Gomez NV, Gorostizaga A, Acquier A, Gonzalez-Calvar SI, Mendez CF, et al. MAP kinase phosphatase-3 (MKP-3) is transcriptionally and post-translationally up-regulated by hCG and modulates cAMP-induced p21 expression in MA-10 Leydig cells. *Mol Cell Endocrinol* (2013) 371:174–81. doi:10.1016/j.mce.2012.12.006
98. Rone MB, Midzak AS, Issop L, Rammouz G, Jagannathan S, Fan J, et al. Identification of a dynamic mitochondrial protein complex driving cholesterol import, trafficking, and metabolism to steroid hormones. *Mol Endocrinol* (2012) 26:1868–82. doi:10.1210/me.2012-1159
99. Jefcoate C. High-flux mitochondrial cholesterol trafficking, a specialized function of the adrenal cortex. *J Clin Invest* (2002) 110:881–90. doi:10.1172/JCI0216771

100. Allen JA, Shankara T, Janus P, Buck S, Diemer T, Hales KH, et al. Energized, polarized, and actively respiring mitochondria are required for acute Leydig cell steroidogenesis. *Endocrinology* (2006) 147:3924–35. doi:10.1210/en.2005-1204
101. Granot Z, Melamed-Book N, Bahat A, Orly J. Turnover of StAR protein: roles for the proteasome and mitochondrial proteases. *Mol Cell Endocrinol* (2007) 265-266:51–8. doi:10.1016/j.mce.2006.12.003
102. Miller WL. Steroid hormone synthesis in mitochondria. *Mol Cell Endocrinol* (2013) 379:62–73. doi:10.1016/j.mce.2013.04.014
103. Granot Z, Kobiler O, Melamed-Book N, Eimerl S, Bahat A, Lu B, et al. Turnover of mitochondrial steroidogenic acute regulatory (StAR) protein by Lon protease: the unexpected effect of proteasome inhibitors. *Mol Endocrinol* (2007) 21:2164–77. doi:10.1210/me.2005-0458
104. Midzak A, Rone M, Aghazadeh Y, Culty M, Papadopoulos V. Mitochondrial protein import and the genesis of steroidogenic mitochondria. *Mol Cell Endocrinol* (2011) 336:70–9. doi:10.1016/j.mce.2010.12.007
105. Bahat A, Perlberg S, Melamed-Book N, Lauria I, Langer T, Orly J. StAR enhances transcription of genes encoding the mitochondrial proteases involved in its own degradation. *Mol Endocrinol* (2014) 28:208–24. doi:10.1210/me.2013-1275
106. Duarte A, Castillo AF, Podesta EJ, Poderoso C. Mitochondrial fusion and ERK activity regulate steroidogenic acute regulatory protein localization in mitochondria. *PLoS One* (2014) 9:e100387. doi:10.1371/journal.pone.0100387
107. Bose HS, Lingappa VR, Miller WL. The steroidogenic acute regulatory protein, StAR, works only at the outer mitochondrial membrane. *Endocr Res* (2002) 28:295–308. doi:10.1081/ERC-120016800
108. Arakane F, Sugawara T, Nishino H, Liu Z, Holt JA, Pain D, et al. Steroidogenic acute regulatory protein (StAR) retains activity in the absence of its mitochondrial import sequence: implications for the mechanism of StAR action. *Proc Natl Acad Sci U S A* (1996) 93:13731–6. doi:10.1073/pnas.93.24.13731
109. Arakane F, Kallen CB, Watari H, Foster JA, Sepuri NB, Pain D, et al. The mechanism of action of steroidogenic acute regulatory protein (StAR). StAR acts on the outside of mitochondria to stimulate steroidogenesis. *J Biol Chem* (1998) 273:16339–45. doi:10.1074/jbc.273.26.16339
110. Martin SJ. Mitochondrial fusion: bax to the fussure. *Dev Cell* (2011) 20:142–3. doi:10.1016/j.devcel.2011.01.016
111. Rizzuto R, Brini M, Pizzo P, Murgia M, Pozzan T. Chimeric green fluorescent protein as a tool for visualizing subcellular organelles in living cells. *Curr Biol* (1995) 5:635–42. doi:10.1016/S0960-9822(95)00128-X
112. de Brito OM, Scorrano L. Mitofusin 2 tethers endoplasmic reticulum to mitochondria. *Nature* (2008) 456:605–10. doi:10.1038/nature07534
113. Vance JE. MAM (mitochondria-associated membranes) in mammalian cells: lipids and beyond. *Biochim Biophys Acta* (2014) 1841:595–609. doi:10.1016/j.bbalip.2013.11.014
114. Sugiura A, Nagashima S, Tokuyama T, Amo T, Matsuki Y, Ishido S, et al. MITOL regulates endoplasmic reticulum-mitochondria contacts via Mitofusin2. *Mol Cell* (2013) 51:20–34. doi:10.1016/j.molcel.2013.04.023
115. Lewin TM, Van Horn CG, Krisans SK, Coleman RA. Rat liver acyl-CoA synthetase 4 is a peripheral-membrane protein located in two distinct subcellular organelles, peroxisomes, and mitochondrial-associated membrane. *Arch Biochem Biophys* (2002) 404:263–70. doi:10.1016/S0003-9861(02)00247-3
116. Merrill RA, Dagda RK, Dickey AS, Cribbs JT, Green SH, Usachev YM, et al. Mechanism of neuroprotective mitochondrial remodeling by PKA/AKAP1. *PLoS Biol* (2011) 9:e1000612. doi:10.1371/journal.pbio.1000612
117. Qi X, Disatnik MH, Shen N, Sobel RA, Mochly-Rosen D. Aberrant mitochondrial fission in neurons induced by protein kinase C{delta} under oxidative stress conditions in vivo. *Mol Biol Cell* (2010) 22:256–65. doi:10.1091/mbc.E10-06-0551
118. Soto EA, Kliman HJ, Strauss JF III, Paavola LG. Gonadotropins and cyclic adenosine 3',5'-monophosphate (cAMP) alter the morphology of cultured human granulosa cells. *Biol Reprod* (1986) 34:559–69. doi:10.1095/biolreprod34.3.559
119. Li D, Sewer MB. RhoA and DIAPH1 mediate adrenocorticotropin-stimulated cortisol biosynthesis by regulating mitochondrial trafficking. *Endocrinology* (2010) 151:4313–23. doi:10.1210/en.2010-0044
120. Fulop L, Szanda G, Enyedi B, Varnai P, Spat A. The effect of OPA1 on mitochondrial Ca(2)(+) signaling. *PLoS One* (2011) 6:e25199. doi:10.1371/journal.pone.0025199
121. Spat A, Fulop L, Szanda G. The role of mitochondrial Ca(2+) and NAD(P)H in the control of aldosterone secretion. *Cell Calcium* (2012) 52:64–72. doi:10.1016/j.ceca.2012.01.009
122. Issop L, Fan J, Lee S, Rone MB, Basu K, Mui J, et al. Mitochondria-associated membrane formation in hormone-stimulated Leydig cell steroidogenesis: role of ATAD3. *Endocrinology* (2015) 156:334–45. doi:10.1210/en.2014-1503
123. Petrescu AD, Gallegos AM, Okamura Y, Strauss JF III, Schroeder F. Steroidogenic acute regulatory protein binds cholesterol and modulates mitochondrial membrane sterol domain dynamics. *J Biol Chem* (2001) 276:36970–82. doi:10.1074/jbc.M101939200
124. Mathieu AP, Fleury A, Ducharme L, Lavigne P, LeHoux JG. Insights into steroidogenic acute regulatory protein (StAR)-dependent cholesterol transfer in mitochondria: evidence from molecular modeling and structure-based thermodynamics supporting the existence of partially unfolded states of StAR. *J Mol Endocrinol* (2002) 29:327–45. doi:10.1677/jme.0.0290327
125. Tsujishita Y, Hurley JH. Structure and lipid transport mechanism of a StAR-related domain. *Nat Struct Biol* (2000) 7:408–14. doi:10.1038/75192
126. Yaworsky DC, Baker BY, Bose HS, Best KB, Jensen LB, Bell JD, et al. pH-dependent Interactions of the carboxyl-terminal helix of steroidogenic acute regulatory protein with synthetic membranes. *J Biol Chem* (2005) 280:2045–54. doi:10.1074/jbc.M410937200
127. Reitz J, Gehrig-Burger K, Strauss JF III, Gimpl G. Cholesterol interaction with the related steroidogenic acute regulatory lipid-transfer (START) domains of StAR (STARD1) and MLN64 (STARD3). *FEBS J* (2008) 275:1790–802. doi:10.1111/j.1742-4658.2008.06337.x
128. Papaleo E, Ranzani V, Tripodi F, Vitriolo A, Cirulli C, Fantucci P, et al. An acidic loop and cognate phosphorylation sites define a molecular switch that modulates ubiquitin charging activity in Cdc34-like enzymes. *PLoS Comput Biol* (2011) 7:e1002056. doi:10.1371/journal.pcbi.1002056
129. Poderoso C, Duarte A, Cooke M, Orlando U, Gottifredi V, Solano AR, et al. The spatial and temporal regulation of the hormonal signal. Role of mitochondria in the formation of a protein complex required for the activation of cholesterol transport and steroids synthesis. *Mol Cell Endocrinol* (2013) 371:26–33. doi:10.1016/j.mce.2012.12.024

13

Signaling Interactions in the Adrenal Cortex

András Spät[1,2], László Hunyady[1,2] and Gergő Szanda[1]*

[1] Department of Physiology, Semmelweis University Medical School, Budapest, Hungary, [2] Laboratory of Molecular Physiology, Hungarian Academy of Sciences, Budapest, Hungary

***Correspondence:**
András Spät
spat@eok.sote.hu*

The major physiological stimuli of aldosterone secretion are angiotensin II (AII) and extracellular K^+, whereas cortisol production is primarily regulated by corticotropin (ACTH) in fasciculata cells. AII triggers Ca^{2+} release from internal stores that is followed by store-operated and voltage-dependent Ca^{2+} entry, whereas K^+-evoked depolarization activates voltage-dependent Ca^{2+} channels. ACTH acts primarily through the formation of cAMP and subsequent protein phosphorylation by protein kinase A. Both Ca^{2+} and cAMP facilitate the transfer of cholesterol to mitochondrial inner membrane. The cytosolic Ca^{2+} signal is transferred into the mitochondrial matrix and enhances pyridine nucleotide reduction. Increased formation of NADH results in increased ATP production, whereas that of NADPH supports steroid production. In reality, the control of adrenocortical function is a lot more sophisticated with second messengers crosstalking and mutually modifying each other's pathways. Cytosolic Ca^{2+} and cGMP are both capable of modifying cAMP metabolism, while cAMP may enhance Ca^{2+} release and voltage-activated Ca^{2+} channel activity. Besides, mitochondrial Ca^{2+} signal brings about cAMP formation within the organelle and this further enhances aldosterone production. Maintained aldosterone and cortisol secretion are optimized by the concurrent actions of Ca^{2+} and cAMP, as exemplified by the apparent synergism of Ca^{2+} influx (inducing cAMP formation) and Ca^{2+} release during response to AII. Thus, cross-actions of parallel signal transducing pathways are not mere intracellular curiosities but rather substantial phenomena, which fine-tune the biological response. Our review focuses on these functionally relevant interactions between the Ca^{2+} and the cyclic nucleotide signal transducing pathways hitherto described in the adrenal cortex.

Keywords: cAMP, Ca^{2+} signal, mitochondria, aldosterone, angiotensin II, ACTH, potassium ion, cortisol

INTRODUCTION

The adrenal cortex contains three zones, of which *glomerulosa* secretes the mineralocorticoid aldosterone, *fasciculata* synthesizes the glucocorticoid cortisol (or corticosterone in rodents), whereas the *reticularis* produces androgens [reviewed in Ref. (1)]. Aldosterone, acting on the distal nephron, augments Na^+ reabsorption as well as K^+ and H^+ excretion. Through changes in sodium balance, it influences the extracellular fluid space and blood pressure, and its importance in cardiovascular, renal, and inflammatory diseases has also been recognized (2–4). Cortisol, among other things, controls intermediary metabolism, modulates immune responses, and is essential for the resistance of the organism to noxious stimuli. Adrenal androgens exert important anabolic effects in females and have substantial clinical significance in adrenal pathologies.

Sodium and/or fluid depletion, hemodynamic changes, and hyperkalemia stimulate aldosterone secretion. When fluid loss is severe, ACTH synergizes with angiotensin II (AII) in stimulating glomerulosa cells. During hypervolemia, atrial natriuretic peptide (ANP) inhibits aldosterone secretion [for reviews, see Ref. (5, 6)]. Cortisol production is governed by ACTH. The regulation of ACTH secretion and the signaling in zona *reticularis* (7) are beyond the scope of this review.

CLASSICAL SIGNALING PATHWAYS IN THE ADRENAL CORTEX

Signaling Pathways in Glomerulosa Cells

The major signaling pathways of ACTH, K^+, and AII, termed "classical" here have been described in several reviews [e.g., Ref. (5, 6, 8, 9)] and are only briefly summarized below.

ACTH binds to the melanocortin-type receptor MC2R, which activates adenylyl cyclase (AC) *via* the heterotrimeric G-protein G_s (10, 11), and subsequent cAMP formation activates protein kinase A (PKA). PKA then phosphorylates and induces the hormone-sensitive lipase (previously "cholesterol ester hydrolase") (12) as well as the steroidogenic acute regulatory protein (StAR), the protein transporting cholesterol into the mitochondria (13, 14). As a result of these, the steroid precursor cholesterol is released from lipid droplets and transported to side-chain cleavage by CYP11A1, located in the inner mitochondrial membrane. This causes the stimulation of adrenal steroidogenesis.

Extracellular K^+ and AII act by generating cytosolic Ca^{2+} signal. Depolarization induced by physiological elevations of $[K^+]$ activates T-type voltage-dependent Ca^{2+} channels the current of which was detected in rat (15–17), bovine (16, 18, 19), and human glomerulosa cells (20). Concomitant cell swelling evoked by K^+ also enhances this T-type current (21, 22).

The unique sensitivity of glomerulosa cells to K^+ (6, 23, 24) may be attributed to their high permeability to K^+ (19, 25–28) and the function of the T-type channel $Ca_v3.2$. The channel's subunit α_{1H} is expressed in rat, murine, and bovine glomerulosa cell (29, 30). In view of the very negative membrane potential of isolated glomerulosa cells (27, 31), basal Ca^{2+} influx was attributed to a steady-state window current (19, 32). The control of $Ca_v3.2$ in glomerulosa cells has recently been analyzed in murine adrenal slices (30), in which cells had a mean resting potential of −82 mV. Spontaneous membrane potential oscillations generated by $Ca_v3.2$ were observed between −87 and −75 mV. Increasing $[K^+]$ up to 5 mM depolarized the membrane and increased oscillation frequency and peak amplitudes, whereas the increased frequency upon AII stimulation was most probably due to a G_i-mediated shift in the voltage dependence of channel activation toward more negative potentials (33). In either cases, the ensuing Ca^{2+} signal (*via* CaMKII and p42/44 MAP kinase) acts on hormone-sensitive lipase (34) and StAR (13, 35, 36) [similarly to the actions of PKA (37)].

Angiotensin II stimulates aldosterone secretion after binding to AT_1 receptors (AT1Rs) (38–40). Acting *via* the G-protein G_q and phospholipase C_β, it induces the formation of inositol 1,4,5-trisphosphate (IP_3) (41–43) which, through specific receptors [IP3Rs (44–46)] generates Ca^{2+} signal. Out of the three receptor isoforms expressed in glomerulosa cells (47), the dominant IP_3R1 exhibits the greatest affinity for IP_3. The initial Ca^{2+} release is followed by Ca^{2+} influx (48, 49) through store-operated (50, 51) and later *via* T-type Ca^{2+} channels (18, 33) [but see Ref. (52)]. In isolated rat glomerulosa cells, AII-induced T-type current is activated by depolarization (19) brought about by the inhibition of the Na^+/K^+ pump (53) and by the two-pore domain K^+ channel TASK (25, 54). In murine cells maintained *in situ*, T-current is enhanced by a G_i-mediated increase in the frequency of oscillating action potentials (30, 33).

Angiotensin II inhibits L-type current (55) and thus attenuates Ca^{2+} signals evoked by high $[K^+]$ (56, 57). This effect of the peptide is mediated by the G-protein G_i, expressed in glomerulosa cells (55, 58).

Due to space limits, this review does not deal with diacylglycerol - protein kinase C (PKC), lipoxygenase, and MAPK pathways [reviewed, e.g., in Ref. (6)].

Signaling in Fasciculata Cells

The physiological stimulus of glucocorticoid synthesis and secretion by fasciculata cells is ACTH, acting *via* MC2R receptors and cAMP. The mode of cAMP action is identical to that described above for glomerulosa cell [for review, see Ref. (59)].

ACTH action on fasciculata cells requires Ca^{2+}. As observed already in the 70s, ACTH induces membrane potential changes (60) due mainly to Ca^{2+} influx (61). Both T-type ($Ca_v3.2$) and L-type ($Ca_v1.3$ and a non-identified) isoforms were characterized in bovine fasciculata cells, and their participation in ACTH- and AII-stimulated cortisol secretion was demonstrated (62). We are not aware of data on Ca^{2+} channels in rat and native human fasciculata cells; however, the observation that rat fasciculata cells were unresponsive to 13 mM K^+ (23) indicates the lack of T-type Ca^{2+} channels. The resting membrane potential in bovine fasciculata cells is set by the background K^+ channel bTREK-1 (63), whereas the TASK-3 background K^+ channel, characteristic for rat glomerulosa cell (26), is undetectable in bovine fasciculata cells (64).

Albeit AT1R is expressed in human, bovine, and ovine fasciculata cells (65–67) data whether AII *alone* stimulates cortisol secretion are conflicting (62, 68–70). Rat *fasciculata* cells do not express detectable amounts of AT1R (71–73) [but see Ref. (74)] or inositol 1,4,5-trisphosphate receptor (IP3R) mRNA (47) and, accordingly, AII does not stimulate steroid production in these cells (23, 74, 75).

The expression of AT1R in fasciculata cells and the stimulation of cortisol secretion by the peptide raise the question whether AII plays any role in the control of cortisol secretion in man. In lack of comprehensive studies, we hypothesize that in stress situations, stimulation of fasciculata cells by AII may contribute to the stimulatory action of ACTH. On the other hand, in case of long-term high AII levels, cortisol secretion is maintained at resting level by the feed-back control of ACTH secretion.

The human adrenocortical cancer-derived H295R cell, a widely used model for studying steroid production, does not express either MC2R receptors (76) or $Ca_v3.2$ T-type Ca^{2+} channels (30) [but see Ref. (77)]. Not surprisingly, these cells are insensitive to ACTH and respond to K^+ at supraphysiological concentrations only (78).

INTERACTION OF SIGNALING PATHWAYS IN ADRENOCORTICAL CELLS

(Auto)Regulation of Ca^{2+} Metabolism by Ca^{2+}

The formation, metabolism, and the action of IP_3 all depend on cytosolic [Ca^{2+}] ([Ca^{2+}]$_c$). Phospholipase C_β, generating IP_3 from PIP_2 (79) and the IP_3 metabolizing IP_3-3 kinase are both activated by Ca^{2+} (80–82). High [Ca^{2+}]$_c$ may reduce IP_3 binding (83), whereas elevation of [Ca^{2+}]$_c$ up to ~300 nM increases the sensitivity of IP_3R1 to IP_3 [reviewed in Ref. (6)]. These characteristics play an important role in the oscillatory pattern of Ca^{2+} release. IP_3R phosphorylation by PKA, PKC, or CaMKII enhances Ca^{2+} release, while calcineurin decreases this phosphorylation state (84). Also, calcium–calmodulin activates the plasmalemmal Ca ATPase (85) and inhibits the Na^+/K^+ ATPase (86, 87), the latter resulting in depolarization and Ca^{2+} influx through T-type channels (see Signaling Pathways in Glomerulosa Cells).

Effects of Ca^{2+} on Cytosolic cAMP

Early reports on K^+-evoked cAMP formation suggested a role for Ca^{2+} in the activation of AC (88, 89). Maintained secretagogue effect of ACTH in rat glomerulosa (90) and bovine fasciculata cells is also Ca^{2+}-dependent (62) with calcium–calmodulin affecting primarily the formation of cAMP (91). In fact, in bovine cells, the effect of ACTH on cAMP formation correlates to extracellular [Ca^{2+}] (92), and ACTH-induced cAMP formation is potentiated by AII in the presence of Ca^{2+} only (69).

Nevertheless, conflicting data were reported concerning the effect of AII on cAMP formation in bovine adrenocortical cells (69, 93–95). Reduced cAMP formation was reported in AII-stimulated rat glomerulosa cells (96, 97), whereas enhanced cAMP formation was observed in the human H295R cell (98). In this respect, the Ca^{2+} sensitivity of different transmembrane adenylyl cyclase isoforms (99, 100) should be considered. The Ca^{2+}-activatable isoform AC1 is expressed in human glomerulosa and fasciculata cells (99); the Ca^{2+}/calmodulin-activatable AC3 was found in human (99), rat (101), and bovine (69) glomerulosa cells. Ca^{2+}-inhibited isoforms (AC5 and AC6) were detected in human (99) and rat glomerulosa cells (102). It should also be kept in mind that Ca^{2+}-activatable AC isoforms are more responsive to store-operated Ca^{2+} entry than to Ca^{2+} release. This phenomenon is due to the colocalization of Ca^{2+} activatable AC isoforms and store-operated Ca^{2+} channels in plasmalemmal lipid rafts (103) and may account for the delayed cAMP response to AII (98).

After the description of G_i in rat glomerulosa cells (58), the reported inhibition of AC by AII was attributed to this inhibitory G-protein (55, 95). Summarizing, the cell-type differences in the effect AII on AC may be attributed to G_i density and the ratio of the various AC isoforms.

The Ca^{2+}-modified signaling pathways are summarized in **Figure 1**.

Effects of cAMP on Ca^{2+} Signaling

ACTH or cell-permeable cAMP analogs may induce a sustained Ca^{2+} signal after a lag time of a few minutes as was shown in rat (104), bovine (92), and human glomerulosa cells (105), as well as in H295R cells (106). Several molecular interactions may warrant such an effect. PKA phosphorylates L-type Ca^{2+} channels (105, 107) [but see Ref. (108)], the ensuing Ca^{2+} current activates phospholipase C_δ, and the generated IP_3 induces Ca^{2+} release from the endoplasmic reticulum (ER). In addition, PKA also phosphorylates and activates IP_3R1 [reviewed in Ref. (6)]. In fact, ACTH evokes a small phosphoinositide response (109) and PKC activation (110) in rat glomerulosa cells. By the same token, 8Br-cAMP enhanced AII-induced IP_3 formation in bovine cells (111). Taken together, cAMP and its downstream effectors may enhance both Ca^{2+} influx and Ca^{2+} release in the adrenals.

The cAMP-modified signaling pathways are summarized in **Figure 2**.

Signaling Modulation by cGMP

Cyclic GMP is formed after the activation of ANP receptors. The nucleotide reduces T-type Ca^{2+} current (112) and inhibits the AC (113). In addition, cGMP activates PDE2A (114–116), one of phosphodiesterase isozymes identified in adrenocortical cells [reviewed by Vezzosi and Bertherat (117)]. By these actions, ANP reduces basal and stimulated aldosterone secretion (112).

Synergistic Effects of Ca^{2+} Release and Ca^{2+} Influx

Moderate hyperkalemia increases the sensitivity and the maximal aldosterone response to AII (118–120). Potassium (4–8 mM) potentiates the secretory response to thapsigargin (evoking net Ca^{2+} release from the ER), whereas the secretory effects of thapsigargin and AII (300 pM) are additive only (119). When net Ca^{2+} release was induced with Ni^{2+}, an inhibitor of microsomal Ca^{2+} uptake, the aldosterone response to physiological concentrations of K^+ was again potentiated (121). These observations indicate that Ca^{2+} release and influx act in synergism on aldosterone secretion.

The synergism between Ca^{2+} release and influx may be explained by the formation of microdomains. Increased subplasmalemmal [Ca^{2+}] (formed around the orifice of Ca^{2+} channels) may activate e.g., Ca^{2+}-dependent AC isoforms and may induce specific gene expression (122, 123). On the other hand, Ca^{2+} release into the perinuclear space may turn on Ca^{2+}-dependent nuclear genes and enhance NAD(P)H formation in ER-vicinal mitochondria (see Ca^{2+} Signal and Mitochondrial Function). In addition, the reduction in exchangeable Ca^{2+} pool during exposure to AII (124) may be counterbalanced by concomitant Ca^{2+} influx.

Angiotensin II-induced initial IP_3 peak is followed by sustained suprabasal IP3 formation (41). Li^+ inhibits the resynthesis of phosphoinositides and precludes the maintained formation of IP_3, and thus attenuates the post-initial phase of AII-induced

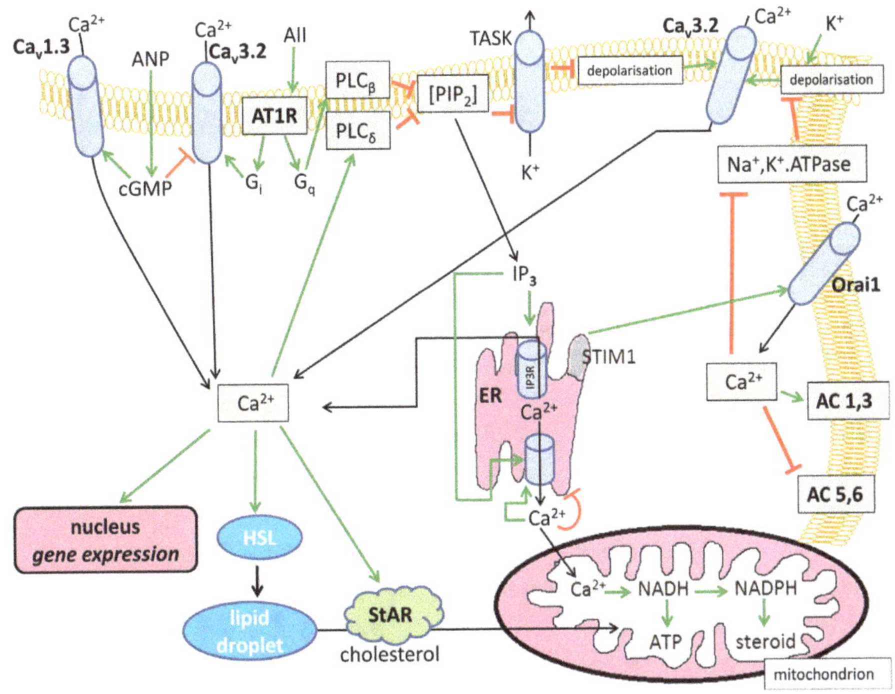

FIGURE 1 | Effects of Ca^{2+} on cytosolic cAMP in glomerulosa cells. Positive modulations are shown with green arrows and negative effects are shown with red blunted arrows. Black arrows indicate substance transport. $Ca_v1.3$, L-type voltage-dependent Ca^{2+} channel; $Ca_v3.2$, T-type voltage-dependent Ca^{2+} channel; ANP, atrial natriuretic peptide; AII, angiotensin II; AT1R, angiotensin II receptor type 1, G_i and G_q, heterotrimeric G-proteins; PIP_2, phosphatidyl inositol 1,4,5-trisphosphate; TASK, KCNK3 or KCNK9-type K^+ channel; AC, transmembrane adenylyl cyclase; ER, endoplasmic reticulum; IP_3, inositol 1,4,5-trisphosphate; IP3R, IP_3 receptor; HSL, hormone-sensitive lipase; StAR, steroidogenic acute regulatory protein.

(but not ACTH-induced) aldosterone output of glomerulosa cells (125). This indicates that sustained suprabasal IP_3 formation, Ca^{2+} release and, probably, store-operated Ca^{2+} entry all support long-lasting aldosterone secretion.

EFFECTS OF CONVERGENT SIGNALING ON GENE EXPRESSION

Both Ca^{2+} and cyclic nucleotide signaling affect the transcriptome of adrenocortical cells (126, 127). Complex transcriptional or epigenetic (128) changes during adrenal zonation, remodeling, and neoplastic transformation are beyond the scope of this study [for review, see, e.g., Ref. (129, 130)]. Instead, we focus on instances where gene expression is modulated by parallel signal transducing pathways. One illustrative example of such an interplay involves the transcriptional regulation of hormone-sensitive lipase and StAR, both of which are induced by the cAMP-PKA (12–14) and by the Ca^{2+} pathway (13, 34–36). Along similar lines, Ca^{2+} and cAMP, through overlapping *cis* regulatory elements, synergistically induce the transcription of aldosterone synthase (CYP11B2) (131) and (as observed in non-adrenal cells) the mitochondrial Ca^{2+} uniporter (MCU, see below) (132). Transcription of type I 3β-hydroxysteroid dehydrogenase (HSD3B1), expressed predominantly in the human zona glomerulosa (133), can be induced by AII but not by K^+ (134). A plausible explanation is that only AII [in part *via* PKC (135, 136)] recruits the nuclear receptor subfamily 4 (NGFI-B), which is also necessary for the induction of HSD3B1. In contrast, both AII and K^+ induce CYP11B2 expression *via* the Ca^{2+}/CaMK and MAP kinase pathways (137).

In vascular smooth muscle cells, both G_s- and G_q-initiated signaling dampen the expression of AT1R through mRNA destabilization (138). Interestingly, to carry out this mRNA degradation, the pathways partially converge on PKA (139). An effect closely reminiscent of such a convergence was observed in H295R cells where forskolin, db-cAMP, and AII all brought about a rapid drop in AT1R message levels. [Nevertheless, long-term AT1R repression was induced with forskolin/db-cAMP only (140).]

Ca^{2+} SIGNAL AND MITOCHONDRIAL FUNCTION

Calcium activates three dehydrogenases in suspended or homogenized mitochondria (141). Ca^{2+}-dependent mitochondrial NADH and NADPH (NAD(P)H) formation in living cells was first demonstrated in K^+-stimulated glomerulosa cells (142). Similar response to AII and vasopressin was also reported (143, 144). The significance of increased NADH and ensuing ATP production (145) in any biological response is obvious, whereas NADPH is a cofactor of steroid biosynthesis (1). Noteworthy, the spatial and temporal pattern of AII-induced cytosolic Ca^{2+} signal depends on mitochondrial metabolism (78).

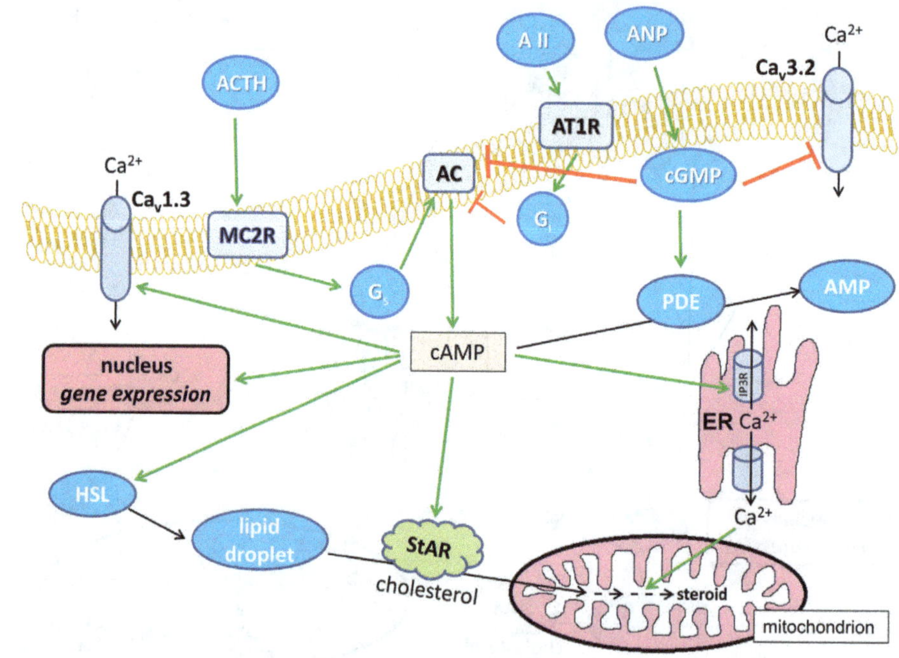

FIGURE 2 | Effects of cAMP on Ca^{2+} signaling in glomerulosa cells. Positive modulations are shown with green arrows and negative effects are shown with red blunted arrows. Black arrows indicate substance transport. $Ca_v1.3$, L-type voltage-dependent Ca^{2+} channel; $Ca_v3.2$, T-type voltage-dependent Ca^{2+} channel; ANP, atrial natriuretic peptide; AII, angiotensin II; AT1R, angiotensin II receptor type 1, G_i and G_q, heterotrimeric G-proteins; AC, transmembrane adenylyl cyclase; ER, endoplasmic reticulum; IP3R, IP_3 receptor; HSL, hormone-sensitive lipase; StAR, steroidogenic acute regulatory protein; ACTH, corticotropin; MC2R, melanocortin receptor type 2, PDE, cAMP phosphodiesterase; AMP, adenosine monophosphate.

The primary event in the mitochondrial response to a cytosolic Ca^{2+} signal is the transfer of the ion into the mitochondrial matrix (146–149). Ca^{2+} transport occurs through the MCU complex, the velocity of which is a sigmoid function of $[Ca^{2+}]_c$ due to the allosteric control of the MCU channel by the regulatory subunits MICU1 and MICU2 [reviewed in Ref. (150)]. IP_3-induced Ca^{2+} release from the ER generates high-Ca^{2+} microdomains between the ER and mitochondria and allows for mitochondrial Ca^{2+} uptake by the low-Ca^{2+}-affinity MCU (151). However, the mitochondria of glomerulosa cells are uniquely sensitive to Ca^{2+} (152) and influx-induced low-Ca^{2+} signals are also effective in elevating mitochondrial $[Ca^{2+}]$ ($[Ca^{2+}]_m$) (153). This responsiveness may be essential for maintained aldosterone secretion in response to long-lasting hyperkalemia, characterized by small elevation of $[Ca^{2+}]_c$.

Increased $[Ca^{2+}]_m$ and the ensuing NAD(P)H formation play an essential role in the stimulation of aldosterone production. Targeted mitochondrial expression of a Ca^{2+} binding protein reduces both $[Ca^{2+}]_m$ and NAD(P)H and ensuing aldosterone production in response to AII (154). The opposite, increased mitochondrial Ca^{2+} uptake after the knockdown of p38 MAPK or the silencing of mitochondrial protein OPA1 results in increased NAD(P)H formation and enhanced aldosterone production (155).

A recently recognized and biologically significant action of Ca^{2+} signaling is the formation of cAMP in mitochondria. In addition to the nine isoforms of transmembrane AC, a soluble isoform (sAC) was prepared from testis (156). Its activity is not influenced by forskolin or G-proteins but increased by bicarbonate (157) and Ca^{2+} (158). The expression of sAC in the mitochondrial matrix together with a degrading mechanism sensitive to phosphodiesterase 2A inhibitors were recently described in HeLa cells (159, 160). The activity of intramitochondrial sAC increased in response to mitochondrial Ca^{2+} signal in HeLa and CHO cells and in rat cardiomyocytes (161). Importantly, mitochondrial cAMP (mt-cAMP) supported ATP formation (160, 161).

The sAC is also expressed in H295R adrenocortical cells, and it is found in the particulate fraction predominantly. In these cells, AII-induced mitochondrial Ca^{2+} signal increased the formation of mt-cAMP, and this response was enhanced by the PDE2A inhibitor EHNA. Mitochondrial cAMP signaling was attenuated with the sAC inhibitor 2-OH-estradiol, after silencing of the sAC gene and by the buffering of mitochondrial Ca^{2+} by S100G protein. All these maneuvers also attenuated aldosterone production, showing the cell-type-specific significance of mt-cAMP for the first time (98).

CONCLUSION

Adrenocortical steroid production is under the control of both Ca^{2+} signaling and cyclic nucleotide metabolism. Importantly, these intracellular pathways are rarely, or probably never, independent. As postulated by Berridge in 1975 (162), cAMP and Ca^{2+} signaling may be antagonistic or synergistic in nature and, as hopefully accentuated by this review, the adrenal cortex is no exception to this rule. As shown in **Figures 1** and **2**, the aforementioned signal transducing pathways have the potential to interact at a number of points and levels of signaling. However, it needs to be stressed that these potential interactions are not enforced all at once but, instead, may be limited temporally and spatially (e.g., to signaling microdomains). Also, significant variance in the expression pattern and intensity of the relevant signaling molecules is to be expected depending on species and on the stimuli the organism is concurrently exposed to.

In spite of the interspecies differences and of the incongruences in some experimental data, it is probably safe to conclude that an adequate biological response necessitates the intricate interplay of parallel signaling pathways. That is to say that, e.g., in glomerulosa cells, sustained aldosterone response evoked by long-lasting tonic stimuli will be satisfactory only if the Ca^{2+} release/influx is accompanied by the sufficient formation of cAMP. Albeit the secretagogues AII and K^+ invoke predominantly Ca^{2+} signaling and the effects of ACTH are mediated chiefly by cAMP, the increase of both factors at the same time may *potentiate* the final response. Thus, the separate intracellular pathways need not be activated to the same extent but nevertheless have to be recruited simultaneously for a sufficient steroid production to follow.

AUTHOR CONTRIBUTIONS

AS and GS compiled the literary data and wrote the manuscript. Data on the control of expression have been discussed with LH.

ACKNOWLEDGMENTS

The authors were supported by the Hungarian Academy of Sciences and by the Hungarian National Science Foundation (OTKA NK100883). GS was also supported by the János Bolyai Research Scholarship of the Hungarian Academy of Sciences. The artwork of the figures was kindly prepared by Ms. Anna Szilágyi.

REFERENCES

1. Vinson GP, Whitehouse B, Hinson J. *The Adrenal Cortex*. Englewood Cliffs, NJ: Prentice Hall (1992). p. 65–139.
2. Gomez-Sanchez CE. Non renal effects of aldosterone. *Steroids* (2014) **91**:1–2. doi:10.1016/j.steroids.2014.10.003
3. Pacurari M, Kafoury R, Tchounwou PB, Ndebele K. The Renin-Angiotensin-aldosterone system in vascular inflammation and remodeling. *Int J Inflam* (2014) **2014**:689360. doi:10.1155/2014/689360
4. Auchus RJ. Classics in cardiovascular endocrinology – aldosterone action beyond electrolytes. *Endocrinology* (2016) **157**(2):429–31. doi:10.1210/en.2015-2061
5. Bollag WB. Regulation of aldosterone synthesis and secretion. *Compr Physiol* (2014) **4**:1017–55. doi:10.1002/cphy.c130037
6. Spät A, Hunyady L. Control of aldosterone secretion: a model for convergence in cellular signaling pathways. *Physiol Rev* (2004) **84**:489–539. doi:10.1152/physrev.00030.2003
7. Parker LN. Control of adrenal androgen secretion. *Endocrinol Metab Clin North Am* (1991) **20**(2):401–21.
8. Hattangady NG, Olala LO, Bollag WB, Rainey WE. Acute and chronic regulation of aldosterone production. *Mol Cell Endocrinol* (2012) **350**:151–62. doi:10.1016/j.mce.2011.07.034
9. Payne AH, Hales DB. Overview of steroidogenic enzymes in the pathway from cholesterol to active steroid hormones. *Endocr Rev* (2004) **25**:947–70. doi:10.1210/er.2003-0030
10. Albano JDM, Brown BL, Ekins RP, Tait SAS, Tait JF. The effects of potassium, 5-hydroxytryptamine, adrenocorticotropin and angiotensin II on the concentration of adenosine 3':5'-cyclic monophosphate in suspensions of dispersed rat adrenal zona glomerulosa and zona fasciculata cells. *Biochem J* (1974) **142**:391–400. doi:10.1042/bj1420391
11. Grahame-Smith DG, Butcher RW, Ney RL, Sutherland EW. Adenosine 3',5'-monophosphate as the intracellular mediator of the action of adrenocorticotropic hormone on the adrenal cortex. *J Biol Chem* (1967) **242**:5535–41.
12. Holm C, Osterlund T, Laurell H, Contreras JA. Molecular mechanisms regulating hormone-sensitive lipase and lipolysis. *Annu Rev Nutr* (2000) **20**:365–93. doi:10.1146/annurev.nutr.20.1.365
13. Kim YC, Ariyoshi N, Artemenko I, Elliott ME, Bhattacharyya KK, Jefcoate CR. Control of cholesterol access to cytochrome P450scc in rat adrenal cells mediated by regulation of the steroidogenic acute regulatory protein. *Steroids* (1997) **62**:10–20. doi:10.1016/S0039-128X(96)00153-5
14. Rone MB, Fan J, Papadopoulos V. Cholesterol transport in steroid biosynthesis: role of protein-protein interactions and implications in disease states. *Biochim Biophys Acta* (2009) **179**:646–58. doi:10.1016/j.bbalip.2009.03.001
15. Durroux T, Gallo-Payet N, Payet MD. Three components of the calcium current in cultured glomerulosa cells from rat adrenal gland. *J Physiol* (1988) **404**:713–29. doi:10.1113/jphysiol.1988.sp017315
16. Quinn SJ, Brauneis U, Tillotson DL, Cornwall MC, Williams GH. Calcium channels and control of cytosolic calcium in rat and bovine zona glomerulosa cells. *Am J Physiol* (1992) **262**:C598–606.
17. Várnai P, Osipenko ON, Vizi ES, Spät A. Activation of calcium current in voltage-clamped rat glomerulosa cells by potassium ions. *J Physiol* (1995) **483**:67–78. doi:10.1113/jphysiol.1995.sp020568
18. Cohen CJ, McCarthy RT, Barrett PQ, Rasmussen H. Ca channels in adrenal glomerulosa cells: K^+ and angiotensin II increase T-type Ca channel current. *Proc Natl Acad Sci U S A* (1988) **85**:2412–6. doi:10.1073/pnas.85.7.2412
19. Lotshaw DP. Role of membrane depolarization and T-type Ca^{2+} channels in angiotensin II and K^+ stimulated aldosterone secretion. *Mol Cell Endocrinol* (2001) **175**:157–71. doi:10.1016/S0303-7207(01)00384-7
20. Payet MD, Durroux T, Bilodeau L, Guillon G, Gallo-Payet N. Characterization of K^+ and Ca^{2+} ionic currents in glomerulosa cells from human adrenal glands. *Endocrinology* (1994) **134**:2589–98. doi:10.1210/endo.134.6.7515004
21. Makara JK, Petheo GL, Tóth A, Spät A. Effect of osmolarity on aldosterone production by rat adrenal glomerulosa cells. *Endocrinology* (2000) **141**:1705–10. doi:10.1210/endo.141.5.7465
22. Makara JK, Koncz P, Petheo GL, Spät A. Role of cell volume in K^+-induced Ca^{2+} signaling by rat adrenal glomerulosa cells. *Endocrinology* (2003) **144**:4916–22. doi:10.1210/en.2003-0383
23. Braley LM, Williams GH. Rat adrenal cell sensitivity to angiotensin II, alpha-1-24-ACTH, and potassium: a comparative study. *Am J Physiol* (1977) **233**:E402–6.
24. Spät A. Glomerulosa cell-a unique sensor of extracellular K^+ concentration. *Mol Cell Endocrinol* (2004) **217**:23–6. doi:10.1016/j.mce.2003.10.046
25. Czirják G, Fischer T, Spät A, Lesage F, Enyedi P. TASK (TWIK-related acid-sensitive K^+ channel) is expressed in glomerulosa cells of rat adrenal cortex and inhibited by angiotensin II. *Mol Endocrinol* (2000) **14**:863–74. doi:10.1210/mend.14.6.0466
26. Czirják G, Enyedi P. TASK-3 dominates the background potassium conductance in rat adrenal glomerulosa cells. *Mol Endocrinol* (2002) **16**:621–9. doi:10.1210/me.16.3.621
27. Quinn SJ, Cornwall MC, Williams GH. Electrical properties of isolated rat adrenal glomerulosa and fasciculata cells. *Endocrinology* (1987) **120**:903–14. doi:10.1210/endo-120-3-903
28. Velarde-Miranda C, Gomez-Sanchez EP, Gomez-Sanchez CE. Regulation of aldosterone biosynthesis by the Kir3.4 (KCNJ5) potassium channel. *Clin Exp Pharmacol Physiol* (2013) **40**(12):895–901. doi:10.1111/1440-1681.12151
29. Schrier AD, Wang H, Talley EM, Perez-Reyes E, Barrett PQ. alpha1H T-type Ca^{2+} channel is the predominant subtype expressed in bovine and rat zona glomerulosa. *Am J Physiol Cell Physiol* (2001) **280**:C265–72.

30. Hu C, Rusin CG, Tan Z, Guagliardo NA, Barrett PQ. Zona glomerulosa cells of the mouse adrenal cortex are intrinsic electrical oscillators. *J Clin Invest* (2012) **122**(6):2046–53. doi:10.1172/JCI61996
31. Várnai P, Petheö GL, Makara JK, Spät A. Electrophysiological study on the high K^+ sensitivity of rat glomerulosa cells. *Pflügers Arch* (1998) **435**:429–31. doi:10.1007/s004240050534
32. Barrett PQ, Ertel EA, Smith MM, Nee JJ, Cohen CJ. Voltage-gated calcium currents have two opposing effects on the secretion of aldosterone. *Am J Physiol Cell Physiol* (1995) **268**:C985–92.
33. Lu HK, Fern RJ, Luthin D, Linden J, Liu LP, Cohen CJ, et al. Angiotensin II stimulates T-type Ca^{2+} channel currents via activation of a G protein, G_i. *Am J Physiol Cell Physiol* (1996) **271**:C1340–9.
34. Cherradi N, Pardo B, Greenberg AS, Kraemer FB, Capponi AM. Angiotensin II activates cholesterol ester hydrolase in bovine adrenal glomerulosa cells through phosphorylation mediated by p42/p44 mitogen-activated protein kinase. *Endocrinology* (2003) **144**:4905–15. doi:10.1210/en.2003-0325
35. Cherradi N, Brandenburger Y, Capponi AM. Mitochondrial regulation of mineralocorticoid biosynthesis by calcium and the StAR protein. *Eur J Endocrinol* (1998) **139**:249–56. doi:10.1530/eje.0.1390249
36. Clark BJ, Combs R. Angiotensin II and cyclic adenosine 3',5'-monophosphate induce human steroidogenic acute regulatory protein transcription through a common steroidogenic factor-1 element. *Endocrinology* (1999) **140**:4390–8. doi:10.1210/en.140.10.4390
37. Capponi AM. The control by angiotensin II of cholesterol supply for aldosterone biosynthesis. *Mol Cell Endocrinol* (2004) **217**:113–8. doi:10.1016/j.mce.2003.10.055
38. Whitebread S, Mele M, Kamber B, De Gasparo M. Preliminary biochemical characterization of two angiotensin II receptor subtypes. *Biochem Biophys Res Commun* (1989) **163**:284–91. doi:10.1016/0006-291X(89)92133-5
39. Balla T, Baukal AJ, Eng S, Catt KJ. Angiotensin II receptor subtypes and biological responses in the adrenal cortex and medulla. *Mol Pharmacol* (1991) **40**:401–6.
40. Hajnóczky G, Csordás G, Bagó A, Chiu AT, Spät A. Angiotensin II exerts its effect on aldosterone production and potassium permeability through receptor subtype AT_1 in rat adrenal glomerulosa cells. *Biochem Pharmacol* (1992) **43**:1009–12. doi:10.1016/0006-2952(92)90606-J
41. Enyedi P, Büki B, Mucsi I, Spät A. Polyphosphoinositide metabolism in adrenal glomerulosa cells. *Mol Cell Endocrinol* (1985) **41**:105–12. doi:10.1016/0303-7207(85)90147-9
42. Rossier MF, Capponi AM, Vallotton MB. Inositol trisphosphate isomers in angiotensin II-stimulated adrenal glomerulosa cells. *Mol Cell Endocrinol* (1988) **57**:163–8. doi:10.1016/0303-7207(88)90071-8
43. Baukal AJ, Balla T, Hunyady L, Hausdorff W, Guillemette G, Catt KJ. Angiotensin II and guanine nucleotides stimulate formation of inositol 1,4,5-trisphosphate and its metabolites in permeabilized adrenal glomerulosa cells. *J Biol Chem* (1988) **263**:6087–92.
44. Baukal AJ, Guillemette G, Rubin R, Spät A, Catt KJ. Binding sites for inositol trisphosphate in the bovine adrenal cortex. *Biochem Biophys Res Commun* (1985) **133**:532–8. doi:10.1016/0006-291X(85)90939-8
45. Guillemette G, Balla T, Baukal AJ, Spät A, Catt KJ. Intracellular receptors for inositol 1,4,5-trisphosphate in angiotensin II target tissues. *J Biol Chem* (1987) **262**:1010–5.
46. Spät A, Bradford PG, McKinney JS, Rubin RP, Putney JW Jr. A saturable receptor for ^{32}P-inositol-1,4,5-triphosphate in hepatocytes and neutrophils. *Nature* (1986) **319**:514–6. doi:10.1038/319514a0
47. Enyedi P, Szabadkai G, Horváth A, Szilágyi L, Gráf L, Spät A. Inositol 1,4,5-trisphosphate receptor subtypes in adrenal glomerulosa cells. *Endocrinology* (1994) **134**:2354–9. doi:10.1210/en.134.6.2354
48. Hunyady L, Rohács T, Bagó A, Deák F, Spät A. Dihydropyridine-sensitive initial component of the ANG II-induced Ca^{2+} response in rat adrenal glomerulosa cells. *Am J Physiol Cell Physiol* (1994) **266**:C67–72.
49. Kramer RE. Angiotensin II-stimulated changes in calcium metabolism in cultured glomerulosa cells. *Mol Cell Endocrinol* (1988) **60**:199–210. doi:10.1016/0303-7207(88)90179-7
50. Burnay MM, Python CP, Vallotton MB, Capponi AM, Rossier MF. Role of the capacitative calcium influx in the activation of steroidogenesis by angiotensin-II in adrenal glomerulosa cells. *Endocrinology* (1994) **135**:751–8. doi:10.1210/en.135.2.751
51. Rohács T, Bagó A, Deák F, Hunyady L, Spät A. Capacitative Ca^{2+} influx in adrenal glomerulosa cells. Possible role in angiotensin II response. *Am J Physiol* (1994) **267**:C1246–52.
52. Rossier MF, Aptel HBC, Python CP, Burnay MM, Vallotton MB, Capponi AM. Inhibition of low threshold calcium channels by angiotensin II in adrenal glomerulosa cells through activation of protein kinase. *J Biol Chem* (1995) **270**:15137–42. doi:10.1074/jbc.270.25.15137
53. Hajnóczky G, Csordás G, Hunyady L, Kalapos MP, Balla T, Enyedi P, et al. Angiotensin-II inhibits Na^+/K^+ pump in rat adrenal glomerulosa cells: possible contribution to stimulation of aldosterone production. *Endocrinology* (1992) **130**:1637–44. doi:10.1210/endo.130.3.1311245
54. Lopes CM, Rohacs T, Czirjak G, Balla T, Enyedi P, Logothetis DE. PIP2 hydrolysis underlies agonist-induced inhibition and regulates voltage gating of two-pore domain K^+ channels. *J Physiol* (2005) **564**:117–29. doi:10.1113/jphysiol.2004.081935
55. Maturana AD, Casal AJ, Demaurex N, Vallotton MB, Capponi AM, Rossier MF. Angiotensin II negatively modulates L-type calcium channels through a pertussis toxin-sensitive G protein in adrenal glomerulosa cells. *J Biol Chem* (1999) **274**:19943–8. doi:10.1074/jbc.274.28.19943
56. Balla T, Holló Z, Várnai P, Spät A. Angiotensin II inhibits potassium-induced calcium signal generation in rat adrenal glomerulosa cells. *Biochem J* (1991) **273**:399–404. doi:10.1042/bj2730399
57. Cirillo M, Quinn SJ, Canessa ML. Early and late effects of angiotensin-II on Ca^{2+} fluxes in bovine adrenal zona glomerulosa cells. *Endocrinology* (1993) **132**:1921–30. doi:10.1210/en.132.5.1921
58. Enyedi P, Mucsi I, Hunyady L, Catt KJ, Spät A. The role of guanyl nucleotide binding proteins in the formation of inositol phosphates in adrenal glomerulosa cells. *Biochem Biophys Res Commun* (1986) **140**:941–7. doi:10.1016/0006-291X(86)90726-6
59. Enyeart JJ. Biochemical and Ionic signaling mechanisms for ACTH-stimulated cortisol production. *Vitam Horm* (2005) **70**:265–9. doi:10.1016/S0083-6729(05)70008-X
60. Matthews EK, Saffran M. Ionic dependence of adrenal steroidogenesis and ACTH-induced changes in the membrane potential of adrenocortical cells. *J Physiol* (1973) **234**:43–64. doi:10.1113/jphysiol.1973.sp010333
61. Lymangrover JR, Matthews EK, Saffran M. Membrane potential changes of mouse adrenal zona fasciculata cells in response to adrenocorticotropin and adenosine 3',5'-monophosphate. *Endocrinology* (1982) **110**:462–8. doi:10.1210/endo-110-2-462
62. Enyeart JJ, Enyeart JA. Adrenal fasciculata cells express T-type and rapidly and slowly activating L-type Ca^{2+} channels that regulate cortisol secretion. *Am J Physiol Cell Physiol* (2015) **308**:C899–918. doi:10.1152/ajpcell.00002.2015
63. Enyeart JJ, Danthi SJ, Liu H, Enyeart JA. Angiotensin II inhibits bTREK-1 K^+ channels in adrenocortical cells by separate Ca^{2+}- and ATP hydrolysis-dependent mechanisms. *J Biol Chem* (2005) **280**:30814–28. doi:10.1074/jbc.M504283200
64. Enyeart JA, Danthi SJ, Enyeart JJ. TREK-1 K^+ channels couple angiotensin II receptors to membrane depolarization and aldosterone secretion in bovine adrenal glomerulosa cells. *Am J Physiol Endocrinol Metab* (2004) **287**:E1154–65. doi:10.1152/ajpendo.00223.2004
65. Naville D, Lebrethon MC, Kermabon AY, Rouer E, Benarous R, Saez JM. Characterization and regulation of the angiotensin II type-1 receptor (binding and mRNA) in human adrenal fasciculata-reticularis cells. *FEBS Lett* (1993) **321**:184–8. doi:10.1016/0014-5793(93)80104-3
66. Dell GC, Morley SD, Mullins JJ, Williams BC, Walker SW. Multiple signal transduction systems regulate angiotensin II type 1 (AT1) receptor mRNA expression in bovine adrenocortical cells. *Endocr Res* (1996) **22**:363–8.
67. Bird IM, Magness RR, Mason JI, Rainey WE. Angiotensin-II acts via the type 1 receptor to inhibit 17 alpha-hydroxylase cytochrome P450 expression in ovine adrenocortical cells. *Endocrinology* (1992) **130**:3113–21. doi:10.1210/endo.130.6.1317775
68. Bird IM, Williams BC, Walker SW. Identification and metabolism of phosphoinositol species formed on angiotensin II stimulation of zona fasciculata-reticularis cells from the bovine adrenal cortex. *Mol Cell Endocrinol* (1992) **83**:29–38. doi:10.1016/0303-7207(92)90192-9
69. Burnay MM, Vallotton MB, Capponi AM, Rossier MF. Angiotensin II potentiates adrenocorticotropic hormone-induced cAMP formation in bovine adrenal glomerulosa cells through a capacitative calcium influx. *Biochem J* (1998) **330**:21–7. doi:10.1042/bj3300021

70. Trnka P, Orellana L, Walsh M, Pool L, Borzi P. Reninoma: an uncommon cause of Renin-mediated hypertension. *Front Pediatr* (2014) **2**:89. doi:10.3389/fped.2014.00089
71. Aguilar F, Lo M, Claustrat B, Saez JM, Sassard J, Li JY. Hypersensitivity of the adrenal cortex to trophic and secretory effects of angiotensin II in Lyon genetically-hypertensive rats. *Hypertension* (2004) **43**:87–93. doi:10.1161/01.HYP.0000107194.44040.d4
72. Healy DP, Maciejewski AR, Printz MP. Autoradiographic localization of [125I]-angiotensin II binding sites in the rat adrenal gland. *Endocrinology* (1985) **116**:1221–3. doi:10.1210/endo-116-3-1221
73. Lehoux JG, Bird IM, Briere N, Martel D, Ducharme L. Influence of dietary sodium restriction on angiotensin II receptors in rat adrenals. *Endocrinology* (1997) **138**:5238–47. doi:10.1210/endo.138.12.5612
74. Whitley GSJ, Hyatt PJ, Tait JF. Angiotensin II-induced inositol phosphate production in isolated rat zona glomerulosa and fasciculata/reticularis cells. *Steroids* (1987) **49**:271–86. doi:10.1016/0039-128X(87)90004-3
75. Braley LM, Menachery AI, Brown EM, Williams GH. Comparative effect of angiotensin II, potassium, adrenocorticotropin, and cyclic adenosine 3',5'-monophosphate on cytosolic calcium in rat adrenal cells. *Endocrinology* (1986) **119**:1010–9. doi:10.1210/endo-119-3-1010
76. Parmar J, Key RE, Rainey WE. Development of an adrenocorticotropin-responsive human adrenocortical carcinoma cell line. *J Clin Endocrinol Metab* (2008) **93**:4542–6. doi:10.1210/jc.2008-0903
77. Rossier MF, Lesouhaitier O, Perrier E, Bockhorn L, Chiappe A, Lalevee N. Aldosterone regulation of T-type calcium channels. *J Steroid Biochem Mol Biol* (2003) **85**:383–8. doi:10.1016/S0960-0760(03)00201-2
78. Szanda G, Koncz P, Várnai P, Spät A. Mitochondrial Ca^{2+} uptake with and without the formation of high-Ca^{2+} microdomains. *Cell Calcium* (2006) **40**:527–38. doi:10.1016/j.ceca.2006.08.019
79. Kim YH, Park TJ, Lee YH, Baek KJ, Suh PG, Ryu SH, et al. Phospholipase C-delta1 is activated by capacitative calcium entry that follows phospholipase C-beta activation upon bradykinin stimulation. *J Biol Chem* (1999) **274**:26127–34. doi:10.1074/jbc.274.37.26127
80. Biden TJ, Altin JG, Karjalainen A, Bygrave FL. Stimulation of hepatic inositol 1,4,5-trisphosphate kinase activity by Ca^{2+}-dependent and -independent mechanisms. *Biochem J* (1988) **256**:697–701. doi:10.1042/bj2560697
81. Balla T, Baukal AJ, Guillemette G, Catt KJ. Multiple pathways of inositol polyphosphate metabolism in angiotensin-stimulated adrenal glomerulosa cells. *J Biol Chem* (1988) **263**:4083–91.
82. Rossier MF, Dentand IA, Lew PD. Interconversion of inositol (1,4,5)-trisphosphate to inositol (1, 3,4,5)-tetrakisphosphate and (1,3,4)-trisphosphate in permeabilized adrenal glomerulosa cells is calcium-sensitive and ATP-dependent. *Biochem Biophys Res Commun* (1986) **139**:259–65. doi:10.1016/S0006-291X(86)80107-3
83. Spät A, Fabiato A, Rubin RP. Binding of inositol trisphosphate by a liver microsomal fraction. *Biochem J* (1986) **233**:929–32. doi:10.1042/bj2330929
84. Poirier SN, Poitras M, Chorvatova A, Payet MD, Guillemette G. FK506 blocks intracellular Ca^{2+} oscillations in bovine adrenal glomerulosa cells. *Biochemistry* (2001) **40**:6486–92. doi:10.1021/bi010207k
85. Carafoli E. Calcium pump of the plasma membrane. *Physiol Rev* (1991) **71**:129–53.
86. Netticadan T, Kato K, Tappia P, Elimban V, Dhalla NS. Phosphorylation of cardiac Na^+-K^+ ATPase by Ca^{2+}/calmodulin dependent protein kinase. *Biochem Biophys Res Commun* (1997) **238**:544–8. doi:10.1006/bbrc.1997.7305
87. Yingst DR, Davis J, Krenz S, Schiebinger RJ. Insights into the mechanism by which inhibition of Na,K-ATPase stimulates aldosterone production. *Metabolism* (1999) **48**:1167–71. doi:10.1016/S0026-0495(99)90133-6
88. Hyatt PJ, Tait JF, Tait SAS. The mechanism of the effect of K^+ on the steroidogenesis of rat zona glomerulosa cells of the adrenal cortex: role of cyclic AMP. *Proc R Soc Lond B Biol Sci* (1986) **227**:21–42. doi:10.1098/rspb.1986.0007
89. Kojima I, Kojima K, Rasmussen H. Intracellular calcium and adenosine 3',5'-cyclic monophosphate as mediators of potassium-induced aldosterone secretion. *Biochem J* (1985) **228**:69–76. doi:10.1042/bj2280069
90. Spät A. Stimulus-secretion coupling in angiotensin-stimulated adrenal glomerulosa cells. *J Steroid Biochem* (1988) **29**:443–53. doi:10.1016/0022-4731(88)90256-7
91. Balla T, Hunyady L, Spät A. Possible role of calcium uptake and calmodulin in adrenal glomerulosa cells: effects of verapamil and trifluoperazine. *Biochem Pharmacol* (1982) **31**:1267–71. doi:10.1016/0006-2952(82)90014-4
92. Kojima I, Kojima K, Rasmussen H. Role of calcium and cAMP in the action adrenocorticotropin on aldosterone secretion. *J Biol Chem* (1985) **260**:4248–56.
93. Begeot M, Langlois D, Penhoat A, Saez JM. Variations in guanine-binding proteins (Gs, Gi) in cultured bovine adrenal cells. Consequences on the effects of phorbol ester and angiotensin II on adrenocorticotropin-induced and cholera-toxin-induced cAMP production. *Eur J Biochem* (1988) **174**:317–21. doi:10.1111/j.1432-1033.1988.tb14100.x
94. Marie J, Jard S. Angiotensin II inhibits adenylate cyclase from adrenal cortex glomerulosa zone. *FEBS Lett* (1983) **159**:97–101. doi:10.1016/0014-5793(83)80424-4
95. Hausdorff WP, Sekura RD, Aguilera G, Catt KJ. Control of aldosterone production by angiotensin II is mediated by two guanine nucleotide regulatory proteins. *Endocrinology* (1987) **120**:1668–78. doi:10.1210/endo-120-4-1668
96. Bell JBG, Tait JF, Tait SAS, Barnes GD, Brown BL. Lack of effect of angiotensin on levels of cyclic AMP in isolated adrenal zona glomerulosa cells from the rat. *J Endocrinol* (1981) **91**:145–54. doi:10.1677/joe.0.0910145
97. Woodcock EA, Johnston CI. Inhibition of adenylate cyclase in rat adrenal glomerulosa cells by angiotensin II. *Endocrinology* (1984) **115**:337–41. doi:10.1210/endo-115-1-337
98. Katona D, Rajki A, Di BG, Pozzan T, Spät A. Calcium-dependent mitochondrial cAMP production enhances aldosterone secretion. *Mol Cell Endocrinol* (2015) **412**:196–204. doi:10.1016/j.mce.2015.05.002
99. Coté M, Guillon G, Payet MD, Gallo-Payet N. Expression and regulation of adenylyl cyclase isoforms in the human adrenal gland. *J Clin Endocrinol Metab* (2001) **86**:4495–503. doi:10.1210/jcem.86.9.7837
100. Cooper DM, Tabbasum VG. Adenylate cyclase-centred microdomains. *Biochem J* (2014) **462**:199–213. doi:10.1042/BJ20140560
101. Nishimoto K, Rainey WE, Bollag WB, Seki T. Lessons from the gene expression pattern of the rat zona glomerulosa. *Mol Cell Endocrinol* (2013) **371**:107–13. doi:10.1016/j.mce.2012.12.023
102. Shen T, Suzuki Y, Poyard M, Best-Belpomme M, Defer N, Hanoune J. Localization and differential expression of adenylyl cyclase messenger ribonucleic acids in rat adrenal gland determined by in situ hybridization. *Endocrinology* (1997) **138**:4591–8. doi:10.1210/en.138.11.4591
103. Willoughby D, Cooper DM. Organization and Ca^{2+} regulation of adenylyl cyclases in cAMP microdomains. *Physiol Rev* (2007) **87**:965–1010. doi:10.1152/physrev.00049.2006
104. Tremblay E, Payet MD, Gallo-Payet N. Effects of ACTH and angiotensin II on cytosolic calcium in cultured adrenal glomerulosa cells. Role of cAMP production in the ACTH effect. *Cell Calcium* (1991) **12**:655–73. doi:10.1016/0143-4160(91)90036-E
105. Gallo-Payet N, Grazzini E, Coté M, Chouinard L, Chorvatova A, Bilodeau L, et al. Role of Ca^{2+} in the action of adrenocorticotropin in cultured human adrenal glomerulosa cells. *J Clin Invest* (1996) **98**:460–6. doi:10.1172/JCI118812
106. Fülöp L, Rajki A, Katona D, Szanda G, Spät A. Extramitochondrial OPA1 and adrenocortical function. *Mol Cell Endocrinol* (2013) **381**:70–9. doi:10.1016/j.mce.2013.07.021
107. Durroux T, Gallo-Payet N, Payet MD. Effects of adrenocorticotropin on action potential and calcium currents in cultured rat and bovine glomerulosa cells. *Endocrinology* (1991) **129**:2139–47. doi:10.1210/endo-129-4-2139
108. Lenglet S, Louiset E, Delarue C, Vaudry H, Contesse V. Activation of 5-HT(7) receptor in rat glomerulosa cells is associated with an increase in adenylyl cyclase activity and calcium influx through T-type calcium channels. *Endocrinology* (2002) **143**:1748–60. doi:10.1210/endo.143.5.8817
109. Hunyady L, Balla T, Nagy K, Spät A. Control of phosphatidylinositol turnover in adrenal glomerulosa cells. *Biochim Biophys Acta* (1982) **713**:352–7. doi:10.1016/0005-2760(82)90253-3
110. Hajnóczky G, Várnai P, Buday L, Faragó A, Spät A. The role of protein kinase-C in control of aldosterone production by rat adrenal glomerulosa cells: activation of protein kinase-C by stimulation with potassium. *Endocrinology* (1992) **130**:2230–6. doi:10.1210/en.130.4.2230
111. Baukal AJ, Hunyady L, Balla T, Ely JA, Catt KJ. Modulation of agonist-induced inositol phosphate metabolism by cyclic adenosine 3',5'-monophosphate in

adrenal glomerulosa cells. *Mol Endocrinol* (1990) **4**:1712–9. doi:10.1210/mend-4-11-1712

112. McCarthy RT, Isales CM, Bollag WB, Rasmussen H, Barrett PQ. Atrial natriuretic peptide differentially modulates T- and L-type calcium channels. *Am J Physiol* (1990) **258**:F473–8.
113. Ganguly A. Atrial natriuretic peptide-induced inhibition of aldosterone secretion: a quest for mediator(s). *Am J Physiol Endocrinol Metab* (1992) **263**:E181–94.
114. Coté M, Payet MD, Rousseau E, Guillon G, Gallo-Payet N. Comparative involvement of cyclic nucleotide phosphodiesterases and adenylyl cyclase on adrenocorticotropin-induced increase of cyclic adenosine monophosphate in rat and human glomerulosa cells. *Endocrinology* (1999) **140**:3594–601. doi:10.1210/endo.140.8.6889
115. MacFarland RT, Zelus BD, Beavo JA. High concentrations of a cGMP-stimulated phosphodiesterase mediate ANP-induced decreases in cAMP and steroidogenesis in adrenal glomerulosa cells. *J Biol Chem* (1991) **266**:136–42.
116. Nikolaev VO, Gambaryan S, Engelhardt S, Walter U, Lohse MJ. Real-time monitoring of the PDE2 activity of live cells: hormone-stimulated cAMP hydrolysis is faster than hormone-stimulated cAMP synthesis. *J Biol Chem* (2005) **280**:1716–9. doi:10.1074/jbc.C400505200
117. Vezzosi D, Bertherat J. Phosphodiesterases in endocrine physiology and disease. *Eur J Endocrinol* (2011) **165**:177–88. doi:10.1530/EJE-10-1123
118. Fredlund P, Saltman S, Kondo T, Douglas J, Catt KJ. Aldosterone production by isolated glomerulosa cells: modulation of sensitivity to angiotensin II and ACTH by extracellular potassium concentration. *Endocrinology* (1977) **100**:481–6. doi:10.1210/endo-100-2-481
119. Hajnóczky G, Várnai P, Holló Z, Christensen SB, Balla T, Enyedi P, et al. Thapsigargin-induced increase in cytoplasmic Ca^{2+} concentration and aldosterone production in rat adrenal glomerulosa cells: interaction with potassium and angiotensin-II. *Endocrinology* (1991) **128**:2639–44. doi:10.1210/endo-128-5-2639
120. Pratt JH, Rothrock JK, Dominguez JH. Evidence that angiotensin-II and potassium collaborate to increase cytosolic calcium and stimulate the secretion of aldosterone. *Endocrinology* (1989) **125**:2463–9. doi:10.1210/endo-125-5-2463
121. Spät A, Balla I, Balla T, Enyedi P, Hajnóczky G, Rohács T. Sustained stimulation of aldosterone production by angiotensin II is potentiated by nickel. *Am J Physiol Endocrinol Metab* (1990) **258**:E555–61.
122. Dolmetsch RE, Pajvani U, Fife K, Spotts JM, Greenberg ME. Signaling to the nucleus by an L-type calcium channel-calmodulin complex through the MAP kinase pathway. *Science* (2001) **294**:333–9. doi:10.1126/science.1063395
123. Kar P, Nelson C, Parekh AB. Selective activation of the transcription factor NFAT1 by calcium microdomains near Ca^{2+} release-activated Ca^{2+} (CRAC) channels. *J Biol Chem* (2011) **286**:14795–803. doi:10.1074/jbc.M111.220582
124. Balla T, Szebeny M, Kanyár B, Spät A. Angiotensin II and FCCP mobilizes calcium from different intracellular pools in adrenal glomerulosa cells; analysis of calcium fluxes. *Cell Calcium* (1985) **6**:327–42. doi:10.1016/0143-4160(85)90003-X
125. Balla T, Enyedi P, Hunyady L, Spät A. Effects of lithium on angiotensin-stimulated phosphatidylinositol turnover and aldosterone production in adrenal glomerulosa cells: a possible causal relationship. *FEBS Lett* (1984) **171**:179–82. doi:10.1016/0014-5793(84)80483-4
126. Xing Y, Parker CR, Edwards M, Rainey WE. ACTH is a potent regulator of gene expression in human adrenal cells. *J Mol Endocrinol* (2010) **45**:59–68. doi:10.1677/JME-10-0006
127. Nogueira EF, Xing Y, Morris CA, Rainey WE. Role of angiotensin II-induced rapid response genes in the regulation of enzymes needed for aldosterone synthesis. *J Mol Endocrinol* (2009) **42**:319–30. doi:10.1677/JME-08-0112
128. Howard B, Wang Y, Xekouki P, Faucz FR, Jain M, Zhang L, et al. Integrated analysis of genome-wide methylation and gene expression shows epigenetic regulation of CYP11B2 in aldosteronomas. *J Clin Endocrinol Metab* (2014) **99**:E536–43. doi:10.1210/jc.2013-3495
129. Pihlajoki M, Dorner J, Cochran RS, Heikinheimo M, Wilson DB. Adrenocortical zonation, renewal, and remodeling. *Front Endocrinol* (2015) **6**:27. doi:10.3389/fendo.2015.00027
130. Drelon C, Berthon A, Mathieu M, Martinez A, Val P. Adrenal cortex tissue homeostasis and zonation: a WNT perspective. *Mol Cell Endocrinol* (2015) **408**:156–64. doi:10.1016/j.mce.2014.12.014
131. Clyne CD, Zhang Y, Slutsker L, Mathis JM, White PC, Rainey WE. Angiotensin II and potassium regulate human CYP11B2 transcription through common cis-elements. *Mol Endocrinol* (1997) **11**:638–49. doi:10.1210/mend.11.5.9920
132. Shanmughapriya S, Rajan S, Hoffman NE, Zhang X, Guo S, Kolesar JE, et al. Ca^{2+} signals regulate mitochondrial metabolism by stimulating CREB-mediated expression of the mitochondrial Ca^{2+} uniporter gene MCU. *Sci Signal* (2015) **8**:ra23. doi:10.1126/scisignal.2005673
133. Doi M, Satoh F, Maekawa T, Nakamura Y, Fustin JM, Tainaka M, et al. Isoform-specific monoclonal antibodies against 3beta-hydroxysteroid dehydrogenase/isomerase family provide markers for subclassification of human primary aldosteronism. *J Clin Endocrinol Metab* (2014) **99**:E257–62. doi:10.1210/jc.2013-3279
134. Yarimizu D, Doi M, Ota T, Okamura H. Stimulus-selective induction of the orphan nuclear receptor NGFIB underlies different influences of angiotensin II and potassium on the human adrenal gland zona glomerulosa-specific 3beta-HSD isoform gene expression in adrenocortical H295R cells. *Endocr J* (2015) **62**:765–76. doi:10.1507/endocrj.EJ15-0211
135. Bassett MH, Suzuki T, Sasano H, White PC, Rainey WE. The orphan nuclear receptors NURR1 and NGFIB regulate adrenal aldosterone production. *Mol Endocrinol* (2004) **18**:279–90. doi:10.1210/me.2003-0005
136. Nogueira EF, Rainey WE. Regulation of aldosterone synthase by activator transcription factor/cAMP response element-binding protein family members. *Endocrinology* (2010) **151**:1060–70. doi:10.1210/en.2009-0977
137. Szekeres M, Turu G, Orient A, Szalai B, Supeki K, Cserzo M, et al. Mechanisms of angiotensin II-mediated regulation of aldosterone synthase expression in H295R human adrenocortical and rat adrenal glomerulosa cells. *Mol Cell Endocrinol* (2009) **302**:244–53. doi:10.1016/j.mce.2008.12.015
138. Wang X, Nickenig G, Murphy TJ. The vascular smooth muscle type I angiotensin II receptor mRNA is destabilized by cyclic AMP-elevating agents. *Mol Pharmacol* (1997) **52**:781–7. doi:10.1124/mol.52.5.781
139. Wang X, Murphy TJ. Inhibition of cyclic AMP-dependent kinase by expression of a protein kinase inhibitor/enhanced green fluorescent fusion protein attenuates angiotensin II-induced type 1 AT1 receptor mRNA down-regulation in vascular smooth muscle cells. *Mol Pharmacol* (1998) **54**:514–24.
140. Bird IM, Mason JI, Rainey WE. Hormonal regulation of angiotensin II type 1 receptor expression and AT1-RmRNA levels in human adrenocortical cells. *Endocr Res* (1995) **21**:169–82. doi:10.3109/07435809509030432
141. McCormack JG, Halestrap AP, Denton RM. Role of calcium ions in regulation of mammalian intramitochondrial metabolism. *Physiol Rev* (1990) **70**:391–425.
142. Pralong WF, Hunyady L, Várnai P, Wollheim CB, Spät A. Pyridine nucleotide redox state parallels production of aldosterone in potassium-stimulated adrenal glomerulosa cells. *Proc Natl Acad Sci U S A* (1992) **89**:132–6. doi:10.1073/pnas.89.1.132
143. Pralong WF, Spät A, Wollheim CB. Dynamic pacing of cell metabolism by intracellular Ca^{2+}. *J Biol Chem* (1994) **269**:27310–4.
144. Rohács T, Nagy G, Spät A. Cytoplasmic Ca^{2+} signalling and reduction of mitochondrial pyridine nucleotides in adrenal glomerulosa cells in response to K^+, angiotensin II and vasopressin. *Biochem J* (1997) **322**:785–92. doi:10.1042/bj3220785
145. Jouaville LS, Pinton P, Bastianutto C, Rutter GA, Rizzuto R. Regulation of mitochondrial ATP synthesis by calcium: evidence for a long-term metabolic priming. *Proc Natl Acad Sci U S A* (1999) **96**:13807–12. doi:10.1073/pnas.96.24.13807
146. Rizzuto R, Simpson AWM, Brini M, Pozzan T. Rapid changes of mitochondrial Ca^{2+} revealed by specifically targeted recombinant aequorin. *Nature* (1992) **358**:325–7. doi:10.1038/358325a0
147. Hajnóczky G, Robb-Gaspers LD, Seitz MB, Thomas AP. Decoding of cytosolic calcium oscillations in the mitochondria. *Cell* (1995) **82**:415–24. doi:10.1016/0092-8674(95)90430-1
148. Brandenburger Y, Kennedy ED, Python CP, Rossier MF, Vallotton MB, Wollheim CB, et al. Possible role for mitochondrial calcium in angiotensin II- and potassium-stimulated steroidogenesis in bovine adrenal glomerulosa cells. *Endocrinology* (1996) **137**:5544–51. doi:10.1210/endo.137.12.8940382
149. Spät A, Pitter JG. The effect of cytoplasmic Ca^{2+} signal on the redox state of mitochondrial pyridine nucleotides. *Mol Cell Endocrin* (2004) **215**:115–8. doi:10.1016/j.mce.2003.11.004

150. Kamer KJ, Mootha VK. The molecular era of the mitochondrial calcium uniporter. *Nat Rev Mol Cell Biol* (2015) **16**:545–53. doi:10.1038/nrm4039
151. Rizzuto R, Brini M, Murgia M, Pozzan T. Microdomains with high Ca^{2+} close to IP_3-sensitive channels that are sensed by neighboring mitochondria. *Science* (1993) **262**:744–7. doi:10.1126/science.8235595
152. Pitter JG, Maechler P, Wollheim CB, Spät A. Mitochondria respond to Ca^{2+} already in the submicromolar range: correlation with redox state. *Cell Calcium* (2002) **31**:97–104. doi:10.1054/ceca.2001.0264
153. Rohács T, Tory K, Dobos A, Spät A. Intracellular calcium release is more efficient than calcium influx in stimulating mitochondrial NAD(P)H formation in adrenal glomerulosa cells. *Biochem J* (1997) **328**:525–8. doi:10.1042/bj3280525
154. Wiederkehr A, Szanda G, Akhmedov D, Mataki C, Heizmann CW, Schoonjans K, et al. Mitochondrial matrix calcium is an activating signal for hormone secretion. *Cell Metab* (2011) **13**:601–11. doi:10.1016/j.cmet.2011.03.015
155. Spät A, Fülöp L, Szanda G. The role of mitochondrial Ca^{2+} and NAD(P)H in the control of aldosterone secretion. *Cell Calcium* (2012) **52**:64–72. doi:10.1016/j.ceca.2012.01.009
156. Buck J, Sinclair ML, Schapal L, Cann MJ, Levin LR. Cytosolic adenylyl cyclase defines a unique signaling molecule in mammals. *Proc Natl Acad Sci U S A* (1999) **96**:79–84. doi:10.1073/pnas.96.1.79
157. Chen Y, Cann MJ, Litvin TN, Iourgenko V, Sinclair ML, Levin LR, et al. Soluble adenylyl cyclase as an evolutionarily conserved bicarbonate sensor. *Science* (2000) **289**:625–8. doi:10.1126/science.289.5479.625
158. Litvin TN, Kamenetsky M, Zarifyan A, Buck J, Levin LR. Kinetic properties of "soluble" adenylyl cyclase. Synergism between calcium and bicarbonate. *J Biol Chem* (2003) **278**:15922–6. doi:10.1074/jbc.M212475200
159. Zippin JH, Chen Y, Nahirney P, Kamenetsky M, Wuttke MS, Fischman DA, et al. Compartmentalization of bicarbonate-sensitive adenylyl cyclase in distinct signaling microdomains. *FASEB J* (2003) **17**:82–4.
160. Acin-Perez R, Salazar E, Kamenetsky M, Buck J, Levin LR, Manfredi G. Cyclic AMP produced inside mitochondria regulates oxidative phosphorylation. *Cell Metab* (2009) **9**:265–76. doi:10.1016/j.cmet.2009.01.012
161. Di Benedetto G, Scalzotto E, Mongillo M, Pozzan T. Mitochondrial Ca^{2+} uptake induces cyclic AMP generation in the matrix and modulates organelle ATP levels. *Cell Metab* (2013) **17**:965–75. doi:10.1016/j.cmet.2013.05.003
162. Berridge MJ. The interaction of cyclic nucleotides and calcium in the control of cell activity. *Adv Cyclic Nucl Res* (1975) **6**:1–98.

14

Aldo-Keto Reductases 1B in Adrenal Cortex Physiology

*Emilie Pastel[1], Jean-Christophe Pointud[2], Antoine Martinez[2] and A. Marie Lefrançois-Martinez[2]**

[1] *Diabetes and Obesity Research Group, University of Exeter Medical School, Exeter, UK,* [2] *CNRS, UMR 6293/INSERM U1103, Génétique, Reproduction et Développement, Clermont Université, Aubière, France*

Correspondence:
A. Marie Lefrançois-Martinez
a-marie.lefrancois-martinez@univ-bpclermont.fr

Aldose reductase (AKR1B) proteins are monomeric enzymes, belonging to the aldo-keto reductase (AKR) superfamily. They perform oxidoreduction of carbonyl groups from a wide variety of substrates, such as aliphatic and aromatic aldehydes or ketones. Due to the involvement of human aldose reductases in pathologies, such as diabetic complications and cancer, AKR1B subgroup enzymatic properties have been extensively characterized. However, the issue of AKR1B function in non-pathologic conditions remains poorly resolved. Adrenal activities generated large amount of harmful aldehydes from lipid peroxidation and steroidogenesis, including 4-hydroxynonenal (4-HNE) and isocaproaldehyde (4-methylpentanal), which can both be reduced by AKR1B proteins. More recently, some AKR1B isoforms have been shown to be endowed with prostaglandin F synthase (PGFS) activity, suggesting that, in addition to possible scavenger function, they could instigate paracrine signals. Interestingly, the adrenal gland is one of the major sites for human and murine AKR1B expression, suggesting that their detoxifying/signaling activity could be specifically required for the correct handling of adrenal function. Moreover, chronic effects of ACTH result in a coordinated regulation of genes encoding the steroidogenic enzymes and some AKR1B isoforms. This review presents the molecular mechanisms accounting for the adrenal-specific expression of some AKR1B genes. Using data from recent mouse genetic models, we will try to connect their enzymatic properties and regulation with adrenal functions.

Keywords: aldose reductase, adrenal physiology, AKR1B

INTRODUCTION

The pituitary adrenocorticotropic hormone is the main regulator of adrenal steroidogenesis acting through the cAMP-dependent protein kinase (PKA) signaling pathway. The fixation of ACTH second messenger, cAMP, on PKA regulatory subunits, leads to the release of catalytic subunits that in turn phosphorylate several targets, including transcription factors, such as the CCAAT enhancer-binding protein (C/EBP) and the cAMP response element-binding protein (CREB). Acting coordinately with tissue-specific factors such as the steroidogenic factor 1 (SF1), they stimulate expression of genes encoding enzymes and proteins involved in cholesterol metabolism, mobilization, and transport. In the adrenal cortex, steroidogenesis activation results in the generation of large amount of lipid aldehydes i.e., isocaproaldehyde (4-methylpentanal) produced by the CYP11A1 cholesterol side-chain cleavage and 4-hydroxynonenal (4-HNE), whose harmfulness has to be supported by coordinately regulated detoxifying enzymes. We and other groups have previously observed that the adrenal gland is one of the main sites of expression of both murine and human AKR1B proteins

(1–3). Aldose reductases are cytosolic monomeric enzymes, belonging to the aldo-keto reductase (AKR) superfamily. This superfamily encompasses more than 150 NAD(P)(H)-dependent oxidoreductases distributed in all prokaryotic and eukaryotic kingdoms, including yeast, plant, invertebrates, and vertebrates. They catalyze the reduction of carbonyl groups from a wide variety of substrates, such as aliphatic and aromatic aldehydes, ketones, keto prostaglandins, ketosteroids, and xenobiotics. Based on sequence identity, these proteins are divided in 15 families termed AKR1–AKR15, each family having less than 40% amino acid sequence identity with the others (4–6).

Among the AKR1 family, the aldose reductase subgroup-designated AKR family 1 member B (AKR1B) is one of the most characterized because of its involvement in human diseases, such as diabetic complications resulting from the ability of the former AKR family 1 member B1 (AKR1B1) to reduce glucose into sorbitol in a NADPH + H^+-dependent manner during hyperglycemia. In addition to glucose conversion, AKR1B proteins display multiple other activities, including reduction of aldehyde group of by-products derived from lipid peroxidation or steroid synthesis, retinoids, xenobiotics, and prostaglandins (1, 7–9). The AKR1B subfamily includes proteins sharing a high degree of similarity (i.e., more than 65% of identity; **Table 1**). They are organized in two subgroups based on their ability to reduce glucose: aldose reductases (AR; AKR1B1-6) and aldose reductase-like proteins (ARLP; Akr1b7-19), respectively (4, 10–12). Their structure, enzymatic properties, and substrate specificities have been the subject of many studies (1, 5, 7, 13–17), emphasizing that in addition to their high percentage of identity, they also display redundant substrate specificities and overlapping expression patterns. These potential redundancies, then, complicate study of their distinct biological functions in specific physiological or pathological processes. Analysis of murine genetic models and identification of the mechanisms regulating their expression are the necessary steps to complete our understanding in AKR1Bs biological function.

This review will provide an updated integrative view on specific regulations of human and murine aldose reductase genes with enzymatic and functional data in the adrenal gland physiology [further information on AKR1Bs in other endocrine functions is reviewed in Ref. (18)]. Since several studies allowed identification of some murine and human aldose reductase genes as orthologs, common features will be presented for each corresponding pair, and individual isoform specificities will be discussed.

TABLE 1 | Comparison of protein sequence identity (%) between human (h) and murine (m) AKR1B proteins.

		Aldose reductases		Aldose reductase-like proteins				
	AKR1	**B1**	**b3**	**b7**	**b8**	**B10**	**B15**	**b16**
Aldose reductases	B1 (h)	100	85.8	71.6	70.7	71	65.1	70.7
	b3 (m)	85.8	100	69.7	69.4	70.7	65.4	70.3
Aldose reductase-like proteins	b7 (m)	71.8	69.7	100	82.3	79.8	72.1	84.8
	b8 (m)	70.7	69.4	82.3	100	82.3	74.9	82.6
	B10 (h)	65.1	70.7	79.8	82.3	100	86	82.9
	B15 (h)	65.1	65.4	72.1	74.9	86	100	76.2
	b16 (m)	70.7	70.3	84.8	82.6	82.9	76.2	100

*The protein sequences were aligned using the Clustal Omega program. The amino acid sequences used to achieve this multiple alignment correspond to the accession numbers listed in **Table 2**.*

The Gray shade highlights the necessary 100% identity between 2 identical protein sequences.

HUMAN AND MURINE AKR1B GENE SYNOPSIS

Human AKR1B Genes

Three human AKR1B genes organized in tandem on chromosome 7q33–35 have been identified (**Table 2**; **Figure 1**): *AKR1B1* [human aldose reductase (19)], *AKR1B10* [also designated as HSI reductase: human small intestine reductase (1, 7)], and *AKR1B15* (20). *AKR1B1* seems to be ubiquitously expressed, whereas *AKR1B10* expression was only reported in small intestine, colon, liver, thymus, and adrenal gland (1, 7). *AKR1B15* gene was recently characterized and identified as closely related to the *AKR1B1* and *AKR1B10* cluster on chromosome 7 (**Figure 1**). *AKR1B15* undergoes alternative splicing, giving rise to two protein isoforms, designated as AK1R1B15.1 and AKR1B15.2, expressed in thyroid gland and testis, respectively, and both in adipose tissue and placenta. *AKR1B15.1* transcript encodes a putative protein sharing 68 and 91% sequence identity with AKR1B1 and AKR1B10, respectively (21). Both *AKR1B15* transcripts were absent from human adrenal (20).

Murine Akr1b Genes

Four murine Akr1b genes have been described: *Akr1b3* (murine aldose reductase), *Akr1b7* [previously named MVDP: mouse vas deferens protein (22)], *Akr1b8* [previously named FR-1: fibroblast growth factor (FGF)-related protein (23)], and *Akr1b16* (21) (**Table 2**). Murine aldose reductase genes are located on chromosome 6 (locus 6B1), and their tandem arrangement suggests (as for the three human *AKR1Bs*) that these four genes arise from an ancestral gene duplication event (10, 12) (**Figure 1**). Several studies had allowed identification of murine *Akr1b3*, *Akr1b8* as the orthologs of the human *AKR1B1* and *AKR1B10*, respectively. However, this phylogenetic analysis between human and mouse AR has some limits and will be commented below. *AKR1B1*, *Akr1b3*, and *Akr1b16* are rather ubiquitously expressed (11, 21), whereas *Akr1b7* and *Akr1b8* exhibit a restricted tissue distribution. Indeed, *Akr1b7* is detected in vas deferens, adrenal glands, gonads, intestine, white adipose tissue, eye, liver, and kidney (2, 22, 24–26) and *Akr1b8* in testis, heart, adrenal glands, intestine, and liver (2, 11, 23).

AKR1B IN ADRENALS: BETWEEN DETOXIFICATION AND PARACRINE SIGNALING

Akr1b3/AKR1B1: Expression Pattern and Relevant Functions

In studies using murine adrenal cell lines (Y1 adrenocortical cells and MPC862L chromaffin cells), we found that Akr1b3 protein

TABLE 2 | Human and murine members of the aldo-keto reductase B1 subgroup (AKR1B).

Symbol	Common associated protein designation	Species	ARN	Protein
AKR1B1	Aldose reductase	Human	NM_001628	NP_001619
Ark1b3	Aldose reductase	Mouse	NM_009658	NP_033788
Akr1b7	Mouse *vas deferens* protein (MVDP)	Mouse	NM_009731	NP_033861
Akr1b8	Fibroblast growth factor-regulated protein 1 (FR-1)	Mouse	NM_008012	NP_032038
AKR1B10	Small intestine reductase (HSI)	Human	NM_020299	NP_064695
AKR1B15	Aldose reductase (putative)	Human	NM_001080538	NP_001074007
Akr1b16	Aldose reductase (putative)	Mouse	NM_172398	NP_765986

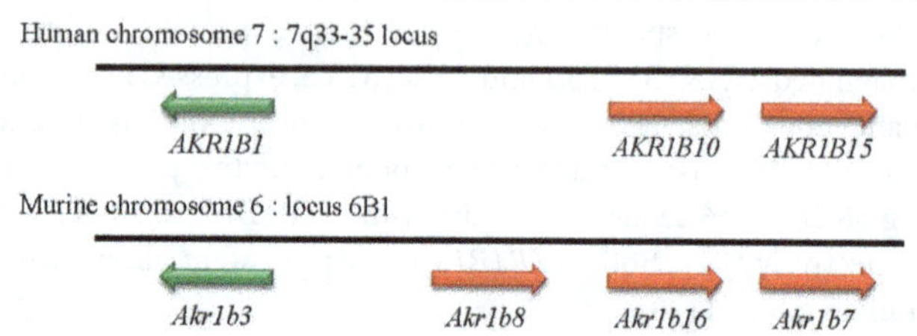

FIGURE 1 | Genomic organization of AKR1B genes in humans and mice. In human and mouse genomes, genes encoding aldose reductase are located on chromosomes 7 and 6, respectively. Whatever the case, these genes are organized in tandem.

accumulates in both adrenal cortex and medulla. Moreover, *in vivo* and *ex vivo* hormonal manipulations demonstrated that unlike the other murine Akr1b7 and Akr1b8 isoforms, Akr1b3 is expressed in the whole gland (27). Finally, cAMP stimulation failed to modulate *Akr1b3* expression in Y1 cell line, confirming that *Akr1b3* was insensitive to ACTH signaling (28) (**Table 3**).

Considering their enzymatic properties and expression levels in murine adrenal cortex, Akr1b7 and Akr1b8 are considered as the main isocaproaldehyde reductase and 4-HNE reductase, respectively, while Akr1b3 could rather participate in the elimination of these toxic compounds in basal physiological conditions (27–29). Moreover, Akr1b3 also displays 9-,11-endoperoxide reductase activity that, when coupled to COX-1 (cyclooxygenase type 1), allows prostaglandin F2α ($PGF_{2\alpha}$) synthesis in adrenal cortex and medulla (see below).

Despite all these evidences upon Akr1b3 involvement in both lipid aldehyde detoxification and $PGF_{2\alpha}$ synthesis, *in vivo Akr1b3* gene invalidation (*Akr1b3*$^{-/-}$ mice) did not highlight any phenotype related to adrenal gland (30, 31). The lack of adrenal dysfunction in *Akr1b3*$^{-/-}$ mice may result from the redundancy of enzymatic properties carried by the other murine isoforms expressed in the gland (Akr1b7 and Akr1b8) that could then compensate Akr1b3 loss.

TABLE 3 | Localization and regulation of AKR1B in adrenal gland.

Isoforms	Localization	Analyses	Control by ACTH/ cAMP	Transcriptional regulators	Reference
Human					
AKR1B1	Cortex	IHC, RNA master blot	+	n.d.	(1, 27)
AKR1B10	Adrenal[a]	RNA master blot	n.d.	n.d.	(1)
AKR1B15	n.d.	n.d.	n.d.	n.d.	–
Mouse					
Akr1b3	Cortex and medulla	WB	No	No	(27, 28)
Akr1b7	Cortex	NB, WB, IHC, ISH	+	Sp1, C/EBPβ, SF1	(2, 27, 28, 55, 58, 67)
Akr1b8	Cortex	WB, ISH	No	No	(2, 27, 28)
Akr1b16	n.d.	n.d.	n.d.	n.d.	–

[a]*Intra-adrenal tissue localization was not specified.*
n.d., not determined; NB, Northern Blot; WB, Western Blot; RT–PCR, reverse transcription–polymerase chain reaction; ISH, in situ hybridization; IHC, immunohistochemistry; n.d., not determined.

In human adrenal gland, *AKR1B1* transcripts have been initially detected using RNA master blot (1) (**Table 3**). Thereafter, using immunohistochemistry, we confirmed those results and demonstrated that AKR1B1 expression pattern is restricted to the cortex of adrenal gland (27). Treatment of the human adrenocortical tumor cells NC1-H295 with forskolin (adenylyl cyclase inducer) allowed us to suggest that similar to the murine isoform Akr1b7, *AKR1B1* expression was sensitive to ACTH (32) (**Table 3**). The molecular mechanisms and *cis*-acting elements responsible for ACTH/cAMP responsiveness of *AKR1B1* gene have not been investigated to date (**Figure 2**). Analysis of *AKR1B1* expression in stress-related disorders was not explored to date. Moreover, analysis of adrenal samples from Cushing's disease (ACTH-producing pituitary tumor) revealed unchanged mRNA levels of *AKR1B1* gene (32).

Based on its enzymatic properties, AKR1B1 has long been considered as the sole isocaproaldehyde reductase in the human adrenal gland (33) (**Figure 3A**; **Table 4**). Interestingly, unlike murine Akr1b7 isoform, NADPH-dependent isocaproaldehyde reductase activity carried by AKR1B1 was inhibited by tolrestat, a potent and specific aldose reductase inhibitor belonging to the carboxylic acids group of AR inhibitors (13, 29, 33). We demonstrated that AKR1B1 was also able to convert PGH_2 into $PGF_{2\alpha}$ (34) (**Figure 3C**; **Table 4**). This 9-,11-endoperoxide reductase activity is also strictly NADPH-dependent and inhibited by tolrestat.

We observed that in the human adrenal gland, AKR1B1 and the cAMP-inducible COX-2 isoform were co-localized in steroidogenic cortical cells (27) (**Table 3**). Then, we can consider that human adrenal cortex has the potential to produce $PGF_{2\alpha}$ in response to ACTH surge. The shared properties of human AKR1B1 and mouse Akr1b7, such as hormonal regulation and reductase activity toward common substrates, prompted us to postulate that they can be considered as functional orthologs

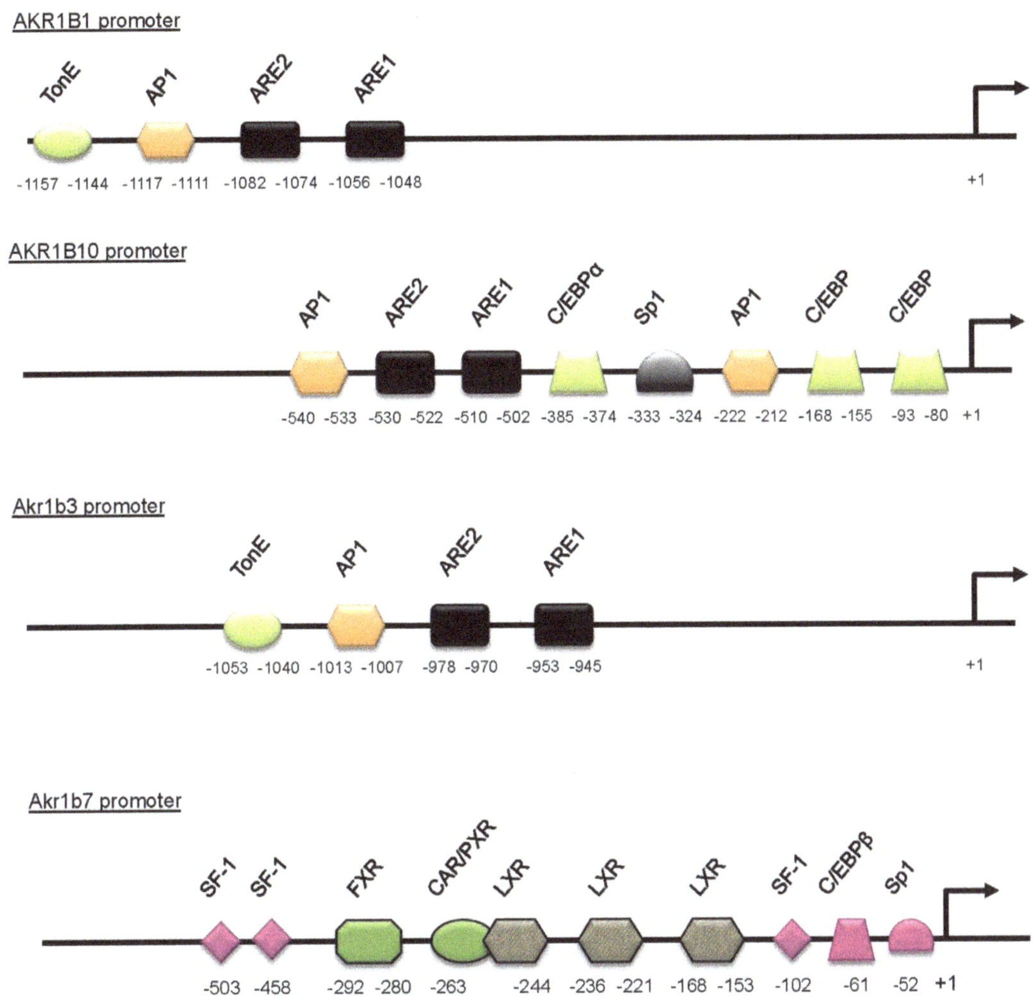

FIGURE 2 | Schematic representation of the *AKR1B1, AKR1B10, Akr1b3,* and *Akr1b7* promoters. *Cis-* and *trans-*acting factors shown to be involved in stress responsiveness are indicated. The DNA-binding site for transcription factors and nuclear receptors required for the *Akr1b7*-specific expression in adrenal gland (pink boxes) are shown. LXR-binding sites are involved in both adrenal and intestine *Akr1b7* expression. TonE, tonicity response element; AP1, activator protein 1 binding site; ARE, antioxidant response element; C/EBP, CCAAT enhancer binding protein binding site; Sp1, selective promoter factor 1 binding site.

at least in the adrenal cortex (32). Moreover, increased levels of *AKR1B1* transcripts in human were observed in adrenocortical adenomas harboring glucocorticoid autonomous hypersecretion (32). The possibility that AKR1B1 prostaglandin F synthase (PGFS) activity could participate in an intra-adrenal feedback loop between endocrine activities of cortex and medulla in human adrenal gland remains to be explored.

Given the high expression of *AKR1B1* in the adrenal cortex, we evaluated alterations in its expression in association with human adrenal disorders. The relative abundance of *AKR1B1* mRNA was decreased in adrenocortical carcinomas (ACC) when compared to benign tumors, Cushing's hyperplasia, or normal adrenals (32). These data were reinforced by de Reyniès et al., who demonstrated that decreased *AKR1B1* expression was associated with malignancy using an unsupervised clustering analysis of the human adrenal tumors transcriptome (35). This identified AKR1B1 as a potential negative marker for adrenocortical malignancy.

Akr1b8/AKR1B10: Phylogeny, Regulation, and Enzymatic Specificities

Akr1b8 mRNA was initially detected in both fetal and adult murine adrenal cortex but remained undetected in the medulla by *in situ* hybridization (2). In fibroblasts as well as in adrenocortical Y1 cell line, *Akr1b8* was previously shown to be controlled by the FGF and phorbol myristate acetate (PMA) (23, 28). On the contrary, dexamethasone-induced ACTH suppression did not influence *Akr1b8* mRNA and protein accumulation (27), suggesting that its biological function did not seem to be related to the ACTH-dependent steroidogenic activity present in adrenocortical cells (**Table 3**). Interestingly, in digestive tract organs, such as liver and small intestine, *Akr1b8* gene was recently showed to be a target of NF-E2-related factor2 (Nrf2), which mediates transcriptional response to oxidative stress by binding to antioxidant response element (ARE) sites (36). As expected, *Akr1b8* expression was downregulated in digestive tract from Nrf2 knockout mice.

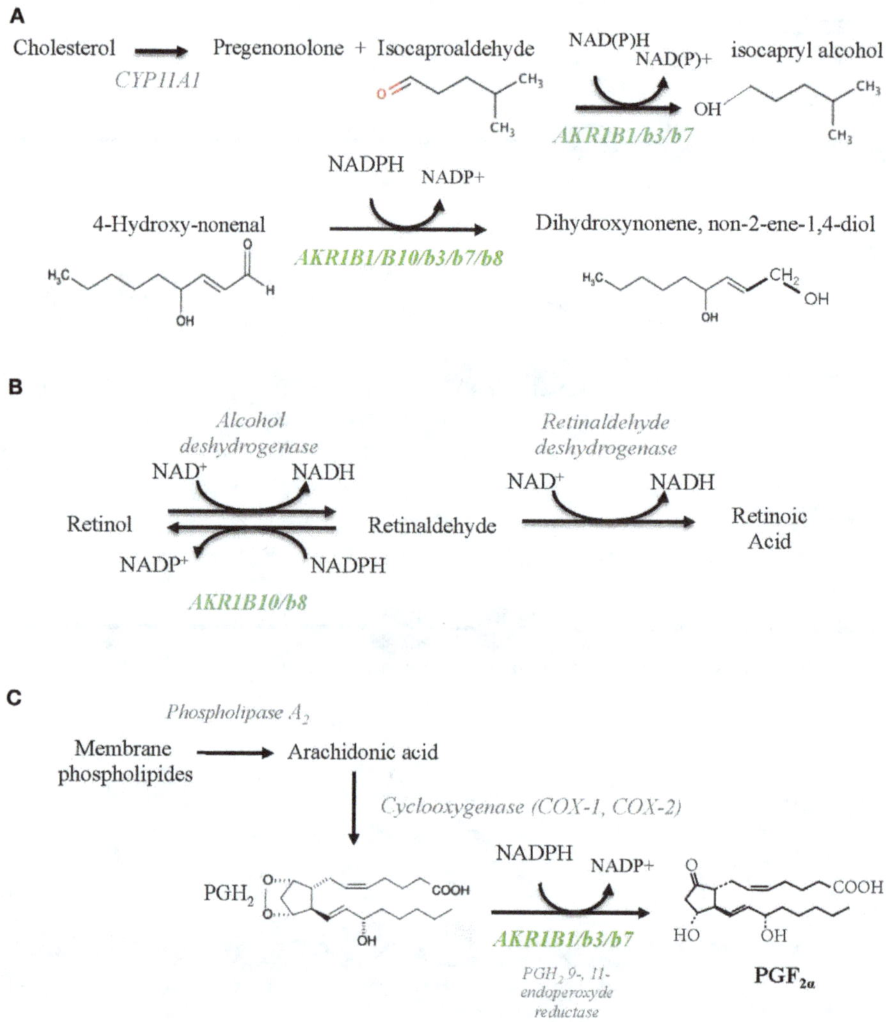

FIGURE 3 | Schematic diagrams of enzymatic reactions illustrating AKR1B involvement toward lipid aldehyde detoxification (A), retinoids (B), and prostaglandins (C) metabolism. All the indicated substrates and enzymatic activities are supposed to coexist in the adrenal glands, but their relative importance in adrenal function remains unknown so far. AKR1B isoforms endowed with each of these activities are indicated in green.

TABLE 4 | Kinetic constants of AKR1B toward isocaproaldehyde, 4-hydroxynonenal, retinaldehyde, and prostaglandin H_2.

Substrates	Isocaproaldehyde		4-hydroxynonenal		All-*trans*-retinaldehyde		Prostaglandin H_2	
	K_m (μM)	k_{cat} (s^{-1})	K_m (μM)	k_{cat} (s^{-1})	K_m (mM)	k_{cat} (min^{-1})	K_m (μM)	V_{max} (nmol/min/mg)
Human								
AKR1B1	1[a]	0.66[a]	716[d]	0.84[d]	1.1[e]	0.35[e]	1.9[f]	44[f]
AKR1B10	330[b]	0.72[b]	31[d]	2.01[d]	0.6[e]	27[e]	No activity[f]	
AKRB15	n.d.		2.2[g]	0.08[g]	1[g]	5.4[g]	n.d.	
Mouse								
Akr1b3	62[c]	1.3[c]	665[g]	0.82[d]	1.0[e]	0.52[e]	26[f]	26[f]
Akr1b7	320[c]	0.38[c]	256[g]	0.1[d]	0.5[e]	0.02[e]	53.4[f]	53.4[f]
Akr1b8	71[c]	0.03[c]	230[g]	3.18[d]	2.1[e]	0.05[e]	No activity[f]	
Akr1b16	n.d.		n.d.		n.d.		n.d.	

n.d., not determined.
Reference: [a](33); [b](40); [c](28); [d](11); [e](12); [f](34); [g](14).

However, no adrenal phenotype was described in these mice, and neither oxidative stress nor Nrf2 have been involved in adrenal *Akr1b8* expression so far.

Previous studies demonstrated that some AKR1B proteins showed efficient catalytic activity for the reduction of the abundant and highly reactive lipid-derived aldehyde 4-hydroxy-2-nonenal and the phospholipid aldehydes (17). In particular, Akr1b8 displays the most efficient phospholipid aldehyde and HNE-reductase activity in mouse tissues (17, 28, 37) (**Figure 3**; **Table 4**). All these enzymatic data suggest that in the adrenal cortex, Akr1b8 isoform could be devoted to detoxify aldehyde lipids abundantly accumulated in this tissue (38). Furthermore, expression of an antisense RNA directed against *Akr1b7* suppressed isocaproaldehyde reductase activity in adrenocortical Y1 cells without any alteration of Akr1b8 protein accumulation (29). In view of its enzymatic features and constitutive expression, Akr1b8 is unlikely to be the principal isocaproaldehyde reductase in the adrenocortical gland (28). *Akr1b8* gene disruption in mice led to reduced lipid synthesis and diminished proliferation of colonic epithelial cells but had no evident effect on general appearance, body weight, and reproduction. However, *in vivo* adrenal Akr1b8 physiological role remains to be examined since *Akr1b8* gene disruption first report did not notice evident effect on the adrenal physiology (39).

Whether *Akr1b8* and human *AKR1B10* gene can be considered as ortholog is still a matter of debate since they share high sequence identity, and proteins display several close structural and enzymatic properties (11) (**Tables 1** and **4**). In contrast to *Akr1b8*, *AKR1B10* gene expression is not controlled by FGF (12). Although *AKR1B10* mRNA was initially detected in adrenal glands using a human RNA Master Blot, to date, there is no more information available on its *in situ* localization and transcriptional control in this organ (1). Moreover, *AKR1B10* gene expression pattern only partially overlaps that of *Akr1b8*, since *AKR1B10* transcripts are absent from heart, lung, or testis (7, 11).

Comparative studies demonstrated that AKR1B10 exhibits higher 4-HNE-reductase activity than AKR1B1, while lower than the murine Akr1b8 (11, 16). *Ex vivo* studies revealed that both human AKR1B1 and -B10 also share the ability to reduce isocaproaldehyde (1, 40). Nevertheless, in a comparative enzymatic study, Hara and colleagues showed that AKR1B1 had a more effective isocaproaldehyde reductase activity than AKR1B10, suggesting that in human steroidogenic organs, the latter was unlikely to play a major role in the detoxification of steroidogenic by-products (41).

The AKR superfamily has been added as a novel group of cytosolic enzymes that could contribute to retinoid–redox conversion. Based on their cofactor specificity (NADPH), AKR work in the reductive direction (42). Retinol (vitamin A) and its derivatives, retinaldehyde and retinoic acid (RA), are essential for the growth and maintenance of many tissues. RA is a key molecule in the development of different vertebrate organs by promoting cell differentiation and apoptosis. The control of retinaldehyde levels is essential in the regulation of RA synthesis and therefore of its signaling role. Once synthesized from β-carotene through the β-carotene 15,15′ monooxygenase 1 (BCO1), retinaldehyde has two alternative fates, its irreversible oxidation to RA (metabolism fate) by the aldehyde dehydrogenases (ADH) or its reduction back to retinol (storage fate) by the retinaldehyde reductase activity of AKR (43) (**Figure 3B**; **Table 4**). Comparative *in vitro* enzymatic studies on murine and human AKRs have fairly evidenced that among AKR1B proteins, AKR1B10 is so far the only retinaldehyde reductase with the highest k_{cat} value for the retinaldehyde reduction (11, 12, 44). *Ex vivo* AKR1B10 overexpression in different cell systems demonstrated its contribution in increasing retinol production (45, 46). In rodent, previous data evidenced that normal adrenal gland may function as an important site of retinoic acid synthesis involving class I- and IV-ADH, thus furthering retinaldehyde metabolism rather than its storage through the AKR activity (47). According to its expression, whether the well-established retinaldehyde reductase activity of AKR1B10 is operated in normal human adrenal physiology remains to be explored.

AKR1B10 expression was initially characterized in hepatocellular carcinoma and subsequently found to be altered by tumorigenesis process in several other organs (7, 48–50). Moreover, *AKR1B10* expression was associated with smoker's non-small cell lung carcinomas (48) and was suggested to be involved in drug resistance (51). A putative mechanism by which the activity of AKR1B enzymes could promote tumor growth is the conversion of retinaldehyde to retinol resulting in RA deprivation and blockage of its differentiating effect, promoting cell proliferation and fostering tumorigenesis (43). Furthermore, recent studies have shown that in breast cancer cells, AKR1B10 associates with acetyl-CoA carboxylase-alpha (ACCA), the rate-limiting enzyme of *de novo* synthesis of long-chain fatty acids, and blocks its ubiquitination and proteasome degradation. Long-chain fatty acids are the building blocks of biomembranes and the precursor of lipid second messengers, playing a critical role in cell growth and proliferation (52). The AKR1B10-mediated regulation on ACCA stability represents a novel regulatory mechanism, in which AKR1B10 promotes cell survival *via* modulating lipid synthesis, mitochondrial function, oxidative stress, and carbonyl levels (53).

Adrenocortical carcinomas are very aggressive and rare malignant tumors with poor prognosis (54). Microarray analysis was used to seek molecular predictors of malignancy and survival in a large cohort of unilateral adrenocortical tumors (http://www.ebi.ac.uk/arrayexpress, experiment E-TABM-311). Unsupervised clustering analysis allowed robust discrimination of malignant and benign tumors. On the basis of this analysis, *AKR1B10* expression was not found to be associated with the ACC group (35).

Akr1b7: Expression Profile, Detoxification Function, and Paracrine Action

High levels of *Akr1b7* transcripts were initially observed by *in situ* hybridization in fetal and adult murine adrenal cortex but were undetectable in the medulla (2). We confirmed these results by immunohistochemistry experiments, which allowed us to further restrict major Akr1b7 expression to the *zona fasciculata* (55). *In vivo*, ACTH suppression with dexamethasone treatment resulted in a marked decrease of *Akr1b7* mRNA levels that were restored when the treated mice were injected with exogenous ACTH. This ACTH/cAMP-induced *Akr1b7* transcription was blocked by a PKA inhibitor (H89) in the murine adrenocortical ATC and Y1 cell lines (55, 56).

In the adrenal gland, basal and ACTH-induced expressions of *Akr1b7* gene depend on three SF1 response element (SFRE) and on other *cis*-elements located in the upstream promoter region (**Figure 3**). Using transgenic mice and transfection experiments, we characterized a cryptic SFRE 102 bp upstream of the transcription start site that supports basal expression of *Akr1b7* in the adrenal cortex. Among the two other SFREs identified further upstream, the site at −458 was a *bona fide* SFRE, essential for both basal and cAMP-stimulated promoter activity. The last SFRE, an Sp1, and C/EBPβ binding sites, respectively, localized at positions −503, −52, and −61 are all involved in cAMP responsiveness (57, 58).

AKR1Bs are capable to handle the large amount of isocaproaldehyde, a toxic by-product coming from the cholesterol side-chain cleavage during the initial step of steroid biosynthesis. Furthermore, isocaproaldehyde accumulation decreased viability of Y1 cells (29). Although Akr1b3, Akr1b7, and Akr1b8 all were able to reduce isocaproaldehyde, the two former seemed to be the more efficient reductases for this substrate (28). However, the silencing of *Akr1b7* gene was sufficient to abolish the cAMP-induced isocaproaldehyde reductase activity in Y1 cells. Therefore, Akr1b7 was the main enzyme in charge of isocaproaldehyde detoxification in the adrenal cortex (29). Altogether, these data showed that in the adrenal cortex, ACTH not only controls expression of enzymes synthetizing steroids but also of proteins scavenging toxic by-products derived from steroidogenesis.

Madore et al. established that the bovine 20α-hydroxysteroid dehydrogenase, AKR1B5 was responsible for $PGF_{2\alpha}$ synthesis in the endometrium (59). Thereafter, we demonstrated by *ex vivo* studies, that AKR1B1, Akr1b3, and Akr1b7 were also able to reduce PGH_2 into $PGF_{2\alpha}$, whereas Akr1b8 and AKR1B10 were devoid of this $PGF_{2\alpha}$ synthase activity (**Table 4**). Due to their recent discovery, this 9-,11-endoperoxide reductase activity has not been investigated yet for Akr1b16 and AKR1B15. Moreover, their enzymatic constants suggested that AKR1B1, Akr1b3, and Akr1b7 had a higher 9-,11-endoperoxide reductase activity than the other PGF synthases already described (34). Prostaglandins are paracrine/autocrine signal molecules produced from a common precursor, PGH_2, which is derived from arachidonic acid by COX-1 or COX-2. Unlike COX-1, which is a constitutively expressed enzyme, COX-2 is not expressed in most organs under basal conditions but can be stimulated by inflammation and various mitogenic factors (60). Following these observations, we carefully examined the $PGF_{2\alpha}$ biosynthetic pathway in the adrenal gland (27).

Prostaglandin F2α was produced by both cortical (steroidogenic cells) and medullary (chromaffin cells) tissue of the adrenal gland. In primary adrenocortical cell culture, $PGF_{2\alpha}$ release was induced 2.5-fold by ACTH treatment. This secretion was correlated with ACTH responsiveness of both COX-2 and Akr1b7. Using *ex vivo* gain- and loss-of-function strategies, we demonstrated the pivotal role of Akr1b7 in ACTH-induced $PGF_{2\alpha}$ release, and it is functionally coupled with COX-2. In the adrenal medulla in which *Akr1b7* was not expressed, $PGF_{2\alpha}$ was produced from the coordinated activities of Akr1b3 and COX-1. Adrenal expression of $PGF_{2\alpha}$-specific receptor (FP) was restricted to the chromaffin cells, suggesting that both autocrine and paracrine mechanisms (within the medulla and between steroidogenic and medulla cells, respectively) were relaying $PGF_{2\alpha}$ action. In agreement with this hypothesis, we demonstrated that $PGF_{2\alpha}$ repressed both basal and glucocorticoid-induced dopamine release in the chromaffin cell line MPC862L. Comparison of the $PGF_{2\alpha}$-responsiveness of isolated cells and whole adrenal tissue cultures showed that $PGF_{2\alpha}$-mediated repression of glucocorticoid release is an indirect mechanism relying on a decrease in catecholamine secretion, which in turn decreased cortical steroidogenesis.

These functional data led us to propose an intra-adrenal feedback loop in which adrenal endocrine activities are regulated through the involvement of AKRs [**Figure 4** and Ref. (18)]. Surprisingly, however, the absence of Akr1b7 *in vivo* did not

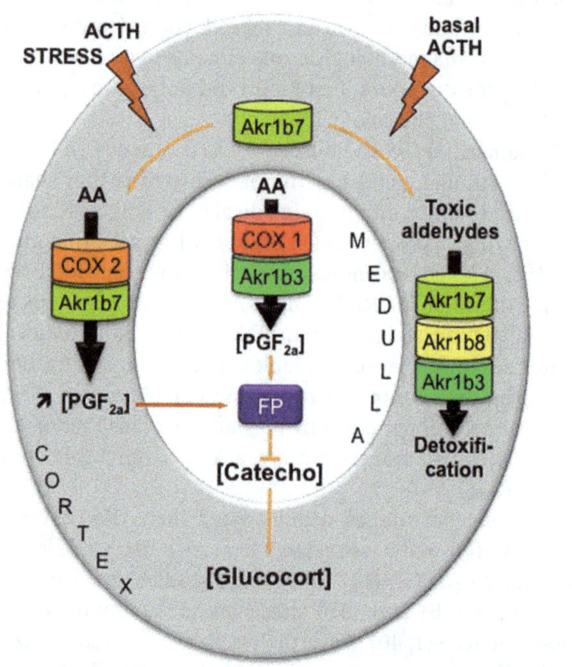

FIGURE 4 | Proposed model integrating dual functions of aldose reductases in the regulation of mouse adrenal endocrine functions [adapted from Ref. (18)]. AKR1B family is endowed with enzymatic activities that at least ensure two metabolic functions: the production of $PGF_{2\alpha}$ and the detoxification of lipid aldehydes. Arachidonic acid (AA) is metabolized into PGH_2, the precursor of all prostanoids, by COX enzymes and then converted into $PGF_{2\alpha}$ by the 9-,11-endoperoxyde reductase activity of PGF synthases of the AKR1B family. AKR1B are also capable to reduce toxic lipid aldehydes resulting from the particularly high prooxidant activities of P450 cytochromes in adrenocortical cells (i.e., isocaproaldehyde and 4-HNE). The mechanism integrating these dual functions was the following: (1) In basal conditions, $PGF_{2\alpha}$ is constitutively secreted by chromaffin cells (by the coupling of COX-1 and Akr1b3), thus regulating catecholamine production and also limiting their paracrine action on steroidogenesis. (2) During a stress situation, ACTH transiently induces COX-2 and Akr1b7 expression, which results in $PGF_{2\alpha}$ production inside the cortex. $PGF_{2\alpha}$ produced in the cortex then represses catecholamine release by the medulla *via* a paracrine action on its FP receptor. Decreased catecholamine release in turn reduces the effect of ACTH on glucocorticoids production (27). After the stress response has ended, COX-2 returns to undetectable levels. The coupling between Akr1b7 and COX-2 does not take place. Then, Akr1b7 together with Akr1b8 and Akr1b3 function only as cortical detoxifying enzymes of the harmful aldehydes produced under chronic/basal stimulation of steroidogenesis. Catecho, catecholamine; Glucocort, glucocorticoids.

affect basal adrenocortical function as illustrated by normal glucocorticoid plasma levels in *Akr1b7*$^{-/-}$ mice (61). Indeed, these mice displayed an obese phenotype that did not rely on adrenal dysfunction but on the lack of Akr1b7-dependent production of $PGF_{2\alpha}$ within the stromal vascular adipose tissue (3, 61). Adrenal expression of Akr1b3 and b8 is not affected in knockout mice and since they all share redundant enzymatic activities regarding detoxification of lipid aldehydes (see Akr1b3/AKR1B1: Expression Pattern and Relevant Functions and Akr1b8/AKR1B10: Phylogeny, Regulation, and Enzymatic Specificities), the remaining isoforms can compensate the absence of Akr1b7 at least in basal conditions. Importantly, Akr1b7 is the only one out of the three adrenal isoforms to be ACTH-responsive (27) and also the most abundantly expressed (3). Taken together, these hallmarks would predict that physiological importance of Akr1b enzymes in adrenal function should be rather explored under stress conditions during which scavenging capacity of constitutive (and less abundant) isoforms should be exhausted.

FUTURE DIRECTIONS

Fighting against oxidative stress is a challenging but mandatory task for adrenocortical cells. Indeed, P450 cytochrome systems involved in steroidogenesis, and in particular glucocorticoid production, contribute very significantly to oxidative stress by cellular reactive oxygen species (ROS) production (62). The redox imbalance due to excessive ROS production can cause adrenal damage that may progress to severe insufficiency, including familial glucocorticoid deficiency (FGD). Therefore, adrenal cortex is well supplied in antioxidant defense genes encoding enzymes of the superoxide dismutase (SOD), glutathione peroxidase (GPX), and peroxiredoxin (PRDX) families [for review, see Ref. (63)]. Since the precursor works of Feige's group showing the ACTH responsiveness of *SOD2* expression, the expected coordinated regulation of antioxidant enzymatic systems and P450s systems producing prooxidant by-products has been somewhat neglected (64). Accordingly, AKR1B enzymes family may be considered as antioxidant defense genes. Among these, ACTH-responsive ones, e.g., *Akr1b7* and *SOD2* genes, could participate in the adaptive response of antioxidant systems of adrenal cortex under stress conditions. Disturbance in redox homeostasis was the most recently discovered cause of FGD and mutations in *NNT* gene (nicotinamide nucleotide transhydrogenase) account for about 10% of cases (65). NNT ensures mitochondrial NADPH supply that is essential to ROS detoxification enzymatic systems. Then, it would be interesting to know whether adrenal-specific deficit in AKR1B enzymes could contribute to cortical damage or adrenal insufficiency in mice carrying a spontaneous *Nnt* mutation (66). This could provide the proof of principle for studying the physiological contribution of AKR1B family in detoxifying function in steroidogenic organs and beyond.

AUTHOR CONTRIBUTIONS

All authors listed have made substantial, direct, and intellectual contribution to the work and approved it for publication.

FUNDING

This work was supported by funds from the Centre National de la Recherche Scientifique, Clermont Université, Institut National de la Santé et de la Recherche Médicale and grant from the Région Auvergne.

REFERENCES

1. Hyndman DJ, Flynn TG. Sequence and expression levels in human tissues of a new member of the aldo-keto reductase family. *Biochim Biophys Acta* (1998) 1399:198–202. doi:10.1016/S0167-4781(98)00109-2
2. Lau ET, Cao D, Lin C, Chung SK, Chung SS. Tissue-specific expression of two aldose reductase-like genes in mice: abundant expression of mouse vas deferens protein and fibroblast growth factor-regulated protein in the adrenal gland. *Biochem J* (1995) 312(Pt 2):609–15. doi:10.1042/bj3120609
3. Pastel E, Pointud JC, Loubeau G, Dani C, Slim K, Martin G, et al. Aldose reductases influence prostaglandin F2α levels and adipocyte differentiation in male mouse and human species. *Endocrinology* (2015) 156:1671–84. doi:10.1210/en.2014-1750
4. Hyndman D, Bauman DR, Heredia VV, Penning TM. The aldo-keto reductase superfamily homepage. *Chem Biol Interact* (2003) 14(3–144):621–31. doi:10.1016/S0009-2797(02)00193-X
5. Jez JM, Bennett MJ, Schlegel BP, Lewis M, Penning TM. Comparative anatomy of the aldo-keto reductase superfamily. *Biochem J* (1997) 326(Pt 3):625–36. doi:10.1042/bj3260625
6. Jez JM, Flynn TG, Penning TM. A new nomenclature for the aldo-keto reductase superfamily. *Biochem Pharmacol* (1997) 54:639–47. doi:10.1016/S0006-2952(97)84253-0
7. Cao D, Fan ST, Chung SS. Identification and characterization of a novel human aldose reductase-like gene. *J Biol Chem* (1998) 273:11429–35. doi:10.1074/jbc.273.19.11429
8. Jin Y, Penning TM. Aldo-keto reductases and bioactivation/detoxication. *Annu Rev Pharmacol Toxicol* (2007) 47:263–92. doi:10.1146/annurev.pharmtox.47.120505.105337
9. Petrash JM. All in the family: aldose reductase and closely related aldo-keto reductases. *Cell Mol Life Sci* (2004) 61:737–49. doi:10.1007/s00018-003-3402-3
10. Ho HT, Jenkins NA, Copeland NG, Gilbert DJ, Winkles JA, Louie HW, et al. Comparisons of genomic structures and chromosomal locations of the mouse aldose reductase and aldose reductase-like genes. *Eur J Biochem* (1999) 259:726–30. doi:10.1046/j.1432-1327.1999.00110.x
11. Joshi A, Rajput S, Wang C, Ma J, Cao D. Murine aldo-keto reductase family 1 subfamily B: identification of AKR1B8 as an ortholog of human AKR1B10. *Biol Chem* (2010) 391:1371–8. doi:10.1515/BC.2010.144
12. Ruiz FX, Moro A, Gallego O, Ardèvol A, Rovira C, Petrash JM, et al. Human and rodent aldo-keto reductases from the AKR1B subfamily and their specificity with retinaldehyde. *Chem Biol Interact* (2011) 191:199–205. doi:10.1016/j.cbi.2011.02.007
13. Barski OA, Tipparaju SM, Bhatnagar A. The aldo-keto reductase superfamily and its role in drug metabolism and detoxification. *Drug Metab Rev* (2008) 40:553–624. doi:10.1080/03602530802431439
14. Giménez-Dejoz J, Kolář MH, Ruiz FX, Crespo I, Cousido-Siah A, Podjarny A, et al. Substrate specificity, inhibitor selectivity and structure-function relationships of aldo-keto reductase 1B15: a novel human retinaldehyde reductase. *PLoS One* (2015) 10:e0134506. doi:10.1371/journal.pone.0134506
15. Penning TM. The aldo-keto reductases (AKRs): overview. *Chem Biol Interact* (2015) 234:236–46. doi:10.1016/j.cbi.2014.09.024
16. Shen Y, Zhong L, Johnson S, Cao D. Human aldo-keto reductases 1B1 and 1B10: a comparative study on their enzyme activity toward electrophilic carbonyl compounds. *Chem Biol Interact* (2011) 191:192–8. doi:10.1016/j.cbi.2011.02.004

17. Spite M, Baba SP, Ahmed Y, Barski OA, Nijhawan K, Petrash JM, et al. Substrate specificity and catalytic efficiency of aldo-keto reductases with phospholipid aldehydes. *Biochem J* (2007) 405:95–105. doi:10.1042/BJ20061743
18. Pastel E, Pointud JC, Volat F, Martinez A, Lefrançois-Martinez AM. Aldo-keto reductases 1B in endocrinology and metabolism. *Front Pharmacol* (2012) 3:148. doi:10.3389/fphar.2012.00148
19. Bohren KM, Bullock B, Wermuth B, Gabbay KH. The aldo-keto reductase superfamily. cDNAs and deduced amino acid sequences of human aldehyde and aldose reductases. *J Biol Chem* (1989) 264:9547–51.
20. Weber S, Salabei JK, Möller G, Kremmer E, Bhatnagar A, Adamski J, et al. Aldo-keto Reductase 1B15 (AKR1B15): a mitochondrial human aldo-keto reductase with activity toward steroids and 3-keto-acyl-CoA conjugates. *J Biol Chem* (2015) 290:6531–45. doi:10.1074/jbc.M114.610121
21. Salabei JK, Li X-P, Petrash JM, Bhatnagar A, Barski OA. Functional expression of novel human and murine AKR1B genes. *Chem Biol Interact* (2011) 191:177–84. doi:10.1016/j.cbi.2011.01.020
22. Pailhoux EA, Martinez A, Veyssiere GM, Jean CG. Androgen-dependent protein from mouse vas deferens. cDNA cloning and protein homology with the aldo-keto reductase superfamily. *J Biol Chem* (1990) 265:19932–6.
23. Donohue PJ, Alberts GF, Hampton BS, Winkles JA. A delayed-early gene activated by fibroblast growth factor-1 encodes a protein related to aldose reductase. *J Biol Chem* (1994) 269:8604–9.
24. Brunskill EW, Sequeira-Lopez MLS, Pentz ES, Lin E, Yu J, Aronow BJ, et al. Genes that confer the identity of the renin cell. *J Am Soc Nephrol* (2011) 22:2213–25. doi:10.1681/ASN.2011040401
25. Schmidt DR, Schmidt S, Holmstrom SR, Makishima M, Yu RT, Cummins CL, et al. AKR1B7 is induced by the farnesoid X receptor and metabolizes bile acids. *J Biol Chem* (2011) 286:2425–32. doi:10.1074/jbc.M110.181230
26. Tirard J, Gout J, Lefrancois-Martinez AM, Martinez A, Begeot M, Naville D. A novel inhibitory protein in adipose tissue, the aldo-keto reductase AKR1B7: its role in adipogenesis. *Endocrinology* (2007) 148:1996–2005. doi:10.1210/en.2006-1707
27. Lambert-Langlais S, Pointud JC, Lefrancois-Martinez AM, Volat F, Manin M, Coudore F, et al. Aldo keto reductase 1B7 and prostaglandin F2alpha are regulators of adrenal endocrine functions. *PLoS One* (2009) 4:e7309. doi:10.1371/journal.pone.0007309
28. Martinez A, Aigueperse C, Val P, Dussault M, Tournaire C, Berger M, et al. Physiological functions and hormonal regulation of mouse vas deferens protein (AKR1B7) in steroidogenic tissues. *Chem Biol Interact* (2001) 13(0–132):903–17. doi:10.1016/S0009-2797(00)00244-1
29. Lefrancois-Martinez AM, Tournaire C, Martinez A, Berger M, Daoudal S, Tritsch D, et al. Product of side-chain cleavage of cholesterol, isocaproaldehyde, is an endogenous specific substrate of mouse vas deferens protein, an aldose reductase-like protein in adrenocortical cells. *J Biol Chem* (1999) 274:32875–80. doi:10.1074/jbc.274.46.32875
30. Aida K, Ikegishi Y, Chen J, Tawata M, Ito S, Maeda S, et al. Disruption of aldose reductase gene (Akr1b1) causes defect in urinary concentrating ability and divalent cation homeostasis. *Biochem Biophys Res Commun* (2000) 277:281–6. doi:10.1006/bbrc.2000.3648
31. Ho HT, Chung SK, Law JW, Ko BC, Tam SC, Brooks HL, et al. Aldose reductase-deficient mice develop nephrogenic diabetes insipidus. *Mol Cell Biol* (2000) 20:5840–6. doi:10.1128/MCB.20.16.5840-5846.2000
32. Lefrancois-Martinez AM, Bertherat J, Val P, Tournaire C, Gallo-Payet N, Hyndman D, et al. Decreased expression of cyclic adenosine monophosphate-regulated aldose reductase (AKR1B1) is associated with malignancy in human sporadic adrenocortical tumors. *J Clin Endocrinol Metab* (2004) 89:3010–9. doi:10.1210/jc.2003-031830
33. Matsuura K, Deyashiki Y, Bunai Y, Ohya I, Hara A. Aldose reductase is a major reductase for isocaproaldehyde, a product of side-chain cleavage of cholesterol, in human and animal adrenal glands. *Arch Biochem Biophys* (1996) 328:265–71. doi:10.1006/abbi.1996.0172
34. Kabututu Z, Manin M, Pointud JC, Maruyama T, Nagata N, Lambert S, et al. Prostaglandin F2{alpha} synthase activities of aldo-keto reductase 1B1, 1B3 and 1B7. *J Biochem* (2009) 145:161–8. doi:10.1093/jb/mvn152
35. de Reyniès A, Assié G, Rickman DS, Tissier F, Groussin L, René-Corail F, et al. Gene expression profiling reveals a new classification of adrenocortical tumors and identifies molecular predictors of malignancy and survival. *J Clin Oncol* (2009) 27:1108–15. doi:10.1200/JCO.2008.18.5678
36. Luo L, Chen Y, Wu D, Shou J, Wang S, Ye J, et al. Butylated hydroxyanisole induces distinct expression patterns of Nrf2 and detoxification enzymes in the liver and small intestine of C57BL/6 mice. *Toxicol Appl Pharmacol* (2015) 288:339–48. doi:10.1016/j.taap.2015.08.006
37. Srivastava S, Chandra A, Ansari NH, Srivastava SK, Bhatnagar A. Identification of cardiac oxidoreductase(s) involved in the metabolism of the lipid peroxidation-derived aldehyde-4-hydroxynonenal. *Biochem J* (1998) 329(Pt 3):469–75. doi:10.1042/bj3290469
38. Burczynski JM, Hayes JR, Longhurst PA, Colby HD. Species differences in adrenal lipid peroxidation: role of alpha-tocopherol. *Free Radic Biol Med* (1999) 26:987–91. doi:10.1016/S0891-5849(98)00289-5
39. Shen Y, Ma J, Yan R, Ling H, Li X, Yang W, et al. Impaired self-renewal and increased colitis and dysplastic lesions in colonic mucosa of AKR1B8-deficient mice. *Clin Cancer Res* (2015) 21:1466–76. doi:10.1158/1078-0432.CCR-14-2072
40. Martin H-J, Maser E. Role of human aldo-keto-reductase AKR1B10 in the protection against toxic aldehydes. *Chem Biol Interact* (2009) 178:145–50. doi:10.1016/j.cbi.2008.10.021
41. Endo S, Matsunaga T, Mamiya H, Ohta C, Soda M, Kitade Y, et al. Kinetic studies of AKR1B10, human aldose reductase-like protein: endogenous substrates and inhibition by steroids. *Arch Biochem Biophys* (2009) 487:1–9. doi:10.1016/j.abb.2009.05.009
42. Crosas B, Cederlund E, Torres D, Jornvall H, Farres J, Pares X. A vertebrate aldo-keto reductase active with retinoids and ethanol. *J Biol Chem* (2001) 276:19132–40. doi:10.1074/jbc.M010478200
43. Ruiz FX, Porté S, Parés X, Farrés J. Biological role of aldo-keto reductases in retinoic acid biosynthesis and signaling. *Front Pharmacol* (2012) 3:58. doi:10.3389/fphar.2012.00058
44. Crosas B, Hyndman DJ, Gallego O, Martras S, Parés X, Flynn TG, et al. Human aldose reductase and human small intestine aldose reductase are efficient retinal reductases: consequences for retinoid metabolism. *Biochem J* (2003) 373:973–9. doi:10.1042/BJ20021818
45. Gallego O, Ruiz FX, Ardèvol A, Domínguez M, Alvarez R, de Lera AR, et al. Structural basis for the high all-trans-retinaldehyde reductase activity of the tumor marker AKR1B10. *Proc Natl Acad Sci U S A* (2007) 104:20764–9. doi:10.1073/pnas.0705659105
46. Wang R, Wang G, Ricard MJ, Ferris B, Strulovici-Barel Y, Salit J, et al. Smoking-induced upregulation of AKR1B10 expression in the airway epithelium of healthy individuals. *Chest* (2010) 138:1402–10. doi:10.1378/chest.09-2634
47. Haselbeck RJ, Ang HL, Deltour L, Duester G. Retinoic acid and alcohol/retinol dehydrogenase in the mouse adrenal gland: a potential endocrine source of retinoic acid during development. *Endocrinology* (1997) 138:3035–41. doi:10.1210/endo.138.7.5274
48. Fukumoto S, Yamauchi N, Moriguchi H, Hippo Y, Watanabe A, Shibahara J, et al. Overexpression of the aldo-keto reductase family protein AKR1B10 is highly correlated with smokers' non-small cell lung carcinomas. *Clin Cancer Res* (2005) 11:1776–85. doi:10.1158/1078-0432.CCR-04-1238
49. Rajkumar T, Vijayalakshmi N, Gopal G, Sabitha K, Shirley S, Raja UM, et al. Identification and validation of genes involved in gastric tumorigenesis. *Cancer Cell Int* (2010) 10:45. doi:10.1186/1475-2867-10-45
50. Yoshitake H, Takahashi M, Ishikawa H, Nojima M, Iwanari H, Watanabe A, et al. Aldo-keto reductase family 1, member B10 in uterine carcinomas: a potential risk factor of recurrence after surgical therapy in cervical cancer. *Int J Gynecol Cancer* (2007) 17:1300–6. doi:10.1111/j.1525-1438.2007.00932.x
51. Matsunaga T, Wada Y, Endo S, Soda M, El-Kabbani O, Hara A. Aldo-keto reductase 1B10 and its role in proliferation capacity of drug-resistant cancers. *Front Pharmacol* (2012) 3:5. doi:10.3389/fphar.2012.00005
52. Ma J, Yan R, Zu X, Cheng JM, Rao K, Liao DF, et al. Aldo-keto reductase family 1 B10 affects fatty acid synthesis by regulating the stability of acetyl-CoA carboxylase-alpha in breast cancer cells. *J Biol Chem* (2008) 283:3418–23. doi:10.1074/jbc.M707650200
53. Wang C, Yan R, Luo D, Watabe K, Liao DF, Cao D. Aldo-keto reductase family 1 member B10 promotes cell survival by regulating lipid synthesis and eliminating carbonyls. *J Biol Chem* (2009) 284:26742–8. doi:10.1074/jbc.M109.022897
54. Libè R, Fratticci A, Bertherat J. Adrenocortical cancer: pathophysiology and clinical management. *Endocr Relat Cancer* (2007) 14:13–28. doi:10.1677/erc.1.01130

55. Aigueperse C, Martinez A, Lefrancois-Martinez AM, Veyssiere G, Jean CI. Cyclic AMP regulates expression of the gene coding for a mouse vas deferens protein related to the aldo-keto reductase superfamily in human and murine adrenocortical cells. *J Endocrinol* (1999) 160:147–54. doi:10.1677/joe.0.1600147
56. Ragazzon B, Lefrancois-Martinez AM, Val P, Sahut-Barnola I, Tournaire C, Chambon C, et al. Adrenocorticotropin-dependent changes in SF-1/DAX-1 ratio influence steroidogenic genes expression in a novel model of glucocorticoid-producing adrenocortical cell lines derived from targeted tumorigenesis. *Endocrinology* (2006) 147:1805–18. doi:10.1210/en.2005-1279
57. Martinez A, Val P, Sahut-Barnola I, Aigueperse C, Veyssiere G, Lefrancois-Martinez AM. Steroidogenic factor-1 controls the aldose reductase akr1b7 gene promoter in transgenic mice through an atypical binding site. *Endocrinology* (2003) 144:2111–20. doi:10.1210/en.2002-220825
58. Val P, Aigueperse C, Ragazzon B, Veyssiere G, Lefrancois-Martinez AM, Martinez A. Adrenocorticotropin/3′,5′-cyclic AMP-mediated transcription of the scavenger akr1-b7 gene in adrenocortical cells is dependent on three functionally distinct steroidogenic factor-1-responsive elements. *Endocrinology* (2004) 145:508–18. doi:10.1210/en.2003-1093
59. Madore E, Harvey N, Parent J, Chapdelaine P, Arosh JA, Fortier MA. An aldose reductase with 20 alpha-hydroxysteroid dehydrogenase activity is most likely the enzyme responsible for the production of prostaglandin f2 alpha in the bovine endometrium. *J Biol Chem* (2003) 278:11205–12. doi:10.1074/jbc.M208318200
60. Ramsay RG, Ciznadija D, Vanevski M, Mantamadiotis T. Transcriptional regulation of cyclo-oxygenase expression: three pillars of control. *Int J Immunopathol Pharmacol* (2003) 16:59–67.
61. Volat FE, Pointud JC, Pastel E, Morio B, Sion B, Hamard G, et al. Depressed levels of prostaglandin F2α in mice lacking Akr1b7 increase basal adiposity and predispose to diet-induced obesity. *Diabetes* (2012) 61:2796–806. doi:10.2337/db11-1297
62. Rapoport R, Sklan D, Hanukoglu I. Electron leakage from the adrenal cortex mitochondrial P450scc and P450c11 systems: NADPH and steroid dependence. *Arch Biochem Biophys* (1995) 317:412–6. doi:10.1006/abbi.1995.1182
63. Prasad R, Kowalczyk JC, Meimaridou E, Storr HL, Metherell LA. Oxidative stress and adrenocortical insufficiency. *J Endocrinol* (2014) 221:R63–73. doi:10.1530/JOE-13-0346
64. Chinn AM, Ciais D, Bailly S, Chambaz E, LaMarre J, Feige JJ. Identification of two novel ACTH-responsive genes encoding manganese-dependent superoxide dismutase (SOD2) and the zinc finger protein TIS11b [tetradecanoyl phorbol acetate (TPA)-inducible sequence 11b]. *Mol Endocrinol* (2002) 16:1417–27. doi:10.1210/mend.16.6.0844
65. Meimaridou E, Kowalczyk J, Guasti L, Hughes CR, Wagner F, Frommolt P, et al. Mutations in NNT encoding nicotinamide nucleotide transhydrogenase cause familial glucocorticoid deficiency. *Nat Genet* (2012) 44:740–2. doi:10.1038/ng.2299
66. Toye AA, Lippiat JD, Proks P, Shimomura K, Bentley L, Hugill A, et al. A genetic and physiological study of impaired glucose homeostasis control in C57BL/6J mice. *Diabetologia* (2005) 48:675–86. doi:10.1007/s00125-005-1680-z
67. Aigueperse C, Val P, Pacot C, Darne C, Lalli E, Sassone-Corsi P, et al. SF-1 (steroidogenic factor-1), C/EBPbeta (CCAAT/enhancer binding protein), and ubiquitous transcription factors NF1 (nuclear factor 1) and Sp1 (selective promoter factor 1) are required for regulation of the mouse aldose reductase-like gene (AKR1B7) expression in adrenocortical cells. *Mol Endocrinol* (2001) 15:93–111. doi:10.1210/mend.15.1.0577

15

Role of ACTH in the Interactive/Paracrine Regulation of Adrenal Steroid Secretion in Physiological and Pathophysiological Conditions

Hervé Lefebvre[1,2,3], Michaël Thomas[1,2], Céline Duparc[1,2], Jérôme Bertherat[4,5] and Estelle Louiset[1,2]*

[1] U982, Laboratory of Neuronal and Neuroendocrine Differentiation and Communication, INSERM, Institute for Research and Innovation in Biomedicine, Mont-Saint-Aignan, France, [2] Normandie Université, UNIROUEN, Rouen, France, [3] Department of Endocrinology, Diabetes and Metabolic Diseases, University Hospital of Rouen, Rouen, France, [4] U1016, INSERM, Institut Cochin, Paris, France, [5] Department of Endocrinology and Metabolic Diseases, Hôpital Cochin, Assistance Publique-Hôpitaux de Paris, Paris, France

***Correspondence:**
Hervé Lefebvre
herve.lefebvre@chu-rouen.fr

In the normal human adrenal gland, steroid secretion is regulated by a complex network of autocrine/paracrine interactions involving bioactive signals released by endothelial cells, nerve terminals, chromaffin cells, immunocompetent cells, and adrenocortical cells themselves. ACTH can be locally produced by medullary chromaffin cells and is, therefore, a major mediator of the corticomedullary functional interplay. Plasma ACTH also triggers the release of angiogenic and vasoactive agents from adrenocortical cells and adrenal mast cells and, thus, indirectly regulates steroid production through modulation of the adrenal blood flow. Adrenocortical neoplasms associated with steroid hypersecretion exhibit molecular and cellular defects that tend to reinforce the influence of paracrine regulatory loops on corticosteroidogenesis. Especially, ACTH has been found to be abnormally synthesized in bilateral macronodular adrenal hyperplasia responsible for hypercortisolism. In these tissues, ACTH is detected in a subpopulation of adrenocortical cells that express gonadal markers. This observation suggests that ectopic production of ACTH may result from impaired embryogenesis leading to abnormal maturation of the adrenogonadal primordium. Globally, the current literature indicates that ACTH is a major player in the autocrine/paracrine processes occurring in the adrenal gland in both physiological and pathological conditions.

Keywords: ACTH, aldosterone, cortisol, Cushing's syndrome, aldosterone-producing adenoma, hyperplasia, adrenocortical cells, VEGF

INTRODUCTION

The adrenal cortex is a heterogeneous tissue that not only contains steroidogenic cells but also hosts various cell types that are able to locally release a wide variety of bioactive signals. This histological organization results in a complex interactive network that participates in the regulation of both basal and ACTH-induced corticosteroidogenesis. The intracortical sources of regulatory factors include chromaffin cells arranged in cords or islets, nerve fibers originating from extraadrenal neurones or cell bodies located in the adrenal medulla, cells of the immune system, including lymphocytes, macrophages/monocytes and mast cells, endothelial cells, and adipocytes. These autocrine/paracrine mechanisms have been extensively reviewed during the past years (1–5). However, their physiological role, especially their exact contribution to the regulation of corticosteroid synthesis remains a matter of debate although some data indicate that intraadrenal regulatory signals may mediate parts of the biological effects of ACTH on the adrenal cortex. Interestingly, adrenocortical neoplasms associated with steroid hypersecretion exhibit molecular and cellular defects that tend to reinforce the potency of paracrine factors to activate corticosteroidogenesis. For instance, abnormal expression of ACTH has been reported in adrenocortical cells in both tumors and hyperplasias responsible for hypercortisolism (6–11).

In the present review article, we have updated the current knowledge on the role of ACTH in the cell-to-cell communication processes occurring in the adrenal cortex in both physiological and pathological conditions. We will also discuss the potential interest of the intraadrenal ACTH regulatory loop for the clinical management of patients with primary adrenal excess of corticosteroids.

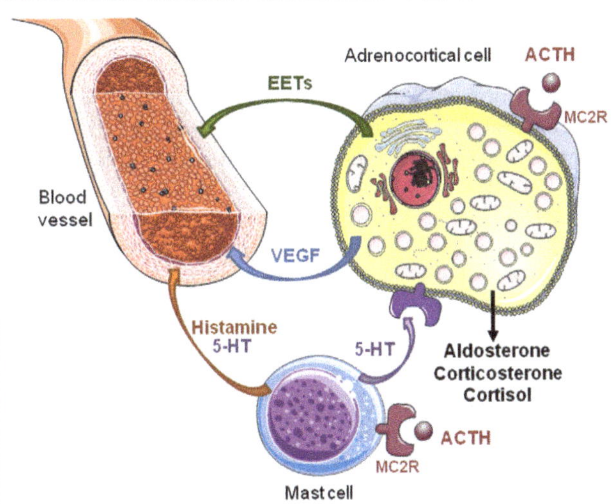

FIGURE 1 | Direct and indirect effects of ACTH on steroidogenesis in the adrenal gland. ACTH exerts a direct stimulatory effect on adrenocortical cells *via* melanocortin type 2 receptors (MC2R). Activation of MC2R increases secretion of steroid hormones, vascular endothelial growth factor (VEGF), and epoxyeicosatrienoic acids (EETs). Angiogenesis induced by VEGF, an endothelial cell-specific mitogen factor, allows adrenal tissue growth in response to ACTH. Increase in adrenal blood flow elicited by EETs, which are potent vasorelaxant agents, favors steroid production. In rats, ACTH also activates adrenal mast cells inducing local release of histamine and serotonin (5-HT). These factors modulate the tonicity of adrenal arterioles and, thus, the adrenal blood flow that indirectly influences the steroidogenesis. In addition, 5-HT stimulates steroid secretion through activation of different 5-HT receptor subtypes expressed by normal and tumor human adrenocortical cells.

EFFECT OF ACTH ON THE ADRENAL VASCULATURE

The adrenal cortex is a richly vascularized organ. This extensive vasculature is essential for delivery of tropic hormone and steroid hormones precursors to the gland and secretion of mature hormones into the blood flow. Furthermore, the establishment of such dense vascular network ensures that every adrenocortical cell is in contact with at least one endothelial cell (12, 13). This remarkable histological organization allows paracrine regulation of adrenocortical cells by endothelial cells through release of endothelins, adrenomedullin, nitric oxide, and prostacyclin (14). For instance, Rossi et al. have shown that endothelin-1 released by endothelial cells is an important regulator of aldosterone secretion, and may then indirectly influence arterial blood pressure (15, 16). The release of endothelin by adrenocortical sinusoids is thought to mediate the modulation of adrenal steroidogenesis by the adrenal blood (17). Interestingly, ACTH appears able to both act on development and maintenance of the adrenal vasculature and regulate the adrenal blood flow (18, 19), influencing thus steroid production through an indirect effect in addition to its intrinsic steroidogenic action on adrenocortical cells (**Figure 1**).

The modulation of adrenal angiogenesis by ACTH may involve several bioactive signals. Thrombospondins (TSPs) represent a wide family of extracellular proteins consisting of five members, TSP1–5, which can bind multiple cell surface molecules, including heparin sulfate proteoglycans, low-density lipoprotein receptor-related protein, integrins, CD36, and CD47 (20). Owing to the great diversity of their binding partners, TSPs are involved in various biological processes, such as cell adhesion, spreading and migration, and angiogenesis (20, 21). In this respect, TSPs are known to inhibit angiogenesis by preventing migration of capillary endothelial cells. Interestingly, adrenocortical cells release high amounts of TSP2 in response to ACTH (22), suggesting that TSP2 may mediate some of the biological actions of ACTH in the adrenal cortex, especially centripetal adrenocortical cell migration, which is a fundamental process in the dynamic organization and remodeling of the adrenal cortex (23). However, the physiological role of TSP2, which is primarily expressed in zona glomerulosa and zona fasciculata, remains unclear since TSP2-null mice exhibit no alteration in corticosteroid secretion or adrenal development (24). In addition, syndromes of ACTH excess, including Cushing's disease and 21-hydroxylase deficiency, are associated with adrenocortical hyperplasia, a process that underlies active angiogenesis. Conversely, several observations indicate that vascular endothelial growth factor (VEGF) plays a pivotal role in the trophic effects of ACTH on the adrenal vasculature (25). VEGF is a widely expressed cytokine that acts as an endothelial cell-specific mitogen and angiogenic factor. In the bovine adrenal gland, VEGF is expressed in zona glomerulosa and zona fasciculata cells and its release is stimulated by ACTH (26). Upregulation of VEGF by ACTH has also been reported in human adrenal (27). The effect of ACTH on adrenal VEGF production involves transcription-independent mechanisms, including stabilization of VEGF mRNA by the HuR protein (28). Conversely, ACTH suppression by dexamethasone in mice results in progressive decrease of VEGF expression in adrenocortical cells and regression of the vascular network (29). Interestingly, ACTH also stimulates VEGF expression in human fetal adrenocortical cells, suggesting that VEGF is an important mediator of the trophic action of ACTH during the adrenal development (30).

Consistently, an increase in VEGF expression in adrenocortical cells has been noticed in the regenerating adrenal cortex in rats (31, 32). It is noteworthy that, in parallel to its effect on adrenal vasculature development *via* local synthesis of VEGF, ACTH also favors adrenal tissue growth through an antiapoptotic action on adrenocortical cells (29) and stimulation of synthesis of growth factors (30). Finally, VEGF may be involved in the capacity of ACTH to induce endothelial fenestration, a phenomenon that favors cell-to-cell interactions (26, 33).

The mechanism by which ACTH modulates the adrenal blood flow is obviously not univocal. Adrenocortical cells themselves are able to release vasorelaxant agents in response to ACTH. These compounds include metabolites of arachidonic acid, such as epoxyeicosatrienoic acids (EETs) (34). In addition, in the rat adrenal gland, capsular mast cells modulate the tonicity of adrenal arterioles and, thus, the adrenal blood flow through local release of histamine and serotonin (5-hydroxytryptamine; 5-HT) (17, 35). Interestingly, rat adrenal mast cells are sensitive to the action of ACTH, suggesting that they may represent an important intermediate in the effect of corticotropin on the adrenal blood flow (35). In humans, the presence of mast cells has been reported in both the subcapsular region of the normal adrenal gland (36) and various types of adrenocortical tumors, including deoxycorticosterone-secreting tumors, aldosterone-producing adenomas (APAs), and adrenocortical carcinomas (37–39). However, there is currently no data reported in the literature indicating that human adrenal mast cells are target cells for ACTH.

INDIRECT EFFECTS OF ACTH ON CORTICOSTEROIDOGENESIS THROUGH ADRENOCORTICAL CELL SECRETORY PRODUCTS

Adrenocortical cells are important sources of bioactive compounds that are able to modulate steroidogenesis through autocrine/paracrine actions. In man, it is doubtful that corticosteroid may affect their own secretion in physiological conditions. Conversely, the adrenal cortex is known to express the diverse components of the renin–angiotensin system, leading to local synthesis of angiotensin II and potential autocrine/paracrine stimulation of aldosterone secretion (40). Interestingly, renin production, which primarily occurs in zona glomerulosa cells, is stimulated by ACTH and reduced by hypophysectomy or dexamethasone administration (41, 42). This observation may explain why plasma renin levels are usually not suppressed in patients with overt ACTH-dependent hypercortisolism (43, 44). In fact, it is conceivable that, in this condition, ACTH-induced adrenal renin secretion may compensate inhibition of renal renin synthesis by hypervolemia and hypertension secondary to cortisol excess.

Adrenocortical cells also synthesize and release various cytokines, such as interleukin-1 (IL-1), IL-3, IL-6, and tumor necrosis factor-α (TNF- α) (1). These signals may influence the steroidogenic and mitogenic activities of adrenocortical cells *via* autocrine/paracrine processes (5). Indeed, ACTH has been shown to modulate cytokine production by adrenocortical cells, either positively (IL-6) or negatively (TNF-α) (45, 46). Intraadrenal cytokines may, thus, represent important effectors of ACTH capable of potentiating or attenuating its action on adrenocortical cells. However, there is currently no evidence that the impact of ACTH on adrenal cytokine synthesis may be involved in the pathogenesis of ACTH-dependent adrenal hyperplasia and/or hypercortisolism.

Several types of adrenocortical neoplasms are associated with illicit neuroendocrine differentiation of adrenocortical cells (47). This is especially true for APAs that have been shown to express synaptophysin, neuronal cell adhesion molecule, neuron specific enolase, and SV2 (48, 49). In addition, we have observed that APA cells may also abnormally synthesize 5-HT that is able to stimulate aldosterone secretion through activation of the overexpressed serotonergic type 4 (5-HT4) receptor (50, 51). Because APA cells also express high amounts of the ACTH receptor, i.e., the melanocortin receptor type 2 (MC2R) (51–53), it is conceivable that locally produced 5-HT may act as an amplifier of the stimulatory effect of ACTH on aldosterone secretion by APA tissues.

Inhibins and activin are dimeric peptides belonging to the TGF-β family. Inhibins are formed by combination of the α-subunit encoded by INHA and A or B isoform of the β-subunit, encoded by *INHBA* and *INHBB*, respectively. Alternatively, activin is a homodimer composed of two β-subunits. The action of activin is mediated by its specific receptors type I and II, and the intracellular proteins SMAD. Inhibins counteract the biological effects of activin by antagonizing activin type II receptor and formation of an inactive complex with the TGFβ type III receptor β-glycan. Adrenocortical cells are able to express both α and β subunits (54–56). In particular, the α-inhibin is expressed in the zona reticularis under the positive control of ACTH, whereas β-subunits are mainly present in the outer cortex. Both activin receptors and the inhibin co-receptor β-glycan are also detected in the adrenal cortex (55, 56). It has been demonstrated that ACTH stimulates secretion of inhibin A and B, without modifying production of activin A (55). These data indicate that ACTH also controls corticosteroidogenesis through modulation of the intraadrenal activins/inhibins ratio.

INDIRECT EFFECTS OF ACTH ON CORTICOSTEROIDOGENESIS THROUGH NON-STEROIDOGENIC ADRENAL CELLS

The adrenal gland is surrounded by adipose tissue and its cortical region contains adipocytes either isolated or arranged in small islets (57). Like cells of the immune system, adipocytes release a wide panel of cytokines, suggesting that they could influence the adrenocortical function through a cell-to-cell communication process. For instance, adipocytes have been shown to activate aldosterone release by secreting soluble bioactive factors, which have not been yet characterized (57–59). Conversely, leptin exerts an inhibitory action on ACTH-induced corticosteroid secretion in human adrenocortical cells without affecting their viability and proliferation (60–63). It is possible that peri- and intraadrenal adipocytes may be controlled by ACTH and, thus, constitute a relay in the action of the hormone on the adrenal cortex. In support of this hypothesis, it has been reported that murine adipocyte cell lines and immortalized adipocytes express the MC2R, and ACTH regulate adipocyte functions in these models (64–66). In addition, patients with congenital adrenal hyperplasia due to 21-hydroxylase deficiency, a condition which is associated with chronically high plasma ACTH levels, can present with adrenal myelolipoma (67–69), suggesting a role of ACTH in the development of lipomatous tissue inclusions in the adrenal glands. However, in contrast to the observations made in murine cells, human mature adipocytes only express low levels of the MC2R and ACTH does not influence lipolysis in the mature human adipose tissue (70).

PARACRINE CONTROL OF ADRENAL STEROIDOGENESIS BY INTRAADRENAL ACTH

In the normal adrenal gland, chromaffin cells release detectable amounts of ACTH that is a major mediator in the corticomedullary functional interaction (71, 72) (**Figure 2**). This secretory process can be activated by corticotropin-releasing hormone (CRH) that is expressed in the adrenal medullary tissue (11). As chromaffin cells are also regulated by splanchnic nerves and proinflammatory cytokines, it seems possible that they may be important intermediates in the activation of the adrenal cortex during stress and inflammation. However, the physiological role of the paracrine control of corticosteroidogenesis by adrenomedullary ACTH remains unclear (3).

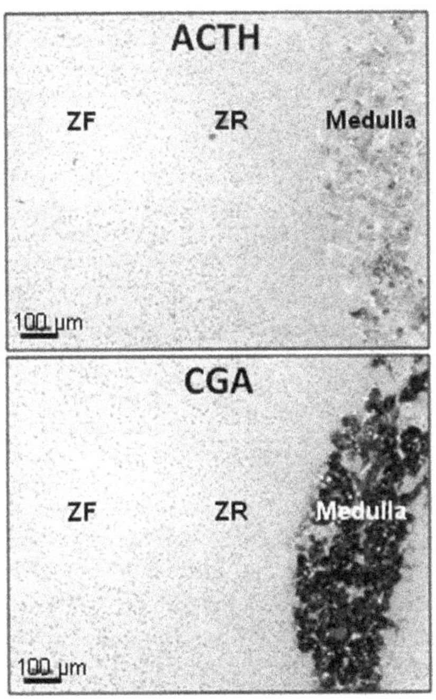

FIGURE 2 | **Presence of ACTH in the normal human adrenal.** ACTH immunoreactivity is exclusively located in some chromaffin cells (high panel), identified as chromogranin A (CGA) immunoreactive cells (low panel), in the medulla. ACTH was detected by using antibodies against the N-terminal region of the peptide. ZF, zona fasciculata; ZR, zona reticularis. Illustration of the data published in Ref. (9).

Conversely, clinicopathological studies have shown that paracrine interactions involving ACTH produced by chromaffin cells may play a role in the pathogenesis of hypercortisolism. Pheochromocytoma can occasionally produce ACTH resulting in ACTH-dependent Cushing's syndrome (73–75). Hypercortisolism seems to be mainly the consequence of the endocrine corticotropic action of ACTH whose plasma levels are typically elevated in this situation (76). Nevertheless, this mechanism may not be exclusive. In fact, hyperplasia of the adrenal cortex adjacent to pheochromocytoma has also been observed, indicating that ACTH originating from the pheochromocytoma tissue can stimulate adrenocortical cells in a paracrine manner (11, 77–80). Such a histological pattern is close to what is observed in corticomedullary mixed tumors that are composed of intermingled adrenocortical and pheochromocytoma tissues (81–84). These rare tumors are sometimes associated with hypercortisolism, suggesting that pheochromocytes release paracrine signals capable of activating glucocorticoid synthesis (81, 84). ACTH could be one of them although it is not excluded that catecholamines may exert a stimulatory action on cortisol production through illicit expression of adrenergic receptors in tumor adrenocortical cells (85, 86).

Alternatively, the occurrence of ectopic production of ACTH in the adrenal cortex has already been reported. Very rarely, ACTH-positive cells in the adrenocortical tissue can reveal adrenal micrometastases of an ACTH-secreting cancer. In the published cases, plasma ACTH levels were strongly elevated, as a result of ACTH secretion by the primary tumor (87–89). More surprisingly, a subpopulation of adrenocortical cells has been shown to produce detectable amounts of ACTH in various types of adrenal neoplasms. A first case of adrenocortical cortisol-secreting adenoma associated with production of ACTH by tumor cells, has been described in 2001 by Hiroi et al. (6). Illicit synthesis of ACTH was considered to result from abnormal pituitary differentiation of the tissue as witnessed by co-expression of 17-hydroxylase and pituitary homeobox factor-1 mRNAs by adrenocortical cells (6). At the ultrastructural level, tumor cells exhibited characteristics of both steroidogenic cells and neuroendocrine cells, and the tumor was, thus, referred to as an adrenocortical–pituitary hybrid adenoma. Bilateral macronodular adrenal hyperplasia (BMAH), a rare cause of primary adrenal hypercortisolism, has also been found to contain ACTH-producing cells. This observation was first reported by Pereira et al. who also noticed that ACTH-positive cells were labeled by antibodies to chromogranin A (CGA), suggesting that these cells may correspond to intracortical chromaffin cells (90). Subsequently, several teams reported expression of proopiomelanocortin (POMC) and ACTH in groups of adrenocortical cells in isolated BMAH cases (8, 10, 91) (**Figure 3**). In one case, it could be shown that ACTH-positive cells also expressed 17-hydroxylase but were negative for pituitary corticotroph markers (8). The role of ACTH in the pathogenesis of BMAH has been more extensively investigated in a large series of 30 cases (9). Adrenal hyperplasia samples expressed POMC mRNA at variable levels. Proconvertase 1, a protease implicated in the maturation of POMC into ACTH, was also visualized in clusters of adrenal cells, indicating that ACTH could be generated from POMC in the BMAH tissues. In agreement with this

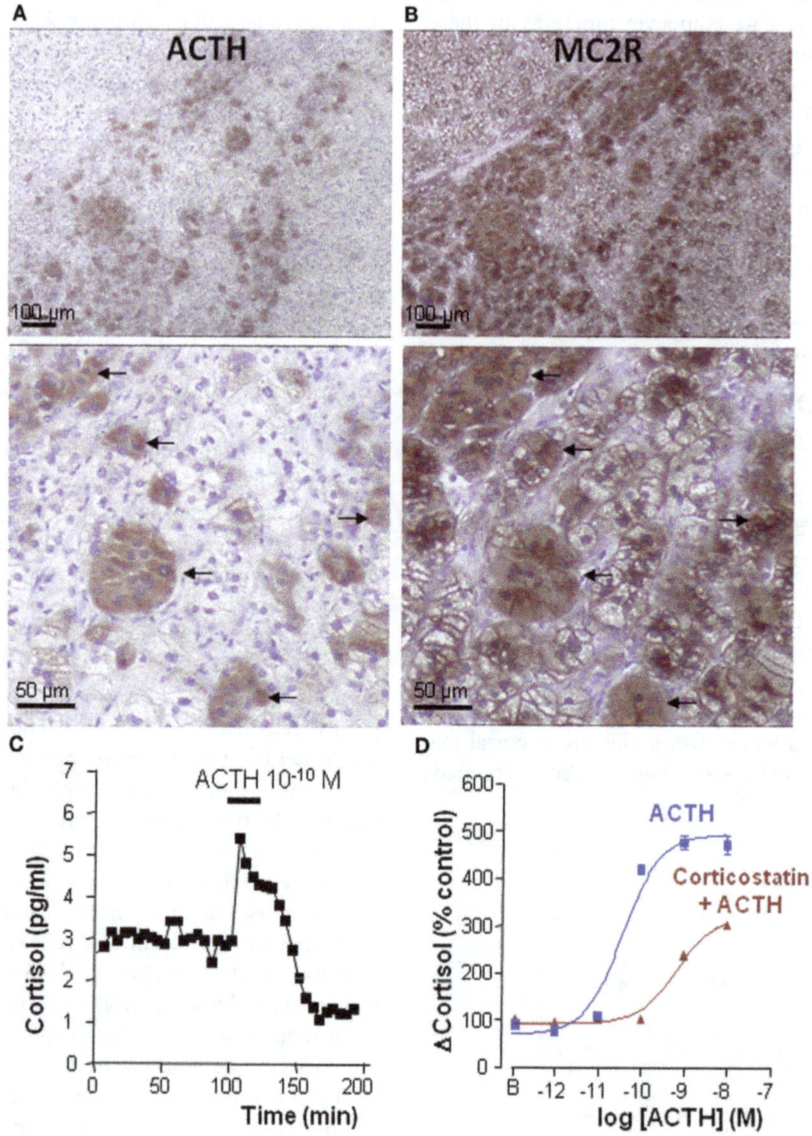

FIGURE 3 | Intraadrenal ACTH regulation of cortisol secretion in bilateral macronodular adrenal hyperplasia (BMAH). (A,B) Consecutive sections of a BMAH tissue labeled with ACTH and MC2R antibodies. **(A)** Heterogeneous distribution of ACTH-producing cell clusters in BMAH. **(B)** The ACTH receptor MC2R is highly expressed in ACTH-producing cells (arrows) and in their vicinity. **(C)** ACTH sensitivity of BMAH tissues. Application of exogenous ACTH stimulated cortisol secretion by perifused BMAH explants. **(D)** Corticostatin, a MC2R antagonist, inhibited *in vitro* the cortisol response of cultured BMAH cells to ACTH. Illustration of the data published in Ref. (9).

finding, ACTH immunoreactivity was detected, as previously noticed, in some adrenocortical cells either isolated or arranged in small groups disseminated in the tissues. The presence of corticotropin can also be seen in some chromaffin cells of the adrenal medulla. Surprisingly, adrenocortical ACTH-positive cells also displayed characteristics of steroidogenic cells, such as the presence of numerous lipid inclusions and several markers of steroidogenic differentiation, including steroidogenic factor 1 (SF1), 17-hydroxylase, and the HDL-cholesterol receptor scavenger receptor B1 (SRB1). It could be, thus, concluded that they constitute a subcategory of adrenocortical steroidogenic cells characterized by an unusual capacity to synthesize ACTH. BMAH specimens were found to express very low levels of T-pit [a transduction factor which controls pituitary corticotrophs differentiation (92)], confirming that ectopic synthesis of ACTH in adrenocortical cells does not result from illicit corticotropic-like differentiation of the latter (9) but may rather be considered as an additional feature of neuroendocrine differentiation of the hyperplastic tissues (47, 93, 94). Interestingly, ACTH-containing cells were also positive for gonadal markers like the gonadal marker insulin-like 3 (INSL3), exhibiting thus a pseudo-gonadal phenotype (8, 9, 95, 96). This observation is concordant with expression of POMC and synthesis of ACTH previously reported in testicular Leydig cells and ovarian granulosa cells (97, 98).

Because the adrenal glands and gonads both originate from a same tissue precursor, the adrenogonadal primordium, it is likely that the occurrence of these pseudo-gonadal cells in BMAH tissues may be the consequence of altered embryogenesis, explaining the bilaterality of the lesions.

Perifusion studies revealed that ACTH is released by BMAH tissues *in vitro* in a pulsatile mode (9), in agreement with older clinical studies showing a clear pulsatility of cortisol secretion in patients with BMAH (99). The ectopic secretion of ACTH by the hyperplastic adrenal glands has also been detected *in vivo* in two patients through adrenal vein catheterization (9). Taken collectively, these data suggested that, in BMAH tissues, intraadrenal ACTH may exert an autocrine/paracrine action to stimulate cortisol secretion, supplying therefore circulating ACTH that is suppressed by cortisol excess. This hypothesis was supported by statistical analyses showing positive correlations between ACTH and cortisol levels in BMAH culture medium. In addition, basal plasma cortisol concentrations measured *in vivo* were positively correlated with both the levels of POMC mRNA and the ACTH histological score in the tissues. Most importantly, MC2R antagonists, such as corticostatin and ACTH (7–38), were found to inhibit *in vitro* spontaneous and ACTH-evoked cortisol secretion by BMAH explants (9) (**Figure 3**). Clinical studies with MC2R antagonists are now mandatory to confirm that cortisol production is actually dependent on intraadrenal ACTH in patients with BMAH.

Bilateral macronodular adrenal hyperplasia tissues also constitute an interesting model for the study of the regulation of MC2R expression in the adrenal cortex. MC2R mRNA is globally underexpressed in BMAH samples versus normal adrenals (100). In fact, we could observe that, at variance with the normal adrenal cortex that is diffusely labeled by anti-MC2R antibodies, BMAH explants exhibit heterogeneous distribution of the receptor that appears highly expressed in the vicinity of clusters of ACTH-producing cells and more weakly at distance (**Figure 3**). Indeed, as previously established in the normal adrenal gland (101–103), MC2R seems to be upregulated by ACTH in BMAH tissues. In fact, MC2R mRNA levels were positively correlated with POMC mRNA rates and MC2R-like immunoreactivity was principally visualized in the vicinity of ACTH-positive cells (9). Interestingly, ACTH-producing cells were also found to express the receptor, suggesting that intraadrenal ACTH possibly exerts autocrine actions in BMAH.

All these data indicate that intraadrenal ACTH plays a pivotal role in the pathogenesis of hypercortisolism associated with BMAH. Deciphering the mode of regulation of ACTH production by BMAHs is, thus, essential for the comprehension of the pathophysiology of the disease. At variance with pituitary ACTH, intraadrenal ACTH does not seem to be regulated by cortisol, as suggested by the lack of action of dexamethasone and the glucocorticoid receptor antagonist RU486 on ACTH release by BMAH explants (9). Conversely, we noticed that ligands of various membrane receptors that are known to be abnormally expressed by BMAH cells, i.e., 5-HT, LH/hCG, and glucose-dependent insulinotropic peptide (GIP), are able to activate ACTH production from BMAH tissues *in vitro* (9). This surprising finding indicated that activation of illicit membrane receptors may stimulate cortisol production *via* two mechanisms, including a direct effect on corticosteroidogenesis, as previously shown in BMAH cell culture (93, 104), and an indirect action mediated by ACTH secretion (9). Consistently, MC2R antagonists were found to partially inhibit *in vitro* the cortisol response evoked by GIP in perifused BMAH samples. Taken together, these results suggest that intraadrenal ACTH may be regarded as a common intermediate and amplifier of the action of several illicit membrane receptors in BMAH tissues. Targeting the MC2R with specific antagonists may, thus, represent an efficient strategy for the treatment of BMAH-associated hypercortisolism. The pathophysiology links between intraadrenal ACTH and abnormally expressed receptors may be more complex and could form a complete auto-amplification loop in the hyperplastic tissues. In fact, although the presence of the LH and GIP receptors in adrenocortical cells may be simply considered as features of pseudo-gonadal differentiation of BMAH tissues, overexpression of some membrane receptors, such as 5-HT receptors, may result from local production from ACTH. This hypothesis is supported by intriguing observations recently performed in another type of adrenal hyperplasia associated with hypercortisolism, namely primary pigmented adrenocortical disease (PPNAD). The disease is caused in most patients by germline inactivating mutations that affect the *PRKAR1A* gene (105), resulting in constitutive activation of protein kinase A (PKA) in adrenocortical cells (106). Since MC2R are positively coupled to the cAMP/PKA pathway, it can be considered that *PRKAR1A* mutations partly mimic the action of ACTH on adrenal steroidogenic cells. Interestingly, PPNAD have been found to overexpress several types of 5-HT receptors, including the

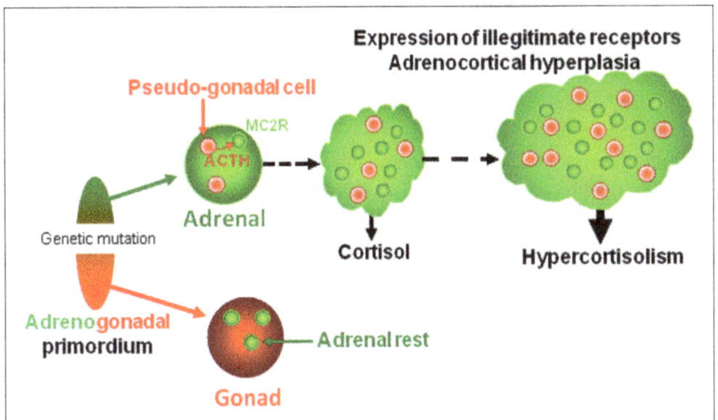

FIGURE 4 | Putative pathophysiological mechanism responsible for bilateral macronodular adrenal hyperplasia. Both gonads and adrenals originate from the adrenogonadal primordium. It can be speculated that the causative genetic mutations may alter differentiation and/or separation of the adrenogonadal primordium leading to the presence of pseudo-gonadal cells in the adrenals. Secretion of ACTH by intraadrenal pseudo-gonadal cells may progressively stimulate, *via* activation of MC2R, both cortisol secretion and growth of the adrenocortical tissue, leading to bilateral adrenal hyperplasia associated with hypercortisolism. In parallel, sustained activation of the PKA pathway consecutive to activation of MC2R by intraadrenal ACTH may activate expression of some illegitimate receptors. Activation of steroidogenesis by ligands of illegitimate receptors further reinforces cortisol hypersecretion through both an intrinsic stimulatory action and an indirect effect *via* local release of ACTH.

5-HT_4 receptor (107). It seems, thus, conceivable that abnormal expression of 5-HT receptors in BMAH tissues may result from exposure of adrenocortical cells to locally produced ACTH whose release is subsequently increased by the 5-HT signaling pathway.

There is now no doubt that BMAH is a genetically determined condition, *ARMC5* being a major susceptibility gene of the disease (108). It is now well established that the development of macronodular adrenal hyperplasia requires inactivation of the two *ARMC5* alleles, respectively, by the first germline mutation and a secondary somatic genetic event. Surprisingly, inactivation of *ARMC5* expression in the human adrenocortical cell line H295R, which reproduces the molecular defects observed in adrenocortical cells of patients with BMAH, results in a decrease in expression of steroidogenic enzymes (108, 109). It seems, thus, that a second line event is necessary for the emergence of hypercortisolism. We hypothesize that *ARMC5* mutations may alter differentiation and/or separation of the adrenogonadal primordium leading to the presence of pseudo-gonadal cells in the adrenal areas. Progressive expression of POMC and ACTH by these cells may then result in cortisol hypersecretion. Because illicit expression of ACTH has also been observed in non-ARMC5-mutated adrenal hyperplasias, it seems that abnormal differentiation of adrenocortical cells is a frequent histological feature in BMAH tissues whatever the causative firstline genetic defect (**Figure 4**).

CONCLUSION

In addition to its well-known action on adrenocortical cells to promote steroidogenesis through activation of the MC2R, ACTH exerts multiple effects through the paracrine communication processes that occur in the adrenal gland in both physiological and pathophysiological conditions. ACTH can also be abnormally produced in adrenal neoplasms in which the hormone acts, thus, as an autocrine/paracrine factor to activate steroid secretion. This new pathophysiological concept opens novel avenues for the development of original pharmacological treatments of primary adrenal syndromes of steroid excess.

AUTHOR CONTRIBUTIONS

HL, MT, and EL: wrote the paper. CD, EL: acquisition, analysis, and interpretation of data. EL: designed the figures. JB: revised the paper and gave intellectual contribution.

ACKNOWLEDGMENTS

This work was supported by Institut National de la Santé et de la Recherche Médicale Unité 982, the Centre Hospitalier Universitaire de Rouen, the Assistance Publique-Hôpitaux de Paris and the Conseil Régional de Normandie, the Société Française d'Endocrinologie (SFE).

REFERENCES

1. Bornstein SR, Rutkowski H, Vrezas I. Cytokines and steroidogenesis. *Mol Cell Endocrinol* (2004) 215:135–41. doi:10.1016/j.mce.2003.11.022
2. Ehrhart-Bornstein M, Hinson JP, Bornstein SR, Scherbaum WA, Vinson GP. Intraadrenal interactions in the regulation of adrenocortical steroidogenesis. *Endocr Rev* (1998) 19:101–43. doi:10.1210/edrv.19.2.0326
3. Haase M, Willenberg HS, Bornstein SR. Update on the corticomedullary interaction in the adrenal gland. *Endocr Dev* (2011) 20:28–37. doi:10.1159/000321211
4. Nussdorfer GG. Paracrine control of adrenal cortical function by medullary chromaffin cells. *Pharmacol Rev* (1996) 48:495–530.
5. Nussdorfer GG, Mazzocchi G. Immune-endocrine interactions in the mammalian adrenal gland: facts and hypotheses. *Int Rev Cytol* (1998) 183:143–84. doi:10.1016/S0074-7696(08)60144-8
6. Hiroi N, Chrousos GP, Kohn B, Lafferty A, Abu-Asab M, Bonat S, et al. Adrenocortical-pituitary hybrid tumor causing Cushing's syndrome. *J Clin Endocrinol Metab* (2001) 86:2631–7. doi:10.1210/jcem.86.6.7590
7. Iwata M, Oki Y, Okazawa T, Ishizawa S, Taka C, Yamazaki K, et al. A rare case of adrenocorticotropic hormone (ACTH)-independent macroadrenal hyperplasia showing ectopic production of ACTH. *Intern Med* (2012) 51:2181–7. doi:10.2169/internalmedicine.51.7547
8. Lefebvre H, Duparc C, Chartrel N, Jegou S, Pellerin A, Laquerriere A, et al. Intraadrenal adrenocorticotropin production in a case of bilateral macronodular adrenal hyperplasia causing Cushing's syndrome. *J Clin Endocrinol Metab* (2003) 88:3035–42. doi:10.1210/jc.2002-030014
9. Louiset E, Duparc C, Young J, Renouf S, Tetsi Nomigni M, Boutelet I, et al. Intraadrenal corticotropin in bilateral macronodular adrenal hyperplasia. *N Engl J Med* (2013) 369:2115–25. doi:10.1056/NEJMoa1215245
10. Mazzuco TL, Thomas M, Martinie M, Cherradi N, Sturm N, Feige J-J, et al. Cellular and molecular abnormalities of a macronodular adrenal hyperplasia causing beta-blocker-sensitive Cushing's syndrome. *Arq Bras Endocrinol Metabol* (2007) 51:1452–62. doi:10.1590/S0004-27302007000900007
11. Vrezas I, Willenberg HS, Mansmann G, Hiroi N, Fritzen R, Bornstein SR. Ectopic adrenocorticotropin (ACTH) and corticotropin-releasing hormone (CRH) production in the adrenal gland: basic and clinical aspects. *Microsc Res Tech* (2003) 61:308–14. doi:10.1002/jemt.10340
12. Kikuta A, Murakami T. Microcirculation of the rat adrenal gland: a scanning electron microscope study of vascular casts. *Am J Anat* (1982) 164:19–28. doi:10.1002/aja.1001640103
13. Sasano H, Ohashi Y, Suzuki T, Nagura H. Vascularity in human adrenal cortex. *Mod Pathol* (1998) 11:329–33.
14. Hinson JP, Kapas S. The role of endothelial cell products in the regulation of adrenocortical function: actions of endothelin, nitric oxide, adrenomedullin and PAMP. *Horm Metab Res* (1998) 30:334–40. doi:10.1055/s-2007-978894
15. Rossi G, Albertin G, Belloni A, Zanin L, Biasolo MA, Prayer-Galetti T, et al. Gene expression, localization, and characterization of endothelin A and B receptors in the human adrenal cortex. *J Clin Invest* (1994) 94:1226–34. doi:10.1172/JCI117440
16. Rossi GP, Andreis PG, Colonna S, Albertin G, Aragona F, Belloni AS, et al. Endothelin-1[1-31]: a novel autocrine-paracrine regulator of human adrenal cortex secretion and growth. *J Clin Endocrinol Metab* (2002) 87:322–8. doi:10.1210/jcem.87.1.8134
17. Hinson JP, Vinson GP, Kapas S, Teja R. The relationship between adrenal vascular events and steroid secretion: the role of mast cells and endothelin. *J Steroid Biochem Mol Biol* (1991) 40:381–9. doi:10.1016/0960-0760(91)90205-J
18. Ansurudeen I, Kopprasch S, Ehrhart-Bornstein M, Bornstein SR, Willenberg HS. Endothelial cell-mediated regulation of aldosterone release from human adrenocortical cells. *Mol Cell Endocrinol* (2007) 26(5–266):150–6. doi:10.1016/j.mce.2006.12.011
19. Ansurudeen I, Kopf PG, Gauthier KM, Bornstein SR, Cowley AW, Campbell WB. Aldosterone secretagogues increase adrenal blood flow in male rats. *Endocrinology* (2014) 155:127–32. doi:10.1210/en.2013-1532
20. Adams JC, Lawler J. The thrombospondins. *Cold Spring Harb Perspect Biol* (2011) 3:a009712. doi:10.1101/cshperspect.a009712
21. Stenina-Adognravi O. Thrombospondins: old players, new games. *Curr Opin Lipidol* (2013) 24:401–9. doi:10.1097/MOL.0b013e3283642912
22. Danik M, Chinn AM, Lafeuillade B, Keramidas M, Aguesse-Germon S, Penhoat A, et al. Bovine thrombospondin-2: complete complementary deoxyribonucleic acid sequence and immunolocalization in the external

zones of the adrenal cortex. *Endocrinology* (1999) 140:2771–80. doi:10.1210/endo.140.6.6835

23. Pihlajoki M, Dörner J, Cochran RS, Heikinheimo M, Wilson DB. Adrenocortical zonation, renewal, and remodeling. *Front Endocrinol* (2015) 6:27. doi:10.3389/fendo.2015.00027
24. Kyriakides TR, Zhu YH, Yang Z, Bornstein P. The distribution of the matricellular protein thrombospondin 2 in tissues of embryonic and adult mice. *J Histochem Cytochem* (1998) 46:1007–15. doi:10.1177/002215549804600904
25. Thomas M, Keramidas M, Monchaux E, Feige J-J. Role of adrenocorticotropic hormone in the development and maintenance of the adrenal cortical vasculature. *Microsc Res Tech* (2003) 61:247–51. doi:10.1002/jemt.10333
26. Gaillard I, Keramidas M, Liakos P, Vilgrain I, Feige JJ, Vittet D. ACTH-regulated expression of vascular endothelial growth factor in the adult bovine adrenal cortex: a possible role in the maintenance of the microvasculature. *J Cell Physiol* (2000) 185:226–34. doi:10.1002/1097-4652(200011)185:2<226::AID-JCP7>3.0.CO;2-E
27. Heikkilä P, Arola J, Voutilainen R, Salmenkivi K, Kahri AI, Liu J. Expression of vascular endothelial growth factor in human adrenals. *Endocr Res* (2000) 26:867–71. doi:10.3109/07435800009048610
28. Cherradi N, Lejczak C, Desroches-Castan A, Feige J-J. Antagonistic functions of tetradecanoyl phorbol acetate-inducible-sequence 11b and HuR in the hormonal regulation of vascular endothelial growth factor messenger ribonucleic acid stability by adrenocorticotropin. *Mol Endocrinol* (2006) 20:916–30. doi:10.1210/me.2005-0121
29. Thomas M, Keramidas M, Monchaux E, Feige J-J. Dual hormonal regulation of endocrine tissue mass and vasculature by adrenocorticotropin in the adrenal cortex. *Endocrinology* (2004) 145:4320–9. doi:10.1210/en.2004-0179
30. Shifren JL, Mesiano S, Taylor RN, Ferrara N, Jaffe RB. Corticotropin regulates vascular endothelial growth factor expression in human fetal adrenal cortical cells. *J Clin Endocrinol Metab* (1998) 83:1342–7. doi:10.1210/jcem.83.4.4730
31. Albertin G, Rucinski M, Carraro G, Forneris M, Andreis P, Malendowicz LK, et al. Adrenomedullin and vascular endothelium growth factor genes are overexpressed in the regenerating rat adrenal cortex, and AM and VEGF reciprocally enhance their mRNA expression in cultured rat adrenocortical cells. *Int J Mol Med* (2005) 16:431–5. doi:10.3892/ijmm.16.3.431
32. Taniguchi A, Tajima T, Nonomura K, Shinohara N, Mikami A, Koyanagi T. Expression of vascular endothelial growth factor and its receptors Flk-1 and Flt-1 during the regeneration of autotransplanted adrenal cortex in the adrenalectomized rat. *J Urol* (2004) 171:2445–9. doi:10.1097/01.ju.0000127755.87490.37
33. Apkarian RP, Curtis JC. Hormonal regulation of capillary fenestrae in the rat adrenal cortex: quantitative studies using objective lens staging scanning electron microscopy. *Scan Electron Microsc* (1986) Pt 4:1381–93.
34. Zhang DX, Gauthier KM, Falck JR, Siddam A, Campbell WB. Steroid-producing cells regulate arterial tone of adrenal cortical arteries. *Endocrinology* (2007) 148:3569–76. doi:10.1210/en.2007-0169
35. Hinson JP, Vinson GP, Pudney J, Whitehouse BJ. Adrenal mast cells modulate vascular and secretory responses in the intact adrenal gland of the rat. *J Endocrinol* (1989) 121:253–60. doi:10.1677/joe.0.1210253
36. Lefebvre H, Contesse V, Delarue C, Feuilloley M, Hery F, Grise P, et al. Serotonin-induced stimulation of cortisol secretion from human adrenocortical tissue is mediated through activation of a serotonin4 receptor subtype. *Neuroscience* (1992) 47:999–1007. doi:10.1016/0306-4522(92)90047-6
37. Aiba M, Iri H, Suzuki H, Kageyama K, Kawai T, Abe O, et al. Numerous mast cells in an 11-deoxycorticosterone-producing adrenocortical tumor. Histologic evaluation of benignancy and comparison with mast cell distribution in adrenal glands and neoplastic counterparts of 67 surgical specimens. *Arch Pathol Lab Med* (1985) 109:357–60.
38. Duparc C, Moreau L, Dzib JFG, Boyer H-G, Tetsi Nomigni M, Boutelet I, et al. Mast cell hyperplasia is associated with aldosterone hypersecretion in a subset of aldosterone-producing adenomas. *J Clin Endocrinol Metab* (2015) 100:E550–60. doi:10.1210/jc.2014-3660
39. Louiset E, Isvi K, Gasc JM, Duparc C, Cauliez B, Laquerrière A, et al. Ectopic expression of serotonin7 receptors in an adrenocortical carcinoma co-secreting renin and cortisol. *Endocr Relat Cancer* (2008) 15:1025–34. doi:10.1677/ERC-08-0085
40. Peters J. Local renin-angiotensin systems in the adrenal gland. *Peptides* (2012) 34:427–32. doi:10.1016/j.peptides.2012.01.023
41. Baba K, Doi Y, Franco-Saenz R, Mulrow PJ. Mechanisms by which nephrectomy stimulates adrenal renin. *Hypertension* (1986) 8:997–1002. doi:10.1161/01.HYP.8.11.997
42. Doi Y, Atarashi K, Franco-Saenz R, Mulrow PJ. Effect of changes in sodium or potassium balance, and nephrectomy, on adrenal renin and aldosterone concentrations. *Hypertension* (1984) 6:I124–9. doi:10.1161/01.HYP.6.2_Pt_2.I124
43. Cui J, Dou J, Yang G, Zang L, Jin N, Chen K, et al. The changes in renin-angiotensin-aldosterone-system in different subtypes of Cushing's syndrome. *Zhonghua Nei Ke Za Zhi* (2015) 54:618–22. doi:10.3760/cma.j.issn.0578-1426.2015.07.010
44. Luton JP, Vidal-Trecan G, Mouveroux F, Bricaire H. Hypertension and Cushing's disease. *Ann Med Interne* (1983) 134:203–8.
45. Barney M, Call GB, McIlmoil CJ, Husein OF, Adams A, Balls AG, et al. Stimulation by interleukin-6 and inhibition by tumor necrosis factor of cortisol release from bovine adrenal zona fasciculata cells through their receptors. *Endocrine* (2000) 13:369–77. doi:10.1385/ENDO:13:3:369
46. Judd AM, MacLeod RM. Differential release of tumor necrosis factor and IL-6 from adrenal zona glomerulosa cells in vitro. *Am J Physiol* (1995) 268:E114–20.
47. Lefebvre H, Prévost G, Louiset E. Autocrine/paracrine regulatory mechanisms in adrenocortical neoplasms responsible for primary adrenal hypercorticism. *Eur J Endocrinol* (2013) 169:R115–38. doi:10.1530/EJE-13-0308
48. Caroccia B, Fassina A, Seccia TM, Recarti C, Petrelli L, Belloni AS, et al. Isolation of human adrenocortical aldosterone-producing cells by a novel immunomagnetic beads method. *Endocrinology* (2010) 151:1375–80. doi:10.1210/en.2009-1243
49. Li Q, Johansson H, Kjellman M, Grimelius L. Neuroendocrine differentiation and nerves in human adrenal cortex and cortical lesions. *APMIS* (1998) 106:807–17. doi:10.1111/j.1699-0463.1998.tb00227.x
50. Cartier D, Jégou S, Parmentier F, Lihrmann I, Louiset E, Kuhn J-M, et al. Expression profile of serotonin4 (5-HT4) receptors in adrenocortical aldosterone-producing adenomas. *Eur J Endocrinol* (2005) 153:939–47. doi:10.1530/eje.1.02051
51. Ye P, Mariniello B, Mantero F, Shibata H, Rainey WE. G-protein-coupled receptors in aldosterone-producing adenomas: a potential cause of hyperaldosteronism. *J Endocrinol* (2007) 195:39–48. doi:10.1677/JOE-07-0037
52. Murakami M, Yoshimoto T, Nakabayashi K, Tsuchiya K, Minami I, Bouchi R, et al. Integration of transcriptome and methylome analysis of aldosterone-producing adenomas. *Eur J Endocrinol* (2015) 173:185–95. doi:10.1530/EJE-15-0148
53. Zwermann O, Suttmann Y, Bidlingmaier M, Beuschlein F, Reincke M. Screening for membrane hormone receptor expression in primary aldosteronism. *Eur J Endocrinol* (2009) 160:443–51. doi:10.1530/EJE-08-0711
54. Arola J, Liu J, Heikkilä P, Voutilainen R, Kahri A. Expression of inhibin alpha in the human adrenal gland and adrenocortical tumors. *Endocr Res* (1998) 24:865–7. doi:10.3109/07435809809032699
55. Vänttinen T, Kuulasmaa T, Liu J, Voutilainen R. Expression of activin/inhibin receptor and binding protein genes and regulation of activin/inhibin peptide secretion in human adrenocortical cells. *J Clin Endocrinol Metab* (2002) 87:4257–63. doi:10.1210/jc.2002-020460
56. Vänttinen T, Liu J, Kuulasmaa T, Kivinen P, Voutilainen R. Expression of activin/inhibin signaling components in the human adrenal gland and the effects of activins and inhibins on adrenocortical steroidogenesis and apoptosis. *J Endocrinol* (2003) 178:479–89. doi:10.1677/joe.0.1780479
57. Ehrhart-Bornstein M, Lamounier-Zepter V, Schraven A, Langenbach J, Willenberg HS, Barthel A, et al. Human adipocytes secrete mineralocorticoid-releasing factors. *Proc Natl Acad Sci U S A* (2003) 100:14211–6. doi:10.1073/pnas.2336140100
58. Krug AW, Vleugels K, Schinner S, Lamounier-Zepter V, Ziegler CG, Bornstein SR, et al. Human adipocytes induce an ERK1/2 MAP kinases-mediated upregulation of steroidogenic acute regulatory protein (StAR) and an angiotensin II-sensitization in human adrenocortical cells. *Int J Obes (Lond)* (2007) 31:1605–16. doi:10.1038/sj.ijo.0803642
59. Schinner S, Willenberg HS, Krause D, Schott M, Lamounier-Zepter V, Krug AW, et al. Adipocyte-derived products induce the transcription of the StAR promoter and stimulate aldosterone and cortisol secretion from

adrenocortical cells through the Wnt-signaling pathway. *Int J Obes (Lond)* (2007) 31:864–70. doi:10.1038/sj.ijo.0803508
60. Glasow A, Bornstein SR. Leptin and the adrenal gland. *Eur J Clin Invest* (2000) 30(Suppl 3):39–45. doi:10.1046/j.1365-2362.2000.0300s3039.x
61. Glasow A, Haidan A, Hilbers U, Breidert M, Gillespie J, Scherbaum WA, et al. Expression of Ob receptor in normal human adrenals: differential regulation of adrenocortical and adrenomedullary function by leptin. *J Clin Endocrinol Metab* (1998) 83:4459–66. doi:10.1210/jcem.83.12.5337
62. Pralong FP, Roduit R, Waeber G, Castillo E, Mosimann F, Thorens B, et al. Leptin inhibits directly glucocorticoid secretion by normal human and rat adrenal gland. *Endocrinology* (1998) 139:4264–8. doi:10.1210/endo.139.10.6254
63. Szücs N, Varga I, Jakab C, Patócs A, Gláz E, Tóth M, et al. Leptin inhibits cortisol and corticosterone secretion in pathologic human adrenocortical cells. *Pituitary* (2001) 4:71–7. doi:10.1023/A:1012990928218
64. Iwen KAH, Senyaman O, Schwartz A, Drenckhan M, Meier B, Hadaschik D, et al. Melanocortin crosstalk with adipose functions: ACTH directly induces insulin resistance, promotes a pro-inflammatory adipokine profile and stimulates UCP-1 in adipocytes. *J Endocrinol* (2008) 196:465–72. doi:10.1677/JOE-07-0299
65. Jun D-J, Na K-Y, Kim W, Kwak D, Kwon E-J, Yoon JH, et al. Melanocortins induce interleukin 6 gene expression and secretion through melanocortin receptors 2 and 5 in 3T3-L1 adipocytes. *J Mol Endocrinol* (2010) 44:225–36. doi:10.1677/JME-09-0161
66. Kim NS, Kim Y-J, Cho SY, Lee TR, Kim SH. Transcriptional activation of melanocortin 2 receptor accessory protein by PPARγ in adipocytes. *Biochem Biophys Res Commun* (2013) 439:401–6. doi:10.1016/j.bbrc.2013.08.061
67. German-Mena E, Zibari GB, Levine SN. Adrenal myelolipomas in patients with congenital adrenal hyperplasia: review of the literature and a case report. *Endocr Pract* (2011) 17:441–7. doi:10.4158/EP10340.RA
68. Nermoen I, Rørvik J, Holmedal SH, Hykkerud DL, Fougner KJ, Svartberg J, et al. High frequency of adrenal myelolipomas and testicular adrenal rest tumours in adult Norwegian patients with classical congenital adrenal hyperplasia because of 21-hydroxylase deficiency. *Clin Endocrinol (Oxf)* (2011) 75:753–9. doi:10.1111/j.1365-2265.2011.04151.x
69. Almeida MQ, Kaupert LC, Brito LP, Lerario AM, Mariani BMP, Ribeiro M, et al. Increased expression of ACTH (MC2R) and androgen (AR) receptors in giant bilateral myelolipomas from patients with congenital adrenal hyperplasia. *BMC Endocr Disord* (2014) 14:42. doi:10.1186/1472-6823-14-42
70. Kiwaki K, Levine JA. Differential effects of adrenocorticotropic hormone on human and mouse adipose tissue. *J Comp Physiol B* (2003) 173:675–8. doi:10.1007/s00360-003-0377-1
71. Ehrhart-Bornstein M, Haidan A, Alesci S, Bornstein SR. Neurotransmitters and neuropeptides in the differential regulation of steroidogenesis in adrenocortical-chromaffin co-cultures. *Endocr Res* (2000) 26:833–42. doi:10.3109/07435800009048606
72. Suda T, Tomori N, Tozawa F, Demura H, Shizume K, Mouri T, et al. Immunoreactive corticotropin and corticotropin-releasing factor in human hypothalamus, adrenal, lung cancer, and pheochromocytoma. *J Clin Endocrinol Metab* (1984) 58:919–24. doi:10.1210/jcem-58-5-919
73. Ballav C, Naziat A, Mihai R, Karavitaki N, Ansorge O, Grossman AB. Mini-review: pheochromocytomas causing the ectopic ACTH syndrome. *Endocrine* (2012) 42:69–73. doi:10.1007/s12020-012-9646-7
74. Cohade C, Broussaud S, Louiset E, Bennet A, Huyghe E, Caron P. Ectopic Cushing's syndrome due to a pheochromocytoma: a new case in the post-partum and review of literature. *Gynecol Endocrinol* (2009) 25:624–7. doi:10.1080/09513590903015411
75. Oh HC, Koh J-M, Kim MS, Park JY, Shong YK, Lee K-U, et al. A case of ACTH-producing pheochromocytoma associated with pregnancy. *Endocr J* (2003) 50:739–44. doi:10.1507/endocrj.50.739
76. Newell-Price J, Bertagna X, Grossman AB, Nieman LK. Cushing's syndrome. *Lancet* (2006) 367:1605–17. doi:10.1016/S0140-6736(06)68699-6
77. Erem C, Hacihasanoglu A, Ersöz HO, Reis AK, Calik A, Ukinç K, et al. Pheochromocytoma combined with pre-clinical Cushing's syndrome in the same adrenal gland. *J Endocrinol Invest* (2005) 28:561–5. doi:10.1007/BF03347247
78. Inoue J, Oishi S, Naomi S, Umeda T, Sato T. Pheochromocytoma associated with adrenocortical adenoma: case report and literature review. *Endocrinol Jpn* (1986) 33:67–74. doi:10.1507/endocrj1954.33.67
79. Takizawa N, Muguruma K, Sasano H. Pheochromocytoma and subclinical Cushing's syndrome with focal adrenocortical hyperplasia. *Int J Urol* (2011) 18:548–9. doi:10.1111/j.1442-2042.2011.02759.x
80. Yoshioka M, Saito H, Kawakami Y, Mineyama H, Sekiya M. Adrenomedullary hyperplasia associated with cortisol producing adenoma. *Endocr J* (1993) 40:467–71. doi:10.1507/endocrj.40.467
81. Alexandraki KI, Michail OP, Nonni A, Diamantis D, Giannopoulou I, Kaltsas GA, et al. Corticomedullary mixed adrenal tumor: case report and literature review. *Endocr J* (2009) 56:817–24. doi:10.1507/endocrj.K09E-010
82. Kaneko T, Matsushima H, Homma Y. Dopamine-secreting corticomedullary mixed tumor of the adrenal gland. *Int J Urol* (2012) 19(12):1123–4. doi:10.1111/j.1442-2042.2012.03107.x
83. Lau SK, Chu PG, Weiss LM. Mixed cortical adenoma and composite pheochromocytoma-ganglioneuroma: an unusual corticomedullary tumor of the adrenal gland. *Ann Diagn Pathol* (2011) 15:185–9. doi:10.1016/j.anndiagpath.2010.02.005
84. Wieneke JA, Thompson LD, Heffess CS. Corticomedullary mixed tumor of the adrenal gland. *Ann Diagn Pathol* (2001) 5:304–8. doi:10.1053/adpa.2001.28297
85. Hirata Y, Uchihashi M, Sueoka S, Matsukura S, Fujita T. Presence of ectopic beta-adrenergic receptors on human adrenocortical cortisol-producing adenomas. *J Clin Endocrinol Metab* (1981) 53:953–7. doi:10.1210/jcem-53-5-953
86. Lacroix A, Tremblay J, Rousseau G, Bouvier M, Hamet P. Propranolol therapy for ectopic beta-adrenergic receptors in adrenal Cushing's syndrome. *N Engl J Med* (1997) 337:1429–34. doi:10.1056/NEJM199711133372004
87. Guha P, Sahai SS, Sarkar D, Sardar P, Mandal B, Das BK, et al. Gastric adenocarcinoma associated with lymphangitis carcinomatosa, adrenal metastasis with ectopic ACTH syndrome and malignant common bile duct stricture. *Arab J Gastroenterol* (2012) 13:31–4. doi:10.1016/j.ajg.2011.07.010
88. Sand M, Uecker S, Bechara FG, Gelos M, Sand D, Wiese TH, et al. Simultaneous ectopic adrenocorticotropic hormone syndrome and adrenal metastasis of a medullary thyroid carcinoma causing paraneoplastic Cushing's syndrome. *Int Semin Surg Oncol* (2007) 4:15. doi:10.1186/1477-7800-4-15
89. Satoh H, Saito R, Hisata S, Shiihara J, Taniuchi S, Nakamura Y, et al. An ectopic ACTH-producing small cell lung carcinoma associated with enhanced corticosteroid biosynthesis in the peritumoral areas of adrenal metastasis. *Lung Cancer* (2012) 76:486–90. doi:10.1016/j.lungcan.2011.12.007
90. Pereira MAA, Araújo RS, Bisi H. Síndrome de Cushing Associada à Hiperplasia Macronodular das Adrenais. Apresentação de um Caso e Revisão da Literatura. *Arq Bras Endocrinol Metab* (2001) 45:619–27. doi:10.1590/S0004-27302001000600015
91. Mijnhout GS, Danner SA, van de Goot FRW, van Dam EWCM. Macronodular adrenocortical hyperplasia in a postmenopausal woman. *Neth J Med* (2004) 62:454–5.
92. Pulichino A-M, Vallette-Kasic S, Tsai JP-Y, Couture C, Gauthier Y, Drouin J. Tpit determines alternate fates during pituitary cell differentiation. *Genes Dev* (2003) 17:738–47. doi:10.1101/gad.1065703
93. Bertherat J, Contesse V, Louiset E, Barrande G, Duparc C, Groussin L, et al. In vivo and in vitro screening for illegitimate receptors in adrenocorticotropin-independent macronodular adrenal hyperplasia causing Cushing's syndrome: identification of two cases of gonadotropin/gastric inhibitory polypeptide-dependent hypercortisolism. *J Clin Endocrinol Metab* (2005) 90:1302–10. doi:10.1210/jc.2004-1256
94. Louiset E, Contesse V, Groussin L, Cartier D, Duparc C, Barrande G, et al. Expression of serotonin7 receptor and coupling of ectopic receptors to protein kinase A and ionic currents in adrenocorticotropin-independent macronodular adrenal hyperplasia causing Cushing's syndrome. *J Clin Endocrinol Metab* (2006) 91:4578–86. doi:10.1210/jc.2006-0538
95. Ivell R, Heng K, Anand-Ivell R. Insulin-like factor 3 and the HPG axis in the male. *Front Endocrinol* (2014) 5:6. doi:10.3389/fendo.2014.00006
96. Pelusi C, Fanelli F, Pariali M, Zanotti L, Gambineri A, Pasquali R. Parallel variations of insulin-like peptide 3 (INSL3) and antimüllerian hormone (AMH) in women with the polycystic ovary syndrome according to menstrual cycle pattern. *J Clin Endocrinol Metab* (2013) 98:E1575–82. doi:10.1210/jc.2013-1107

97. de Keyzer Y, Lenne F, Massias JF, Vieau D, Luton JP, Kahn A, et al. Pituitary-like proopiomelanocortin transcripts in human Leydig cell tumors. *J Clin Invest* (1990) 86:871–7. doi:10.1172/JCI114787
98. Lacaze-Masmonteil T, de Keyzer Y, Luton JP, Kahn A, Bertagna X. Characterization of proopiomelanocortin transcripts in human nonpituitary tissues. *Proc Natl Acad Sci U S A* (1987) 84:7261–5. doi:10.1073/pnas.84.20.7261
99. van Aken MO, Pereira AM, van Thiel SW, van den Berg G, Frölich M, Veldhuis JD, et al. Irregular and frequent cortisol secretory episodes with preserved diurnal rhythmicity in primary adrenal Cushing's syndrome. *J Clin Endocrinol Metab* (2005) 90:1570–7. doi:10.1210/jc.2004-1281
100. Assie G, Louiset E, Sturm N, René-Corail F, Groussin L, Bertherat J, et al. Systematic analysis of G protein-coupled receptor gene expression in adrenocorticotropin-independent macronodular adrenocortical hyperplasia identifies novel targets for pharmacological control of adrenal Cushing's syndrome. *J Clin Endocrinol Metab* (2010) 95:E253–62. doi:10.1210/jc.2009-2281
101. Lebrethon MC, Naville D, Begeot M, Saez JM. Regulation of corticotropin receptor number and messenger RNA in cultured human adrenocortical cells by corticotropin and angiotensin II. *J Clin Invest* (1994) 93:1828–33. doi:10.1172/JCI117168
102. Mountjoy KG, Bird IM, Rainey WE, Cone RD. ACTH induces up-regulation of ACTH receptor mRNA in mouse and human adrenocortical cell lines. *Mol Cell Endocrinol* (1994) 99:R17–20. doi:10.1016/0303-7207(94)90160-0
103. Xing Y, Parker CR, Edwards M, Rainey WE. ACTH is a potent regulator of gene expression in human adrenal cells. *J Mol Endocrinol* (2010) 45:59–68. doi:10.1677/JME-10-0006
104. Lacroix A, Bourdeau I, Lampron A, Mazzuco TL, Tremblay J, Hamet P. Aberrant G-protein coupled receptor expression in relation to adrenocortical overfunction. *Clin Endocrinol (Oxf)* (2010) 73:1–15. doi:10.1111/j.1365-2265.2009.03689.x
105. Stratakis CA, Boikos SA. Genetics of adrenal tumors associated with Cushing's syndrome: a new classification for bilateral adrenocortical hyperplasias. *Nat Clin Pract Endocrinol Metab* (2007) 3:748–57. doi:10.1038/ncpendmet0648
106. Groussin L, Kirschner LS, Vincent-Dejean C, Perlemoine K, Jullian E, Delemer B, et al. Molecular analysis of the cyclic AMP-dependent protein kinase A (PKA) regulatory subunit 1A (PRKAR1A) gene in patients with Carney complex and primary pigmented nodular adrenocortical disease (PPNAD) reveals novel mutations and clues for pathophysiology: augmented PKA signaling is associated with adrenal tumorigenesis in PPNAD. *Am J Hum Genet* (2002) 71:1433–42. doi:10.1086/344579
107. Bram Z, Renouf S, Duparc C, Ragazzon B, Libe R, Martinez A, et al. Activation of the PKA pathway triggers formation of an illicit serotonergic regulatory loop in primary pigmented nodular adrenal disease (PPNAD) tissues associated with Cushing's syndrome. *Endocrine Abstracts 29 OC7.2.* Florence, Italy: (2012).
108. Assié G, Libé R, Espiard S, Rizk-Rabin M, Guimier A, Luscap W, et al. ARMC5 mutations in macronodular adrenal hyperplasia with Cushing's syndrome. *N Engl J Med* (2013) 369:2105–14. doi:10.1056/NEJMoa1304603
109. Drougat L, Espiard S, Bertherat J. Genetics of primary bilateral macronodular adrenal hyperplasia: a model for early diagnosis of Cushing's syndrome? *Eur J Endocrinol* (2015) 173:M121–31. doi:10.1530/EJE-15-0532

16

Role of ACTH and Other Hormones in the Regulation of Aldosterone Production in Primary Aldosteronism

Nada El Ghorayeb, Isabelle Bourdeau and André Lacroix*

Department of Medicine, Division of Endocrinology, Centre de Recherche du Centre hospitalier de l'Université de Montréal (CRCHUM), Université de Montréal, Montréal, QC, Canada

Correspondence:
André Lacroix
andre.lacroix@umontreal.ca

The major physiological regulators of aldosterone production from the adrenal zona glomerulosa are potassium and angiotensin II; other acute regulators include adrenocorticotropic hormone (ACTH) and serotonin. Their interactions with G-protein coupled hormone receptors activate cAMP/PKA pathway thereby regulating intracellular calcium flux and CYP11B2 transcription, which is the specific steroidogenic enzyme of aldosterone synthesis. In primary aldosteronism (PA), the increased production of aldosterone and resultant relative hypervolemia inhibits the renin and angiotensin system; aldosterone secretion is mostly independent from the suppressed renin–angiotensin system, but is not autonomous, as it is regulated by a diversity of other ligands of various eutopic or ectopic receptors, in addition to activation of calcium flux resulting from mutations of various ion channels. Among the abnormalities in various hormone receptors, an overexpression of the melanocortin type 2 receptor (MC2R) could be responsible for aldosterone hypersecretion in aldosteronomas. An exaggerated increase in plasma aldosterone concentration (PAC) is found in patients with PA secondary either to unilateral aldosteronomas or bilateral adrenal hyperplasia (BAH) following acute ACTH administration compared to normal individuals. A diurnal increase in PAC in early morning and its suppression by dexamethasone confirms the increased role of endogenous ACTH as an important aldosterone secretagogue in PA. Screening using a combination of dexamethasone and fludrocortisone test reveals a higher prevalence of PA in hypertensive populations compared to the aldosterone to renin ratio. The variable level of MC2R overexpression in each aldosteronomas or in the adjacent zona glomerulosa hyperplasia may explain the inconsistent results of adrenal vein sampling between basal levels and post ACTH

Abbreviations: β-AR, β-adrenergic receptors; 5-HT_4R, serotonin receptor; AC, adenylate cyclase; ACTH, adrenocorticotropin hormone; APA, aldosterone-producing adenoma; APA, aldosterone-producing adenoma; APCCs, aldosterone-producing cell clusters; AT-1 receptor, angiotensin II type 1 receptor; ATP, adenosine triphosphate; AVS, adrenal venous sampling; BAH, bilateral adrenal hyperplasia; cAMP, cyclic adenosine monophosphate; CREB, cAMP response element binding protein; CYP11B1, cytochrome P450 family 11 subfamily B member 1 encodes 11-beta hydroxylase; CYP11B2, cytochrome P450 family 11 subfamily B member 2 encodes aldosterone synthetase; ET, endothelin-1; FH, familial hyperaldosteronism; FST, fludrocortisone suppression test; GIP, glucose-dependent insulinotropic peptide; GPCR, G-protein-coupled receptor; GRA, glucocorticoid-remediable aldosteronism; Gs-α, G stimulatory α subunit; LH–hCG, luteinizing hormone/human chorionic gonadotropin; MC2R, melanocortin type 2 receptor; mRNA, messenger ribonucleic acid; PA, primary aldosteronsim; PAC, plasma aldosterone; PKA, protein kinase; RAS, rennin–angiotensin system; RT-PCR, reverese transcriptase-polymerase chain reaction; StAR, steroidogenic acute regulatory protein; TRH, thyrotropin releasing hormone; UA, unilateral adrenalectomy; V1-AVPR, vasopressin receptor type 1; ZF, zona fasciculata; ZG, zona glomerulosa.

administration in the determination of source of aldosterone excess. In the rare cases of glucocorticoid remediable aldosteronism, a chimeric CYP11B2 becomes regulated by ACTH activating its chimeric CYP11B1 promoter of aldosterone synthase in bilateral adrenal fasciculate-like hyperplasia. This review will focus on the role of ACTH on excess aldosterone secretion in PA with particular focus on the aberrant expression of MC2R in comparison with other aberrant ligands and their GPCRs in this frequent pathology.

Keywords: ACTH, aldosterone regulation, melanocortin type 2 receptor, aberrant G-protein coupled receptors, primary aldosteronism

INTRODUCTION

Primary aldosteronism (PA) was first described in patients with unilateral aldosterone-producing adenomas (1). It is characterized by increased aldosterone secretion causing salt retention, increased urinary potassium excretion, relative hypervolemia, suppressed plasma renin activity (PRA), and hypertension. PA is the most common curable form of secondary hypertension as it affects 4.3% of the general hypertensive population, 9.5% of patients referred to hypertension clinics (2), and up to 20% of those with resistant hypertension (3). PA is most often secondary to bilateral adrenal hyperplasia (BAH; 50–70% of cases) or to an aldosterone-producing adenoma (APA; 30–50% of cases) (4). The classical concept that a unique unilateral aldosteronoma is the causative lesion responsible for a high proportion of this surgically curable form of PA was recently challenged by the identification of zona glomerulosa (ZG) hyperplasia and nodulation adjacent to aldosteronomas when resected adrenals are examined carefully (5–7).

In order to prevent cardiovascular, metabolic and renal morbidities, early diagnosis and management of PA are mandatory (8–10). Unilateral adrenalectomy (UA) provides superior benefit compared to medical therapy in lateralized PA in terms of cardiovascular outcomes (11, 12), quality of life (12), and all-cause mortality (13); however, in BAH, pharmacological blockade of aldosterone excess using mineralocorticoid receptor antagonists, such as spironolactone or eplerenone, is the recommended treatment (4). Therefore, subtyping of PA is required to direct patients to surgical vs. medical therapy (4). To date, adrenal vein sampling (AVS) is the gold standard to differentiate lateralized from bilateral sources of PA (4) because adrenal imaging provides poor specificity in detecting lateralized cases (14) except in patients <35 years old (15).

In PA excess, plasma aldosterone concentration (PAC), despite suppressed renin activity, is not really autonomous, as frequently stated. It could be autonomous if it was solely or constitutively regulated by somatic and germline mutations of various ion channels genes regulating intracellular ionic homeostasis and cell membrane potential as reviewed elsewhere (16). In fact, several autocrine/paracrine hormones and regulatory mechanisms (17) activate variable levels of aberrant eutopic or ectopic receptors (18), which regulate aldosterone secretion either in unilateral adenomas or in BAH. In this review, we will focus on the role of one of these hormones, the adrenocorticotropic hormone (ACTH), in stimulating aldosterone secretion in normal and pathologic conditions and briefly mention others which play similar roles in PA.

NORMAL PHYSIOLOGY OF THE RENIN–ANGIOTENSIN SYSTEM

Renin is an enzyme produced primarily by the juxtaglomerular apparatus of the kidney and its release is the rate-limiting step in the regulation of the RAS (19, 20); it is controlled by four factors: (1) the macula densa comprises chemoreceptors for monitoring the sodium and chloride loads present in the distal tubule, (2) juxtaglomerular cells acting as pressure transducers that sense stretch of the afferent arteriolar wall and thus renal perfusion pressure, (3) the sympathetic nervous system (SNS), which increases the release of renin, particularly in response to upright posture, in addition to (4) inhibiting factors, including K^+, Ca^{++}, angiotensin II, and atrial natriuretic peptides (19).

The action of renin on angiotensinogen, synthesized in the liver, generates angiotensin I (19). Angiotensin-converting enzyme (ACE), localized in cell membranes particularly of the lung, cleaves angiotensin I into angiotensin II, which is the main biologically active angiotensin (19). Angiotensin II functions through the AT-1 receptor (AT1R) to maintain normal extracellular volume and blood pressure by increasing aldosterone secretion from the ZG *via* increased transcription of CYP11B2 (aldosterone synthase) (**Figure 1**) as well as constricting vascular smooth muscle, releasing norepinephrine, and epinephrine from the adrenal medulla, enhancing the activity of the SNS and finally promoting the release of vasopressin (19).

Zona glomerulosa cells are organized in rosette structures that spontaneously generate periodic depolarizing changes in membrane potential that are modulated in frequency by angiotensin II and extracellular K^+ (21, 22); Angiotensin II induces cell membrane depolarization most probably due to a Gi-mediated shift in the voltage dependence of channel activation toward more negative potentials thereby increasing intracellular Ca^{2+} signal, which stimulates hormone-sensitive lipase and steroidogenic acute regulatory protein (StAR). Another mechanism by which angiotensin II binding to AT1R stimulates aldosterone secretion implicates activating the phospholipase C/inositol 1,4,5-trisphosphate pathway, releasing Ca^{2+} stores from the endoplasmic reticulum, and activation of T-type voltage-gated Ca^{2+} channels (23) (**Figure 1**).

Dopamine, atrial natriuretic peptide, and heparin inhibit aldosterone secretion. The secretion of aldosterone is restricted

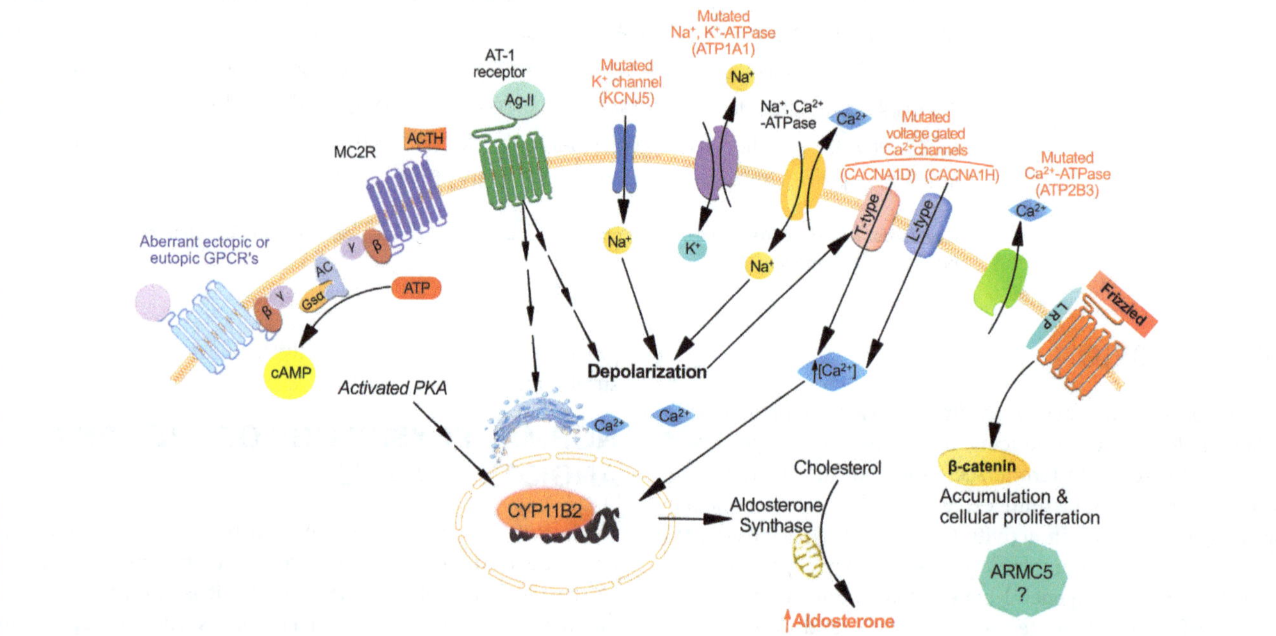

FIGURE 1 | Mechanisms responsible for aldosterone synthesis in zona glomerulosa cells under normal physiological conditions and excess production in primary aldosteronism. The strongly negative resting membrane potential of zona glomerulosa (ZG) cells under resting physiological conditions is maintained by the concentration gradient of K^+ between the intracellular and extracellular space, which is generated by the activity of the Na^+, K^+-ATPase. Angiotensin II and increased K^+ lead to cell membrane depolarization, which opens voltage-dependent Ca^{2+} channels. Furthermore, Angiostensin II acts through the Angiotensin II type 1 receptor (AT1R) inducing Ca^{2+} release from the endoplasmic reticulum. Consequently, the increase in intracellular Ca^{2+} concentration activates the calcium signaling pathway, which triggers activation of CYP11B2 transcription. The role for ACTH in the regulation of aldosterone secretion whether in normal physiology or in PA is in part determined by the level of expression of ACTH receptors (MC2R) in ZG cells. MC2R which is a GPCR coupled to the stimulatory Gsα subunit may induce an increase of intracellular cAMP concentration which activates protein kinase A thereby increasing CREB phosphorylation and CYP11B2 transcription. Aberrant expression of other GPCR may also be responsible for aldosterone excess despite a suppressed renin angiotensin system: eutopic GPCR include those for serotonin (5-HT_4R); ectopic GPCR include those for glucose-dependent insulinotropic peptide (GIPR), luteinizing hormone/human chorionic gonadotropin (LH-hCG R), β-adrenergic receptors (β-AR), vasopressin (V1-AVPR) glucagon (glucagon receptor), TRH (TRH R), and Endothelin-1 ET_A and ET_B receptors. Other mechanisms implicated in PA involve somatic and germline mutations in ion channels genes regulating intracellular ionic homeostasis and cell membrane potentials: increase intracellular Na^+ concentrations and cell membrane depolarization result from *KCNJ5* gain-of-function mutations affecting GIRK4 and *ATP1A1* mutations of the Na^+, K^+-ATPase. Direct increase of intracellular Ca^{2+} concentrations could also result from mutations in *ATP2B3* encoding for the plasma membrane Ca^{2+}-ATPase, mutations in *CACNA1D* affecting the Cav1.3 subunit of the L-type voltage-gated calcium channel or *CACNA1H* affecting the Cav3.2 subunit of the voltage-gated calcium channel. Finally dysregulation in cellular proliferation/apoptosis accelerating adenoma formation could be due either to activation of the Wnt/β-catenin pathway or to gene mutations such as *ARMC5* although the mechanism of the latter mutation is not fully elucidated.

to the ZG because of zone-specific expression of aldosterone synthase (CYP11B2), which is regulated by the activation of calcium signaling (24).

PATHOPHYSIOLOGY OF PRIMARY ALDOSTERONISM

The binding of free aldosterone to the mineralocorticoid receptor in the cytosol of epithelial cells (24), principally in the kidney, controls potassium homeostasis and maintains normal intravascular volume by increasing intestinal and renal Na^+ and Cl^- absorption and reabsorption, respectively. Increased production of aldosterone in PA results in sodium retention, hypertension, and can also result in hypokalemia (20). In addition to the two most common subtypes of PA (BAH in 50–70% of the cases and APA in 30–50%), less frequent causes include primary (unilateral) adrenal hyperplasia (5%), aldosterone-producing adrenocortical carcinoma (<1%), familial hyperaldosteronism (1%), and ectopic aldosterone-producing adenoma or carcinoma (<0.1%). The mechanisms implicated in the pathophysiology of PA are not fully elucidated. Somatic and germline mutations in ion channels genes regulating intracellular ionic homeostasis and cell membrane potential were described in sporadic APA and type-III familial PA (25–28) (**Figure 1**). Somatic mutations in the potassium channel gene *KCNJ5* are found in almost 30–40% of aldosteronomas and alter channel selectivity allowing enhanced Na^+ conductance. Na^+ influx results in cell depolarization, the activation of voltage-gated Ca^{2+} channels, aldosterone production, and cell proliferation (25, 29). Somatic and germline mutations in *CACNA1D* gene encoding a voltage-gated calcium channel result in channel activation and less depolarized potentials causing increased Ca^{2+} influx, aldosterone production and cell proliferation in affected ZG cells (27, 30). Mutations in *ATP1A1* gene (encoding the Na^+/K^+ ATPase α subunit) and *ATP2B3* gene (encoding the plasma membrane Ca^{2+} ATPase) were identified in 5.2 and 1.6%, respectively of patients in a series of APA (26). Mutations in *CACNA1H* gene, which encodes a voltage-gated calcium channel (Cav3.2) were discovered in children with PA; they result in impaired channel inactivation and activation at more hyperpolarized potentials, producing increased intracellular Ca^{2+} and aldosterone excess (31). Different mutations in the genes described above are found in different aldosterone-producing nodules from the same adrenal, suggesting that somatic mutations are independent events (32, 33).

No mutations of any of the above ion channel genes were found in BAH or in ZG hyperplasia adjacent to the dominant aldosteronomas (26, 29, 32, 33); these findings suggest that nodule formation and excess aldosterone production are two dissociated events, implying a two-hit hypothesis for APA formation (16, 34). The first hit causing a unilateral aldosteronoma or a dominant nodule adjacent to ZG hyperplasia may result from a somatic mutation in one of the genes described above, at least in approximately 60% of cases. Possible causes of the second hit that results in dysregulation in cellular proliferation/apoptosis accelerating adenoma formation could be due either to activation of the Wnt/β-catenin pathway (35, 36), PKA pathway, or to gene mutations such as *ARMC5* (37) (**Figure 1**). However, the pathophysiology of progression from normal adrenal to APA and the causes of diffuse bilateral hyperplasias, either as BAH or in mild form adjacent to the dominant aldosteronoma, are still unknown. Aldosterone-producing cell clusters (APCCs), which have increased expression of CYP11B2, are nests of cells below the adrenal capsule. They protrude into cortisol-producing cells that are usually negative for CYP11B2 expression. Nishimoto et al. found that APCCs are common in normal adrenals, and they harbor a different mutational spectrum compared to APA suggesting that APCCs could be a precursor for APA (38). In addition, several hormones activating variable levels of eutopic or ectopic aberrant receptors (18) (**Figure 1**) as well as autocrine and paracrine regulatory mechanisms (17) can increase aldosterone secretion in PA (either APA or BAH) independently from the suppressed RAS (see later section).

ROLE OF ACTH IN ALDOSTERONE PRODUCTION IN NORMAL PHYSIOLOGY

Adrenocorticotropic hormone can stimulate aldosterone secretion acutely and transiently under normal conditions, but to a lesser extent than angiotensin II and potassium. ACTH is a 39-amino-acid peptide, which results from the cleavage of its proopiomelanocortin (POMC) precursor by prohormone convertases PC1/3 and may be further cleaved by PC2 to generate α-melanocyte-stimulating hormone (α-MSH) (39, 40). It is mainly produced in the anterior pituitary corticotropes, but is also produced in brain, adrenal medulla, skin, and placenta (41–43). ACTH can induce aldosterone production at lower doses than the ones needed for cortisol and DHEA production (44). Furthermore, ACTH stimulates aldosterone production acutely and sometimes chronically.

Acute Effects of ACTH

The initial binding of ACTH to its specific melanocortin type 2 receptor (MC2R) stimulates both cortisol and aldosterone secretion. MC2R (45) is a seven transmembrane domain receptor that belongs to the family of melanocortin receptors (MCRs) (45). Five MCRs constitute a distinct family of G-protein coupled hormone receptors (GPCR); MC2R is the smallest MCR and GPCR (45, 46). MC2R is expressed in zona fasciculata (ZF) and ZG cells (47). The binding of ACTH to its MC2R induces the dissociation of Gs-α subunit and activation of adenylate cyclase (AC) that generates cAMP from ATP (48) (**Figure 1**). cAMP molecules bind to specific domains of the regulatory subunits of protein kinase A (PKA) thereby dissociating the tetramer and releasing the catalytic subunit (PRKACA) from its inactivating regulatory subunits. Activated PRKACA phosphorylates and activates steroidogenic acute regulatory protein (StAR) as well as cAMP response element binding protein (CREB), thereby increasing StAR expression. On the other hand, activation of the PKA pathway induces a slow but sustained calcium influx through the L-type calcium channels. The subsequent increase in intracellular calcium activates calcium/calmodulin-dependent protein kinase and steroidogenesis (49, 50).

Chronic Effects of ACTH

In contrast to *in vivo* studies that suggest that ACTH is a short-term stimulator of aldosterone production, *in vitro* studies showed that ACTH can act as a major stimulus of aldosterone secretion. Continuous intravenous infusion of ACTH leads to a transient stimulation of aldosterone secretion, whereas its pulsatile administration leads to a sustained stimulation of aldosterone up to 72 h (51). Moreover, chronic exposure to ACTH (2 days or more) leads to transformation of ZG cells into ZF-like cells with elongated mitochondria with lamellar and tubular cristae becoming round with ovoid cristae; at the functional level, the synthesis of angiotensin II receptors, steroidogenic enzymes, and their products is altered (52–56).

ROLE OF ACTH IN EXCESS ALDOSTERONE SECRETION IN PA

Diurnal Rhythmicity of Aldosterone

In recumbent normal subjects on a regular diet, the circadian rhythm of PAC is regulated by the activity of plasma renin independently of ACTH (57). In contrast, patients with PA have a circadian rhythm of PAC mediated by changes in ACTH rather than by the suppressed plasma renin–angiotensin II levels (58). Several groups described that PAC falls following overnight sleep when ACTH levels are low despite upright posture or angiotensin II infusion. Similarly, they noted a marked increase in PAC shortly after ACTH administration (59–63), which was higher compared to normal controls or patients with essential hypertension (64, 65). Furthermore, abolition of diurnal rhythm by dexamethasone in PA demonstrates the impact of ACTH on adrenal steroidogenesis (66). Administration of dexamethasone 0.75–2.0 mg per day for 2 days decreased aldosterone levels by a mean of 49% in a group of 15 patients with aldosteronomas; in 33%, the suppression was greater than 80% (67).

ACTH Role in Familial Hyperaldosteronism

Familial hyperaldosteronism (FH) type-1, previously known as glucocorticoid-remediable aldosteronism (GRA), was first described as a form of hyperaldosteronism relieved by dexamethasone (68). It is suspected in young PA patients whose relatives suffer from cerebrovascular accidents. It is an autosomal dominant disease whereby the promoter of the chimeric 11β-hydroxylase/aldosterone synthase gene belongs to the 5′ end of CYP11 B1 (11β hydroxylase) and drives the expression of the 3′ end of CYP11 B2 (aldosterone synthase) ectopically in ZF cells under the main regulation by ACTH (69); in these patients, dexamethasone usually decreases aldosterone secretion by more than 80% or to <4 ng/dL (67), but the diagnosis is now performed using genetic analysis. In contrast to FH type-1, FH type-2 is defined as PA in a patient with a first-degree relative (parent/sibling/offspring) with established PA but without FH type-1 gene rearrangement. Linkage analysis has mapped FH type-2 to chromosome 7p22 but no responsible gene has been identified yet (70). The prevalence of FH type-2 in PA is higher (1.2–6%) than FH type-1 (≤1%). The FH type-3 and -4 are not regulated by ACTH stimulation, but they are caused by germline mutations in *KCNJ5* (71) and *CACNA1D/CACNA1H* (30, 31) genes, respectively.

ACTH Suppression or Stimulation Tests Can Reveal the Presence of PA

Based on the rationale that ACTH plays a more important role in PA than in normal subjects or those with essential hypertension, investigators in Athens compared the classical saline infusion test (SIT) to postdexamethasone SIT in 151 patients with single adrenal adenomas and detected almost double rate of aldosterone hypersecretion following dexamethasone administration (24 vs. 12%) (72). Similarly, they used a combined fludrocortisone–dexamethasone suppression test (FDST), which is a modification of the classic confirmatory fludrocortisone suppression test (FST) for the diagnosis of PA; it involves the administration of dexamethasone to hypertensives patients at midnight of the last day of the FST in order to eliminate the stimulatory effect of ACTH on aldosterone secretion. They demonstrated that the prevalence of PA rises from 5 to 13% with the usual diagnostic tests to 28.7–31% when using FDST; mineralocorticoid receptor blockade resulted in significant improvement in blood pressure in these patients (73–75). The same group administered an ultralow-dose (0.03 μg) ACTH to 113 hypertensives without PA: the 30 patients (27%) who exhibited an aldosterone hyperresponse had significantly higher PAC, ARR, and PAC/ACTH ratio in the treadmill test; normalization of blood pressure by mineralocorticoid antagonists in these patients was also evident compared to the group of hypertensive not sensitive to ACTH/stress (76). Therefore, the benefit of mineralocorticoid blockade could extend even to hypertensive patients without confirmed PA who present an aldosterone hyperreseponse to ACTH/stress, this category of hypertenives harboring a mild form of BAH. In contrast, another group examining the diagnostic accuracy of ACTH test in 158 hypertensive patients found that it was not very effective in differentiating between APA patients and non-PA patients (77).

Use of ACTH to Identify the Source of Aldosterone Excess

Many efforts were conducted to find an easier and cheaper test than adrenal vein sampling (AVS), which is available only in tertiary care center with experienced angioradiologists to distinguish between lateralized and bilateral sources of aldosterone. Differential increase in PAC during upright posture was suggested to be a valuable tool to distinguish APA from BAH, but further studies showed that several APA and BAH had similar rise in PAC to upright posture (78). APA whether responsive or not to angiotensin II was found to be more sensitive to ACTH stimulation resulting in larger increase of PAC than in patients with BAH or essential hypertension (79–81). BAH patients also displayed increased response of PAC to ACTH administration than normal subjects or patients with essential hypertension (82). PAC increased more after ACTH bolus in the APA group compared with BAH group, which had an intermediate increase compared to normal controls (18, 66). A study in which patients received dexamethasone (1 mg) the evening before receiving i.v. injection of 50 IU of ACTH showed that the exaggerated PAC response was higher after 120 min in patients with APA than in BAH (83). It was suggested that this could be used for identifying the etiology subtype; however, significant overlap was present between APA, unilateral hyperplasia, and BAH cases and using an optimal cutoff value of the aldosterone >78 ng/dL for APA, provided a sensitivity of 76.8% and a specificity of 87.2% (83).

Kline et al. studied 65 patients with confirmed PA who were divided by histology into confirmed lateralized and non-lateralized; PAC in inferior vena cava (IVC) sampled during AVS before and after cosyntropin infusion was analyzed. Baseline and peak IVC aldosterone was higher in lateralized patients (APA) but incremental aldosterone rise was much greater in subjects with bilateral hyperplasia (84). This shows that ACTH can regulate APA as well as BAH, but that the effects are more pronounced in APA.

Role of ACTH Stimulation during Adrenal Venous Sampling

The usefulness of ACTH stimulation in the conduct of AVS procedure is controversial and remains a matter of debate because of conflicting results. Some centers use cosyntropin infusion or bolus in order to minimize stress-induced or spontaneous fluctuations in aldosterone secretion when performing sequential non-simultaneous AVS, to maximize the gradient of cortisol from the adrenal vein to the inferior vena cava, and to maximize aldosterone secretion from an APA (85). In contrast, other groups found that ACTH-stimulation of aldosterone production from the contralateral gland or adjacent hyperplasia may reduce the gradient of aldosterone production resulting in incorrect lateralization (86, 87). The effect of both continuous ACTH infusion and bolus on the performance and interpretation of AVS in confirmed PA patients was investigated (88). Both methods lead to a significant increase in selectivity index for the right adrenal vein and ACTH bolus for the left adrenal vein. Lateralization index was not significantly affected after continuous ACTH infusion and i.v. bolus. In 88 and 78% of the patients, the diagnosis obtained was the same before and after ACTH infusion and i.v. bolus, respectively (88). Recently, our group demonstrated that ACTH increased selectivity on both sides from 66.7% in basal samples to 91.8% poststimulation. A discordance of lateralization between basal and post-ACTH values was observed in 28% of cases, mostly lateralized cases basally that became bilateral post ACTH (87). The variation in the response to ACTH stimulation could be due to the variable expression of MC2R in APA (see later) (18). Careful examination of the levels of aldosterone in the adrenal vein contralateral to the dominant or lateralized APA and pathology confirmed the frequent presence of bilateral background hyperplasia and this could predict less favorable post-operative outcome with residual hypertension (35, 87).

INCREASED BUT VARIABLE EXPRESSION OF MC2R IN PA

The explanation for the increased role of ACTH in the regulation of aldosterone in PA may be secondary to the overexpression and function of MC2R in this condition. The expression of MC2R mRNA was shown to be upregulated in human adrenocortical neoplasms specifically in functional adenomas in contrast to non-functioning adenomas and carcinomas (89). More specifically, a few studies have demonstrated increased eutopic expression of MC2R assessed by RT-PCR or transcriptome studies in resected aldosteronomas as compared to cortisol-secreting adenomas, non-functional adenomas, and adrenocortical carcinomas (90–92). A particularly pertinent informative study included 15 adrenal tumors (14 APA and 1 BAH); MC2R mRNA levels were increased by a mean of 3.9-fold in those tissues compared to normal adrenal (18). However great variability existed in the level of expression in each tumor as 4 had lower levels than normal (0.3-fold to 0.7-fold), while those with increased expression varied between 1.4- and 20.6-fold compared to normal. The data are limited to mRNA expression without available measurements at the protein levels (no good specific MC2R antibody), but correlated well with the *in vivo* increased response to ACTH administration. There is almost no data on MC2R expression in BAH as those patients are usually not operated, but in the only case with BAH studied by this group MC2R was 20-fold increased. These data appear to be compatible with the findings that the majority of patients stimulated with ACTH during AVS will have concordant results before and after ACTH as the majority overexpress MC2R; however, the 28% of discordant results we found (87) may be explained by cases where MC2R are relatively decreased in the dominant adenoma but is present in adjacent hyperplasia. This hypothesis remains to be validated in prospective studies.

OTHER HORMONES AND ABERRANT RECEPTORS REGULATING ALDOSTERONE SECRETION IN PRIMARY ALDOSTERONISM

Adrenocorticotropin hormone is not the exclusive trigger of aldosterone secretion since several other hormones have a role in the pathophysiology of PA in addition to the ion channels mutations. Serotonin plays a significant role in aldosterone synthesis in normal physiological and in PA. The administration of serotonin 5-HT_4 agonists such as metoclopramide, cisapride, and tegaserod resulted in higher stimulation of aldosterone in PA as compared to the physiological moderate increase in normal individuals (18, 93, 94). Whereas non-specific inhibitors of 5-HT such as cyproheptadine and ketanserin produced only minor and transient inhibition of aldosterone secretion in aldosteronomas (95, 96), specific 5-HT_4R antagonists such as GR113808 were potent inhibitors of basal- and cisapride-induced aldosterone secretion (93). Chromaffin cells, endothelial cells, nerve terminals, and cells of the immune system are localized in the immediate vicinity of ZG cells and can secrete various factors to control aldosterone secretion (97). Local release of 5-HT by perivascular mast cells (MC) can activate 5-HT_4R expressed in ZG cells and consequently stimulate aldosterone production (98). A role of MC in tumorigenesis was proposed (99, 100). The density of MC was found to be increased in APA tissues compared with normal adrenals (101). As the 5-HT_4R have been found to be overexpressed in the majority of APA (but variable as MC2R) (17, 18, 102) and the ligand may be locally overexpressed also, a paracrine loop of regulation of aldosterone production appears to be present.

The compelling evidence supporting that various aberrant GPCR are frequently expressed in bilateral macronodular adrenal hyperplasia and Cushing's syndrome (103) led many researchers to investigate the presence of aberrant GPCR in PA. Adrenal production of aldosterone in APA and BAH was found to be under the influence of aberrant GPCR and their ligands, as demonstrated by *in vivo* and *in vitro* studies (104, 105). The expression of ectopic receptors, which are usually not expressed at significant levels in normal ZG cells include those for glucose-dependent insulinotropic peptide (GIPR) (106), luteinizing hormone/human chorionic gonadotropin (LH–hCG R) (18, 106–112), β-adrenergic receptors (β-AR) (113), vasopressin (V1-AVPR) (18, 106, 114, 115), glucagon (glucagon receptor), TRH (TRH R) (18, 112, 116) and Endothelin-1 ET_A and ET_B receptors (117). Using a microarray approach in 10 aldosteronomas compared with five normal adrenals and 13 cortisol-secreting adenomas, the six GCPRs with highest increase in expression included LHCGR, 5-HT_4R, GnRHR, glutamate receptor metabotropic 3, endothelin receptor ET_B receptors, and MC2R (92). **Table 1** summarizes the different types of aberrant eutopic or ectopic GPCR involved in aldosterone excess in PA. Co-expression of multiple aberrant GPCR was also reported; renin-independent stimulation of aldosterone secretion was observed *in vivo* following mixed meal, oral glucose, or administration of GIP, vasopressin, and tegaserod in a patient with unilateral source of PA (106). On the other hand, co-secretion of aldosterone and cortisol due to aberrant expression of GPCR was noted; in a patient with BMAH and β-AR-aberrant expression, isoproterenol stimulated both cortisol and aldosterone production (113).

Activating somatic *CTNNB1* (β-catenin) mutations have now been identified in tumors of three women with APAs, two who presented during pregnancy and one after menopause (118). All three had heterozygous activating mutations of *CTNNB1* and expressed aberrant LHCG and GNRH receptors at levels 100-fold

TABLE 1 | Types of GPCR involved in aldosterone hypersecretion in patients with PA.

Aberrant receptor	Phenotype	*In vivo* screening protocol	Targeted medical therapy
MC2R (eutopic) (90–92)	ACTH-dependent hyperaldosteronism	Cosyntropin	
GIP receptor (ectopic) (102)	Food-dependent hyperaldosteronism	Mixed meal Oral glucose	Octreotide, pasireotide GIPR antagonist
Vasopressin receptor (ectopic) (18, 102, 114, 115)	Upright posture-dependent hyperaldosteronism	Upright posture AVP/desmopressin	Specific AVP receptors antagonist
β-adrenergic receptor (ectopic) (113)	Upright posture Insulin-induced hypoglycemia Exercise/stress test hyperaldosteronism	Upright posture Isoproterenol (β1-agonist)	β-blockers
GnRH receptor, LH/hCG receptor (ectopic) (18, 102, 107–112)	Luteal phase of ovarian cycle/Pregnancy (transient) Postmenopausal (persistent)-dependent hyperaldosteronism	GnRH, hCG, Recombinant LH	Long-acting GnRH agonist (leuprolide acetate)
5-HT$_4$ receptor (eutopic) (18, 93, 94, 102)	Serotonin-dependent dependent	5-HT$_4$ receptor agonists (metoclopramide, cisapride, tegaserod)	5-HT$_4$ receptor antagonist (GR113808)
Glucagon receptor (ectopic) (18)	Hypoglycemia?	Intravenous glucagon	Octreotide
TRH receptor (ectopic) (18, 112, 116)	Hypothyroidism		
Endothelin-1 A and B receptors (ectopic) (117)			

higher than in other APAs. It was shown that the *CTNNB1* mutation led to activation of the WNT pathway; it was suggested that could be the cause of dedifferentiation of gonadal progenitor cells present in the adrenal tissues with increased expression of gonadal receptors. It is thought that the high levels of endogenous human chorionic gonadotropin (hCG) during pregnancy and of gonadotropin-releasing hormone (GnRH) and luteinizing hormone (LH) after menopause led to the identification of APAs in these patients (118).

It is currently unclear whether these aberrant regulatory secretory mechanisms by ACTH and other hormones and the overexpression of their GPCR in PA are secondary to unknown proliferative mechanisms or are primary and at least partially responsible for the abnormal proliferation, the initiation of diffuse BAH. However, they clearly play a role in aldosterone secretion which is not autonomous.

CONCLUSION

Our understanding of the increased occurrence and complexity of molecular etiology and unique signature in each case of PA has progressed greatly in recent years. The increased role of ACTH, of the variable expression of MC2R, and of other aberrant GPCR in PA should receive further attention in the future. The development of effective antagonists to MC2R and other aberrant GPCR could eventually offer interesting alternatives in patients with bilateral sources of excess aldosterone in combination with better antagonists of the mineralocorticoid receptor.

AUTHOR CONTRIBUTIONS

NG, IB, and AL contributed to the conception and design of the manuscript as well as to drafting the review article and they all provided final approval of the version to be published.

FUNDING

This work is supported by grant 201209NMD from the Canadian Institutes of Health Research to AL and IB. NG fellowship support was also provided in part by Novartis Canada. IB receives a salary Grant from FRQS (Fonds de la recherche du Québec-Santé).

REFERENCES

1. Conn JW. Presidential address. I. Painting background. II. Primary aldosteronism, a new clinical syndrome. *J Lab Clin Med* (1955) 45(1):3–17.
2. Hannemann A, Wallaschofski H. Prevalence of primary aldosteronism in patient's cohorts and in population-based studies – a review of the current literature. *Horm Metab Res* (2012) 44(3):157–62. doi:10.1055/s-0031-1295438
3. Calhoun DA. Is there an unrecognized epidemic of primary aldosteronism? Pro. *Hypertension* (2007) 50(3):447–453; discussion 447–453. doi:10.1161/HYPERTENSIONAHA.106.086116
4. Funder JW, Carey RM, Fardella C, Gomez-Sanchez CE, Mantero F, Stowasser M, et al. Case detection, diagnosis, and treatment of patients with primary aldosteronism: an endocrine society clinical practice guideline. *J Clin Endocrinol Metab* (2008) 93(9):3266–81. doi:10.1210/jcem.93.9.9998
5. Boulkroun S, Samson-Couterie B, Dzib JF, Lefebvre H, Louiset E, Amar L, et al. Adrenal cortex remodeling and functional zona glomerulosa hyperplasia in primary aldosteronism. *Hypertension* (2010) 56(5):885–92. doi:10.1161/HYPERTENSIONAHA.110.158543
6. Nishimoto K, Nakagawa K, Li D, Kosaka T, Oya M, Mikami S, et al. Adrenocortical zonation in humans under normal and pathological conditions. *J Clin Endocrinol Metab* (2010) 95(5):2296–305. doi:10.1210/jc.2009-2010
7. Duan K, Mete O. Clinicopathologic correlates of primary aldosteronism. *Arch Pathol Lab Med* (2015) 139(7):948–54. doi:10.5858/arpa.2014-0156-RS
8. Catena C, Colussi G, Nadalini E, Chiuch A, Baroselli S, Lapenna R, et al. Cardiovascular outcomes in patients with primary aldosteronism after treatment. *Arch Intern Med* (2008) 168(1):80–5. doi:10.1001/archinternmed.2007.33

9. Mulatero P, Monticone S, Bertello C, Viola A, Tizzani D, Iannaccone A, et al. Long-term cardio- and cerebrovascular events in patients with primary aldosteronism. *J Clin Endocrinol Metab* (2013) 98(12):4826–33. doi:10.1210/jc.2013-2805
10. Savard S, Amar L, Plouin PF, Steichen O. Cardiovascular complications associated with primary aldosteronism: a controlled cross-sectional study. *Hypertension* (2013) 62(2):331–6. doi:10.1161/HYPERTENSIONAHA.113.01060
11. Catena C, Colussi G, Lapenna R, Nadalini E, Chiuch A, Gianfagna P, et al. Long-term cardiac effects of adrenalectomy or mineralocorticoid antagonists in patients with primary aldosteronism. *Hypertension* (2007) 50(5):911–8. doi:10.1161/HYPERTENSIONAHA.107.095448
12. Ahmed AH, Gordon RD, Sukor N, Pimenta E, Stowasser M. Quality of life in patients with bilateral primary aldosteronism before and during treatment with spironolactone and/or amiloride, including a comparison with our previously published results in those with unilateral disease treated surgically. *J Clin Endocrinol Metab* (2011) 96(9):2904–11. doi:10.1210/jc.2011-0138
13. Reincke M, Fischer E, Gerum S, Merkle K, Schulz S, Pallauf A, et al. Observational study mortality in treated primary aldosteronism: the German Conn's registry. *Hypertension* (2012) 60(3):618–24. doi:10.1161/HYPERTENSIONAHA.112.197111
14. Magill SB, Raff H, Shaker JL, Brickner RC, Knechtges TE, Kehoe ME, et al. Comparison of adrenal vein sampling and computed tomography in the differentiation of primary aldosteronism. *J Clin Endocrinol Metab* (2001) 86(3):1066–71. doi:10.1210/jc.86.3.1066
15. Lim V, Guo Q, Grant CS, Thompson GB, Richards ML, Farley DR, et al. Accuracy of adrenal imaging and adrenal venous sampling in predicting surgical cure of primary aldosteronism. *J Clin Endocrinol Metab* (2014) 99(8):2712–9. doi:10.1210/jc.2013-4146
16. Lalli E, Barhanin J, Zennaro MC, Warth R. Local control of aldosterone production and primary aldosteronism. *Trends Endocrinol Metab* (2016). doi:10.1016/j.tem.2016.01.003
17. Lefebvre H, Prévost G, Louiset E. Autocrine/paracrine regulatory mechanisms in adrenocortical neoplasms responsible for primary adrenal hypercorticism. *Eur J Endocrinol* (2013) 169(5):R115–38. doi:10.1530/EJE-13-0308
18. Zwermann O, Suttmann Y, Bidlingmaier M, Beuschlein F, Reincke M. Screening for membrane hormone receptor expression in primary aldosteronism. *Eur J Endocrinol* (2009) 160(3):443–51. doi:10.1530/EJE-08-0711
19. Hall JE. Historical perspective of the renin-angiotensin system. *Mol Biotechnol* (2003) 24(1):27–39. doi:10.1385/MB:24:1:27
20. Spat A, Hunyady L. Control of aldosterone secretion: a model for convergence in cellular signaling pathways. *Physiol Rev* (2004) 84(2):489–539. doi:10.1152/physrev.00030.2003
21. Hu C, Rusin CG, Tan Z, Guagliardo NA, Barrett PQ. Zona glomerulosa cells of the mouse adrenal cortex are intrinsic electrical oscillators. *J Clin Invest* (2012) 122(6):2046–53. doi:10.1172/JCI61996
22. Barrett PQ, Guagliardo NA, Klein PM, Hu C, Breault DT, Beenhakker MP. Role of voltage-gated calcium channels in the regulation of aldosterone production from zona glomerulosa cells of the adrenal cortex. *J Physiol* (2016). doi:10.1113/JP271896
23. Spät A, Hunyady L, Szanda G. Signaling interactions in the adrenal cortex. *Front Endocrinol* (2016) 7:17. doi:10.3389/fendo.2016.00017
24. Arlt W, Stewart PM. Adrenal corticosteroid biosynthesis, metabolism, and action. *Endocrinol Metab Clin North Am* (2005) 34(2):293–313, viii. doi:10.1016/j.ecl.2005.01.002
25. Choi M, Scholl UI, Yue P, Björklund P, Zhao B, Nelson-Williams C, et al. K+ channel mutations in adrenal aldosterone-producing adenomas and hereditary hypertension. *Science* (2011) 331(6018):768–72. doi:10.1126/science.1198785
26. Beuschlein F, Boulkroun S, Osswald A, Wieland T, Nielsen HN, Lichtenauer UD, et al. Somatic mutations in ATP1A1 and ATP2B3 lead to aldosterone-producing adenomas and secondary hypertension. *Nat Genet* (2013) 45(4):.e441–2. doi:10.1038/ng.2550
27. Scholl UI, Goh G, Stölting G, de Oliveira RC, Choi M, Overton JD, et al. Somatic and germline CACNA1D calcium channel mutations in aldosterone-producing adenomas and primary aldosteronism. *Nat Genet* (2013) 45(9):1050–4. doi:10.1038/ng.2695
28. Fernandes-Rosa FL, Williams TA, Riester A, Steichen O, Beuschlein F, Boulkroun S, et al. Genetic spectrum and clinical correlates of somatic mutations in aldosterone-producing adenoma. *Hypertension* (2014) 64(2):354–61. doi:10.1161/HYPERTENSIONAHA.114.03419
29. Boulkroun S, Beuschlein F, Rossi GP, Golib-Dzib JF, Fischer E, Amar L, et al. Prevalence, clinical, and molecular correlates of KCNJ5 mutations in primary aldosteronism. *Hypertension* (2012) 59(3):592–8. doi:10.1161/HYPERTENSIONAHA.111.186478
30. Scholl UI, Nelson-Williams C, Yue P, Grekin R, Wyatt RJ, Dillon MJ, et al. Hypertension with or without adrenal hyperplasia due to different inherited mutations in the potassium channel KCNJ5. *Proc Natl Acad Sci U S A* (2012) 109(7):2533–8. doi:10.1073/pnas.1121407109
31. Scholl UI, Stölting G, Nelson-Williams C, Vichot AA, Choi M, Loring E, et al. Recurrent gain of function mutation in calcium channel CACNA1H causes early-onset hypertension with primary aldosteronism. *Elife* (2015) 4:e06315. doi:10.7554/eLife.06315
32. Fernandes-Rosa F, Giscos-Douriez I, Amar L, Gomez-Sanchez CE, Meatchi T, Boulkroun S, et al. PP.09.27: genetic abnormalities in lateralized multinodular primary aldosteronism. *J Hypertens* (2015) 33:e215–6. doi:10.1097/01.hjh.0000468004.04564.fb
33. Fernandes-Rosa FL, Giscos-Douriez I, Amar L, Gomez-Sanchez CE, Meatchi T, Boulkroun S, et al. Different somatic mutations in multinodular adrenals with aldosterone-producing adenoma. *Hypertension* (2015) 66(5):1014–22. doi:10.1161/HYPERTENSIONAHA.115.05993
34. Gomez-Sanchez CE, Gomez-Sanchez EP. Mutations of the potassium channel KCNJ5 causing aldosterone-producing adenomas: one or two hits? *Hypertension* (2012) 59(2):196–7. doi:10.1161/HYPERTENSIONAHA.111.186205
35. Boulkroun S, Samson-Couterie B, Golib-Dzib JF, Amar L, Plouin PF, Sibony M, et al. Aldosterone-producing adenoma formation in the adrenal cortex involves expression of stem/progenitor cell markers. *Endocrinology* (2011) 152(12):4753–63. doi:10.1210/en.2011-1205
36. El Wakil A, Lalli E. The Wnt/beta-catenin pathway in adrenocortical development and cancer. *Mol Cell Endocrinol* (2011) 332(1–2):32–7. doi:10.1016/j.mce.2010.11.014
37. Zilbermint M, Xekouki P, Faucz FR, Berthon A, Gkourogianni A, Schernthaner-Reiter MH, et al. Primary aldosteronism and ARMC5 variants. *J Clin Endocrinol Metab* (2015) 100(6):E900–9. doi:10.1210/jc.2014-4167
38. Nishimoto K, Tomlins SA, Kuick R, Cani AK, Giordano TJ, Hovelson DH, et al. Aldosterone-stimulating somatic gene mutations are common in normal adrenal glands. *Proc Natl Acad Sci U S A* (2015) 112(33):E4591–9. doi:10.1073/pnas.1505529112
39. Raffin-Sanson ML, de Keyzer Y, Bertagna X. Proopiomelanocortin, a polypeptide precursor with multiple functions: from physiology to pathological conditions. *Eur J Endocrinol* (2003) 149(2):79–90. doi:10.1530/eje.0.1490079
40. Dores RM, Londraville RL, Prokop J, Davis P, Dewey N, Lesinski N. Molecular evolution of GPCRs: melanocortin/melanocortin receptors. *J Mol Endocrinol* (2014) 52(3):T29–42. doi:10.1530/JME-14-0050
41. Vrezas I, Willenberg HS, Mansmann G, Hiroi N, Fritzen R, Bornstein SR. Ectopic adrenocorticotropin (ACTH) and corticotropin-releasing hormone (CRH) production in the adrenal gland: basic and clinical aspects. *Microsc Res Tech* (2003) 61(3):308–14. doi:10.1002/jemt.10340
42. Bicknell AB. The tissue-specific processing of pro-opiomelanocortin. *J Neuroendocrinol* (2008) 20(6):692–9. doi:10.1111/j.1365-2826.2008.01709.x
43. Evans JF, Fernando A, Ragolia L. Functional melanocortin-2 receptors are expressed by mouse aorta-derived mesenchymal progenitor cells. *Mol Cell Endocrinol* (2012) 355(1):60–70. doi:10.1016/j.mce.2012.01.019
44. Daidoh H, Morita H, Mune T, Murayama M, Hanafusa J, Ni H, et al. Responses of plasma adrenocortical steroids to low dose ACTH in normal subjects. *Clin Endocrinol (Oxf)* (1995) 43(3):311–5. doi:10.1111/j.1365-2265.1995.tb02037.x
45. Mountjoy KG, Robbins LS, Mortrud MT, Cone RD. The cloning of a family of genes that encode the melanocortin receptors. *Science* (1992) 257(5074):1248–51. doi:10.1126/science.1325670
46. Cone RD, Mountjoy KG, Robbins LS, Nadeau JH, Johnson KR, Roselli-Rehfuss L, et al. Cloning and functional characterization of a family of receptors for the melanotropic peptides. *Ann N Y Acad Sci* (1993) 680:342–63. doi:10.1111/j.1749-6632.1993.tb19694.x

47. Chan LF, Metherell LA, Clark AJ. Effects of melanocortins on adrenal gland physiology. *Eur J Pharmacol* (2011) 660(1):171–80. doi:10.1016/j.ejphar.2010.11.041
48. de Joussineau C, Sahut-Barnola I, Levy I, Saloustros E, Val P, Stratakis CA, et al. The cAMP pathway and the control of adrenocortical development and growth. *Mol Cell Endocrinol* (2012) 351(1):28–36. doi:10.1016/j.mce.2011.10.006
49. Hattangady NG, Olala LO, Bollag WB, Rainey WE. Acute and chronic regulation of aldosterone production. *Mol Cell Endocrinol* (2012) 350(2):151–62. doi:10.1016/j.mce.2011.07.034
50. Gallo-Payet N. Adrenal and extra-adrenal functions of ACTH. *J Mol Endocrinol* (2016) 56(4):135–56. doi:10.1530/JME-15-0257
51. Seely EW, Conlin PR, Brent GA, Dluhy RG. Adrenocorticotropin stimulation of aldosterone: prolonged continuous versus pulsatile infusion. *J Clin Endocrinol Metab* (1989) 69(5):1028–32. doi:10.1210/jcem-69-5-1028
52. Aguilera G, Fujita K, Catt KJ. Mechanisms of inhibition of aldosterone secretion by adrenocorticotropin. *Endocrinology* (1981) 108(2):522–8. doi:10.1210/endo-108-2-522
53. Crivello JF, Gill GN. Induction of cultured bovine adrenocortical zona glomerulosa cell 17-hydroxylase activity by ACTH. *Mol Cell Endocrinol* (1983) 30(1):97–107. doi:10.1016/0303-7207(83)90204-6
54. Bird IM, Pasquarette MM, Rainey WE, Mason JI. Differential control of 17 alpha-hydroxylase and 3 beta-hydroxysteroid dehydrogenaseg expression in human adrenocortical H295R cells. *J Clin Endocrinol Metab* (1996) 81(6): 2171–8. doi:10.1210/jc.81.6.2171
55. Corander MP, Coll AP. Melanocortins and body weight regulation: glucocorticoids, Agouti-related protein and beyond. *Eur J Pharmacol* (2011) 660(1):111–8. doi:10.1016/j.ejphar.2010.10.103
56. Gallo-Payet N, Battista MC. Steroidogenesis-adrenal cell signal transduction. *Compr Physiol* (2014) 4(3):889–964. doi:10.1002/cphy.c130050
57. Williams GH, Tuck ML, Rose LI, Dluhy RG, Underwood RH. Studies of the control of plasma aldosterone concentration in normal man. 3. Response to sodium chloride infusion. *J Clin Invest* (1972) 51(10):2645–52. doi:10.1172/JCI106974
58. Kem DC, Gomez-Sanchez C, Kramer NJ, Holland OB, Higgins JR. Plasma aldosterone and renin activity response to ACTH infusion in dexamethasone-suppressed normal and sodium-depleted man. *J Clin Endocrinol Metab* (1975) 40(1):116–24. doi:10.1210/jcem-40-1-116
59. Wolfe LK, Gordon RD, Island DP, Liddle GW. An analysis of factors determining the circadian pattern of aldosterone excretion. *J Clin Endocrinol Metab* (1966) 26(11):1261–6. doi:10.1210/jcem-26-11-1261
60. Newton MA, Laragh JH. Effects of glucocorticoid administration on aldosterone excretion and plasma renin in normal subjects, in essential hypertension and in primary aldosteronism. *J Clin Endocrinol Metab* (1968) 28(7):1014–22. doi:10.1210/jcem-28-7-1006
61. Schambelan M, Brust NL, Chang BC, Slater KL, Biglieri EG. Circadian rhythm and effect of posture on plasma aldosterone concentration in primary aldosteronism. *J Clin Endocrinol Metab* (1976) 43(1):115–31. doi:10.1210/jcem-43-1-115
62. Guthrie GP Jr. Multiple plasma steroid responses to graded ACTH infusions in patients with primary aldosteronism. *J Lab Clin Med* (1981) 98(3):364–73.
63. Stowasser M, Gordon RD, Klemm SA, Tunny TJ. Renin-aldosterone response to dexamethasone in glucocorticoid-suppressible hyperaldosteronism is altered by coexistent renal artery stenosis. *J Clin Endocrinol Metab* (1993) 77(3):800–4. doi:10.1210/jcem.77.3.8396580
64. Kem DC, Weinberger MH, Higgins JR, Kramer NJ, Gomez-Sanchez C, Holland OB. Plasma aldosterone response to ACTH in primary aldosteronism and in patients with low renin hypertension. *J Clin Endocrinol Metab* (1978) 46(4):552–60. doi:10.1210/jcem-46-4-552
65. Saruta T, Okuno T, Eguchi T, Nakamura R, Saito I, Kondo K, et al. Responses of aldosterone-producing adenomas to ACTH and angiotensins. *Acta Endocrinol (Copenh)* (1979) 92(4):702–9.
66. Sonoyama T, Sone M, Tamura N, Honda K, Taura D, Kojima K, et al. Role of endogenous ACTH on circadian aldosterone rhythm in patients with primary aldosteronism. *Endocr Connect* (2014) 3(4):173–9. doi:10.1530/EC-14-0086
67. Litchfield WR, New MI, Coolidge C, Lifton RP, Dluhy RG. Evaluation of the dexamethasone suppression test for the diagnosis of glucocorticoid-remediable aldosteronism. *J Clin Endocrinol Metab* (1997) 82(11):3570–3. doi:10.1210/jcem.82.11.4381
68. Sutherland DJ, Ruse JL, Laidlaw JC. Hypertension, increased aldosterone secretion and low plasma renin activity relieved by dexamethasone. *Can Med Assoc J* (1966) 95(22):1109–19.
69. Lifton RP, Dluhy RG, Powers M, Rich GM, Gutkin M, Fallo F, et al. Hereditary hypertension caused by chimaeric gene duplications and ectopic expression of aldosterone synthase. *Nat Genet* (1992) 2(1):66–74. doi:10.1038/ng0992-66
70. Sukor N, Mulatero P, Gordon RD, So A, Duffy D, Bertello C, et al. Further evidence for linkage of familial hyperaldosteronism type II at chromosome 7p22 in Italian as well as Australian and South American families. *J Hypertens* (2008) 26(8):1577–82. doi:10.1097/HJH.0b013e3283028352
71. Geller DS, Zhang J, Wisgerhof MV, Shackleton C, Kashgarian M, Lifton RP. A novel form of human mendelian hypertension featuring nonglucocorticoid-remediable aldosteronism. *J Clin Endocrinol Metab* (2008) 93(8):3117–23. doi:10.1210/jc.2008-0594
72. Piaditis GP, Kaltsas GA, Androulakis II, Gouli A, Makras P, Papadogias D, et al. High prevalence of autonomous cortisol and aldosterone secretion from adrenal adenomas. *Clin Endocrinol (Oxf)* (2009) 71(6):772–8. doi:10.1111/j.1365-2265.2009.03551.x
73. Gouli A, Kaltsas G, Tzonou A, Markou A, Androulakis II, Ragkou D, et al. High prevalence of autonomous aldosterone secretion among patients with essential hypertension. *Eur J Clin Invest* (2011) 41(11):1227–36. doi:10.1111/j.1365-2362.2011.02531.x
74. Markou A, Pappa T, Kaltsas G, Gouli A, Mitsakis K, Tsounas P, et al. Evidence of primary aldosteronism in a predominantly female cohort of normotensive individuals: a very high odds ratio for progression into arterial hypertension. *J Clin Endocrinol Metab* (2013) 98(4):1409–16. doi:10.1210/jc.2012-3353
75. Papanastasiou L, Markou A, Pappa T, Gouli A, Tsounas P, Fountoulakis S, et al. Primary aldosteronism in hypertensive patients: clinical implications and target therapy. *Eur J Clin Invest* (2014) 44(8):697–706. doi:10.1111/eci.12286
76. Markou A, Sertedaki A, Kaltsas G, Androulakis II, Marakaki C, Pappa T, et al. Stress-induced aldosterone hyper-secretion in a substantial subset of patients with essential hypertension. *J Clin Endocrinol Metab* (2015) 100(8):2857–64. doi:10.1210/jc.2015-1268
77. Terui K, Kageyama K, Nigawara T, Moriyama T, Sakihara S, Takayasu S, et al. Evaluation of the (1-24) adrenocorticotropin stimulation test for the diagnosis of primary aldosteronism. *J Renin Angiotensin Aldosterone Syst* (2016) 17(1). doi:10.1177/1470320315625703
78. Tunny TJ, Klemm SA, Stowasser M, Gordon RD. Angiotensin-responsive aldosterone-producing adenomas: postoperative disappearance of aldosterone response to angiotensin. *Clin Exp Pharmacol Physiol* (1993) 20(5):306–9. doi:10.1111/j.1440-1681.1993.tb01690.x
79. Mantero F, Gion M, Armanini D, Opocher G. Aldosterone regulation in primary aldosteronism: differences between adenoma and bilateral hyperplasia. *Clin Sci Mol Med Suppl* (1976) 3:329s–32s.
80. Stowasser M, Klemm SA, Tunny TJ, Gordon RD. Plasma aldosterone response to ACTH in subtypes of primary aldosteronism. *Clin Exp Pharmacol Physiol* (1995) 22(6–7):460–2. doi:10.1111/j.1440-1681.1995.tb02044.x
81. Sonoyama T, Sone M, Miyashita K, Tamura N, Yamahara K, Park K, et al. Significance of adrenocorticotropin stimulation test in the diagnosis of an aldosterone-producing adenoma. *J Clin Endocrinol Metab* (2011) 96(9):2771–8. doi:10.1210/jc.2011-0573
82. Biglieri EG, Irony I, Kater CE. Identification and implications of new types of mineralocorticoid hypertension. *J Steroid Biochem* (1989) 32(1B):199–204. doi:10.1016/0022-4731(89)90164-7
83. Jiang Y, Zhang C, Wang W, Su T, Zhou W, Jiang L, et al. Diagnostic value of ACTH stimulation test in determining the subtypes of primary aldosteronism. *J Clin Endocrinol Metab* (2015) 100(5):1837–44. doi:10.1210/jc.2014-3551
84. Kline GA, Pasieka JL, Harvey A, So B, Dias VC. A marked proportional rise in IVC aldosterone following cosyntropin administration during AVS is a signal to the presence of adrenal hyperplasia in primary aldosteronism. *J Hum Hypertens* (2014) 28(5):298–302. doi:10.1038/jhh.2013.116
85. Young WF, Stanson AW. What are the keys to successful adrenal venous sampling (AVS) in patients with primary aldosteronism? *Clin Endocrinol (Oxf)* (2009) 70(1):14–7. doi:10.1111/j.1365-2265.2008.03450.x

86. Seccia TM, Miotto D, De Toni R, Pitter G, Mantero F, Pessina AC, et al. Adrenocorticotropic hormone stimulation during adrenal vein sampling for identifying surgically curable subtypes of primary aldosteronism: comparison of 3 different protocols. *Hypertension* (2009) 53(5):761–6. doi:10.1161/HYPERTENSIONAHA.108.128553
87. El Ghorayeb N, Mazzuco TL, Bourdeau I, Mailhot JP, Shi Zhu P, Therasse E, et al. Basal and post ACTH aldosterone and its ratios are useful during adrenal vein sampling in primary aldosteronism. *J Clin Endocrinol Metab* (2016) 101(4):1826–35. doi:10.1210/jc.2015-3915
88. Monticone S, Satoh F, Giacchetti G, Viola A, Morimoto R, Kudo M, et al. Effect of adrenocorticotropic hormone stimulation during adrenal vein sampling in primary aldosteronism. *Hypertension* (2012) 59(4):840–6. doi:10.1161/HYPERTENSIONAHA.111.189548
89. Reincke M, Beuschlein F, Latronico AC, Arlt W, Chrousos GP, Allolio B. Expression of adrenocorticotrophic hormone receptor mRNA in human adrenocortical neoplasms: correlation with P450scc expression. *Clin Endocrinol (Oxf)* (1997) 46(5):619–26. doi:10.1046/j.1365-2265.1997.1991009.x
90. Arnaldi G, Mancini V, Costantini C, Giovagnetti M, Petrelli M, Masini A, et al. ACTH receptor mRNA in human adrenocortical tumors: overexpression in aldosteronomas. *Endocr Res* (1998) 24(3–4):845–9. doi:10.3109/07435809809032695
91. Schubert B, Fassnacht M, Beuschlein F, Zenkert S, Allolio B, Reincke M. Angiotensin II type 1 receptor and ACTH receptor expression in human adrenocortical neoplasms. *Clin Endocrinol (Oxf)* (2001) 54(5):627–32. doi:10.1046/j.1365-2265.2001.01253.x
92. Ye P, Mariniello B, Mantero F, Shibata H, Rainey WE. G-protein-coupled receptors in aldosterone-producing adenomas: a potential cause of hyperaldosteronism. *J Endocrinol* (2007) 195(1):39–48. doi:10.1677/JOE-07-0037
93. Lefebvre H, Cartier D, Duparc C, Lihrmann I, Contesse V, Delarue C, et al. Characterization of serotonin(4) receptors in adrenocortical aldosterone-producing adenomas: in vivo and in vitro studies. *J Clin Endocrinol Metab* (2002) 87(3):1211–6. doi:10.1210/jcem.87.3.8327
94. Cartier D, Jégou S, Parmentier F, Lihrmann I, Louiset E, Kuhn JM, et al. Expression profile of serotonin4 (5-HT4) receptors in adrenocortical aldosterone-producing adenomas. *Eur J Endocrinol* (2005) 153(6):939–47. doi:10.1530/eje.1.02051
95. Gross MD, Grekin RJ, Gniadek TC, Villareal JZ. Suppression of aldosterone by cyproheptadine in idiopathic aldosteronism. *N Engl J Med* (1981) 305(4):181–5. doi:10.1056/NEJM198107233050401
96. Mantero F, Rocco S, Opocher G, Armanini D, Boscaro M, D'Agostino D. Effect of ketanserin in primary aldosteronism. *J Cardiovasc Pharmacol* (1985) 7(Suppl 7):S172–5. doi:10.1097/00005344-198500077-00048
97. Ehrhart-Bornstein M, Hinson JP, Bornstein SR, Scherbaum WA, Vinson GP. Intraadrenal interactions in the regulation of adrenocortical steroidogenesis. *Endocr Rev* (1998) 19(2):101–43. doi:10.1210/edrv.19.2.0326
98. Lefebvre H, Compagnon P, Contesse V, Delarue C, Thuillez C, Vaudry H, et al. Production and metabolism of serotonin (5-HT) by the human adrenal cortex: paracrine stimulation of aldosterone secretion by 5-HT. *J Clin Endocrinol Metab* (2001) 86(10):5001–7. doi:10.1210/jcem.86.10.7917
99. Soucek L, Lawlor ER, Soto D, Shchors K, Swigart LB, Evan GI. Mast cells are required for angiogenesis and macroscopic expansion of Myc-induced pancreatic islet tumors. *Nat Med* (2007) 13(10):1211–8. doi:10.1038/nm1649
100. Maltby S, Khazaie K, McNagny KM. Mast cells in tumor growth: angiogenesis, tissue remodelling and immune-modulation. *Biochim Biophys Acta* (2009) 1796(1):19–26. doi:10.1016/j.bbcan.2009.02.001
101. Duparc C, Moreau L, Dzib JF, Boyer HG, Tetsi Nomigni M, Boutelet I, et al. Mast cell hyperplasia is associated with aldosterone hypersecretion in a subset of aldosterone-producing adenomas. *J Clin Endocrinol Metab* (2015) 100(4):jc20143660. doi:10.1210/jc.2014-3660
102. Lampron A, Bourdeau I, Oble S, Godbout A, Schürch W, Arjane P, et al. Regulation of aldosterone secretion by several aberrant receptors including for glucose-dependent insulinotropic peptide in a patient with an aldosteronoma. *J Clin Endocrinol Metab* (2009) 94(3):750–6. doi:10.1210/jc.2008-1340
103. El Ghorayeb N, Bourdeau I, Lacroix A. Multiple aberrant hormone receptors in Cushing's syndrome. *Eur J Endocrinol* (2015) 173(4):M45–60. doi:10.1530/EJE-15-0200
104. Lacroix A, Bourdeau I, Lampron A, Mazzuco TL, Tremblay J, Hamet P. Aberrant G-protein coupled receptor expression in relation to adrenocortical overfunction. *Clin Endocrinol (Oxf)* (2010) 73(1):1–15. doi:10.1111/j.1365-2265.2009.03689.x
105. Mazzuco TL, Grunenwald S, Lampron A, Bourdeau I, Lacroix A. Aberrant hormone receptors in primary aldosteronism. *Horm Metab Res* (2010) 42(6):416–23. doi:10.1055/s-0029-1243602
106. Lampronti I, Bianchi N, Zuccato C, Dall'acqua F, Vedaldi D, Viola G, et al. Increase in gamma-globin mRNA content in human erythroid cells treated with angelicin analogs. *Int J Hematol* (2009) 90(3):318–27. doi:10.1007/s12185-009-0422-2
107. Sealey JE, Itskovitz-Eldor J, Rubattu S, James GD, August P, Thaler I, et al. Estradiol- and progesterone-related increases in the renin-aldosterone system: studies during ovarian stimulation and early pregnancy. *J Clin Endocrinol Metab* (1994) 79(1):258–64. doi:10.1210/jcem.79.1.8027239
108. Chidambaram M, Duncan JA, Lai VS, Cattran DC, Floras JS, Scholey JW, et al. Variation in the renin angiotensin system throughout the normal menstrual cycle. *J Am Soc Nephrol* (2002) 13(2):446–52.
109. Saner-Amigh K, Mayhew BA, Mantero F, Schiavi F, White PC, Rao CV, et al. Elevated expression of luteinizing hormone receptor in aldosterone-producing adenomas. *J Clin Endocrinol Metab* (2006) 91(3):1136–42. doi:10.1210/jc.2005-1298
110. Szmuilowicz ED, Adler GK, Williams JS, Green DE, Yao TM, Hopkins PN, et al. Relationship between aldosterone and progesterone in the human menstrual cycle. *J Clin Endocrinol Metab* (2006) 91(10):3981–7. doi:10.1210/jc.2006-1154
111. Albiger NM, Sartorato P, Mariniello B, Iacobone M, Finco I, Fassina A, et al. A case of primary aldosteronism in pregnancy: do LH and GNRH receptors have a potential role in regulating aldosterone secretion? *Eur J Endocrinol* (2011) 164(3):405–12. doi:10.1530/EJE-10-0879
112. Nicolini G, Balzan S, Morelli L, Iacconi P, Sabatino L, Ripoli A, et al. LH, progesterone, and TSH can stimulate aldosterone in vitro: a study on normal adrenal cortex and aldosterone producing adenoma. *Horm Metab Res* (2014) 46(5):318–21. doi:10.1055/s-0033-1358733
113. Lacroix A, Tremblay J, Rousseau G, Bouvier M, Hamet P. Propranolol therapy for ectopic beta-adrenergic receptors in adrenal Cushing's syndrome. *N Engl J Med* (1997) 337(20):1429–34. doi:10.1056/NEJM199711133372004
114. Mune T, Murase H, Yamakita N, Fukuda T, Murayama M, Miura A, et al. Eutopic overexpression of vasopressin v1a receptor in adrenocorticotropin-independent macronodular adrenal hyperplasia. *J Clin Endocrinol Metab* (2002) 87(12):5706–13. doi:10.1210/jc.2002-020067
115. Perraudin V, Delarue C, Lefebvre H, Do Rego JL, Vaudry H, Kuhn JM. Evidence for a role of vasopressin in the control of aldosterone secretion in primary aldosteronism: in vitro and in vivo studies. *J Clin Endocrinol Metab* (2006) 91(4):1566–72. doi:10.1210/jc.2005-1453
116. Fommei E, Iervasi G. The role of thyroid hormone in blood pressure homeostasis: evidence from short-term hypothyroidism in humans. *J Clin Endocrinol Metab* (2002) 87(5):1996–2000. doi:10.1210/jcem.87.5.8464
117. Rossi GP, Ganzaroli C, Cesari M, Maresca A, Plebani M, Nussdorfer GG, et al. Endothelin receptor blockade lowers plasma aldosterone levels via different mechanisms in primary aldosteronism and high-to-normal renin hypertension. *Cardiovasc Res* (2003) 57(1):277–83. doi:10.1016/S0008-6363(02)00658-2
118. Teo AE, Garg S, Shaikh LH, Zhou J, Karet Frankl FE, Gurnell M, et al. Pregnancy, primary aldosteronism, and adrenal CTNNB1 mutations. *N Engl J Med* (2015) 373(15):1429–36. doi:10.1056/NEJMoa1504869

17

Alterations of Phosphodiesterases in Adrenocortical Tumors

Fady Hannah-Shmouni†, Fabio R. Faucz and Constantine A. Stratakis*

Program on Developmental Endocrinology and Genetics (PDEGEN), Section on Endocrinology and Genetics (SEGEN), National Institute of Child Health and Human Development (NICHD), National Institutes of Health (NIH), Bethesda, MD, USA

***Correspondence:**
Constantine A. Stratakis
stratakc@mail.nih.gov

†Submitting author:
Fady Hannah-Shmouni,
fady.hannah-shmouni@nih.gov

Alterations in the cyclic (c)AMP-dependent signaling pathway have been implicated in the majority of benign adrenocortical tumors (ACTs) causing Cushing syndrome (CS). Phosphodiesterases (PDEs) are enzymes that regulate cyclic nucleotide levels, including cyclic adenosine monophosphate (cAMP). Inactivating mutations and other functional variants in *PDE11A* and *PDE8B*, two cAMP-binding PDEs, predispose to ACTs. The involvement of these two genes in ACTs was initially revealed by a genome-wide association study in patients with micronodular bilateral adrenocortical hyperplasia. Thereafter, *PDE11A* or *PDE8B* genetic variants have been found in other ACTs, including macronodular adrenocortical hyperplasias and cortisol-producing adenomas. In addition, downregulation of *PDE11A* expression and inactivating variants of the gene have been found in hereditary and sporadic testicular germ cell tumors, as well as in prostatic cancer. PDEs confer an increased risk of ACT formation probably through, primarily, their action on cAMP levels, but other actions might be possible. In this report, we review what is known to date about *PDE11A* and *PDE8B* and their involvement in the predisposition to ACTs.

Keywords: phosphodiesterases, adrenocortical tumors, adrenal hyperplasia, Cushing syndrome, genetics, Carney complex, cAMP

INTRODUCTION

The development and function of the endocrine system is highly dependent on second messengers in hormonal signaling. Advances in molecular and genetic studies and appreciation for the impact of second messengers on endocrine physiology and disease sparked important discoveries in signal pathway research especially over the past decades. The first second messenger to be identified was cyclic adenosine monophosphate (cAMP), described in 1958 by Earl Sutherland (1). The production and degradation of cAMP is regulated by adenyl cyclases (AC) and phosphodiesterases (PDEs),

---

Abbreviations: AC, adenyl cyclase; ACTH, adrenocorticotropic hormone; AIMAH, ACTH-independent macronodular adrenal hyperplasia; AMP/ATP, adenosine monophosphate/adenosine triphosphate; Alleles, alternative forms of a gene; cAMP, cyclic adenosine monophosphate; CNC, Carney complex; CS, Cushing syndrome; CREB, cAMP-response element-binding protein; GMP/GDP/GTP, guanosine monophosphate/guanosine diphosphate/guanosine triphosphate; Genes, units of inheritance at specific locations (loci) on a chromosome; GPCRs, G protein-coupled receptors; GWA, genome-wide association; heterozygous, a genotype with two different alleles of a gene for a particular trait; homozygous, a genotype with the same allele of a gene for a particular trait; MMAD, massive macronodular adrenocortical disease; mutations, alteration of genetic material producing a new variation; PBAD, primary bimorphic adrenocortical disease; PBMAH, primary bilateral macronodular adrenocortical hyperplasia; PDEs, phosphodiesterases; phenotype, detectable expression of a genotype; PKA, protein kinase A; PPNAD, primary pigmented micronodular adrenal disease; PRKAR1A, protein kinase A regulatory subunit type 1.

respectively (**Figure 1**) (1, 2). Recent studies have demonstrated a link between genetic alterations in PDEs and increased predisposition of tumor formation, particularly in the prostate, testis, and the adrenal cortex (3, 4). In primary bilateral macronodular adrenocortical hyperplasia (PBMAH), aberrant expression of several non-mutated G-protein-coupled receptors (GPCRs) showed that cAMP signaling could be increased without genetic mutations (5). In primary pigmented nodular adrenocortical disease (PPNAD), germline inactivating mutations of the protein kinase A regulatory subunit type 1 (*PRKAR1A*)-linked cAMP-dependent protein kinase (PKA) to adrenocortical tumors (ACTs) (6). Indeed, cAMP signaling dysregulation through expression defects or mutations appears to underlie the pathogenesis of most benign ACTs (5, 7).

Phosphodiesterases exist in over 100 isoforms and are derived from 21 genes separated into 11 *PDE* gene families (summarized in **Table 1**) (8–10). PDEs function through the hydrolyzation of cAMP (PDEs isoform 4, 7, and 8) and cyclic guanosine monophosphate (cGMP) (PDEs isoforms 5, 6, and 9) into AMP and GMP, respectively (8, 9). Dual-specificity PDEs (acting on both cAMP and cGMP with varying affinities) include the PDE1, PDE2, PDE3, PDE10, and PDE11 enzymes. All PDEs share a major structural feature; a conserved catalytic domain with about 300 amino acids located near the C-terminal regions, and a variable regulatory domain located in the N-terminal regions. PDEs vary in a number of ways, including a difference in substrate selectivity, tissue distribution, kinetic, and tissue expression (**Table 1**). The adrenal cortex expresses several isoforms of PDEs, including PDE2A

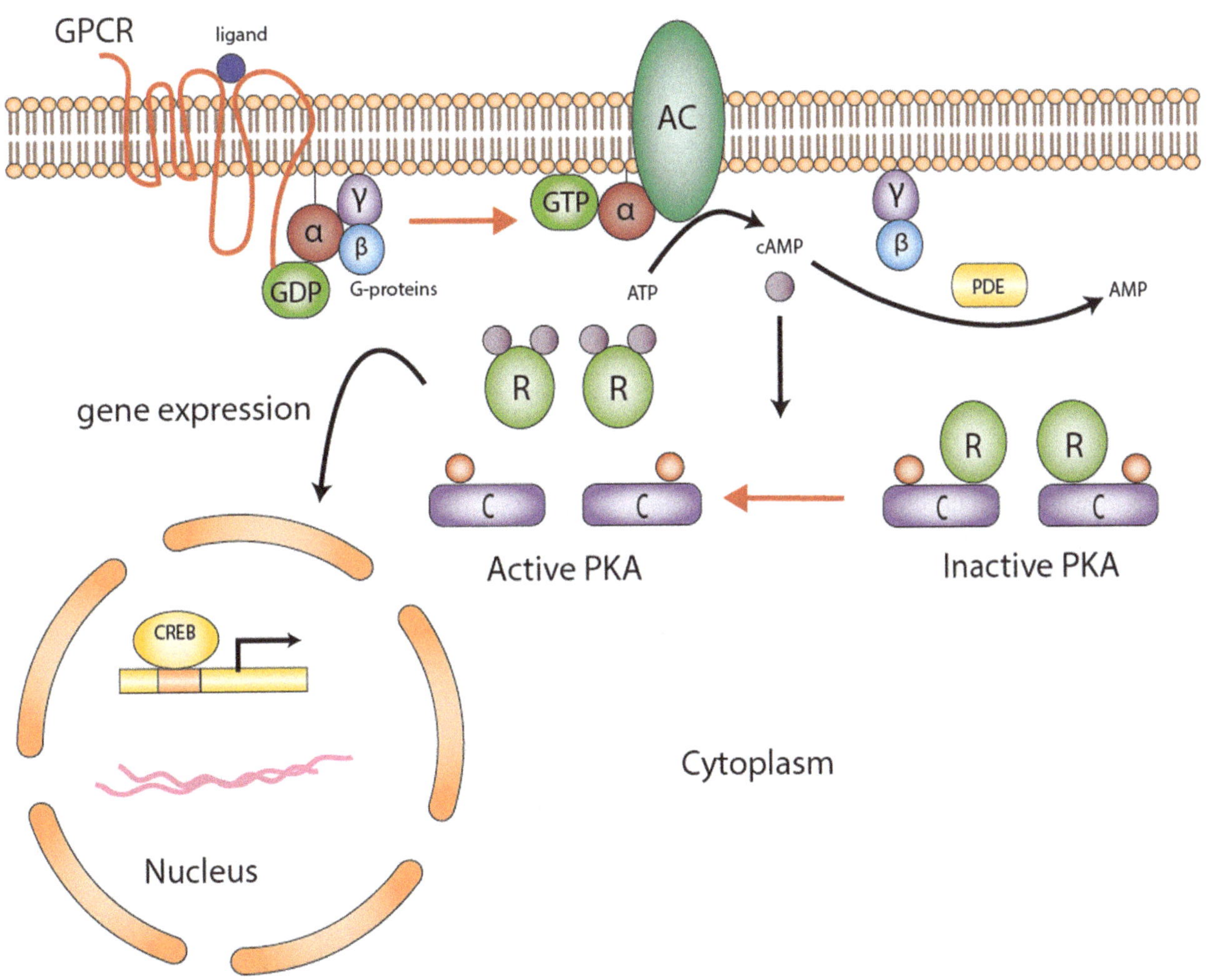

FIGURE 1 | The cyclic AMP-dependent signaling pathway. G protein-coupled receptors (GPCRs) undergo conformational changes in response to various extracellular stimuli. Gsα subunit (G-proteins) exchanges GDP for GTP that activates adenylyl cyclase (AC), converting ATP to cAMP. Elevated cAMP levels, regulated by PDEs (also responsible for degradation of cGMP to GMP), then activate protein kinase A (PKA). PKA consists of a tetramer of two homo- or heterodimers regulatory subunits (*R*) and two catalytic subunits (*C*) responsible for the phosphorylation of several enzymes and transcription factors downstream [e.g., cAMP-response element-binding protein (CREB)]. The end product is gene expression to mediate cell growth and differentiation. Abbreviations: α, β, γ, G_s-protein subunits; AC, adenyl cyclase; C, catalytic subunit of protein kinase A; cAMP, cyclic AMP; CREB, cyclic AMP response element-binding protein, a transcription factor; GPCR, G-protein-coupled receptor; PDE, phosphodiesterase; PKA, protein kinase A; R, the regulatory subunits of protein kinase. Courtesy of Stratakis Lab, NICHD, NIH.

TABLE 1 | Characteristics of phosphodiesterases (PDEs).

PDEs	Gene(s)	Locus	Substrate	Major functions/regulations
PDE1	*PDE1A* *PDE1B* *PDE1C*	2q32.1 12q13.2 17p14.3	cAMP > cGMP cAMP > cGMP cAMP = cGMP	• Vascular smooth muscle contraction, sperm function • Dopaminergic signaling, immune cell activation • Vascular smooth muscle cell proliferation, sperm function
PDE2	*PDE2A*	11q13.4	cAMP = cGMP	• Aldosterone and ACTH secretion, long-term memory
PDE3	*PDE3A* *PDE3B*	12p12.2 11p15.2	cAMP > cGMP	• Cardiac contractility, platelet aggregation, vascular smooth muscle contraction, oocyte maturation, and regulation of renin release • Impact on lipolysis, glycogenolysis, insulin secretion, and cardiac function
PDE4	*PDE4A* *PDE4B* *PDE4C* *PDE4D*	19p13.2 1p31.3 19p13.11 5q11.2–q12.1	cAMP	• Brain function, monocyte and macrophage activation, neutrophil infiltration, vascular smooth muscle proliferation, fertility • Regulate β-adrenergic signaling and excitation–contraction coupling in the heart and thus play a role in vasodilatation and cardiac contractility
PDE5	*PDE5A*	4q26	cGMP > cAMP	• Modulate NO/cGMP effects in vascular smooth muscles, platelets, and lower urinary tract organs • Cardiac stress response
PDE6	*PDE6A* *PDE6B* *PDE6C*	5q32 4p16.3 10q23.33	cGMP > cAMP	• Primary effector enzyme in the phototransduction cascade • Regulate cGMP concentration in rod and cone photoreceptors
PDE7	*PDE7A* *PDE7B*	8q13.1 6q23.3	cAMP	• Play a critical role in the regulation of the human T-cells function
PDE8	*PDE8A* *PDE8B*	15q25.3 5q13.3	cAMP	• Play a role in T-cell activation • Regulate adrenal steroidogenesis • Regulate TSH levels • Control of LH signaling and steroidogenesis in Leydig cells
PDE9	*PDE9A*	21q22.3	cGMP > cAMP	• Energy balance
PDE10	*PDE10A*	6q27	cAMP > cGMP	• Play a role in striatal activation and behavioral activity
PDE11	*PDE11A*	2q31.2	cAMP = cGMP	• Only the A4 splice variant is expressed in adrenal tissue • Sperm production

ACTH, adrenocorticotropic hormone; cAMP, cyclic adenosine monophosphate; cGMP, cyclic guanine monophosphate; LH, luteinizing hormone; PDE11A, phosphodiesterase 11A gene; NO, nitric oxide; TSH, thyroid-stimulating hormone.
Adapted from Ref. (10).

that has been implicated in the downregulation of aldosterone production in adrenal zona glomerulosa cells and the regulation of the adrenocorticotropic hormone (ACTH)-induced increase in intracellular cAMP in the zona fasciculata cells (11).

Recent studies have demonstrated inactivating mutations and other germline variants in *PDE11A* and *PDE8B* in ACT causing Cushing syndrome (CS) (12–17). Here, we present a brief overview of the alterations of PDEs in ACTs. Given the breadth of this topic, we begin with a discussion of the cAMP-dependent signaling pathway in physiology, describe the current classification of ACTs, and then proceed with a discussion of PDE alterations in ACTs.

THE cAMP-DEPENDENT SIGNALING PATHWAY

Briefly, GPCRs undergo conformational changes in response to various extracellular stimuli, such as ACTH (**Figure 1**). The first step in cAMP activation in adrenal cortex is the action of ACTH on its seven-transmembrane receptor, ACTHR [e.g., melanocortin 2 receptor (MC2R)]. This activation leads to the dissociation of the Gsα subunit (encoded by the *GNAS* gene) from the heterotrimeric G-proteins, activation of AC, generation of cAMP, and activating PKA (**Figure 1**). PKA exists as a tetrameric complex of two regulatory subunits (alpha and beta type 1 or alpha and beta type 2, encoded by *PRKAR1A*, *PRKAR2A*, *PRKAR1B*, and *PRKAR2B*) and two catalytic subunits (catalytic alpha and catalytic beta, encoded by *PRKACA* and *PRKACB*, respectively); the latter subunits are responsible for the phosphorylation of several enzymes and transcription factors downstream, including the cAMP-response element-binding protein (CREB). Abnormalities in some of these genes predispose to the formation of cortisol-producing ACTs (**Figure 2**) and increased steroid hormone secretion. The latter is often mediated by secondary factors regulated by PKA; in one study, silencing p54(nrb)/NONO expression in H295R human adrenocortical cells decreased the ability of the cells to increase intracellular cAMP production and subsequent cortisol biosynthesis in response to ACTH (18). The expression of multiple PDE isoforms, including PDE2A, PDE3A, PDE3B, PDE4A, PDE4D, and PDE11A, was induced in p54(nrb)/NONO knockdown cells, which suggests that these proteins may be responsible for the splicing and degradation of *PDE* transcripts (18). Studies in knockout mice (**Table 2**) have also pointed out to the significance of cAMP signaling-regulating genes in ACT formation.

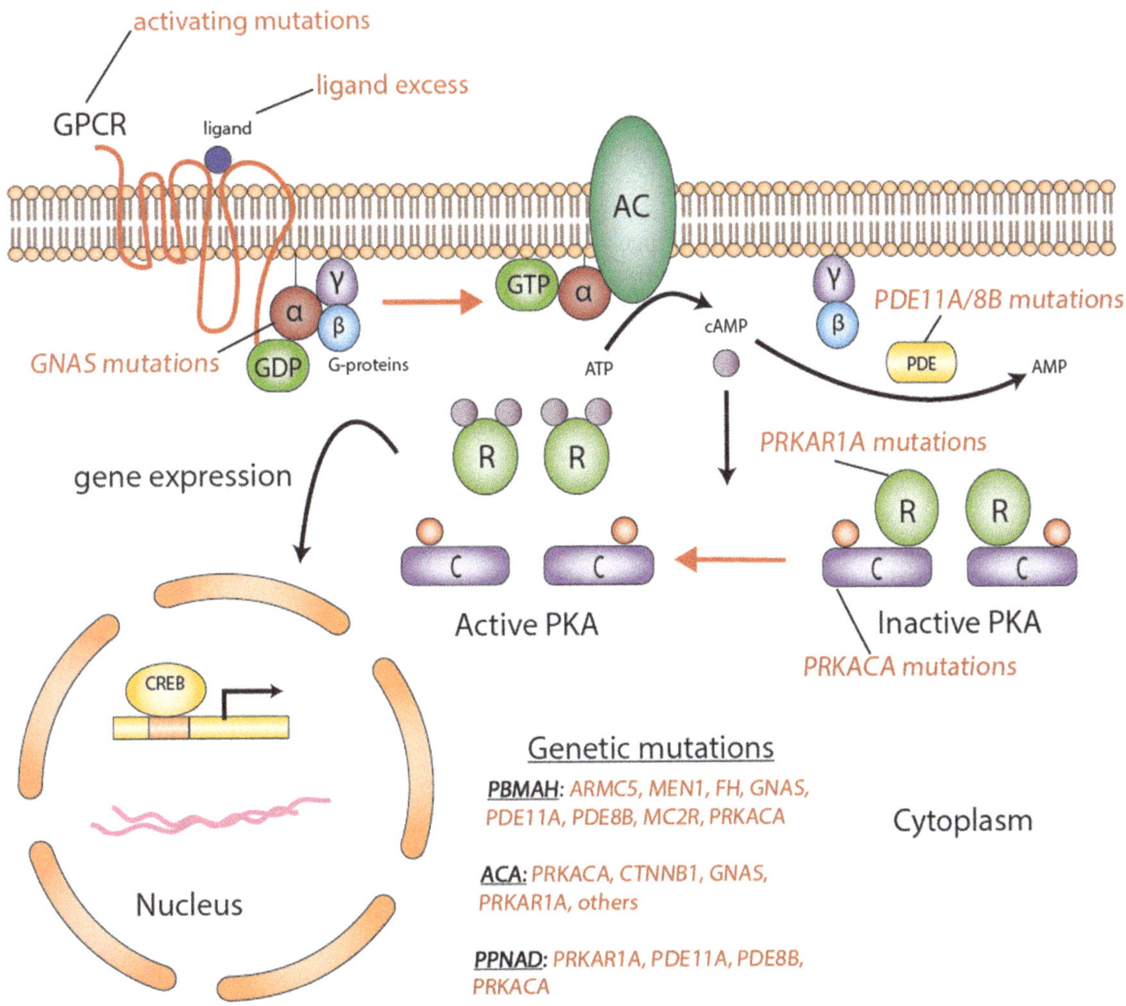

FIGURE 2 | Aberrations in the cyclic AMP-dependent signaling pathway in adrenocortical tumors. Mutations such as activating mutations of *GNAS*, in McCune–Albright syndrome; inactivating germline mutations in *PDE11A* in primary pigmented nodular adrenocortical hyperplasia (PPNAD); and inactivating germline mutations of *PRKAR1A* in Carney's complex, all predispose to the formation of adrenocortical tumors through a cyclic AMP-dependent process. Abbreviations: α, β, γ, G_s-protein subunits; AC, adenyl cyclase; ACA, adrenocortical adenoma; C, catalytic subunit of protein kinase A; cAMP, cyclic AMP; CREB, cyclic AMP response element-binding protein, a transcription factor; GPCR, G-protein-coupled receptor; PBMAH, bilateral macronodular adrenocortical hyperplasia; PDE, phosphodiesterase; PKA, protein kinase A; R, the regulatory subunits of protein kinase; PPNAD, primary pigmented nodular adrenocortical disease. Courtesy of Stratakis Lab, NICHD, NIH.

A HISTORICAL PERSPECTIVE AND NOMENCLATURE OF ADRENOCORTICAL TUMORS

In 1912, Cushing described the pituitary tumors that cause the condition that today bears his name (19). The causes of CS are broadly divided into ACTH-dependent and ACTH-independent disease. In 1984, the first description of Carney complex, a multiple neoplasia syndrome associated with spotty skin pigmentation, cardiac myxomas, pituitary tumors, and CS caused by PPNAD, provided the first insight into the genetic forms of ACT (20). In 1991, Weinstein et al. (21) described Gsα subunit (*GNAS*) mutations in individuals with McCune-Albright syndrome (MAS); MAS is classically associated with polyostotic fibrous dysplasia, café-au-lait skin spots, and precocious puberty but also with adrenal hyperplasia and/or tumors (21). MAS, albeit rare, appears to be the most frequent cause of CS among ACTH-independent adrenal hyperplasia in the infantile period (22).

TABLE 2 | Adrenocortical phosphodiesterases mouse models and phenotypes.

Gene	Model	Phenotype
PDE2	Pde2a^{tm1Dgen} Pde2a^{tm1Dtst}	Homozygous for knockout allele exhibit lethality early in gestation therefore difficult to study (58)
PDE8	Pde8b^{tm1Dgen}	Homozygous for null allele with increased urine corticosterone, decreased serum ACTH, and decreased sensitivity to a PDE8-selective inhibitor (39)
PDE11	Pde11a^{tm1Lex}	No adrenal phenotype. Homozygous for null allele have reduced sperm concentration (45)

Kirschner et al. (23, 24) identified the regulatory subunit type 1A (R1α) of PKA (encoded by the *PRKAR1A* gene on chromosome 17q22-24) as the cause of PPNAD and CNC (25). PPNAD is the most frequent endocrine manifestation in CNC.

In 2006, the first association between *PDE* mutations and ACT, using a genome-wide association (GWA) study approach, was identified in patients with CS with PPNAD but without *GNAS* or *PRKAR1A* mutations (12). Three inactivating mutations in *PDE11A* were identified initially in patients, predominantly children, with micronodular adrenocortical hyperplasia (iMAD), a rare form of bilateral adrenocortical hyperplasia (BAH) leading to CS. Subsequent studies found other *PDE* mutations or functional variants, including alterations in *PDE8B*, in other ACTs, including PBMAH (14–17, 26, 27).

The new genetic findings influenced the diagnostic classification of these ACTs (5). In brief, three major ACTH-independent ACT subtypes exist: bilateral hyperplasias (BAH), adrenocortical adenomas (ACA), and adrenocortical cancer (ACC) (5). PBMAH, a form of BAH, is estimated to affect ~2% of patients with endogenous CS (5). This disease should be distinguished from secondary adrenocortical hyperplasia, which can occur after long-term stimulation by ACTH in Cushing disease (CS in the context of an ACTH-producing pituitary tumor) or ectopic ACTH secretion, predominantly from a neuroendocrine tumor (28). PBMAH is usually sporadic, but familial forms have been described (29). Cortisol-producing adenoma (CPA) is a benign subset of ACAs causing adrenal CS.

Bilateral adrenocortical hyperplasias can be broadly classified on the basis of the size of their nodules into micronodular (<1 cm in diameter) or macrocronodular (>1 cm in diameter) (5). The micronodular subtype is divided into pigmented (c-PPNAD, familial seen in CNC, or isolated, i-PPNAD) and not pigmented (e.g., iMAD) (5). PBMAH is the most common macronodular BAH [previously referred to as massive macronodular adrenocortical disease (MMAD) and ACTH-independent macronodular adrenocortical hyperplasia (AIMAH)] and is largely caused by mutations of the *ARMC5* gene (30); several genes have been implicated in other forms of macronodular BAH, including *GNAS*, *APC*, and *MEN1*. Patients with MAS may develop a form of macronodular bilateral adrenal hyperplasia, called primary bimorphic adrenocortical disease (PBAD).

PDEs IN ADRENOCORTICAL TUMORS

Mutations and variants in ACTs that lead to functional abnormalities of cAMP signaling have been reported in the *GNAS*, *PRKAR1A*, *PDE11A*, and *PDE8B* genes (9). Mutation-negative disease with activation of the cAMP pathway has been reported (31), suggesting that additional genetic (or perhaps epigenetic) "hits" may play a role in the pathogenesis of ACT.

PDE2A

The predominant PDE isoform in adrenal tissue is PDE2A (32). Three PDE2A isoforms exist: PDE2A1, PDE2A2, and PDE2A3, and exhibit higher affinity for cGMP than cAMP (33). PDE2A is implicated in the downregulation of aldosterone production in adrenal zona glomerulosa cells and the regulation of the ACTH-induced increase in intracellular cAMP (11). This ACTH response is described as a rapid and sustained activation of AC followed by a biphasic effect of ACTH on PDE2 activity with an initial and rapid inhibition, followed by a delayed activation (11). In one study, PDE2 involvement was observed to be more important in rat than in human adrenal glomerulosa cells, whereas AC was more stimulated in human than in rat glomerulosa cells (34). Thus, PDE2 activity is involved in the regulation of cAMP accumulation induced by ACTH and suggests that ACTH inhibits this activity. However, no studies to date have reported an association between alterations in PDE2 and ACTs. PDE2A has been shown to be upregulated in beta-catenin (*CTNNB1*)-mutated ACTs (35). However, it has not been studied in individuals with PPNAD that also have somatic mutations in *CTNNB1* (36, 37). Importantly, *Pde2a* knockout mice do not survive past 17–18 days gestation (38); *Pde2a* heterozygote mice are not known to develop ACTs or even hypertension.

PDE8

The PDE8 family of proteins includes two genes, *PDE8A* and *PDE8B*, which encode for two highly specific enzymes responsible for the highest affinity of the PDEs to degrade cAMP (32). Through negative modulation, these isomers play an important role in adrenal, ovarian, and testicular steroidogenesis (32, 39). Although homologous in structure and function, *PDE8B* is the major regulator of one or more pools of cAMP in steroidogenesis and carries the highest expression across zona fasciculata compared to other PDEs (14, 32, 39). PDE8A is expressed from a small population of zona fasciculata cells that lie adjacent to zona glomerulosa (32), while *PDE8B* is expressed throughout the zona fasciculata. The *PDE8B* locus, like that of other PDEs, is quite complex and encodes multiple isoforms, arising mainly from alternative splicing and displaying tissue-specific expression (32, 40, 41). Tsai et al. (39) demonstrated that *Pde8b* knockout mice showed elevated urinary corticosterone as a result of adrenal hypersensitivity toward ACTH (39), pointing to PDE8B's possible role in regulating steroidogenesis. However, the investigators also demonstrated that these mice do not develop adrenal hyperplasia or increased adrenal size.

A GWA study identified a link between the 5q13 locus harboring the *PDE8B* gene and iMAD (12). A novel missense mutation was found in *PDE8B* (c.914A > C, p.P305H) in a 2-year-old girl with iMAD where her father carried the same genetic defect with subclinical disease (15); this pattern of an unaffected male passing on the disease to an affected female was also seen in other alterations of PDEs (12, 42). The p.P305H mutation led to higher levels of cAMP when introduced in HEK293 cells (15).

A more recent study of ACTs found several variations in *PDE8B*: missense substitutions p.H391A, p.P660L, and p.V697I and the c.1365-5G>A splice variant in *PDE8B* were identified (43). Interestingly, one patient with ACC had both the missense p.R121H and the splice c.1365-5G>A variations, while the other germline *PDE8B* mutations were found in samples including PBMAH, PPNAD, and secreting and even non-secreting ACAs (43).

Perhaps, the most important recent finding confirming PDE8B's role in ACT pathogenesis was the genome-wide transcriptomic work by Wilmot Roussel et al. (44). Among over 3000 genes that showed correlation with cortisol secretion in 22 unilateral ACAs (5 non-secreting, 6 subclinical cortisol producing, and 11 cortisol producing), *PDE8B* showed the strongest positive correlation (44). Accordingly, there was marked increase of the PKA activity to cAMP ratio in secreting adenomas compared to non-secreting adenomas (44).

PDE11A

PDE11A is located on chromosome 2q31.2 and encodes a dual-specificity PDE that degrades both cAMP and cGMP (32). This gene is highly polymorphic in the general population (42) and was the first of the PDEs to be linked with an inherited condition associated with ACTs. Four different transcript variants exist (**Table 1**), with only the *PDE11A4* detected in adrenal tissues (32). *Pde11a* knockout mice show impaired sperm function and spermatogenesis (45), but no adrenal phenotype has been described for the knock out or heterozygote mouse. Several studies have reported conflicting results with regard to the adrenal expression of PDE11A, suggesting that its expression may only be driven in the diseased adrenal gland (46, 47). The exact role of *PDE11A* in regulating adrenocortical cAMP levels also remains largely unknown.

Horvath et al. (12) published the first GWA single-nucleotide polymorphism (SNP) association between *PDE11A* mutations and ACTs in patients with CS from PPNAD or iMAD without known genetic defects (12). Three inactivating mutations in *PDE11A* were identified. These tumors showed 2q31–2q35 loss of heterozygosity (LOH) and elevated cAMP levels (12), supporting *PDE11A*'s role in tumor formation. Three of the four patients had PPNAD; a mother and her daughter with the same *PDE11A* gene mutation, and a third unrelated patient with a different *PDE11A* mutation, in which the adrenal glands were described as small (largest total adrenal weight = 6.9 g and normal = 8–9 g) with very minor involvement of the superficial cortex evidenced by a few transcapsular cortical extensions into the peri-adrenal fat (48). The fourth patient's adrenal glands were slightly enlarged owing to hyperplasia of the superficial cortex with a few PPNAD-type nodules in the deep cortex (48). The *PDE11A* mutation was inherited from her father who had an enlarged right adrenal gland but no CS (48).

In another study, Horvath et al. (42) examined two relatively frequent variants of *PDE11A* in ACTs and the general population (42). Twelve of 745 controls had these variants, with a lower frequency in patients with ACTs (1.6%; $\chi^2 = 14.62$, $P < 0.0001$). *In vitro* data demonstrated elevated cAMP levels in HeLa and HEK293 cells, particularly when the p.R804H mutation was studied (42). Another study showed the p.R867G *PDE11A* gene variant in one patient with familial PBMAH (49). The mechanism by which partially inactivated *PDE11A* causes adrenocortical overgrowth is largely unclear; the most likely explanation is chronic (albeit modest) elevations of cAMP levels in adrenocortical tissues. Collectively, these experiments suggest that genetic variations in *PDE11A* may be low-penetrance alleles that occur relatively frequently in the general population and may predispose to the development of ACTs.

The association of *PDE11A* variants and ACTs was studied further in larger cohorts. Libé et al. (27) examined the role of the *PDE11A* in a large cohort of ACT, and found an inactivating mutation (p.R307*) in one ACC, with a significant difference between ACC and controls for a polymorphism in exon 6 (p.E421E; OR, 2.1; $P = 0.03$) (27). Three associated polymorphisms located in intron 10–exon 11–intron 11 were also significant in these tumors (OR, 0.5; $P = 0.01$) (27). Other variants in the study included 22 germline missense variants (18.8%) in ACA, compared to only 11 missense variants (5.7%) in controls (16 versus 10% in ACC, 19 versus 10% in ACA, and 24 versus 9% in PBMAH; OR, 3.53; $P = 0.05$) (27). This study suggested a higher frequency of mutations in ACTs, especially PBMAH, when compared to controls. In another study that examined a large cohort of patients with PBMAH, the frequency of all *PDE11A* variants (e.g., p.D609N or p.M878V) was significantly higher among patients with PBMAH (28%) than controls (7.2%) ($P = 5 \times 10^{-5}$) (17). These variants were also studied in HEK293 cells, where the mutant *PDE11A*-transfected cells had higher cAMP levels than the wild-type ones ($P < 0.05$), suggesting that these mutants exhibit diminished cAMP hydrolytic activity (17).

These experiments pointed to several important points about the possible *PDE11A*'s role in adrenocortical tumorigenesis. First, the spectrum of ACTs varies from benign to malignant. Second, bilateral disease is favored. Third, the allelic losses of the wild-type allele in ACC with missense mutations supports *PDE11A* role as a tumor suppressor gene. Fourth, *PDE11A* sequence defects may underlie at least part of the commonly found adrenocortical incidentalomas.

Alterations in PDEs may also be involved in modifying the expression of syndromic diseases associated with ACTs. CNC is caused by *PRKAR1A* mutations, as discussed earlier (23). In one study of 150 patients with CNC, a higher frequency of *PDE11A* variants was observed when compared with healthy controls (25.3 versus 6.8%, $P < 0.0001$), particularly in men (30.8 versus 13%, $P = 0.025$, PPNAD subgroup) (16). Importantly, these men had a higher incidence of large-cell calcifying Sertoli cell tumors, as well (16). Moreover, simultaneous *in vitro* inactivation of *PRKAR1A* and *PDE11A* by small inhibitory RNA led to increased PKA activity and/or cAMP signaling (16). Thus, it is conceivable that *PDE11A*-inactivating variants act in concert with other genes in disease predisposition and/or progression.

ABERRATIONS IN THE cAMP-DEPENDENT SIGNALING PATHWAY IN CORTISOL-PRODUCING ADENOMAS

Several genetic aberrations in the cAMP-dependent signaling pathway have been implicated in CPA. The most common genetic aberration in CPA is a somatic-activating mutations of *PRKACA* (c.617A>G/p.L206R) with an estimated incidence of ~42% (86 of 206 tumors studied to date) (50–52), with a predilection to younger patients with overt CS, suggesting a driver mutation role in tumorigenesis (44). Somatic mutations in *GNAS* were identified in 5–17% of CPA (53). The somatic allelic losses of *PRKAR1A* were described in 23% of CPA; these tumors were smaller in size and had a paradoxical increase in urinary cortisol levels after dexamethasone suppression (54), due to increased glucocorticoid receptor expression in ACT (55), as often observed in patients with c-PPNAD. Defects in *Wnt*-signaling have been reported in CPA, with *CTNNB1* (p.S45P, p.S45F) in ~23% of cases (56). There are still many unknown genetic defects that lead to CPA formation.

FUTURE DIRECTIONS

There has been significant progress in PDE-related research over the past two decades. Genetic testing has uncovered several adrenocortical conditions that were linked to aberrations in *PDE*, often preceded by a long and insidious pre-diagnostic course. This has allowed earlier identification and better management of these lesions. However, there are several unanswered questions. PDE-related research is hampered by inherent (i.e., complexity of their structures, many intracellular interactions, and largely unknown function) and technical issues (e.g., there is lack of specific antibodies for the multiple isoform of each PDE). In addition to improving the characterization of PDE expression and function, future studies should also focus on the characterization of patients with various ACT phenotypes and PDE genotypes.

Preliminary results in using recombinant compounds to activate or inhibit the PDE11A structure may have important implications for drug development. Jäger et al. (47) produced approximately fourfold to fivefold increase in PDE11A-mediated hydrolysis of both cAMP and cGMP, with some degree of PDE11A specificity, with a cGMP analog (Rp-8-pCPTPET-cGMPS) bound to the PDE11A4 GAF domain (47). Furthermore, Ceyhan et al. (57) showed that BC11-28 and BC11-38 (potent and selective PDE11A inhibitors) in both yeast-based and enzyme assays had a >350-fold selectivity for inhibiting PDE11's cGMP hydrolytic activity versus all other PDEs, while only BC11-38 inhibited PDE11A cAMP hydrolytic activity in H295R cells (57). Thus, a targeted molecular therapy approach for lesions related to defects in PDE may aid in the future management of affected or at risk patients.

CONCLUSION

Alterations in PDEs that lead to dysregulation of the cAMP-dependent signaling pathway have been linked to the development of ACT. These lesions are usually benign and represent an important group of genetic disorders causing CS. As genetic technology continues to revolutionize the field of endocrine genetics and as we continue to discover novel disease-causing genes on an unprecedented scale, new methods to rapidly assess the functional significance of *PDE* variants singly, or in combination, will evolve. In this review, we focused our discussion on the various genotypes and phenotypes of ACT due to alterations in *PDE*, particularly mutations in *PDE8B* and *PDE11A*. Although there has been significant progress in PDE-related research over the past two decades, there are as yet unidentified molecular causes for all of these lesions. We hope that one day targeted molecular therapies will replace adrenalectomy as the treatment of choice for these lesions.

AUTHOR CONTRIBUTIONS

All authors contributed equally to the conception or design of the work; or the acquisition, analysis, or interpretation of data for the work; drafting the work or revising it critically for important intellectual content; final approval of the version to be published; agreement to be accountable for all aspects of the work in ensuring that questions related to the accuracy or integrity of any part of the work are appropriately investigated and resolved.

FUNDING

This work was supported by the intramural program of the *Eunice Kennedy Shriver* National Institute of Child Health and Human Development, National Institutes of Health (NIH), protocol HD008920.

REFERENCES

1. Rall TW, Sutherland EW. Formation of a cyclic adenine ribonucleotide by tissue particles. *J Biol Chem* (1958) 232(2):1065–76.
2. Butcher RW, Sutherland EW. Adenosine 3',5'-phosphate in biological materials. I. Purification and properties of cyclic 3',5'-nucleotide phosphodiesterase and use of this enzyme to characterize adenosine 3',5'-phosphate in human urine. *J Biol Chem* (1962) 237:1244–50.
3. Horvath A, Korde L, Greene MH, Libe R, Osorio P, Faucz FR, et al. Functional phosphodiesterase 11A mutations may modify the risk of familial and bilateral testicular germ cell tumors. *Cancer Res* (2009) 69(13):5301–6. doi:10.1158/0008-5472.CAN-09-0884
4. de Alexandre RB, Horvath AD, Szarek E, Manning AD, Leal LF, Kardauke F, et al. Phosphodiesterase sequence variants may predispose to prostate cancer. *Endocr Relat Cancer* (2015) 22(4):519–30. doi:10.1530/ERC-15-0134
5. Stratakis CA, Boikos SA. Genetics of adrenal tumors associated with Cushing's syndrome: a new classification for bilateral adrenocortical hyperplasias. *Nat Clin Pract Endocrinol Metab* (2007) 3(11):748–57. doi:10.1038/ncpendmet0648
6. Stratakis CA, Kirschner LS, Carney JA. Clinical and molecular features of the Carney complex: diagnostic criteria and recommendations for patient evaluation. *J Clin Endocrinol Metab* (2001) 86(9):4041–6. doi:10.1210/jcem.86.9.7903
7. Horvath A, Stratakis CA. Unraveling the molecular basis of micronodular adrenal hyperplasia. *Curr Opin Endocrinol Diabetes Obes* (2008) 15(3):227–33. doi:10.1097/MED.0b013e3282fe7416
8. Francis SH, Blount MA, Corbin JD. Mammalian cyclic nucleotide phosphodiesterases: molecular mechanisms and physiological functions. *Physiol Rev* (2011) 91(2):651–90. doi:10.1152/physrev.00030.2010
9. Azevedo MF, Faucz FR, Bimpaki E, Horvath A, Levy I, de Alexandre RB, et al. Clinical and molecular genetics of the phosphodiesterases (PDEs). *Endocr Rev* (2014) 35(2):195–233. doi:10.1210/er.2013-1053
10. Vezzosi D, Bertherat J. Phosphodiesterases in endocrine physiology and disease. *Eur J Endocrinol* (2011) 165(2):177–88. doi:10.1530/EJE-10-1123
11. Spiessberger B, Bernhard D, Herrmann S, Feil S, Werner C, Luppa PB, et al. cGMP-dependent protein kinase II and aldosterone secretion. *FEBS J* (2009) 276(4):1007–13. doi:10.1111/j.1742-4658.2008.06839.x
12. Horvath A, Boikos S, Giatzakis C, Robinson-White A, Groussin L, Griffin KJ, et al. A genome-wide scan identifies mutations in the gene encoding

phosphodiesterase 11A4 (PDE11A) in individuals with adrenocortical hyperplasia. *Nat Genet* (2006) 38(7):794–800. doi:10.1038/ng1809
13. Boikos SA, Horvath A, Heyerdahl S, Stein E, Robinson-White A, Bossis I, et al. Phosphodiesterase 11A expression in the adrenal cortex, primary pigmented nodular adrenocortical disease, and other corticotropin-independent lesions. *Horm Metab Res* (2008) 40(5):347–53. doi:10.1055/s-2008-1076694
14. Horvath A, Giatzakis C, Tsang K, Greene E, Osorio P, Boikos S, et al. A cAMP-specific phosphodiesterase (PDE8B) that is mutated in adrenal hyperplasia is expressed widely in human and mouse tissues: a novel PDE8B isoform in human adrenal cortex. *Eur J Hum Genet* (2008) 16(10):1245–53. doi:10.1038/ejhg.2008.85
15. Horvath A, Mericq V, Stratakis CA. Mutation in PDE8B, a cyclic AMP-specific phosphodiesterase in adrenal hyperplasia. *N Engl J Med* (2008) 358(7):750–2. doi:10.1056/NEJMc0706182
16. Libé R, Horvath A, Vezzosi D, Fratticci A, Coste J, Perlemoine K, et al. Frequent phosphodiesterase 11A gene (PDE11A) defects in patients with Carney complex (CNC) caused by PRKAR1A mutations: PDE11A may contribute to adrenal and testicular tumors in CNC as a modifier of the phenotype. *J Clin Endocrinol Metab* (2011) 96(1):E208–14. doi:10.1210/jc.2010-1704
17. Vezzosi D, Libé R, Baudry C, Rizk-Rabin M, Horvath A, Levy I, et al. Phosphodiesterase 11A (PDE11A) gene defects in patients with acth-independent macronodular adrenal hyperplasia (AIMAH): functional variants may contribute to genetic susceptibility of bilateral adrenal tumors. *J Clin Endocrinol Metab* (2012) 97(11):E2063–9. doi:10.1210/jc.2012-2275
18. Lu JY, Sewer MB. p54nrb/NONO regulates cyclic AMP-dependent glucocorticoid production by modulating phosphodiesterase mRNA splicing and degradation. *Mol Cell Biol* (2015) 35(7):1223–37. doi:10.1128/MCB.00993-14
19. Cushing H. The basophil adenomas of the pituitary body and their clinical manifestations (pituitary basophilism). 1932. *Obes Res* (1994) 2(5):486–508. doi:10.1002/j.1550-8528.1994.tb00097.x
20. Stratakis CA. Clinical genetics of multiple endocrine neoplasias, Carney complex and related syndromes. *J Endocrinol Invest* (2001) 24(5):370–83. doi:10.1007/BF03343875
21. Weinstein LS, Shenker A, Gejman PV, Merino MJ, Friedman E, Spiegel AM. Activating mutations of the stimulatory G protein in the McCune-Albright syndrome. *N Engl J Med* (1991) 325(24):1688–95. doi:10.1056/NEJM199112123252403
22. Kirk JM, Brain CE, Carson DJ, Hyde JC, Grant DB. Cushing's syndrome caused by nodular adrenal hyperplasia in children with McCune-Albright syndrome. *J Pediatr* (1999) 134(6):789–92. doi:10.1016/S0022-3476(99)70302-1
23. Kirschner LS, Carney JA, Pack SD, Taymans SE, Giatzakis C, Cho YS, et al. Mutations of the gene encoding the protein kinase A type I-alpha regulatory subunit in patients with the Carney complex. *Nat Genet* (2000) 26(1):89–92. doi:10.1038/79238
24. Kirschner LS, Sandrini F, Monbo J, Lin JP, Carney JA, Stratakis CA. Genetic heterogeneity and spectrum of mutations of the PRKAR1A gene in patients with the Carney complex. *Hum Mol Genet* (2000) 9(20):3037–46. doi:10.1093/hmg/9.20.3037
25. Rothenbuhler A, Stratakis CA. Clinical and molecular genetics of Carney complex. *Best Pract Res Clin Endocrinol Metab* (2010) 24(3):389–99. doi:10.1016/j.beem.2010.03.003
26. Horvath A, Faucz F, Finkielstain GP, Nikita ME, Rothenbuhler A, Almeida M, et al. Haplotype analysis of the promoter region of phosphodiesterase type 8B (PDE8B) in correlation with inactivating PDE8B mutation and the serum thyroid-stimulating hormone levels. *Thyroid* (2010) 20(4):363–7. doi:10.1089/thy.2009.0260
27. Libé R, Fratticci A, Coste J, Tissier F, Horvath A, Ragazzon B, et al. Phosphodiesterase 11A (PDE11A) and genetic predisposition to adrenocortical tumors. *Clin Cancer Res* (2008) 14(12):4016–24. doi:10.1158/1078-0432.CCR-08-0106
28. Lacroix A. Heredity and cortisol regulation in bilateral macronodular adrenal hyperplasia. *N Engl J Med* (2013) 369(22):2147–9. doi:10.1056/NEJMe1312792
29. Lacroix A. ACTH-independent macronodular adrenal hyperplasia. *Best Pract Res Clin Endocrinol Metab* (2009) 23(2):245–59. doi:10.1016/j.beem.2008.10.011
30. Assié G, Libé R, Espiard S, Rizk-Rabin M, Guimier A, Luscap W, et al. ARMC5 mutations in macronodular adrenal hyperplasia with Cushing's syndrome. *N Engl J Med* (2013) 369(22):2105–14. doi:10.1056/NEJMoa1304603
31. Bimpaki EI, Nesterova M, Stratakis CA. Abnormalities of cAMP signaling are present in adrenocortical lesions associated with ACTH-independent Cushing syndrome despite the absence of mutations in known genes. *Eur J Endocrinol* (2009) 161(1):153–61. doi:10.1530/EJE-09-0027
32. Lakics V, Karran EH, Boess FG. Quantitative comparison of phosphodiesterase mRNA distribution in human brain and peripheral tissues. *Neuropharmacology* (2010) 59(6):367–74. doi:10.1016/j.neuropharm.2010.05.004
33. Beavo JA, Hardman JG, Sutherland EW. Stimulation of adenosine 3',5'-monophosphate hydrolysis by guanosine 3',5'-monophosphate. *J Biol Chem* (1971) 246(12):3841–6.
34. Côté M, Payet MD, Rousseau E, Guillon G, Gallo-Payet N. Comparative involvement of cyclic nucleotide phosphodiesterases and adenylyl cyclase on adrenocorticotropin-induced increase of cyclic adenosine monophosphate in rat and human glomerulosa cells. *Endocrinology* (1999) 140(8):3594–601. doi:10.1210/endo.140.8.6889
35. Durand J, Lampron A, Mazzuco TL, Chapman A, Bourdeau I. Characterization of differential gene expression in adrenocortical tumors harboring beta-catenin (CTNNB1) mutations. *J Clin Endocrinol Metab* (2011) 96(7):E1206–11. doi:10.1210/jc.2010-2143
36. Tadjine M, Lampron A, Ouadi L, Horvath A, Stratakis CA, Bourdeau I. Detection of somatic beta-catenin mutations in primary pigmented nodular adrenocortical disease (PPNAD). *Clin Endocrinol (Oxf)* (2008) 69(3):367–73. doi:10.1111/j.1365-2265.2008.03273.x
37. Gaujoux S, Tissier F, Groussin L, Libé R, Ragazzon B, Launay P, et al. Wnt/beta-catenin and 3',5'-cyclic adenosine 5'-monophosphate/protein kinase A signaling pathways alterations and somatic beta-catenin gene mutations in the progression of adrenocortical tumors. *J Clin Endocrinol Metab* (2008) 93(10):4135–40. doi:10.1210/jc.2008-0631
38. Stephenson DT, Coskran TM, Wilhelms MB, Adamowicz WO, O'Donnell MM, Muravnick KB, et al. Immunohistochemical localization of phosphodiesterase 2A in multiple mammalian species. *J Histochem Cytochem* (2009) 57(10):933–49. doi:10.1369/jhc.2009.953471
39. Tsai LC, Shimizu-Albergine M, Beavo JA. The high-affinity cAMP-specific phosphodiesterase 8B controls steroidogenesis in the mouse adrenal gland. *Mol Pharmacol* (2011) 79(4):639–48. doi:10.1124/mol.110.069104
40. Hayashi M, Shimada Y, Nishimura Y, Hama T, Tanaka T. Genomic organization, chromosomal localization, and alternative splicing of the human phosphodiesterase 8B gene. *Biochem Biophys Res Commun* (2002) 297(5):1253–8. doi:10.1016/S0006-291X(02)02371-9
41. Gamanuma M, Yuasa K, Sasaki T, Sakurai N, Kotera J, Omori K. Comparison of enzymatic characterization and gene organization of cyclic nucleotide phosphodiesterase 8 family in humans. *Cell Signal* (2003) 15(6):565–74. doi:10.1016/S0898-6568(02)00146-8
42. Horvath A, Giatzakis C, Robinson-White A, Boikos S, Levine E, Griffin K, et al. Adrenal hyperplasia and adenomas are associated with inhibition of phosphodiesterase 11A in carriers of PDE11A sequence variants that are frequent in the population. *Cancer Res* (2006) 66(24):11571–5. doi:10.1158/0008-5472.CAN-06-2914
43. Rothenbuhler A, Horvath A, Libé R, Faucz FR, Fratticci A, Raffin Sanson ML, et al. Identification of novel genetic variants in phosphodiesterase 8B (PDE8B), a cAMP-specific phosphodiesterase highly expressed in the adrenal cortex, in a cohort of patients with adrenal tumours. *Clin Endocrinol (Oxf)* (2012) 77(2):195–9. doi:10.1111/j.1365-2265.2012.04366.x
44. Wilmot Roussel H, Vezzosi D, Rizk-Rabin M, Barreau O, Ragazzon B, René-Corail F, et al. Identification of gene expression profiles associated with cortisol secretion in adrenocortical adenomas. *J Clin Endocrinol Metab* (2013) 98(6):E1109–21. doi:10.1210/jc.2012-4237
45. Wayman C, Phillips S, Lunny C, Webb T, Fawcett L, Baxendale R, et al. Phosphodiesterase 11 (PDE11) regulation of spermatozoa physiology. *Int J Impot Res* (2005) 17(3):216–23. doi:10.1038/sj.ijir.3901307
46. Yuasa K, Kotera J, Fujishige K, Michibata H, Sasaki T, Omori K. Isolation and characterization of two novel phosphodiesterase PDE11A variants showing unique structure and tissue-specific expression. *J Biol Chem* (2000) 275(40):31469–79. doi:10.1074/jbc.M003041200

47. Jäger R, Russwurm C, Schwede F, Genieser HG, Koesling D, Russwurm M. Activation of PDE10 and PDE11 phosphodiesterases. *J Biol Chem* (2012) 287(2):1210–9. doi:10.1074/jbc.M111.263806
48. Carney JA, Gaillard RC, Bertherat J, Stratakis CA. Familial micronodular adrenocortical disease, Cushing syndrome, and mutations of the gene encoding phosphodiesterase 11A4 (PDE11A). *Am J Surg Pathol* (2010) 34(4):547–55. doi:10.1097/PAS.0b013e3181d31f49
49. Hsiao HP, Kirschner LS, Bourdeau I, Keil MF, Boikos SA, Verma S, et al. Clinical and genetic heterogeneity, overlap with other tumor syndromes, and atypical glucocorticoid hormone secretion in adrenocorticotropin-independent macronodular adrenal hyperplasia compared with other adrenocortical tumors. *J Clin Endocrinol Metab* (2009) 94(8):2930–7. doi:10.1210/jc.2009-0516
50. Beuschlein F, Fassnacht M, Assié G, Calebiro D, Stratakis CA, Osswald A, et al. Constitutive activation of PKA catalytic subunit in adrenal Cushing's syndrome. *N Engl J Med* (2014) 370(11):1019–28. doi:10.1056/NEJMoa1310359
51. Cao Y, He M, Gao Z, Peng Y, Li Y, Li L, et al. Activating hotspot L205R mutation in PRKACA and adrenal Cushing's syndrome. *Science* (2014) 344(6186):913–7. doi:10.1126/science.1249480
52. Goh G, Scholl UI, Healy JM, Choi M, Prasad ML, Nelson-Williams C, et al. Recurrent activating mutation in PRKACA in cortisol-producing adrenal tumors. *Nat Genet* (2014) 46(6):613–7. doi:10.1038/ng.2956
53. Fragoso MC, Domenice S, Latronico AC, Martin RM, Pereira MA, Zerbini MC, et al. Cushing's syndrome secondary to adrenocorticotropin-independent macronodular adrenocortical hyperplasia due to activating mutations of GNAS1 gene. *J Clin Endocrinol Metab* (2003) 88(5):2147–51. doi:10.1210/jc.2002-021362
54. Bertherat J, Groussin L, Sandrini F, Matyakhina L, Bei T, Stergiopoulos S, et al. Molecular and functional analysis of PRKAR1A and its locus (17q22-24) in sporadic adrenocortical tumors: 17q losses, somatic mutations, and protein kinase A expression and activity. *Cancer Res* (2003) 63(17):5308–19.
55. Louiset E, Stratakis CA, Perraudin V, Griffin KJ, Libé R, Cabrol S, et al. The paradoxical increase in cortisol secretion induced by dexamethasone in primary pigmented nodular adrenocortical disease involves a glucocorticoid receptor-mediated effect of dexamethasone on protein kinase A catalytic subunits. *J Clin Endocrinol Metab* (2009) 94(7):2406–13. doi:10.1210/jc.2009-0031
56. Thiel A, Reis AC, Haase M, Goh G, Schott M, Willenberg HS, et al. PRKACA mutations in cortisol-producing adenomas and adrenal hyperplasia: a single-center study of 60 cases. *Eur J Endocrinol* (2015) 172(6):677–85. doi:10.1530/EJE-14-1113
57. Ceyhan O, Birsoy K, Hoffman CS. Identification of biologically active PDE11-selective inhibitors using a yeast-based high-throughput screen. *Chem Biol* (2012) 19(1):155–63. doi:10.1016/j.chembiol.2011.12.010
58. Reed TM, Repaske DR, Snyder GL, Greengard P, Vorhees CV. Phosphodiesterase 1B knock-out mice exhibit exaggerated locomotor hyperactivity and DARPP-32 phosphorylation in response to dopamine agonists and display impaired spatial learning. *J Neurosci* (2002) 22(12):5188–97.

18

Intracellular Molecular Differences in Aldosterone-Compared to Cortisol-Secreting Adrenal Cortical Adenomas

*Eric Seidel and Ute I. Scholl**

Department of Nephrology, University Hospital Düsseldorf, Heinrich Heine University, Düsseldorf, Germany

***Correspondence:**
Ute I. Scholl
ute.scholl@med.uni-duesseldorf.de

The adrenal cortex is a major site of steroid hormone production. Two hormones are of particular importance: aldosterone, which is produced in the zona glomerulosa in response to volume depletion and hyperkalemia, and cortisol, which is produced in the zona fasciculata in response to stress. In both cases, acute stimulation leads to increased hormone production, and chronic stimulation causes hyperplasia of the respective zone. Aldosterone- and cortisol-producing adenomas (APAs and CPAs) are benign tumors of the adrenal cortex that cause excess hormone production, leading to primary aldosteronism and Cushing's syndrome, respectively. About 40% of the APAs carry somatic heterozygous gain-of-function mutations in the K^+ channel *KCNJ5*. These mutations lead to sodium permeability, depolarization, activation of voltage-gated Ca^{2+} channels, and Ca^{2+} influx. Mutations in the Na^+/K^+-ATPase subunit *ATP1A1* and the plasma membrane Ca^{2+}-ATPase *ATP2B3* similarly cause Na^+ or H^+ permeability and depolarization, whereas mutations in the Ca^{2+} channel *CACNA1D* directly lead to increased calcium influx. One in three CPAs carries a recurrent gain-of-function mutation (L206R) in the *PRKACA* gene, encoding the catalytic subunit of PKA. This mutation causes constitutive PKA activity by abolishing the binding of the inhibitory regulatory subunit to the catalytic subunit. These mutations activate pathways that are relatively specific to the respective cell type (glomerulosa versus fasciculata), and there is little overlap in mutation spectrum between APAs and CPAs, but co-secretion of both hormones can occur. Mutations in *CTNNB1* (beta-catenin) and *GNAS* (Gsα) are exceptions, as they can cause both APAs and CPAs through pathways that are incompletely understood.

Keywords: ***KCNJ5*, *CACNA1D*, *ATP1A1*, *ATP2B3*, *CTNNB1***

INTRODUCTION

Adrenal masses are common tumors in humans. Adrenal incidentalomas may be found in more than 4% of computed tomography series (1), and about 7% are malignant (2). Among hormone-producing lesions, besides pheochromocytomas, cortisol-producing and aldosterone-producing adenomas (CPAs and APAs) of the adrenal cortex are frequently diagnosed (2). Aldosterone and cortisol are physiologically synthesized in the two outer layers of the adrenal cortex (zonae glomerulosa and fasciculata, respectively) from their common precursor cholesterol. The two main stimuli of aldosterone production are angiotensin II (ATII) and hyperkalemia. ATII levels rise in states of volume depletion, *via* activation of the renin–angiotensin system. Binding of ATII to the AT1 receptor, a G protein-coupled receptor in the glomerulosa membrane, leads to the inhibition of potassium channels, depolarization and activation of voltage-gated calcium channels, and the release of calcium from intracellular stores (**Figure 1**). Other factors that physiologically regulate aldosterone release in concert with ATII and K^+ are corticotropin (ACTH, stimulatory) and atrial natriuretic peptide (ANP, inhibitory) (3). Binding of aldosterone to the mineralocorticoid receptor leads to the increased activity of downstream effectors, such as the Na^+/K^+-ATPase or the epithelial sodium channel (ENaC) (4). The increased activity of these pumps and channels in kidney and intestine causes increased sodium and water reabsorption and an increase in systemic blood pressure.

Cortisol is released from the zona fasciculata upon stimulation by pituitary ACTH, in response to stress. ACTH binds to the melanocortin receptor 2, a G protein-coupled receptor, which activates adenylate cyclase (6). As a result, cAMP is produced, which binds to the regulatory subunit of protein kinase A (PKA), causing release of its catalytic subunit. The catalytic subunit then phosphorylates target proteins, such as CREB and ATF, which lead to cortisol production and proliferation (7) (**Figure 1**).

Cortisol influences a variety of biological processes, including skeletal growth, immune response, glucose and lipid metabolism, cognition, and reproduction (8–10).

Cortisol-producing adenomas and APAs feature the compelling combination of both hormone production and proliferation, suggesting that they carry genetic changes that activate both processes. Such changes have been identified over the past 5 years through exome sequencing. Comparing DNA sequences from tumor specimens and corresponding normal tissue (such as blood or adjacent tissue) can reveal tumor-specific (somatic) mutations, which are candidates for disease causation (11). This review will discuss recent genetic discoveries in APAs and CPAs and the underlying pathways.

KCNJ5 MUTATIONS IN PRIMARY ALDOSTERONISM

Primary aldosteronism (PA) features autonomous production of aldosterone from the adrenal gland and accounts for about 10% of hypertension in referral centers. The two most common causes are APAs and bilateral adrenal hyperplasia. Other causes, such as unilateral hyperplasia, malignant tumors, or familial hyperaldosteronism, are rare (12–16).

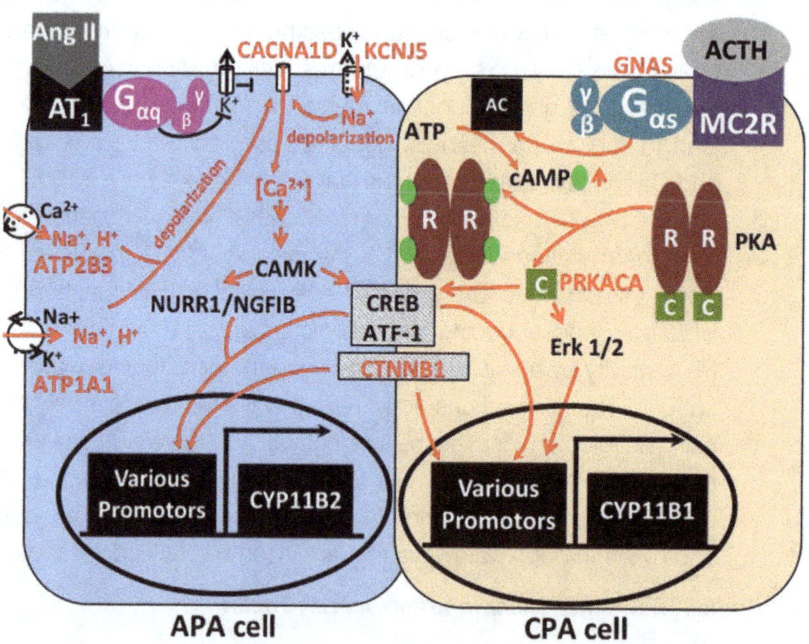

FIGURE 1 | Signaling pathways affected by mutations in APAs and CPAs. In zona glomerulosa, binding of angiotensin II (AngII) to its receptor inhibits potassium channels *via* G protein signaling. This leads to depolarization and opening of voltage-gated calcium channels. Increased intracellular calcium results in the activation of Ca^{2+}/calmodulin-dependent protein kinase (CAMK) and the activation of transcription factors, such as NURR1/NGFIB, CREB, and ATF-1. As a consequence, genes involved in proliferation and aldosterone production (e.g., aldosterone synthase, *CYP11B2*) are activated (5). Mutations in *KCNJ5*, *ATP1A1*, and *ATP2B3* lead to abnormal permeability for sodium or protons, which causes cellular depolarization and activation of the same pathways. Similarly, mutations in the calcium channel gene *CACNA1D* lead to increased calcium influx. In the zona fasciculata, binding of corticotropin (ACTH) to the melanocortin receptor (MC2R) causes activation of adenylate cyclase (AC) by the $G_{\alpha s}$ subunit (encoded by *GNAS*). Binding of cAMP to the regulatory subunit ("R") of protein kinase A (PKA) leads to release of the catalytic subunit ("C," encoded by *PRKACA*) from the complex. Transcription factors CREB, ATF-1, and Erk 1/2 cause increased expression of genes involved in proliferation and cortisol production, such as 11β-hydroxylase (*CYP11B1*). Hypercortisolism can occur due to activating mutations in *GNAS* and *PRKACA*. Activating mutations in β-catenin (*CTNNB1*) are found in both APAs and CPAs; the underlying mechanisms are incompletely understood.

In the first exome sequencing study of APAs, Choi et al. analyzed four tumors and corresponding blood samples (11). This revealed only two to three somatic mutations per tumor. One gene (*KCNJ5*) was mutated in two tumors, with one tumor carrying a heterozygous G151R mutation, and the second carrying a heterozygous L168R mutation. By Sanger sequencing, these two mutations were found in 6 of 18 additional APAs. *KCNJ5* encodes an inward rectifier potassium channel, Kir3.4, or GIRK4. The G151 and L168 residues are located within or close to the selectivity filter of the channel (17), which allows only potassium, but not the smaller sodium ions, to pass through the channel. This suggested an effect of the variants on potassium selectivity. Accordingly, by electrophysiology, mutant channels were found to be permeable to sodium and cause cellular depolarization. These effects were inferred to contribute to aldosterone production and proliferation through the activation of voltage-gated calcium channels and calcium entry (3, 11) (**Figure 1**). Additional support for the notion that *KCNJ5* mutations are sufficient to cause aldosterone production and proliferation came from the discovery of heterozygous germ line *KCNJ5* mutations in families with early-onset PA and massive bilateral adrenal hyperplasia (11, 18–20). The high frequency of *KCNJ5* mutations in APAs (about 35% in European cohorts, more than 60% in Asian cohorts) has subsequently been confirmed in large cohorts (21–29) (**Table 1**). A higher prevalence in Asian cohorts may be due to selection bias; individuals with *KCNJ5* mutations tend to have a more florid presentation at least in some cohorts. Interestingly, *KCNJ5* mutations are more prevalent in females than in males, which could account for the higher overall prevalence of APAs in females, a finding that remains unexplained. *In vitro* studies in the aldosterone-producing human adrenocortical cancer cell line HAC15 have demonstrated that gain-of-function mutations in *KCNJ5* lead to increased expression of aldosterone synthase and increased aldosterone production (30–32). Lastly, a recent study confirmed the role of *CYP11B2* transcriptional regulators NURR1 and ATF2 in mutant *KCNJ5*-induced aldosterone production (33) (**Figure 1**).

KCNJ5 MUTATIONS AND GLUCOCORTICOIDS

Interestingly, tumors with *KCNJ5* mutations tend to be larger than other tumors and have fasciculata-like features by histopathology and gene expression analysis, which may have implications for the radiological diagnosis of these tumors (34–36). Another line of evidence pointing to a more fasciculata-like or mixed glomerulosa–fasciculata phenotype of *KCNJ5*-positive APAs is the finding that heterologous expression of a *KCNJ5* variant in HAC15 cells causes not only upregulation of *CYP11B2* expression but also increased expression of *CYP11B1* and synthesis of hybrid steroids 18-hydroxycorticsol and 18-oxocortisol, as well as corticosterone (31, 33). This raises the question whether *KCNJ5*-positive APAs produce clinically relevant amounts of glucocorticoids. Interestingly, hypersecretion of cortisol and aldosterone are not

TABLE 1 | Mutation frequencies in APAs, A/CPAs, and CPAs.

Reference	*N*	APA						A/CPA		CPA		
		CACNA1D	*KCNJ5*	*ATP2B3*	*ATP1A1*	*GNAS*	*CTNNB1*	*KCNJ5*	*GNAS*	*GNAS*	*PRKACA*	*CTNNB1*
Beuschlein et al. (66)	99	–	–	–	–	–	–	–	–	N/A	22.2	N/A
Goh et al. (69)	55	–	–	–	–	–	–	–	–	5.5	23.6	16.4
Cao et al. (67)	87	–	–	–	–	–	–	–	–	N/A	65.5	N/A
Sato et al. (68)	65	–	–	–	–	–	–	–	–	16.9	52.3	N/A
Di Dalmazi et al. (71)	100	–	–	–	–	–	–	–	–	N/A	22.0	N/A
Thiel et al. (41)	52	–	–	–	–	–	–	–	–	7.7	23.1	25.0
Thiel et al. (41)	4	–	–	–	–	–	–	50.0	NA	–	–	–
Yamada et al. (40)	3	–	–	–	–	–	–	66.7	NA	–	–	–
Nakajima et al. (42)	10	–	–	–	–	–	–	60.0	20.0	–	–	–
Xekouki et al. (84)	53	N/A	30.2	N/A	N/A	N/A	N/A	–	–	–	–	–
Taguchi et al. (28)	23	N/A	65.2	N/A	N/A	N/A	N/A	–	–	–	–	–
Kitamoto et al. (85)	108	1.9	69.4	2.8		N/A	N/A	–	–	–	–	–
Boulkroun et al. (86)	380	N/A	33.9	N/A	N/A	N/A	N/A	–	–	–	–	–
Azizan et al. (87)	73	N/A	41.1	N/A	N/A	N/A	N/A	–	–	–	–	–
Cheng et al. (88)	69	N/A	37.7	N/A	N/A	N/A	N/A	–	–	–	–	–
Kuppusamy et al. (89)	195	N/A	24.6	N/A	N/A	N/A	N/A	–	–	–	–	–
Zheng et al. (27)	168	0.6	76.8	0.6	2.4	N/A	N/A	–	–	–	–	–
Scholl et al. (36)	97	10.3	37.1	3.1	8.2	N/A	2.1	–	–	–	–	–
Scholl et al. (45)	64	7.8	32.8	3.1	1.6	N/A	3.1	–	–	–	–	–
Nakajima et al. (42)	33	N/A	72.3	N/A	N/A	6.1	N/A	–	–	–	–	–
Beuschlein et al. (47)	308	N/A	38.3	1.6	5.2	N/A	N/A	–	–	–	–	–
Williams et al. (24)	112	N/A	39.3	0.9	6.3	N/A	N/A	–	–	–	–	–
Akerstrom et al. (22)	348	N/A	45.1	N/A	N/A	N/A	N/A	–	–	–	–	–
Fernandes-Rosa et al. (23)	474	9.3	38.0	1.7	5.3	N/A	N/A	–	–	–	–	–
Akerstrom et al. (83)	198	1.5	46.5	1.5	3.0	N/A	5.1	–	–	–	–	–
Hong et al. (29)	66	0.0	71.2	0.0	0.0	N/A	N/A	–	–	–	–	–
Wu et al. (25)	148	0.0	59.5	0.7	1.4	N/A	N/A	–	–	–	–	–

N, number of study subjects; N/A, not available.

mutually exclusive in adrenal adenomas, and cases of aldosterone and cortisol co-secreting adenomas (A/CPAs) have been reported (37–40). This phenotype may be underdiagnosed due to incomplete screening for subclinical Cushing's syndrome (CS) in patients with APAs; many of these patients will not receive dexamethasone suppression tests. Yamada et al. reported three female patients with hypertension and hypokalemia who were diagnosed with A/CPAs. Two had *KCNJ5* mutations (G151R and L168R) (40). Thiel et al. reported *KCNJ5* mutations (G151R and L168R) in two of four A/CPAs, and no mutations in *PRKACA*, *ATP1A1*, *ATP2B3*, and *CACNA1D* were found (41). Lastly, Nakajima et al. demonstrated *KCNJ5* mutations in 6 of 10 A/CPAs (42). This suggests that *KCNJ5* mutations may cause excess secretion of not only aldosterone but also glucocorticoids, leading to PA with discrete features of CS. Potential explanations include the overlapping role of transcriptional regulators CREB and ATF in the regulation of both aldosterone and cortisol production (**Figure 1**) as well as a potential role of Ca^{2+} in cAMP formation (43).

In summary, *KCNJ5* mutations have been extensively studied in the context of PA. However, the physiological role of *KCNJ5* in human adrenal glomerulosa remains largely undetermined, and animal studies have been hampered by extremely low or absent expression of *KCNJ5* in rodents (44).

CACNA1D MUTATIONS IN PRIMARY ALDOSTERONISM

The gene with the second highest somatic mutation burden in APAs is *CACNA1D*, with frequencies of about 8–11% described in the initial exome sequencing studies and similar findings in a large follow-up study (23, 35, 45) (**Table 1**). Similar to *KCNJ5* mutations, *CACNA1D* mutations are heterozygous. However, mutations are more scattered throughout the protein. *CACNA1D* encodes an L-type voltage-gated calcium channel ($Ca_V1.3$). Mutant *CACNA1D* channels show activation at more hyperpolarized membrane potentials and, in some cases, reduced channel inactivation compared to wild-type channels (45). In line with the notion that these effects will lead to increased calcium entry, expression of mutant *CACNA1D* channels causes increased aldosterone production in the adrenocortical cancer cell line H295R (46). Again, similar to *KCNJ5* variants, additional evidence for a role of *CACNA1D* in PA came from the discovery of germ line variants at the same positions found to be mutated in tumors (45). Among 100 unrelated subjects with early-onset PA and hypertension, two carried *de novo* mutations in *CACNA1D*. Interestingly, these subjects had a multi-organ phenotype, including primary aldosteronism, seizures, and neurologic abnormalities (PASNA) (45). The discovery of mutations in calcium channels as a cause of PA may suggest that specific calcium channel blockers could be useful in patients carrying such mutations (46).

ATPase MUTATIONS IN PRIMARY ALDOSTERONISM

Additional somatic mutations in APAs without corresponding germ line mutations have been identified. Beuschlein et al. first described heterozygous or hemizygous somatic mutations in the *ATP1A1* and *ATP2B3* genes in 5.2 and 1.6% of APAs, respectively. *ATP1A1* encodes a sodium/potassium ATPase subunit, whereas *ATP2B3* encodes the plasma membrane calcium ATPase. Mutations in both ATPases cluster within the M4 helix, again suggesting a gain-of-function mechanism (47). Azizan et al. subsequently demonstrated that *ATP1A1* mutations cause an ouabain-sensitive, voltage-dependent inward Na^+ or H^+ current, respectively. Heterologous expression of mutant *ATP1A1* in human adrenocortical H295R cells led to increased aldosterone production and *CYP11B2* expression levels (35), consistent with a role of mutant *ATP1A1* in cellular depolarization and activation of voltage-gated calcium channels, as with mutated *KCNJ5*. Similarly, a mutation in *ATP2B3* was shown to induce a pathological Na^+ permeability, with increased intracellular Ca^{2+} levels and aldosterone production in H295R cells (48).

SPECIFIC FEATURES AND ORIGIN OF *CACNA1D*- AND ATPase-MUTANT APAs

Azizan and colleagues first suggested an association of *CACNA1D* and *ATP1A1* mutations with a glomerulosa-like phenotype (35), whereas other groups reported mixed histological phenotypes (23, 36). Glomerulosa-like features in *CACNA1D* and *ATP1A1*-positive tumors could suggest that these tumors are derived from zona glomerulosa cells. Indeed, Nishimoto et al. recently studied 42 normal adrenal glands from kidney donors and identified so-called aldosterone-producing cell clusters (APCCs), nests of cells just below the adrenal capsule that feature high expression of aldosterone synthase and protrude into cortisol-producing cells (49). Remarkably, targeted next-generation sequencing of DNA from 23 APCCs identified known somatic *CACNA1D* mutations in six cases and known somatic *ATP1A1* mutations in two cases, suggesting that APCCs may represent precursors of a subtype of APAs. These results also support the presence of APCCs and potentially subclinical PA in a substantial number of apparently healthy individuals, which is interesting, given that prior clinical studies identified a higher risk of developing hypertension in individuals with increased aldosterone levels within the physiologic range (50). No somatic *KCNJ5* mutations were identified in APCCs, suggesting that APAs carrying such mutations may arise from cells of the zona fasciculata or may grow more rapidly, with precursors evading detection in apparently healthy individuals.

INVESTIGATIONS OF MULTINODULAR TUMORS

Even though the classical presentation of aldosterone-producing adenoma is that of a uninodular lesion, many cases feature associated hyperplasia or multiple secondary nodules, many of which do not show increased expression of aldosterone synthase. Investigations of individual nodules revealed the presence of characteristic APA mutations in aldosterone-producing nodules, whereas non-producing nodules do not carry such mutations (51). Some individuals carry different aldosterone-driver mutations in different nodules, suggesting that independent mutation events account for the development of multiple nodules (52, 53). Whether germ line susceptibility variants promote the formation of multiple tumors remain to be determined. Interestingly, some adenomas appear to show intra-tumoral heterogeneity, indicating that the somatic events underlying APA formation can also occur in the context of preexisting nodules (53). This has led to the proposal of a two-hit model of adenoma development, with one hit being responsible for proliferation and another hit causing hormone production (54). However, the rarity of such findings and the absence of second hits explaining proliferation in the exomes of tumors carrying aldosterone-driver mutations suggest that APA driver mutations alone are sufficient to cause proliferation and hormone production in the majority of APAs.

CACNA1H MUTATIONS IN FAMILIAL HYPERALDOSTERONISM

One additional ion channel gene implicated in PA to date has been found to be mutated in the germ line only, but not in APAs. A novel germ line heterozygous variant in the *CACNA1H* gene (M1549V) was found in 5 of 40 unrelated subjects with PA and hypertension diagnosed at age 10 or below (55). Microscopic glomerulosa hyperplasia without macroscopic enlargement was demonstrated in one subject who had undergone unilateral adrenalectomy, suggesting a limited proliferative effect of the variant. *CACNA1H* encodes the low-voltage-activated T-type calcium channel $Ca_V3.2$ (56). $Ca_V3.2$ has been hypothesized to be responsible for fine adjustments in the aldosterone production when activated by small changes in potassium or ATII levels and appears to be necessary for glomerulosa membrane potential oscillations (55, 57, 58). The observed M1549V variant causes impaired channel inactivation and a slight shift of activation to more hyperpolarized potentials (55), as well as increased *CYP11B2* expression (59), suggesting a pathophysiology similar to that of *CACNA1D* variants.

SOMATIC MUTATIONS IN ADRENAL CUSHING'S SYNDROME

Cushing's syndrome features hypercortisolism and is associated with a plethora of signs and symptoms, including weight gain, hypertension, diabetes mellitus, lethargy, acne, depression, hirsutism, and increased mortality (60, 61). CPAs are less frequent than ACTH-secreting pituitary tumors (62), but still account for up to 10% of endogenous CS (60, 63, 64). Somatic *PRKAR1A* loss-of-function mutations were identified as a cause of sporadic CPAs in a hypothesis-driven approach (65).

Following the description of somatic mutations in PA, using exome sequencing, four groups independently identified somatic mutations in the *PRKACA* gene as a cause of CS (66–69). *PRKACA* encodes the catalytic subunit of protein kinase A involved in the regulation of adrenal cortisol production (see Introduction and **Figure 1**). Beuschlein and colleagues sequenced the exomes of 10 CPAs and identified heterozygous somatic *PRKACA* mutations in eight, with a frequency of 37% in the entire cohort of CPAs associated with overt CS. No *PRKACA* variants were found in CPAs associated with subclinical CS, APAs, or inactive adenomas, and the presence of *PRKACA* variants was associated with a more severe phenotype (66). All but one tumor carried a single variant, L206R, suggesting a gain-of-function effect. L206 is located in the highly conserved interaction site between the regulatory and the catalytic subunits of PKA, and binding of the regulatory subunit at this position prevents substrate phosphorylation. Molecular modeling and functional analysis of PKA activity suggested that the L206R mutation would lead to a steric hindrance and prevent inhibition of catalytic activity by the regulatory subunit (70). Somatic *PRKACA* variants other than L206R are exceedingly rare (71). Further support for the causative role of increased PKA activity in CS came from the discovery of germ line *PRKACA* duplications in subjects with bilateral adrenal hyperplasia and CS (66).

These results were confirmed in independent cohorts. Cao et al. reported an L205R variant (equivalent to L206R in the initial report) in the *PRKACA* gene in 27 of 39 CPAs. Further, two *GNAS* ($G_{\alpha s}$) mutations and a *CTNNB1* (β-catenin) mutation were found (see below) (67). Sato et al. screened tumors of 65 patients with ACTH-independent CS. They identified $PRKACA^{L206R}$ mutations in 52.3% and *GNAS* mutations in 16.9% of the tumors. In addition, they provided evidence of an association of $PRKACA^{L206R}$ with smaller tumor size and a more severe phenotype (68). Lastly, Goh et al. reported a $PRKACA^{L206R}$ mutation in 24% of CPAs (35% of cases with overt CS). They also reported *CTNNB1* mutations in 16% and *GNAS* mutations in 6% of tumors (69). Similar results were found in additional cohorts (39, 41, 71) (**Table 1**). Functionally, L206R has been shown to enhance the phosphorylation of PKA downstream effectors CREB and ATF in cell culture and tumor tissue samples (69) (**Figure 1**).

MUTATIONS IN *GNAS* AND *CTNNB1* IN CUSHING'S SYNDROME AND PRIMARY ALDOSTERONISM

Mutations in *GNAS* have long been known to inhibit GTPase activity of the $G_{\alpha s}$ subunit and thereby cause constitutive $G_{\alpha s}$ activation, abnormal cAMP signaling, endocrine hyperfunction, and tumor formation; postzygotic *GNAS* mutations are found in McCune–Albright syndrome, which can be associated with CS (72, 73). The discovery of mutually exclusive somatic gain-of-function mutations of *PRKACA* and *GNAS* in CPAs (see above) has further demonstrated that increased cAMP signaling is sufficient to cause tumorigenesis and cortisol hypersecretion. However, somewhat unexpectedly, given the absence of *PRKACA* mutations in APAs, *GNAS* variants were also reported in A/CPAs in two instances (42). On a molecular level, given the accessory role of ACTH in stimulating aldosterone secretion, increased cAMP signaling may play a role.

CTNNB1 encodes β-catenin of the Wnt/β–catenin pathway, which is known to play an important role in adrenocortical development and cancer (74). Activating mutations are not only found in benign and malignant adrenal tumors (75) but also in tumors of other organs. Such mutations prevent β-catenin degradation and cause proliferation. Even though such events have been shown to trigger benign aldosterone-secreting and cortisol-secreting tumor development as well as malignancy in a mouse model and human tissue samples (36, 45, 69, 75–77), the exact mechanisms underlying hormone secretion in *CTNNB1* positive tumors remain to be determined.

In this context, a common pathway of *PRKACA*, *GNAS*, and *CTNNB1* has been suggested (78). However, it has been shown that *GNAS* and *CTNNB1* mutations are not always mutually exclusive in CPAs, and that mutations of *CTNNB1* are also present in non-secreting adrenal tumors (79). A recent study described an association with pregnancy in two of three cases with APAs and *CTNNB1* mutations and suggested that the manifestation may be mediated by *CTNNB1*-induced LHCGR expression and increased LH levels in pregnancy (80). However, the absence of an association with pregnancy in previously described female cases (81), the high prevalence of LHCGR overexpression in APAs (82), and the finding of *CTNNB1* mutations in male individuals with APAs (83) suggest a role of additional factors.

CONCLUSION AND OPEN QUESTIONS

Taken together, the recent findings on the genetic causes of APAs and CPAs suggest that both result from gain-of-function mutations that concurrently lead to excess hormone hypersecretion and increased proliferation. In most cases, a single mutation is apparently sufficient for tumor formation and hormone hypersecretion. There is little overlap between CPAs and APAs in terms of the mutational spectrum. While CPAs often carry mutations that lead to increased intracellular cAMP levels, mutations known to cause APAs mostly affect intracellular calcium signaling. Overlapping roles in the function of transcription factors ATF and CREB in glomerulosa and fasciculata function, as well as overlapping roles of signaling downstream of ACTH and calcium in cortisol and aldosterone synthesis, may explain the presence of *KCNJ5* and *GNAS* mutations in tumors secreting both cortisol and aldosterone (**Figure 1**). Open questions include the determinants of the histological phenotype of APAs with certain mutations, the molecular pathways involved in proliferation of both APAs and CPAs, potential additional factors that drive hormone production in tumors with *CTNNB1* mutations, and the pathogenesis of tumors without mutations in known driver genes. In summary, despite significant progress over the past few years, the pathophysiology behind CPAs and APAs has not been fully unraveled. Distinct and common molecular switches appear to exist in both disorders.

AUTHOR CONTRIBUTIONS

All authors listed have made substantial, direct, and intellectual contribution to the work and approved it for publication.

FUNDING

This work was funded by a grant of the Ministry of Innovation, Science and Research of the State of North Rhine-Westphalia (NRW Rückkehrerprogramm to US).

REFERENCES

1. Bovio S, Cataldi A, Reimondo G, Sperone P, Novello S, Berruti A, et al. Prevalence of adrenal incidentaloma in a contemporary computerized tomography series. *J Endocrinol Invest* (2006) 29:298–302. doi:10.1007/BF03344099
2. Young WF Jr. Clinical practice. The incidentally discovered adrenal mass. *N Engl J Med* (2007) 356:601–10. doi:10.1056/NEJMcp065470
3. Spat A, Hunyady L. Control of aldosterone secretion: a model for convergence in cellular signaling pathways. *Physiol Rev* (2004) 84:489–539. doi:10.1152/physrev.00030.2003
4. Masilamani S, Kim GH, Mitchell C, Wade JB, Knepper MA. Aldosterone-mediated regulation of ENaC alpha, beta, and gamma subunit proteins in rat kidney. *J Clin Invest* (1999) 104:R19–23. doi:10.1172/JCI7840
5. Bandulik S, Tauber P, Penton D, Schweda F, Tegtmeier I, Sterner C, et al. Severe hyperaldosteronism in neonatal Task3 potassium channel knockout mice is associated with activation of the intraadrenal renin-angiotensin system. *Endocrinology* (2013) 154:2712–22. doi:10.1210/en.2013-1101
6. Simpson ER, Waterman MR. Regulation of the synthesis of steroidogenic enzymes in adrenal cortical cells by ACTH. *Annu Rev Physiol* (1988) 50:427–40. doi:10.1146/annurev.ph.50.030188.002235
7. Rosenberg D, Groussin L, Jullian E, Perlemoine K, Bertagna X, Bertherat J. Role of the PKA-regulated transcription factor CREB in development and tumorigenesis of endocrine tissues. *Ann N Y Acad Sci* (2002) 968:65–74. doi:10.1111/j.1749-6632.2002.tb04327.x
8. Oakley RH, Cidlowski JA. Cellular processing of the glucocorticoid receptor gene and protein: new mechanisms for generating tissue-specific actions of glucocorticoids. *J Biol Chem* (2011) 286:3177–84. doi:10.1074/jbc.R110.179325
9. Sapolsky RM, Romero LM, Munck AU. How do glucocorticoids influence stress responses? Integrating permissive, suppressive, stimulatory, and preparative actions. *Endocr Rev* (2000) 21:55–89. doi:10.1210/er.21.1.55
10. Barnes PJ. Anti-inflammatory actions of glucocorticoids: molecular mechanisms. *Clin Sci* (1998) 94:557–72. doi:10.1042/cs0940557
11. Choi M, Scholl UI, Yue P, Bjorklund P, Zhao B, Nelson-Williams C, et al. K+ channel mutations in adrenal aldosterone-producing adenomas and hereditary hypertension. *Science* (2011) 331:768–72. doi:10.1126/science.1198785
12. Conn JW. Presidential address. I. Painting background. II. Primary aldosteronism, a new clinical syndrome. *J Lab Clin Med* (1955) 45:3–17.
13. Stowasser M, Gordon RD, Rutherford JC, Nikwan NZ, Daunt N, Slater GJ. Diagnosis and management of primary aldosteronism. *J Renin Angiotensin Aldosterone Syst* (2001) 2:156–69. doi:10.3317/jraas.2001.022
14. Mulatero P, Dluhy RG, Giacchetti G, Boscaro M, Veglio F, Stewart PM. Diagnosis of primary aldosteronism: from screening to subtype differentiation. *Trends Endocrinol Metab* (2005) 16:114–9. doi:10.1016/j.tem.2005.02.007
15. Rossi GP, Bernini G, Caliumi C, Desideri G, Fabris B, Ferri C, et al. A prospective study of the prevalence of primary aldosteronism in 1,125 hypertensive patients. *J Am Coll Cardiol* (2006) 48:2293–300. doi:10.1016/j.jacc.2006.07.059
16. Korah HE, Scholl UI. An update on familial hyperaldosteronism. *Horm Metab Res* (2015) 47:941–6. doi:10.1055/s-0035-1564166
17. Heginbotham L, Lu Z, Abramson T, MacKinnon R. Mutations in the K+ channel signature sequence. *Biophys J* (1994) 66:1061–7. doi:10.1016/S0006-3495(94)80887-2
18. Scholl UI, Nelson-Williams C, Yue P, Grekin R, Wyatt RJ, Dillon MJ, et al. Hypertension with or without adrenal hyperplasia due to different inherited mutations in the potassium channel KCNJ5. *Proc Natl Acad Sci U S A* (2012) 109:2533–8. doi:10.1073/pnas.1121407109
19. Charmandari E, Sertedaki A, Kino T, Merakou C, Hoffman DA, Hatch MM, et al. A novel point mutation in the KCNJ5 gene causing primary hyperaldosteronism and early-onset autosomal dominant hypertension. *J Clin Endocrinol Metab* (2012) 97:E1532–9. doi:10.1210/jc.2012-1334
20. Monticone S, Bandulik S, Stindl J, Zilbermint M, Dedov I, Mulatero P, et al. A case of severe hyperaldosteronism caused by a de novo mutation affecting a

critical salt bridge Kir3.4 residue. *J Clin Endocrinol Metab* (2015) 100:E114–8. doi:10.1210/jc.2014-3636

21. Lenzini L, Rossitto G, Maiolino G, Letizia C, Funder JW, Rossi GP. A meta-analysis of somatic KCNJ5 K channel mutations in 1636 patients with an aldosterone-producing adenoma. *J Clin Endocrinol Metab* (2015) 100:E1089–95. doi:10.1210/jc.2015-2149
22. Akerstrom T, Crona J, Delgado Verdugo A, Starker LF, Cupisti K, Willenberg HS, et al. Comprehensive re-sequencing of adrenal aldosterone producing lesions reveal three somatic mutations near the KCNJ5 potassium channel selectivity filter. *PLoS One* (2012) 7:e41926. doi:10.1371/journal.pone.0041926
23. Fernandes-Rosa FL, Williams TA, Riester A, Steichen O, Beuschlein F, Boulkroun S, et al. Genetic spectrum and clinical correlates of somatic mutations in aldosterone-producing adenoma. *Hypertension* (2014) 64:354–61. doi:10.1161/HYPERTENSIONAHA.114.03419
24. Williams TA, Monticone S, Schack VR, Stindl J, Burrello J, Buffolo F, et al. Somatic ATP1A1, ATP2B3, and KCNJ5 mutations in aldosterone-producing adenomas. *Hypertension* (2014) 63:188–95. doi:10.1161/HYPERTENSIONAHA.113.01733
25. Wu VC, Huang KH, Peng KY, Tsai YC, Wu CH, Wang SM, et al. Prevalence and clinical correlates of somatic mutation in aldosterone producing adenoma-Taiwanese population. *Sci Rep* (2015) 5:11396. doi:10.1038/srep11396
26. Wang B, Li X, Zhang X, Ma X, Chen L, Zhang Y, et al. Prevalence and characterization of somatic mutations in chinese aldosterone-producing adenoma patients. *Medicine (Baltimore)* (2015) 94:e708. doi:10.1097/MD.0000000000000708
27. Zheng FF, Zhu LM, Nie AF, Li XY, Lin JR, Zhang K, et al. Clinical characteristics of somatic mutations in Chinese patients with aldosterone-producing adenoma. *Hypertension* (2015) 65:622–8. doi:10.1161/HYPERTENSIONAHA.114.03346
28. Taguchi R, Yamada M, Nakajima Y, Satoh T, Hashimoto K, Shibusawa N, et al. Expression and mutations of KCNJ5 mRNA in Japanese patients with aldosterone-producing adenomas. *J Clin Endocrinol Metab* (2012) 97:1311–9. doi:10.1210/jc.2011-2885
29. Hong AR, Kim JH, Song YS, Lee KE, Seo SH, Seong MW, et al. Genetics of aldosterone-producing adenoma in Korean patients. *PLoS One* (2016) 11:e0147590. doi:10.1371/journal.pone.0147590
30. Monticone S, Hattangady NG, Nishimoto K, Mantero F, Rubin B, Cicala MV, et al. Effect of KCNJ5 mutations on gene expression in aldosterone-producing adenomas and adrenocortical cells. *J Clin Endocrinol Metab* (2012) 97:E1567–72. doi:10.1210/jc.2011-3132
31. Oki K, Plonczynski MW, Lam ML, Gomez-Sanchez EP, Gomez-Sanchez CE. The potassium channel, Kir3.4 participates in angiotensin II-stimulated aldosterone production by a human adrenocortical cell line. *Endocrinology* (2012) 153:4328–35. doi:10.1210/en.2012-1241
32. Oki K, Plonczynski MW, Luis Lam M, Gomez-Sanchez EP, Gomez-Sanchez CE. Potassium channel mutant KCNJ5 T158A expression in HAC-15 cells increases aldosterone synthesis. *Endocrinology* (2012) 153:1774–82. doi:10.1210/en.2011-1733
33. Hattangady NG, Karashima S, Yuan L, Ponce-Balbuena D, Jalife J, Gomez-Sanchez CE, et al. Mutated KCNJ5 activates the acute and chronic regulatory steps in aldosterone production. *J Mol Endocrinol* (2016). doi:10.1530/JME-15-0324
34. Azizan EA, Lam BY, Newhouse SJ, Zhou J, Kuc RE, Clarke J, et al. Microarray, qPCR, and KCNJ5 sequencing of aldosterone-producing adenomas reveal differences in genotype and phenotype between zona glomerulosa- and zona fasciculata-like tumors. *J Clin Endocrinol Metab* (2012) 97:E819–29. doi:10.1210/jc.2011-2965
35. Azizan EA, Poulsen H, Tuluc P, Zhou J, Clausen MV, Lieb A, et al. Somatic mutations in ATP1A1 and CACNA1D underlie a common subtype of adrenal hypertension. *Nat Genet* (2013) 45:1055–60. doi:10.1038/ng.2716
36. Scholl UI, Healy JM, Thiel A, Fonseca AL, Brown TC, Kunstman JW, et al. Novel somatic mutations in primary hyperaldosteronism are related to the clinical, radiological and pathological phenotype. *Clin Endocrinol (Oxf)* (2015) 83:779–89. doi:10.1111/cen.12873
37. Adachi J, Hirai Y, Terui K, Nakano T, Fukuda Y, Suda T, et al. A report of 7 cases of adrenal tumors secreting both cortisol and aldosterone. *Intern Med* (2003) 42:714–8. doi:10.2169/internalmedicine.42.714
38. Willenberg HS, Spath M, Maser-Gluth C, Engers R, Anlauf M, Dekomien G, et al. Sporadic solitary aldosterone- and cortisol-co-secreting adenomas: endocrine, histological and genetic findings in a subtype of primary aldosteronism. *Hypertens Res* (2010) 33:467–72. doi:10.1038/hr.2010.18
39. Nakajima Y, Okamura T, Gohko T, Satoh T, Hashimoto K, Shibusawa N, et al. Somatic mutations of the catalytic subunit of cyclic AMP-dependent protein kinase (PRKACA) gene in Japanese patients with several adrenal adenomas secreting cortisol [Rapid Communication]. *Endocr J* (2014) 61:825–32. doi:10.1507/endocrj.EJ14-0282
40. Yamada M, Nakajima Y, Taguchi R, Okamura T, Ishii S, Tomaru T, et al. KCNJ5 mutations in aldosterone- and cortisol-co-secreting adrenal adenomas [Rapid Communication]. *Endocr J* (2012) 59:735–41. doi:10.1507/endocrj.EJ12-0247
41. Thiel A, Reis AC, Haase M, Goh G, Schott M, Willenberg HS, et al. PRKACA mutations in cortisol-producing adenomas and adrenal hyperplasia: a single-center study of 60 cases. *Eur J Endocrinol* (2015) 172:677–85. doi:10.1530/EJE-14-1113
42. Nakajima Y, Okamura T, Horiguchi K, Gohko T, Miyamoto T, Satoh T, et al. GNAS mutations in adrenal aldosterone-producing adenomas [Rapid Communication]. *Endocr J* (2016) 63:199–204. doi:10.1507/endocrj.EJ15-0642
43. Spät A, Hunyady L, Szanda G. Signaling interactions in the adrenal cortex. *Front Endocrinol (Lausanne)* (2016) 7:17. doi:10.3389/fendo.2016.00017
44. Chen AX, Nishimoto K, Nanba K, Rainey WE. Potassium channels related to primary aldosteronism: expression similarities and differences between human and rat adrenals. *Mol Cell Endocrinol* (2015) 417:141–8. doi:10.1016/j.mce.2015.09.011
45. Scholl UI, Goh G, Stolting G, de Oliveira RC, Choi M, Overton JD, et al. Somatic and germline CACNA1D calcium channel mutations in aldosterone-producing adenomas and primary aldosteronism. *Nat Genet* (2013) 45:1050–4. doi:10.1038/ng.2695
46. Xie CB, Haris Shaikh L, Garg S, Tanriver G, Teo AE, Zhou J, et al. Regulation of aldosterone secretion by Cav1.3. *Sci Rep* (2016) 6:24697. doi:10.1038/srep24697
47. Beuschlein F, Boulkroun S, Osswald A, Wieland T, Nielsen HN, Lichtenauer UD, et al. Somatic mutations in ATP1A1 and ATP2B3 lead to aldosterone-producing adenomas and secondary hypertension. *Nat Genet* (2013) 45:440–4. doi:10.1038/ng.2550
48. Tauber P, Aichinger B, Christ C, Stindl J, Rhayem Y, Beuschlein F, et al. Cellular pathophysiology of an adrenal adenoma-associated mutant of the plasma membrane Ca^{2+}-ATPase ATP2B3. *Endocrinology* (2016) 157(6):2489–99. doi:10.1210/en.2015-2029
49. Nishimoto K, Tomlins SA, Kuick R, Cani AK, Giordano TJ, Hovelson DH, et al. Aldosterone-stimulating somatic gene mutations are common in normal adrenal glands. *Proc Natl Acad Sci U S A* (2015) 112:E4591–9. doi:10.1073/pnas.1505529112
50. Vasan RS, Evans JC, Larson MG, Wilson PW, Meigs JB, Rifai N, et al. Serum aldosterone and the incidence of hypertension in nonhypertensive persons. *N Engl J Med* (2004) 351:33–41. doi:10.1056/NEJMoa033263
51. Dekkers T, ter Meer M, Lenders JW, Hermus AR, Schultze Kool L, Langenhuijsen JF, et al. Adrenal nodularity and somatic mutations in primary aldosteronism: one node is the culprit? *J Clin Endocrinol Metab* (2014) 99:E1341–51. doi:10.1210/jc.2013-4255
52. Fernandes-Rosa FL, Giscos-Douriez I, Amar L, Gomez-Sanchez CE, Meatchi T, Boulkroun S, et al. Different somatic mutations in multinodular adrenals with aldosterone-producing adenoma. *Hypertension* (2015) 66:1014–22. doi:10.1161/HYPERTENSIONAHA.115.05993
53. Nanba K, Chen AX, Omata K, Vinco M, Giordano TJ, Else T, et al. Molecular heterogeneity in aldosterone-producing adenomas. *J Clin Endocrinol Metab* (2016) 101:999–1007. doi:10.1210/jc.2015-3239
54. Lalli E, Barhanin J, Zennaro MC, Warth R. Local control of aldosterone production and primary aldosteronism. *Trends Endocrinol Metab* (2016) 27:123–31. doi:10.1016/j.tem.2016.01.003
55. Scholl UI, Stölting G, Nelson-Williams C, Vichot AA, Choi M, Loring E, et al. Recurrent gain of function mutation in calcium channel CACNA1H causes early-onset hypertension with primary aldosteronism. *Elife* (2015) 4:e06315. doi:10.7554/eLife.06315
56. Perez-Reyes E. Molecular physiology of low-voltage-activated t-type calcium channels. *Physiol Rev* (2003) 83:117–61. doi:10.1152/physrev.00018.2002
57. Felizola SJ, Maekawa T, Nakamura Y, Satoh F, Ono Y, Kikuchi K, et al. Voltage-gated calcium channels in the human adrenal and primary

aldosteronism. *J Steroid Biochem Mol Biol* (2014) 144 Pt B:410–6. doi:10.1016/j.jsbmb.2014.08.012
58. Hu C, Rusin CG, Tan Z, Guagliardo NA, Barrett PQ. Zona glomerulosa cells of the mouse adrenal cortex are intrinsic electrical oscillators. *J Clin Invest* (2012) 122:2046–53. doi:10.1172/JCI61996
59. Reimer EN, Walenda G, Seidel E, Scholl UI. CACNA1H^{M1549V} mutant calcium channel causes autonomous aldosterone production in HAC15 cells and is inhibited by Mibefradil. *Endocrinology* (2016). doi:10.1210/en.2016-1170
60. Newell-Price J, Trainer P, Besser M, Grossman A. The diagnosis and differential diagnosis of Cushing's syndrome and pseudo-Cushing's states. *Endocr Rev* (1998) 19:647–72. doi:10.1210/edrv.19.5.0346
61. Lindholm J, Juul S, Jorgensen JO, Astrup J, Bjerre P, Feldt-Rasmussen U, et al. Incidence and late prognosis of Cushing's syndrome: a population-based study. *J Clin Endocrinol Metab* (2001) 86:117–23. doi:10.1210/jc.86.1.117
62. Nieman LK, Biller BM, Findling JW, Newell-Price J, Savage MO, Stewart PM, et al. The diagnosis of Cushing's syndrome: an Endocrine Society Clinical Practice Guideline. *J Clin Endocrinol Metab* (2008) 93:1526–40. doi:10.1210/jc.2008-0125
63. Newell-Price J, Bertagna X, Grossman AB, Nieman LK. Cushing's syndrome. *Lancet* (2006) 367:1605–17. doi:10.1016/S0140-6736(06)68699-6
64. Orth DN. Cushing's syndrome. *N Engl J Med* (1995) 332:791–803. doi:10.1056/NEJM199503233321207
65. Bertherat J, Groussin L, Sandrini F, Matyakhina L, Bei T, Stergiopoulos S, et al. Molecular and functional analysis of PRKAR1A and its locus (17q22-24) in sporadic adrenocortical tumors: 17q losses, somatic mutations, and protein kinase A expression and activity. *Cancer Res* (2003) 63:5308–19. doi:10.1016/s0889-8529(05)70113-4
66. Beuschlein F, Fassnacht M, Assie G, Calebiro D, Stratakis CA, Osswald A, et al. Constitutive activation of PKA catalytic subunit in adrenal Cushing's syndrome. *N Engl J Med* (2014) 370:1019–28. doi:10.1056/NEJMoa1310359
67. Cao Y, He M, Gao Z, Peng Y, Li Y, Li L, et al. Activating hotspot L205R mutation in PRKACA and adrenal Cushing's syndrome. *Science* (2014) 344:913–7. doi:10.1126/science.1249480
68. Sato Y, Maekawa S, Ishii R, Sanada M, Morikawa T, Shiraishi Y, et al. Recurrent somatic mutations underlie corticotropin-independent Cushing's syndrome. *Science* (2014) 344:917–20. doi:10.1126/science.1252328
69. Goh G, Scholl UI, Healy JM, Choi M, Prasad ML, Nelson-Williams C, et al. Recurrent activating mutation in PRKACA in cortisol-producing adrenal tumors. *Nat Genet* (2014) 46:613–7. doi:10.1038/ng.2956
70. Calebiro D, Hannawacker A, Lyga S, Bathon K, Zabel U, Ronchi C, et al. PKA catalytic subunit mutations in adrenocortical Cushing's adenoma impair association with the regulatory subunit. *Nat Commun* (2014) 5:5680. doi:10.1038/ncomms6680
71. Di Dalmazi G, Kisker C, Calebiro D, Mannelli M, Canu L, Arnaldi G, et al. Novel somatic mutations in the catalytic subunit of the protein kinase A as a cause of adrenal Cushing's syndrome: a European multicentric study. *J Clin Endocrinol Metab* (2014) 99:E2093–100. doi:10.1210/jc.2014-2152
72. Landis CA, Masters SB, Spada A, Pace AM, Bourne HR, Vallar L. GTPase inhibiting mutations activate the alpha chain of Gs and stimulate adenylyl cyclase in human pituitary tumours. *Nature* (1989) 340:692–6. doi:10.1038/340692a0
73. Weinstein LS, Shenker A, Gejman PV, Merino MJ, Friedman E, Spiegel AM. Activating mutations of the stimulatory G protein in the McCune-Albright syndrome. *N Engl J Med* (1991) 325:1688–95. doi:10.1056/NEJM199112123252403
74. El Wakil A, Lalli E. The Wnt/beta-catenin pathway in adrenocortical development and cancer. *Mol Cell Endocrinol* (2011) 332:32–7. doi:10.1016/j.mce.2010.11.014
75. Tadjine M, Lampron A, Ouadi L, Bourdeau I. Frequent mutations of beta-catenin gene in sporadic secreting adrenocortical adenomas. *Clin Endocrinol (Oxf)* (2008) 68:264–70. doi:10.1111/j.1365-2265.2007.03033.x
76. Berthon A, Sahut-Barnola I, Lambert-Langlais S, de Joussineau C, Damon-Soubeyrand C, Louiset E, et al. Constitutive beta-catenin activation induces adrenal hyperplasia and promotes adrenal cancer development. *Hum Mol Genet* (2010) 19:1561–76. doi:10.1093/hmg/ddq029
77. Gaujoux S, Tissier F, Groussin L, Libe R, Ragazzon B, Launay P, et al. Wnt/beta-catenin and 3′,5′-cyclic adenosine 5′-monophosphate/protein kinase A signaling pathways alterations and somatic beta-catenin gene mutations in the progression of adrenocortical tumors. *J Clin Endocrinol Metab* (2008) 93:4135–40. doi:10.1210/jc.2008-0631
78. Wilson CH, McIntyre RE, Arends MJ, Adams DJ. The activating mutation R201C in GNAS promotes intestinal tumourigenesis in Apc(Min/+) mice through activation of Wnt and ERK1/2 MAPK pathways. *Oncogene* (2010) 29:4567–75. doi:10.1038/onc.2010.202
79. Bonnet S, Gaujoux S, Launay P, Baudry C, Chokri I, Ragazzon B, et al. Wnt/beta-catenin pathway activation in adrenocortical adenomas is frequently due to somatic CTNNB1-activating mutations, which are associated with larger and nonsecreting tumors: a study in cortisol-secreting and -nonsecreting tumors. *J Clin Endocrinol Metab* (2011) 96:E419–26. doi:10.1210/jc.2010-1885
80. Teo AE, Garg S, Haris Shaikh L, Zhou J, Karet Frankl FE, Gurnell M, et al. Pregnancy, primary aldosteronism, and adrenal CTNNB1 mutations. *N Engl J Med* (2015) 373(15):1429–36. doi:10.1056/NEJMoa1504869
81. Murtha TD, Carling T, Scholl UI. Pregnancy, primary aldosteronism, and somatic CTNNB1 mutations. *N Engl J Med* (2016) 374:1492–3. doi:10.1056/NEJMc1514508
82. Teo AED, Garg S, Haris Shaikh L, Zhou J, Karet Frankl FE, Gurnell M, et al. Pregnancy, primary aldosteronism, and adrenal CTNNB1 mutations. *N Engl J Med* (2015) 373:1429–36. doi:10.1056/NEJMoa1504869
83. Akerstrom T, Maharjan R, Sven Willenberg H, Cupisti K, Ip J, Moser A, et al. Activating mutations in CTNNB1 in aldosterone producing adenomas. *Sci Rep* (2016) 6:19546. doi:10.1038/srep19546
84. Xekouki P, Hatch MM, Lin L, Rodrigo de A, Azevedo M, de la Luz Sierra M, et al. KCNJ5 mutations in the National Institutes of Health cohort of patients with primary hyperaldosteronism: an infrequent genetic cause of Conn' syndrome. *Endocr Relat Cancer* (2012) 19:255–60. doi:10.1530/ERC-12-0022
85. Kitamoto T, Suematsu S, Matsuzawa Y, Saito J, Omura M, Nishikawa T. Comparison of cardiovascular complications in patients with and without KCNJ5 gene mutations harboring aldosterone-producing adenomas. *J Atheroscler Thromb* (2015) 22:191–200. doi:10.5551/jat.24455
86. Boulkroun S, Beuschlein F, Rossi GP, Golib-Dzib JF, Fischer E, Amar L, et al. Prevalence, clinical, and molecular correlates of KCNJ5 mutations in primary aldosteronism. *Hypertension* (2012) 59:592–8. doi:10.1161/HYPERTENSIONAHA.111.186478
87. Azizan EA, Murthy M, Stowasser M, Gordon R, Kowalski B, Xu S, et al. Somatic mutations affecting the selectivity filter of KCNJ5 are frequent in 2 large unselected collections of adrenal aldosteronomas. *Hypertension* (2012) 59:587–91. doi:10.1161/HYPERTENSIONAHA.111.186239
88. Cheng CJ, Sung CC, Wu ST, Lin YC, Sytwu HK, Huang CL, et al. Novel KCNJ5 mutations in sporadic aldosterone-producing adenoma reduce Kir3.4 membrane abundance. *J Clin Endocrinol Metab* (2015) 100:E155–63. doi:10.1210/jc.2014-3009
89. Kuppusamy M, Caroccia B, Stindl J, Bandulik S, Lenzini L, Gioco F, et al. A novel KCNJ5-insT149 somatic mutation close to, but outside, the selectivity filter causes resistant hypertension by loss of selectivity for potassium. *J Clin Endocrinol Metab* (2014) 99:E1765–73. doi:10.1210/jc.2014-1927

Permissions

All chapters in this book were first published by Frontiers; hereby published with permission under the Creative Commons Attribution License or equivalent. Every chapter published in this book has been scrutinized by our experts. Their significance has been extensively debated. The topics covered herein carry significant findings which will fuel the growth of the discipline. They may even be implemented as practical applications or may be referred to as a beginning point for another development.

The contributors of this book come from diverse backgrounds, making this book a truly international effort. This book will bring forth new frontiers with its revolutionizing research information and detailed analysis of the nascent developments around the world.

We would like to thank all the contributing authors for lending their expertise to make the book truly unique. They have played a crucial role in the development of this book. Without their invaluable contributions this book wouldn't have been possible. They have made vital efforts to compile up to date information on the varied aspects of this subject to make this book a valuable addition to the collection of many professionals and students.

This book was conceptualized with the vision of imparting up-to-date information and advanced data in this field. To ensure the same, a matchless editorial board was set up. Every individual on the board went through rigorous rounds of assessment to prove their worth. After which they invested a large part of their time researching and compiling the most relevant data for our readers.

The editorial board has been involved in producing this book since its inception. They have spent rigorous hours researching and exploring the diverse topics which have resulted in the successful publishing of this book. They have passed on their knowledge of decades through this book. To expedite this challenging task, the publisher supported the team at every step. A small team of assistant editors was also appointed to further simplify the editing procedure and attain best results for the readers.

Apart from the editorial board, the designing team has also invested a significant amount of their time in understanding the subject and creating the most relevant covers. They scrutinized every image to scout for the most suitable representation of the subject and create an appropriate cover for the book.

The publishing team has been an ardent support to the editorial, designing and production team. Their endless efforts to recruit the best for this project, has resulted in the accomplishment of this book. They are a veteran in the field of academics and their pool of knowledge is as vast as their experience in printing. Their expertise and guidance has proved useful at every step. Their uncompromising quality standards have made this book an exceptional effort. Their encouragement from time to time has been an inspiration for everyone.

The publisher and the editorial board hope that this book will prove to be a valuable piece of knowledge for researchers, students, practitioners and scholars across the globe.

List of Contributors

Ewelina Stelcer
Department of Histology and Embryology, Poznan University of Medical Sciences, Poznan, Poland
Radiobiology Lab, Greater Poland Cancer Centre, Poznan, Poland
Department of Electroradiology, Poznan University of Medical Sciences, Poznan, Poland

Paulina Milecka, Karol Jopek, Marianna Tyczewska, Marta Szyszka, Marta Lesniczak, Beata Szczepaniak, Witold Sza larski, Piotr Celichowski, Ludwik K. Malendowicz and Marcin Rucinski
Department of Histology and Embryology, Poznan University of Medical Sciences, Poznan, Poland

Hanna Komarowska and Marek Ruchala
Department of Endocrinology, Metabolism and Internal Medicine, Poznan University of Medical Sciences, Poznan, Poland

Wiktoria Suchorska
Radiobiology Lab, Greater Poland Cancer Centre, Poznan, Poland
Department of Electroradiology, Poznan University of Medical Sciences, Poznan, Poland

Karlygash Bekova
West Kazakhstan Marat Ospanov Medical University, Aktobe, Kazakhstan

Marek Karczewski
Department of General and Transplantation Surgery, Poznan University of Medical Sciences, Poznan, Poland

Tomasz Wierzbicki
Department of General, Endocrinological and Gastroenterological Surgery, Poznan University of Medical Sciences, Poznan, Poland

Gavin P. Vinson
School of Biological and Chemical Sciences, Queen Mary University of London, London, UK

Claudimara Ferini Pacicco Lotfi and Pedro O. R. de Mendonca
Department of Anatomy, Institute of Biomedical Science, University of São Paulo, São Paulo, Brazil

Andrew Midzak
Research Institute of the McGill University, Montreal, QC, Canada

William C. Engeland, J. Marina Yoder, Carley A. Karsten and Paulo Kofuji
Department of Neuroscience, University of Minnesota, Minneapolis, MN, USA

Adrian John Clark, Mashal Hussain and Li Chan
Centre for Endocrinology, William Harvey Research Institute, Queen Mary University of London, London, UK

Rachel Forfar, Jeff Jerman, Ed McIver and Debra Taylor
Centre for Therapeutics Discovery, MRC Technology, Stevenage, UK

Davids Fridmanis, Ance Roga and Janis Klovins
Latvian Biomedical Research and Study Centre, Riga, Latvia

Robert M. Dores
Department of Biological Sciences, University of Denver, Denver, CO, USA

Wen-Jun Shen, Salman Azhar and Fredric B. Kraemer
The Division of Endocrinology, Stanford University, Stanford, CA, USA
Geriatric Research, Education and Clinical Center, Veterans Affairs Palo Alto Health Care System, Palo Alto, CA, USA

Vassilios Papadopoulos
Research Institute of the McGill University, Montreal, QC, Canada
Department of Biochemistry, McGill University, Montreal, QC, Canada
Department of Pharmacology and Therapeutics, McGill University, Montreal, QC, Canada

Cristina Paz, Fabiana Cornejo Maciel, Alejandra Gorostizaga, Ana F. Castillo, M. Mercedes Mori Sequeiros García, Paula M. Maloberti, Ulises D. Orlando, Pablo G. Mele, Cecilia Poderoso and Ernesto J. Podesta
Departamento de Bioquímica Humana, Facultad de Medicina, Instituto de Investigaciones Biomédicas (INBIOMED), Universidad de Buenos Aires (UBA-CONICET), Ciudad Autónoma de Buenos Aires, Argentina

Carmen Ruggiero and Enzo Lalli
Institut de Pharmacologie Moléculaire et Cellulaire CNRS UMR 7275, Valbonne, France
Laboratoire International Associé (LIA) CNRS NEOGENEX, Valbonne, France
Université de Nice, Valbonne, France

András Spät and László Hunyady
Department of Physiology, Semmelweis University Medical School, Budapest, Hungary
Laboratory of Molecular Physiology, Hungarian Academy of Sciences, Budapest, Hungary

Gergő Szanda
Department of Physiology, Semmelweis University Medical School, Budapest, Hungary

Emilie Pastel
Diabetes and Obesity Research Group, University of Exeter Medical School, Exeter, UK

Jean-Christophe Pointud, Antoine Martinez and A. Marie Lefrançois-Martinez
CNRS, UMR 6293/INSERM U1103, Génétique, Reproduction et Développement, Clermont Université, Aubière, France

Hervé Lefebvre
U982, Laboratory of Neuronal and Neuroendocrine Differentiation and Communication, INSERM, Institute for Research and Innovation in Biomedicine, Mont-Saint-Aignan, France
Normandie Université, UNIROUEN, Rouen, France
Department of Endocrinology, Diabetes and Metabolic Diseases, University Hospital of Rouen, Rouen, France

Michaël Thomas, Céline Duparc and Estelle Louiset
U982, Laboratory of Neuronal and Neuroendocrine Differentiation and Communication, INSERM, Institute for Research and Innovation in Biomedicine, Mont-Saint-Aignan, France
Normandie Université, UNIROUEN, Rouen, France

Jérôme Bertherat
U1016, INSERM, Institut Cochin, Paris, France
Department of Endocrinology and Metabolic Diseases, Hôpital Cochin, Assistance Publique- Hôpitaux de Paris, Paris, France

Nada El Ghorayeb, Isabelle Bourdeau and André Lacroix
Department of Medicine, Division of Endocrinology, Centre de Recherche du Centre hospitalier de l'Université de Montréal (CRCHUM), Université de Montréal, Montréal, QC, Canada

Fady Hannah-Shmouni, Fabio R. Faucz and Constantine A. Stratakis
Program on Developmental Endocrinology and Genetics (PDEGEN), Section on Endocrinology and Genetics (SEGEN), National Institute of Child Health and Human Development (NICHD), National Institutes of Health (NIH), Bethesda, MD, USA

Eric Seidel and Ute I. Scholl
Department of Nephrology, University Hospital Düsseldorf, Heinrich Heine University, Düsseldorf, Germany

Index

www.ingramcontent.com/pod-product-compliance
Lightning Source LLC
LaVergne TN
LVHW060550210926
848485LV00005B/1294
* 9 7 8 1 6 3 9 2 7 8 5 3 4 *